The HANDBOOK *of* HEALTH BEHAVIOR CHANGE

Kristin A. Riekert, PhD, is an Associate Professor of Medicine in the Division of Pulmonary and Critical Care Medicine, Department of Medicine at the Johns Hopkins University and Co-Director of the Johns Hopkins Adherence Research Center (JHARC). Dr. Riekert received her PhD in Clinical Psychology from Case Western Reserve University where she specialized in pediatric psychology. She completed postdoctoral training in health psychology at the Johns Hopkins University. Dr. Riekert is Principal Investigator or Co-Investigator on several National Institutes of Health and foundation sponsored intervention trials focused on improving adherence and health outcomes in cystic fibrosis, asthma, chronic kidney disease, sickle cell disease, and secondhand smoke reduction.

Judith K. Ockene, PhD, MEd, MA, is a tenured Professor of Medicine and Chief of the Division of Preventive and Behavioral Medicine, University of Massachusetts Medical School. She holds the Barbara Helen Smith Chair in Preventive and Behavioral Medicine and is Associate Vice Provost for Gender and Equity. Dr. Ockene is the recipient of numerous National Institutes of Health grants funding research in the prevention of illness and disability and the promotion of health and quality of life for individuals and communities. Much of her research addresses the risk behaviors of tobacco, alcohol, and diet; women's health; and training physicians and medical students in counseling patients for behavior change. She also teaches medical, graduate, and public health students and clinicians how to help patients make lifestyle changes. Dr. Ockene has over 250 peer-reviewed publications and was a scientific editor of two Surgeon General's Reports on Smoking and Health. She is a past member of the U.S. Preventive Services Task Force and past President of the Society of Behavioral Medicine. Dr. Ockene has received several school, state, and national mentoring awards, including the Society of Behavioral Medicine Distinguished Mentor Award in 2009.

Lori Pbert, PhD, is a Professor of Medicine and Associate Chief of the Division of Preventive and Behavioral Medicine in the Department of Medicine at the University of Massachusetts Medical School (UMMS). She is Director of the Center for Tobacco Treatment Research and Training (CTTRT) and of the UMMS Tobacco Treatment Specialist Training and Certification Program. Dr. Pbert is a clinical and translational researcher with over 25 years of experience conducting clinical and community-based trials. She is the recipient of numerous grants from National Institutes of Health funding research in the design and evaluation of behavioral interventions for health promotion and risk behavior change in real-world settings. Dr. Pbert teaches medical and graduate students, physicians, and other health care providers in the theory and practice of health behavior change. She is a fellow in the Society of Behavioral Medicine and a founding member of the American Academy of Pediatrics Center for Child Health Research Tobacco Consortium.

The HANDBOOK of HEALTH BEHAVIOR CHANGE

FOURTH EDITION

KRISTIN A. RIEKERT, PhD
JUDITH K. OCKENE, PhD, MEd, MA
LORI PBERT, PhD

Editors

SPRINGER PUBLISHING COMPANY

NEW YORK

Springer Publishing Company, LLC
11 West 42nd Street
New York, NY 10036
www.springerpub.com

Acquisitions Editor: Sheri W. Sussman
Composition: Exeter Premedia Services Private Ltd.

ISBN: 978-0-8261-9935-5
e-book ISBN: 978-0-8261-9936-2

14 15 16 / 5 4 3

The author and the publisher of this Work have made every effort to use sources believed to be reliable to provide information that is accurate and compatible with the standards generally accepted at the time of publication. The author and publisher shall not be liable for any special, consequential, or exemplary damages resulting, in whole or in part, from the readers' use of, or reliance on, the information contained in this book. The publisher has no responsibility for the persistence or accuracy of URLs for external or third-party Internet websites referred to in this publication and does not guarantee that any content on such websites is, or will remain, accurate or appropriate.

Library of Congress Cataloging-in-Publication Data
Handbook of health behavior change / edited by Kristin A. Riekert, Judith K. Ockene, Lori Pbert.—4th edition.
    p. ; cm.
  Includes bibliographical references and index.
  ISBN 978-0-8261-9935-5—ISBN 978-0-8261-9936-2 (e-book)
  I. Riekert, Kristin A., editor of compilation.   II. Ockene, Judith K., editor of compilation.
  III. Pbert, Lori, editor of compilation.
  [DNLM: 1. Health Promotion. 2. Behavior Therapy. 3. Health Behavior. 4. Patient Compliance.   WA 590]
  RA776.9
  613–dc23
                                                                                    2013034868

Special discounts on bulk quantities of our books are available to corporations, professional associations, pharmaceutical companies, health care organizations, and other qualifying groups. If you are interested in a custom book, including chapters from more than one of our titles, we can provide that service as well.

For details, please contact:
Special Sales Department, Springer Publishing Company, LLC
11 West 42nd Street, 15th Floor, New York, NY 10036-8002
Phone: 877-687-7476 or 212-431-4370; Fax: 212-941-7842
E-mail: sales@springerpub.com

Printed in the United States of America by McNaughton & Gunn.

This book is dedicated to all the people and families who work hard to maintain a healthy lifestyle and take care of their loved ones' health in the midst of multiple personal, social, and cultural challenges, and to the health care professionals who work tirelessly to help their patients and communities live healthier lives.

Contents

Contributors

Claire Abraham, BA   Department of Social Sciences and Health Policy, Wake Forest School of Medicine, Winston-Salem, North Carolina

Jennifer D. Allen, ScD, MPH, RN   Department of Medical Oncology, Dana Farber Cancer Institute, Harvard Medical School, Boston, Massachusetts

Laura H. Bachmann, MD, MPH   Department of Internal Medicine, Wake Forest Baptist Medical Center, Winston-Salem, North Carolina

Jamie S. Bodenlos, PhD   Department of Psychology, Hobart and William Smith Colleges, Geneva, New York

Deborah J. Bowen, PhD   Department of Community Health Sciences, Boston University, Boston, Massachusetts

Matthew M. Burg, PhD   Yale University School of Medicine and Columbia University Medical Center, New York, New York

Lora E. Burke, PhD, MPH, RN   Department of Health and Community Systems, University of Pittsburgh School of Nursing, Pittsburgh, Pennsylvania

David Cella, PhD   Department of Medical Social Sciences, Feinberg School of Medicine, Northwestern University, Chicago, Illinois

Noreen M. Clark, PhD   Center for Managing Chronic Disease, University of Michigan, Ann Arbor, Michigan

Angie L. Cradock, ScD   Department of Social and Behavioral Sciences, Harvard School of Public Health, Boston, Massachusetts

M. Robin DiMatteo, PhD   Department of Psychology, University of California–Riverside, Riverside, California

Anne C. Dobmeyer, PhD, ABPP   Department of Defense, Deployment Health Clinical Center, Walter Reed National Military Medical Center, Bethesda, Maryland

Ellen A. Dornelas, PhD   Helen & Harry Gray Cancer Center, Hartford Hospital and University of Connecticut School of Medicine, Farmington, Connecticut

Dustin T. Duncan, ScD   Department of Social and Behavioral Sciences, Harvard School of Public Health, Boston, Massachusetts

Michelle N. Eakin, PhD   Department of Medicine, Division of Pulmonary and Critical Care Medicine, Johns Hopkins Adherence Research Center, Johns Hopkins University School of Medicine, Baltimore, Maryland

Barbara Estabrook, MSPH, CHES   Department of Medicine, Division of Preventive and Behavioral Medicine, University of Massachusetts Medical School, Worcester, Massachusetts

Marian L. Fitzgibbon, PhD   Department of Medicine and University of Illinois Cancer Center, University of Illinois at Chicago, Chicago, Illinois

Gary D. Foster, PhD   Center for Obesity Research and Education, Temple University, Philadelphia, Pennsylvania

Jonathan Gallagher, MPsychSc   Department of Psychology, Beaumont Hospital, Dublin, Ireland

Russell E. Glasgow, PhD   Division of Cancer Control and Population Sciences, National Cancer Institute, Rockville, Maryland

Jeffrey L. Goodie, PhD, ABPP   Department of Family Medicine, Uniformed Services University of the Health Sciences, Bethesda, Maryland

Steven L. Gortmaker, PhD   Department of Family Medicine, Uniformed Services University of the Health Sciences, Bethesda, Maryland

Lauren A. Grieco, PhD   Stanford Prevention Research Center, Department of Medicine, Stanford University, Stanford, California

Michael A. Harris, PhD   Department of Pediatrics, Oregon Health & Science University, Portland, Oregon

Kelly B. Haskard-Zolnierek, PhD   Department of Psychology, Texas State University, San Marcos, Texas

Rashelle B. Hayes, PhD   Department of Medicine, Division of Preventive and Behavioral Medicine, University of Massachusetts Medical School, Worcester, Massachusetts

Laura L. Hayman, PhD, RN   Department of Nursing, University of Massachusetts–Boston, Boston, Massachusetts

Marisa E. Hilliard, PhD   Department of Pediatrics, Psychology Section, Baylor College of Medicine and Texas Children's Hospital, Houston, Texas

Korey K. Hood, PhD   Department of Pediatrics, Madison Clinic for Pediatric Diabetes, University of California, San Francisco, San Francisco, California

Christopher L. Hunter, PhD, ABPP   Department of Defense, Office of the Chief Medical Officer, TRICARE Management Activity, Defense Health Headquarters, Falls Church, Virginia

Mary R. Janevic, PhD   Center for Managing Chronic Disease, University of Michigan, Ann Arbor, Michigan

David M. Janicke, PhD   Department of Clinical and Health Psychology, University of Florida, Gainesville, Florida

Denise Jolicoeur, MPH, CHES   Division of Preventive and Behavioral Medicine, University of Massachusetts Medical School, Worcester, Massachusetts

Eileen Kaner, PhD   Institute of Health and Society, Newcastle University, Newcastle Upon Tyne, UK

Abby C. King, PhD   Departments of Health Research and Policy and Medicine, Stanford Prevention Research Center, Stanford University School of Medicine, Stanford, California

Angela Kong, PhD, MPH, RD   Institute for Health Research and Policy and University of Illinois Cancer Center, University of Illinois at Chicago, Chicago, Illinois

Rebekka M. Lee, ScD   Department of Social and Behavioral Sciences, Harvard School of Public Health, Boston, Massachusetts

Stephenie C. Lemon, PhD   Department of Medicine, Division of Preventive and Behavioral Medicine, University of Massachusetts Medical School, Worcester, Massachusetts

Crystal S. Lim, PhD   Department of Clinical and Health Psychology, University of Florida, Gainesville, Florida

Ruth McGovern, PhD   Institute of Health and Society, Newcastle University, Newcastle Upon Tyne, UK

Monika M. Mruk, BSN   Department of Nursing, University of Massachusetts–Boston, Boston, Massachusetts

Judith K. Ockene, PhD   Department of Medicine, Division of Preventive and Behavioral Medicine, University of Massachusetts Medical School, Worcester, Massachusetts

Sherry L. Pagoto, PhD   Department of Medicine, Division of Preventive and Behavioral Medicine, University of Massachusetts Medical School, Worcester, Massachusetts

Lori Pbert, PhD   Department of Medicine, Division of Preventive and Behavioral Medicine, University of Massachusetts Medical School, Worcester, Massachusetts

Amy H. Peterman, PhD   Department of Psychology, Health Psychology PhD Program, University of North Carolina at Charlotte, Charlotte, North Carolina

Janice M. Prochaska, PhD Pro-Change Behavior Systems, Inc., South Kingstown, Rhode Island

James O. Prochaska, PhD Department of Psychology, Cancer Prevention Research Center, University of Rhode Island, Kingston, Rhode Island

Judith J. Prochaska, PhD, MPH Stanford Prevention Research Center, Department of Medicine, Stanford University, Stanford, California

Cynthia S. Rand, PhD Department of Medicine, Division of Pulmonary and Critical Care Medicine, Johns Hopkins Adherence Research Center, Johns Hopkins University School of Medicine, Baltimore, Maryland

Jennifer K. Raymond, MD Department of Pediatrics, Oregon Health & Science University, Portland, Oregon

Scott D. Rhodes, PhD, MPH Department of Social Sciences and Health Policy, Wake Forest School of Medicine, Winston-Salem, North Carolina

Kristin A. Riekert, PhD Department of Medicine, Division of Pulmonary and Critical Care Medicine, Johns Hopkins Adherence Research Center, Johns Hopkins University School of Medicine, Baltimore, Maryland

Milagros C. Rosal, PhD Department of Medicine, Division of Preventive and Behavioral Medicine, University of Massachusetts Medical School, Worcester, Massachusetts

Elizabeth Schneider, PhD Department of Clinical and Health Psychology, University of Florida, Gainesville, Florida,

Kristin L. Schneider, PhD Department of Medicine, Division of Preventive and Behavioral Medicine, University of Massachusetts Medical School, Worcester, Massachusetts

Jylana L. Sheats, PhD Stanford Prevention Research Center, Department of Medicine, Stanford University, Stanford, California

Kurt C. Stange, MD, PhD Department of Family Medicine, Case Western Reserve University, Cleveland, Ohio

Cynthia A. Thomson, PhD, RD Mel & Enid Zuckerman College of Public Health, Canyon Ranch Center for Prevention & Health Promotion, University of Arizona, Tucson, Arizona

Melanie W. Turk, PhD, RN Duquesne University School of Nursing, Pittsburgh, Pennsylvania

Lisa Tussing-Humphreys, PhD, RD Department of Medicine and University of Illinois Cancer Center, University of Illinois at Chicago, Chicago, IL

David Victorson, PhD Department of Medical Social Sciences, Feinberg School of Medicine, Northwestern University, Chicago, Illinois

Monica L. Wang, ScD   Department of Medicine, Division of Preventive and Behavioral Medicine, University of Massachusetts Medical School, Worcester, Massachusetts; Department of Social and Behavioral Sciences, Harvard School of Public Health, Boston, Massachusetts

Josie S. Welkom, PhD   Department of Medicine, Division of Pulmonary and Critical Care Medicine, Johns Hopkins Adherence Research Center, Johns Hopkins University School of Medicine, Baltimore, Maryland

Aimee M. Wilkin, MD, MPH   Department of Internal Medicine, Wake Forest Baptist Medical Center, Winston-Salem, North Carolina

Summer L. Williams, PhD   Department of Psychology, Westfield State University, Westfield, Massachusetts

Sandra J. Winter, PhD   Stanford Prevention Research Center, Department of Medicine, Stanford University, Stanford, California

Preface

The adoption and maintenance of healthy lifestyle behaviors and adhering to prescribed therapies are key to optimal health. Four lifestyle behaviors in particular—getting regular physical activity, eating a healthy diet, not smoking, and limiting alcohol consumption—contribute to a longer and healthier life. Indeed, people who engage in all four of these behaviors are significantly less likely to die early from cancer, cardiovascular disease, and other causes compared to people who do not (Ford, Zhao, Tsai, & Li, 2011). Unfortunately, in 2010, 51% of noninstitutionalized American adults had at least one chronic illness; 26% had two or more (Ward & Schiller, 2013). Moreover, chronic illnesses comprised 7 of the top 10 causes of death in 2008 including heart disease, cancer, chronic lower respiratory diseases, stroke, Alzheimer's disease, diabetes, and kidney disease. Together, these 7 chronic illnesses accounted for approximately 67% of all deaths in the United States (Heron, 2012). It is clear that increased attention to the adoption and maintenance of behaviors for optimal health can have significant public health impact.

The overarching goal of the fourth edition *The Handbook of Health Behavior Change* is to inform health care providers, policy makers, health services, and behavioral, and social science researchers of the most current theories, challenges, and interventions for supporting health behavior change, including lifestyle behaviors and chronic disease management. *The Handbook of Health Behavior Change* was first published in 1988 and with each edition there has been growing appreciation for the critical role health behavior plays in maintaining health and well-being. Research has evolved from a primary focus on understanding predictors of engaging in positive health behaviors and the impact of health behaviors on the onset, progression, and exacerbation of diseases to the evaluation of interventions in controlled clinical trials. Now 25 years later, the themes of the previous editions continue to be relevant. In addition, the fourth edition includes new chapters that reflect current practices in the field of health behavior change, including an emphasis on the need to implement and disseminate interventions in real-world settings and a call for a focus on eliminating ever growing health disparities.

Understanding theoretical frameworks that guide the development of strategies and interventions to achieve change in behaviors and inform health behavior research is the first step in supporting meaningful and lasting health behavior change. Therefore *Section I: Chapters 1 to 3* focus on the most frequently used theoretical models in health behavior change research. While each theory is unique, there are many commonalities among them as well. As such, for the fourth edition this section has been reorganized based on the level at which the theories are operating: individual theories, community and population-based models, and health system models. This new organization allows the reader to better understand the strengths and weaknesses of each model relative to other theories operating on the same level.

Section II: Chapters 4 to 6 provide updated reviews of the factors that predict or serve as obstacles to lifestyle change and adherence. The authors in this section consider individual characteristics, psychosocial factors, and the family, community, and broader social and cultural context. Specific challenges faced by vulnerable populations such as children, adolescents, and the elderly and considerations for interventions at different developmental stages are presented. In addition, the interrelationships among culture, health disparities, and health behavior change and the need to take these into account when designing health behavior change programs and policies are addressed in the context of the growing cultural diversity in the United States.

Lifestyle changes, including the big four noted above (physical activity, nutrition, and tobacco and alcohol use), are the topics of *Chapters 7 to 12 in Section III*. This section provides updated reviews of the challenges in maintaining and changing these behaviors as well as the efficacy of various intervention strategies. Beyond these four lifestyle behaviors, there is a chapter on stress management, given the increasingly recognized role of stress in contributing to the development of chronic illnesses, such as cardiovascular disease and cancer, as well as overall mortality. This chapter provides a review of a variety of approaches for addressing stress that are often integrated into other behavior change interventions. Recognizing that risky lifestyle behaviors most often co-occur and are best considered within the context of their interdependence, the final chapter in this section tackles the complexities of multiple-risk behavior change.

Section IV: Chapters 13 to 18 address the challenges of adhering to lifelong medical regimens. The chapters focus on many of the most prevalent chronic illnesses that contribute to avoidable mortality including cardiovascular disease, diabetes, respiratory diseases (specifically asthma and chronic obstructive pulmonary disease [COPD]), infectious diseases (including HIV, other sexually transmitted diseases, and tuberculosis), cancer, and obesity. These chapters highlight the prevalence of nonadherence to regimen components as well as review the efficacy of interventions to support and improve treatment adherence.

New to the handbook, *Section V: Chapters 19 to 22* focus on the development and evaluation of behavior change interventions implemented within a variety of contexts including community settings such as schools and work places, health care systems, and the built environment. This focus on the environments in which behavior change interventions may take place highlights the opportunities and challenges of working within these systems. It also reflects the growing recognition of the importance of implementation science—that interventions must be developed and evaluated in the contexts in which they will ultimately be disseminated.

Section VI: Chapters 23 and 24 flow nicely from the preceding sections and highlights methodological innovations in health behavior change research. The first chapter focuses on the technological innovations in behavior measurement that have occurred since the third edition. Many new opportunities now exist to objectively measure behavior with less burden and more precision. These innovations are allowing health care providers to begin using these tools in clinical care to shape and modify behavior. Perhaps more than any other innovation, the ongoing development and influence of dissemination and implementation of science theories and methodologies have greatly influenced health behavior research. The final chapter of the handbook highlights the importance of conducting translational research and sets out a framework and set of recommendations for moving the field of behavior change research forward to enhance population health.

Across the different behaviors, illnesses, systems, and populations discussed in each chapter, several cross-cutting themes emerge to guide future research directions. First, interventions need to be developed that are informed by and advance theoretical models in order to understand the mechanism of change and translate the application of successful interventions to other settings, populations, and behaviors. Second, new and updated theories, interventions, and research methodologies are needed to tackle the complexity of addressing multiple behaviors and challenges concurrently, reflecting the reality that rarely does a person need to change one behavior to improve health or manage a chronic illness and it is uncommon that there is only one challenge to behavior change. Third, given the profound racial and economic health disparities seen worldwide, it is not surprising that a common theme across the chapters is the need to reduce health disparities. This needs to be accomplished by not only providing culturally sensitive behavior change interventions, but also reducing external barriers by improving access to resources such as health care, nutritious foods, and recreational facilities, and decreasing disproportionate exposure to environmental toxins that cause illnesses or exacerbate symptoms. Fourth, a common theme throughout the handbook is that the most efficacious interventions are multicomponent; however, an equally prevalent theme and future direction are needed to make interventions more accessible. Innovative approaches to harmonize these two seemingly opposite themes are needed. Fifth, technology is proposed in many chapters as a potential solution to this challenge, but currently most technology-based solutions are simplistic and much more work is needed in this area. And finally, in addition to specific chapters targeting dissemination of interventions to community and care settings, most chapters note this as a critical area of future research. If we cannot effectively deliver interventions to target audiences, we cannot improve the health of our population.

In total, the fourth edition of *The Handbook of Health Behavior Change* represents an updated and thorough examination of the factors that influence people's ability to change behaviors to enhance their health and the intrapersonal, interpersonal, sociocultural, environmental, systems, and policy factors that can both positively and negatively affect the choices one makes and one's ability to achieve a desired behavior goal. Beyond understanding predictors, the handbook provides comprehensive reviews of the empirical evidence for various intervention approaches that have been evaluated and offers recommendations for next steps in research to continue to move the field forward. In addition to new and updated information, the fourth edition has been substantially revised to remove redundancy between chapters, and to provide content in a more concise and accessible manner including the addition of learning objectives at the start of each chapter. This book is particularly valuable to students at the graduate and advanced undergraduate level in the fields of public or population health, health communications, medical sociology and anthropology, preventive medicine, and health psychology. The content of the handbook will also be informative to clinical investigators, behavioral and social scientists, and health care practitioners who grapple with the challenges of supporting individuals in their efforts to make well-informed decisions regarding their health-related behaviors, change difficult health habits, and adopt and maintain new behaviors.

REFERENCES

Ford, E. S., Zhao, G., Tsai, J., & Li, C. (2011). Low-risk lifestyle behaviors and all-cause mortality: Findings from the National Health and Nutrition Examination Survey III Mortality Study. *American Journal of Public Health, 101*, 1922–1929.

Heron, M. (2012). Deaths: Leading causes for 2008. *National Vital Statistics Reports, 60*, 1–94.

Ward, B. W., & Schiller, J. S. (2013). Prevalence of multiple chronic conditions among US adults: Estimates from the National Health Interview Survey, 2010. *Preventing Chronic Disease, 10*, E65.

Acknowledgments

The editors warmly acknowledge Charlotte Gerczak, Communications Associate and Assistant to the Editors for *The Handbook of Health Behavior Change*, Fourth Edition, for her unwavering commitment to keeping this new edition on track by reminding them of deadlines and tasks that needed to be done, corresponding with authors, proofreading chapters, and tackling organizational challenges.

I
Theoretical Models of
Health Behavior Change

Theories attempt to explain cause–effect relationships and help to provide a basis for understanding and predicting the occurrence of health-related behaviors, behavior change, and maintenance of change. Therefore, they also help to frame the development of strategies and interventions to achieve change in behaviors and guide health behavior research. No single theory is all encompassing, often making it necessary to use multiple theories to understand how to promote specific behavior change. Using a socio-ecological framework as described in Chapter 2 by Fitzgibbon et al. and colleagues we understand that theories are also needed to address each of the multiple levels of influence on behavior, encompassing the levels of genetics, the individual, the population, or environment, community entities such as the health care system, and policies.

Chapters in Section I provide a detailed review of a wide variety of theories and models of behavior and behavior change, including theories addressing factors on the individual level (Chapter 1), on the community or population level (Chapter 2), and those factors in health care systems affecting the health behaviors of patients and the treatment-delivery behaviors of clinicians (Chapter 3). Each chapter emphasizes that none of these levels that affect behavior act on their own; rather, they do so within the context of the others. Therefore, in order to tackle our public health challenges described throughout this book, behavior change depends on a comprehensive approach of intervening on multiple levels.

Chapter 1, "Individual Theories" by Clark and Janevic, provides an overview of six commonly used individual-level theories and models: social cognitive theory, self regulation model, health belief model, theory of planned action, transtheoretical model, and relapse prevention model. It concludes by asking researchers and clinicians to consider "the need for more rigorous testing and subsequent theory modification to move the field forward" and describes how we might do this. The authors call for "taking theory testing and development in new directions to help ensure the relevance of individual-level theories in an environment where a strong evidence base and multi-level, multi-disciplinary approaches are viewed as critical to addressing today's biggest public health challenges."

Chapter 2, "Understanding Population Health From Multi-Level and Community-Based Models" by Fitzgibbon, Kong, and Tussing-Humphreys, addresses how socio-ecological models that address the multiple levels of influence on behavior can be used for developing interventions that support healthy lifestyles. The authors note that we must pay attention to the communities in which people live and work, and they discuss the benefits and challenges of implementing community-based participatory research. They also note how the RE-AIM evaluation framework that identifies the importance of assessing reach, effectiveness, adoption, implementation, and maintenance when translating multi-level research to action can be applied to the evaluation of health behavior change trials.

Chapter 3, "Health System Models" by Glasgow and Stange, notes that the behaviors of health care practitioners and their patients occur in a multi-level context and discusses key elements of these contexts and three widely used models or frameworks for facilitating and understanding the impact of health systems: the chronic care (and expanded chronic care) model, the practice change, complex adapter system models, and the RE-AIM/PRISM models. The authors note the need to "study and identify the most cost-effective strategies to implement these models in different health care settings." The frameworks provided in this chapter are important in the new and continuously evolving field of implementation science necessary for translating research findings into real-world applications.

Even though there are many theories and models available, there is still much we have not been able to explain about why and how people make changes in health-related behaviors and, even more challenging, how they maintain those changes. To fill in the black box of behavior change, we must be able to move outside of it. Theories can be used to guide us but should not constrain our creativity. It is important for us to be open to integrating, expanding, and testing our theories to help us build on our base of knowledge and to apply what we learn from practice to modify and add to our theories. We must also be mindful of the importance of studying how to implement and disseminate our work using implementation science methodology and theories.

1

Individual Theories

NOREEN M. CLARK
MARY R. JANEVIC

LEARNING OBJECTIVES

- Describe how individual theories of health behavior change are used to guide both observational and intervention-based health behavior research, and the prominent role that these theories have played in health behavior research over more than two decades.
- Discuss the major components and applications of some of the most commonly cited individual theories, including Social Cognitive Theory, the Self-Regulation Model, the Health Belief Model (HBM), the Theory of Planned Behavior (TPB), the Transtheoretical Model (TTM), and the Relapse Prevention (RP) Model.
- Comment on the current state of individual-level theory development, and describe proposals for moving the field forward in ways that increase the value of theories to researchers and practitioners.

The ultimate success of efficacious preventive and curative regimens depends upon individuals' willingness to undertake and maintain the required behaviors. Unfortunately, data indicate that poor adherence to professional advice often occurs wherever some form of discretionary action or self-administration is involved. Scheduled appointments for treatment are missed about 35% of the time and significant numbers of patients do not take prescribed medications in accordance with instructions (DiMatteo, 2004). Adherence to recommended changes in habitual behaviors is disappointing (e.g., smoking cessation programs are considered to be unusually effective if more than one third of the entrants have stopped smoking by the end of 6 months; dietary restrictions are often not observed; and large percentages drop out of weight-control programs).

Given the extensive documentation of suboptimal public participation in screening, immunization, and other preventive health efforts, as well as low levels of individual adherence to prescribed medical therapies (Benner et al., 2002; DiMatteo, 2004; Fotheringham & Sawyer, 1995; Kimmel et al., 2007; Osterberg & Blaschke, 2005; Sackett & Snow, 1979), it is not surprising that behavioral scientists devote extensive conceptual and empirical effort to the explanation and prediction of individuals' health-related decisions. This has resulted in the development and widespread application, over the last four decades, of numerous individual-level behavior-change theories.

Such theories tend to focus on cognitive variables, such as attitudes, beliefs, and expectations, and the factors that influence these variables. They are "rational" in that they assume that individuals wish to maximize positive health outcomes. In spite of increasing attention to multi-level frameworks and theories that account for broader influences on health behavior, individual-level theories remain the most widely used in the research literature (Noar & Mehrotra, 2011; Painter, Borba, Hynes, Mays, & Glanz, 2008). A close examination of how these theories are applied to empirical work reveals considerable variation, however. Theory-based studies range from those that are merely "informed by theory" to those that actually test, or attempt to build, theory (Painter et al., 2008). Michie and Prestwich (2010) report on the development of a useful coding scheme to rate the extent to which behavioral interventions are theory based. While several individual theories have remained consistently popular for decades (Painter et al., 2008), they are being applied in new ways as modes of intervention delivery have evolved, for example, as part of Internet-based behavioral interventions (Webb, Joseph, Yardley, & Michie, 2010).

The appeal of individual theories lies in their potentially powerful applications to health research. For instance, they can form a blueprint for intervention development and evaluation by aiding in the identification of key determinants of health behavior to influence and measure. They can also be used to predict future health actions and, more generally, to help us sift through the complexity of human health-related behavior. Mitigating the potential value of these theories, however, is the reality of incomplete and unclear evidence about the utility and aptness of each theory for a given health behavior or setting, as well as considerable overlap in constructs or components across theories with varying terminology—circumstances that may make the existing menu of theories "overwhelming" to researchers and practitioners (Munro, Lewin, Swart, & Volmink, 2007; Noar & Zimmerman, 2005). Recent writings have addressed these and other issues pertinent to the current state of affairs in health behavior theory; these will be returned to in the final section of this chapter.

The overall goal for this chapter is to give a "snapshot" look at the field of individual health behavior theory. To this end, we provide an overview of six commonly used theories: Social Cognitive Theory and the related Self-Regulation Model; the Health Belief Model (HBM); the Theory of Planned Behavior (TPB), the Transtheoretical Model (TTM; Stages of Change), and the Relapse Prevention (RP) Model. A summary of the origins and primary components will be provided for each of these theories. We will also describe their empirical use and the results of meta-analyses or reviews that lend insight into their value or application. Finally, we will make note, where applicable, of critical attention that a theory has received, including noteworthy limitations or recommendations for future directions. The chapter will conclude with a discussion of recent observations on the state of health behavior theory research.

SOCIAL COGNITIVE THEORY

The underlying concept in social cognitive theory is the reciprocal nature of influences that produce behavior. Personal factors, existing behaviors, and the social and physical environments all interact and as a result of their reciprocal influences shape new behavior. Bandura's (1986, 1999, 2001, 2004, 2011) discussion of social cognitive theory and how individuals learn attempts to explain and predict development of behavior using several key concepts: incentives, outcome expectations, and efficacy expectations. Bandura (1977) outlined the roles of these concepts in a paradigm that assumes that a person with given beliefs, information, attitudes, and needs functioning in given social and physical environments will engage in a behavior that will have a consequent outcome. In this explanation, behavior change and maintenance of behavior are largely a function of (a) expectations about the outcomes that will result from engaging in behavior and (b) expectations about one's ability to engage in or execute the behavior. Thus, "outcome expectations" consist of beliefs about whether given behaviors will lead to given outcomes, whereas "efficacy expectations" consist of beliefs about how capable one is of performing the behavior that leads to those outcomes. The two have been shown to be linked in predicting, for example, exercise behavior (Hallam & Petosa, 2004) and self-management of diabetes (Ianotti et al., 2006; Martin, Dutton, & Brantley, 2012; Shi, Ostwald, & Wang, 2010). It should be emphasized that both outcome and efficacy expectations reflect a person's beliefs about capabilities and the connections between behavior and outcome. It is these perceptions, then, and not necessarily "true" capabilities, that influence behavior. In addition, it is important to understand that the concept of self-efficacy relates to beliefs about capabilities of performing specific behaviors in particular situations (Marks, Allegrante, & Lorig, 2005; Schunk & Carbonari, 1984); self-efficacy does not refer to a personality characteristic or to a global trait that operates independently of contextual factors (Bandura, 1986, 1997). This means that individuals' efficacy expectations will vary greatly depending on the particular task and context that confronts them.

Bandura (1997, 2002) argued that perceived self-efficacy influences all aspects of behavior, including the acquisition of new behaviors (e.g., a sexually active young adult learning how to use a particular contraceptive device), inhibition of existing behaviors (e.g., decreasing or stopping cigarette smoking), and disinhibition of behaviors (e.g., resuming sexual activity after a myocardial infarction). Self-efficacy also affects people's choices of task-change settings, the amount of effort they will expend on a task, and the length of time they will persist in the face of obstacles. Finally, self-efficacy affects people's emotional reactions, such as anxiety and distress and thought patterns. Thus, individuals with low self-efficacy about a particular task may ruminate about their personal deficiencies, rather than thinking about accomplishing or attending to the task at hand; this, in turn, impedes successful performance of the task.

According to Bandura, efficacy expectations vary along dimensions of magnitude, strength, and generality. "Magnitude" refers to the ordering of tasks by difficulty level. Persons having low-magnitude expectations feel capable of performing only the simpler of a graded series of tasks, while those with high-magnitude expectations feel capable of performing even the most difficult tasks in the series. "Strength" refers to judgment regarding how certain one is of one's ability to perform a specific task (Bandura, 1984). "Generality" concerns the extent to which efficacy expectations about a particular situation or experience generalize to other situations. For example, the beliefs of post-myocardial infarction patients about their endurance capabilities generated during supervised exercise testing may or may not generalize to unsupervised exercising at home.

Efficacy expectations are learned from four major sources (Bandura, 1977, 1986, 1997). The first, termed "performance accomplishments," refers to learning through personal experience where one achieves mastery over a difficult or previously feared task and thereby enjoys an increase in self-efficacy. Performance accomplishments attained through personal experience are the most potent source of efficacy expectations.

The second source is "vicarious experience," which includes learning that occurs through observation of events or other people. These events or people are referred to as "models" when they display a set of behaviors or stimulus array that illustrates a certain principle, rule, or response. In order for modeling to affect an observer's self-efficacy positively, however, it is important that the model is viewed as overcoming difficulties through determined effort rather than with ease, and that the model is similar to the observer with regard to other characteristics (e.g., age and gender). Additionally, modeled behaviors presented with clear rewarding outcomes are more effective than modeling with unclear or unrewarded outcomes.

"Verbal persuasion" constitutes the third source of efficacy expectations. This method is quite familiar to all health workers who have exhorted patients to persevere in their efforts to change behavior.

Finally, one's "physiological state" provides information that can influence efficacy expectations. Bandura has noted that because high physiological arousal usually impairs performance, people are more likely to expect failure when they are very tense and viscerally agitated. For example, people who experience extremely sweaty palms, a racing heartbeat, and trembling knees prior to giving a talk find that their self-efficacy plummets; to someone just beginning an exercise program, fatigue and mild aches and pains may be mistakenly interpreted as a sign of physical inefficacy. Self-efficacy has been shown to be associated with asthma outcomes (Mancuso, Rincon, McCulloch, & Charlson, 2001), exercise behavior among arthritis patients (Gyurcsik, Estabrooks, & Frahm-Templar, 2003), self-care behaviors and glycosylated hemoglobin (HbA1c) levels among young adults with diabetes (Johnston-Brooks, Lewis, & Garg, 2002), tobacco use cessation (Ockene, Benfari, Nuttall, Hurwitz, & Ockene, 1982), adherence in type 2 diabetes (Sevick et al., 2009), and exercise training (Pozehl, Duncan, Hertzog, & Norman, 2010).

It is important to distinguish self-efficacy from a number of other concepts with which it is sometimes linked and frequently confused. This confusion occurs in part because the personality traits, states, and processes that these concepts represent can influence efficacy expectations or be influenced by them.

"Health locus of control" refers to a generalized expectation about whether one's health is controlled by one's own behavior or by forces external to oneself (Wallston & Wallston, 1984) and has been a focus of many studies (see, e.g., Burker, Evon, Galanko, & Egan, 2005; Chen, 1995; Hong, Oddone, Dudley, & Bosworth, 2006; Ziff, Conrad, & Lachman, 1995). Health is an outcome, while self-efficacy focuses on beliefs about the capacity to undertake behavior(s) that may or may not lead to desired outcomes (such as health). Bandura (1986) illustrated the importance of the distinction between locus of control and self-efficacy by noting that the conviction that outcomes (e.g., good health) are determined by one's own action can have any number of effects on self-efficacy and behavior. For example, people who view their health as personally determined, but who believe they lack the skills needed to carry out the behaviors that would result in good health, would experience low self-efficacy and approach those activities with a sense of futility.

"Self-esteem" refers to liking and respect for oneself that has some realistic basis (Crandall, 1978) and is a construct that has received considerable attention in the health literature (see, e.g., Franklin, Denyer, Steinbeck, Caterson, & Hill, 2006; Ireys Gross, Werthamer-Larsson, & Kolodner, 1994; Strauss, 2000; Torres, Fernandez, & Maceira, 1995). Thus, self-esteem is concerned with an evaluation of self-worth, while self-efficacy relates to an evaluation of specific capabilities in specific situations. Bandura (1984) highlighted the distinction between the two concepts by pointing out that people can have high self-efficacy for a task from which they derive no self-pride (e.g., being able to brush one's teeth well) or have low self-efficacy for a task but have no loss of self-worth (e.g., not being able to ride a unicycle). However, he observes that people often try to develop self-efficacy in activities that give them a sense of self-worth, so that the two concepts are frequently intertwined.

While this presentation of social cognitive theory emphasizes its cognitive–perceptual dimensions, the importance of the social environment in the theory should be noted (Bandura, 1986, 2004). Although cognitive–motivational aspects have received the most attention, situational determinants are essential to the theory as well. A number of studies support the idea of the influences of the social environment as explicated in social cognitive theory. These include the influence on behavior of social support (Gallant, 2003), role models (Stanton-Salazar & Spina, 2003), norms and cultural practices (Eisenberg, Neumark-Sztainer, Story, & Perry, 2005; Larkey, Hecht, Miller, & Alatorre, 2001), and other dimensions of social interaction (Unger et al., 2006).

Social cognitive theory, especially as articulated by Bandura, has become widely accepted, giving rise to a number of salient constructs and models of behavior change. Several health-related models (for example, the Health Belief Model (HBM) and the Stages of Change Model) attempt to predict health behavior but do not explain how one, for example, comes to have certain beliefs, or develops readiness for change. Social cognitive theory is valued in part because it both predicts and explains behavior change. In this regard, it is a rich and robust theory from which to draw principles of change. Some criticism of social cognitive theory has been raised regarding its focus on individual behavior and its basis in and emphasis on cognition and perception as opposed to greater acknowledgment of "ecological" determinants, including social, economic, and political factors (Bronfenbrenner, 1979). These criticisms, however, have been few and infrequent and it remains a highly regarded theory guiding work in health behavior change (Bandura, 2004; Tierney et al., 2011; Short, James, & Plotnikoff, 2013).

SELF-REGULATION

Self-regulation is a principle directly drawn from social cognitive theory. It is a dimension related to how individuals develop understanding of their own behavior and evolve their outcome and efficacy expectations. Self-regulation has received considerable attention in academic learning (Zimmerman, 1998).

SELF-REGULATION AS A FEEDBACK SYSTEM AND ADHERENCE TO MEDICAL REGIMENS

Leventhal and colleagues (1980, 1998) were among the first to apply the self-regulation construct to health behavior. They view self-regulation as a solution to the basic problem of locus of control in medication adherence. The fundamental notion is that the individual functions as a feedback system. He or she establishes behavioral goals, generates plans and responses to reach these goals, and establishes criteria for monitoring the effects of his or her responses on movement toward or away from the goal. This information is then used to alter coping techniques, set new criteria for evaluating response outputs, and revise goals. The individual is, therefore, an information processing system that regulates his or her relationship to the environment (Bandura, 1980). They posit that people are active problem solvers. Individuals see and define their worlds, select and elaborate coping procedures to manage threats, and change the way they represent problems when they obtain disconfirming feedback. Problem-solving processes occur in a given context and the energy expended or motivation to enhance health and to prevent and cure disease is directed to what is perceived to be the most immediate and urgent threat and is limited by resources and a satisfaction rule (Leventhal et al., 1998). The analogy provided is one of the person acting as if he were a scientist—formulating hypotheses about physiology and the effects of illness and creating a mental picture of his or her ability to take actions to prevent or cure illness.

Leventhal's self-regulation model contains components that depict a process: (1) extracting information from the environment; (2) generating a representation of the illness as dangerous to oneself; and (3) planning and acting, which involve imagining response alternatives to deal with the problem and emotions it generates, and then taking selected actions to achieve specific effects. The feedback loop is achieved by the last step: (4) monitoring or appraising how one's coping reactions affected the environmental problem and oneself. "Each component is a set of processes, each operated within its own set of rules, each has its own potentials" (Leventhal et al., 1980, p. 35).

In this iteration of self-regulation, patients' adherence to a regimen is thought to be influenced by their perceptions and evaluations of the presence or absence of health threats (for example, symptoms). Halm, Mora, and Leventhal (2006) have shown that individuals who conceptualized asthma as an acute, episodic illness were significantly more likely to report lower rates of adherence to inhaled corticosteroids at three separate time periods and after controlling for factors thought to affect medication adherence. Similarly, Brewer, Chapman, Brownlee, and Leventhal (2002) have demonstrated relationships between LDL cholesterol control and the degree to which patients' mental models of disease were similar to that of experts' (i.e., physician-like).

In a study of 366 men and women using a clinic of a university hospital, Cameron, E. Leventhal, and H. Leventhal (1995) found that care-seeking was a function of the characteristics of the symptoms patients identified as distinctive signs of illness, and not of the level of life stresses they experience. E. Leventhal, Hansell, Diefenbach, H. Leventhal, and Glass (1996) have shown mood state to be related to physical symptom reports for patients. Also, this model relies to a fair degree on Bandura's formulations regarding reciprocal determinism and self-regulation, and both this work and Bandura's (1986) social cognitive theory arise from a common theoretical heritage that strongly suggests the importance of the approach to understanding adherence behaviors.

THE ELEMENTS OF SELF-REGULATION AND THEIR RELATIONSHIP TO HEALTH BEHAVIORS

Drawing from the work of Zimmerman in academic learning and Leventhal in medication adherence, Clark and colleagues have undertaken studies to explicate the discrete elements of self-regulation and their relationship to health behavior and health outcomes (Clark et al., 1988; Clark & Starr-Schneidkraut, 1994; Clark & Gong, 2000; Clark, Gong, & Kaciroti, 2001). They have proposed a framework for conceptualizing disease management by patients with chronic conditions designed to explain self-regulatory relationships and guide the development of interventions. In their model (see Figure 1.1), self-regulation is viewed as a means by which patients determine what is effective and what is not, given specific goals. They make these determinations influenced by their social context and according to the resources they have available. The model is based on three assumptions. First, several factors predispose one to manage a disease. Second, management is the conscious use of strategies to manipulate situations to reduce the impact of disease on daily life. One learns which strategies do or do not work through processes of self-regulation. Third, a person is motivated to be self-regulating by a desired goal or end point; the more salient the goal, the more self-regulating a person will try to be. The model is also predicated on the idea that the processes comprising self-regulation are continuous and reciprocal. Information, behavior, feelings, and conclusions generated from any one element of self-regulation as defined in the model (i.e., observation, judging, and reacting) continually influence the other elements.

FIGURE 1.1 The Model of Management of Chronic Disease through self-regulation processes. (Based on the model from Clark, Gong, & Kaciroti, 2001)

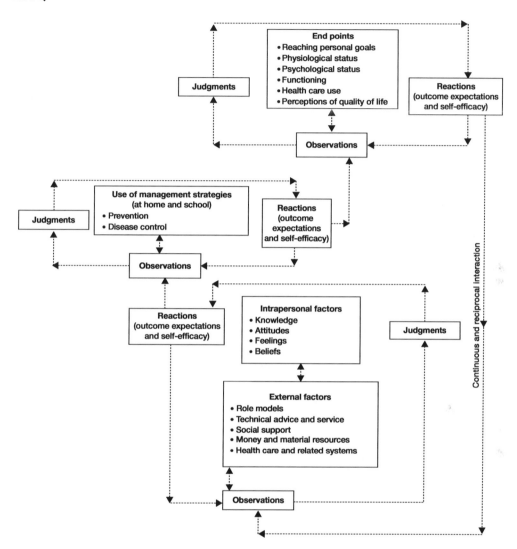

The model posits that when taking a disease management action, an individual is influenced by internal factors, that is, information and beliefs he or she has concerning the specific problem. The action is also influenced by what the person believes to be the benefits of engaging in the behavior to reach his or her personal goal and his or her beliefs that the benefits outweigh the costs. The extent to which the person holds the requisite knowledge and beliefs to support an action depends, in part, on a range of external factors. These include interpersonal relationships through which emotional and instrumental (social) support is given and received. Almost certainly involved is technical advice from a clinician who provides therapeutic recommendations. Availability of money and other resources (e.g., the price of medicine and way to get to a pharmacy) also will influence the person's behavior. It must also be noted that while knowledge, attitudes, and feelings are the basis for action, these can also change as a result of behavior (Bandura, 1986).

Management strategies comprise the individual's means to keep the disease and its effects under control (Clark, 1998). These strategies may be effective or ineffective and may be consistent with clinicians' recommendations or not. Strategies evolve from the person's observations, judgments, and reactions, given the aforementioned internal and external factors. Others can influence the strategy chosen, but in the end, the individual's personal goals, combined internal and external resources, and degree of self-regulation will dictate which management strategy will be derived and further employed.

An example would be a child who wants to play full-court basketball who believes he is susceptible to respiratory problems, thinks medicines will help and so uses them preventively, works out a procedure for taking a breather when active, seeks moral support from his or her friends and coaches, and uses other strategies that enable him or her to reach the personal goal. The child learns which strategies are effective through self-regulation. Self-regulation may be particularly important in diseases where there is no surefire formula an individual can use to control symptoms or deal with crucial interpersonal relationships. In these illnesses, patients (and families) must exercise a high level of decisionmaking in the absence of health professionals. The self-regulatory processes in which they engage entail observing situations where the disease contributes to problems in reaching their goals; judging what types of actions might ameliorate the situation; using management strategies, that is, trying out new behaviors; and drawing conclusions or reacting to the effects of the behavior. Two important reactions are that the behavior resulted in the desired effect and that one can effectively carry out the behavior, that is, self-efficacy (as defined by Bandura, 1997, 2002). Using strategies to prevent symptoms, manage them effectively, and manage the interpersonal relationships needed to control the effects of the disease should lead to important outcomes.

The motivating factor in taking disease management action is a personal goal. Goals are highly idiosyncratic. When an educator or clinician (or any other person attempting to assist with disease management) has a different goal than the individual, the opportunity for successful goal attainment is attenuated. Usually, the clinician has a clinical goal, but this end point is not likely to be as important to the patient as his or her personal goal. When clinician and educator focus on achieving the patient's personal goal, the chances are greater that the therapeutic regimen will appeal to the interests of the patient and be implemented by him or her. The assumption of the model presented here is that enabling people to be the best managers of their disease requires helping them to improve their self-regulation skills and modifying external factors, so that these influences enhance one's ability to be self-regulating. Elements of the model have been shown to be predictive of disease self-management outcomes (Cabana et al., 2006; Clark, Evans, Zimmerman, Levison, & Mellins, 1994; Clark et al., 2001; Janz, Wren, Schottenfeld, & Guire, 2003).

A number of health-related intervention studies have used the concepts associated with self-regulation focusing primarily on the self-monitoring dimensions of available models. These investigations have included failure to respond to a computer-tailored asthma management program, eating behavior and weight loss; hypoglycemia monitoring; blood glucose symptom recognition; representations of heart disease risk; functioning among patients with coronary heart disease and managing diabetes (Joseph et al., 2010; Rejeski, Mihalko, Ambrosius, Bearon, & McClelland, 2011; Barnard, Parkin, Young, & Ashraf, 2012; Kirk et al., 2011; Lee, Cameron, Wunsche, & Steven, 2011; Kubzansky, Park, Peterson, Vokonas, & Sparrow, 2011; Sevick et al., 2008).

Few criticisms have been offered regarding self-regulation as an important concept in explaining health behavior change and predicting health outcomes. Deficiencies mentioned likely reside more in the emphasis of work to date discussing and examining self-regulation than in the construct itself. In this regard, observations similar to those raised about social cognitive theory in general can be made. Self-regulation, especially as described by Clark and colleagues (2001), is based on perceptions developed as a result of observation and personal judgments resulting from them. It relies on change that can occur from an individual's actions based on those perceptions and perforce those things within the control of an individual to influence. More attention has been given in studies to factors in the immediate circle of family and friends that an individual can modify than to wider influences in the social and physical environments, such as community infrastructure, economic conditions, health-related policies, and political dynamics. These latter factors are generally beyond the ability of one individual to change. It has been posited that a combination of interventions based on individual self-regulation with ecological and community development models aimed at a broader system-wide change are required to modify behavior and achieve important health outcomes on a large scale (Clark, 2000).

THE HEALTH BELIEF MODEL

The Health Belief Model (HBM) was developed in the early 1950s by a group of social psychologists at the U.S. Public Health Service (Rosenstock, 1974) in an attempt to understand "the widespread failure of people to accept disease preventives or screening tests for the early detection of asymptomatic disease"; it was later applied to patients' responses to symptoms (Kirscht, 1974) and to adherence to prescribed medical regimens (Becker, 1974).

The basic components of the HBM are derived from a well-established body of psychological and behavioral theory. The antecedents are the same as those giving rise to social cognitive theory; in early iterations these antecedent concepts were called "social learning theory" (Miller & Dollard, 1941; Rosenstock, Strecher, & Becker, 1988). The direction taken in the HBM emphasizes personal belief over the wider range of factors accounted for in social cognitive theory and the construct of self-regulation. The hypothesis is that behavior depends mainly upon two variables: (1) the value placed by an individual on a particular goal and (2) the individual's estimate of the likelihood that a given action will achieve that goal (Maiman & Becker, 1974). When these variables were conceptualized in the context of health-related behavior, the correspondences were: (1) the desire to avoid illness (or if ill, to get well) and (2) the belief that a specific health action will prevent (or ameliorate) illness (i.e., the individual's estimate of the threat of illness and of the likelihood of being able, through personal action, to reduce that threat).

Specifically, HBM consists of the following dimensions (Figure 1.2): *Perceived susceptibility,* or one's subjective perception of the risk of contracting a condition; *perceived severity,* or feelings concerning the seriousness of contracting an illness (or of leaving it untreated); while low perceptions of seriousness might provide insufficient motivation for behavior, very high perceived severity might inhibit action; *perceived benefits,* or beliefs regarding the effectiveness of the various actions available to reduce disease threat; *perceived barriers,* or the potential negative aspects of a particular health action that may act as impediments to undertaking the recommended behavior; and *cues to action,* or stimuli to trigger the decision-making process.

In the HBM context, it is understood that diverse demographic, personal, structural, and social factors have the potential to influence health behaviors. However, these variables are believed to work through their effects on the individual's health motivations and subjective perceptions, rather than functioning as direct causes of health action (Becker et al., 1977).

FIGURE 1.2 The Health Belief Model. (From Becker, Drachman, & Kirscht, 1974. Copyright 1974 by the American Public Health Association. Reprinted with permission)

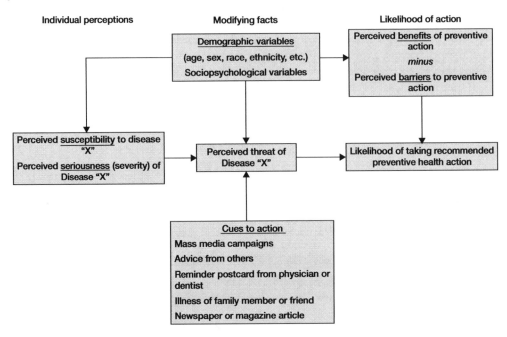

The HBM has received extensive research attention. A large body of evidence has accumulated in support of the HBM's ability to account for undertaking preventive health actions, seeking diagnoses, and following prescribed medical advice (i.e., adherence to regimens), although the variance in difference it accounts for has not always been great. A review (Janz & Becker, 1984) summarized findings from 46 HBM-related investigations (18 prospective and 28 retrospective). Twenty-four studies examined preventive health behaviors (PHB); 19 explored sick-role behaviors (SRB); and 3 addressed clinic utilization. A "significant ratio" was constructed that divides the number of positive, statistically significant findings for an HBM dimension by the total number of studies reporting significance levels for that dimension.

In the preponderance of cases, each HBM dimension was found to be significantly associated with the health-related behaviors under study; overall, the significance ratio orderings (in descending order) were "barriers" (89%), "susceptibility" (81%), "benefits" (78%), and "severity" (65%). Findings from prospective studies were at least as favorable as those obtained from retrospective research. Also, the model has been shown to be associated with a range of preventive behaviors and influential as part of health-related interventions; examples include cancer screening (Champion et al., 2002; Janz et al., 2003), condom use (Hounton, Carabin, & Henderson, 2005), vaccination (de Wit, Vet, Schutten, & van Steenbergen, 2005), and malaria chemoprophylaxis (Farquharson, Noble, Barker, & Beherns, 2004; Pine et al., 2000). It also has been associated with disease management, including heart disease (George & Shalansky, 2007; Pinto, Lively, Siganga, Holiday-Goodman, & Kamm, 2006), HIV disease (Barclay et al., 2007), calcium intake (Jung, Martin Ginis, Phillips, & Lordon, 2011), health-seeking behavior (Venmans, Gorter, Hak, & Rutten, 2008; Venmans et al., 2011), and colon cancer awareness (Holt, Roberts et al., 2009; Holt, Shipp et al., 2009).

Across a wide range of topical areas of study, HBM has provided relatively limited explanations of the variance in findings. Investigators have tried to boost the effects of

HBM by combining constructs with others from social cognitive theory, specifically self-efficacy. Clark and colleagues (1988) added self-efficacy to dimensions of the HBM and found that the variance explained in the management of asthma by school-aged children did not increase significantly. Adih and Alexander (1999), however, found that self-efficacy along with constructs from the HBM were significant predictors of condom use among youth, although the relative contribution of each construct was not specified.

Along similar lines, criticisms of the HBM have included that despite the body of findings relating HBM dimensions to health actions, the HBM as a psychosocial model is limited to accounting for as much of the variance in individuals' health-related behaviors as can be explained by their attitudes and beliefs. It is clear that other forces influence health actions as well; for example: (a) some behaviors (e.g., cigarette smoking and brushing teeth) have a substantial habitual component, obviating any ongoing psychosocial decision-making process; (b) many health-related behaviors are undertaken for what are ostensibly non-health-related reasons (e.g., dieting to appear more attractive and stopping smoking or jogging to attain social approval); and (c) economic or environmental factors may prevent the individual from undertaking a preferred course of action (e.g., a worker in a hazardous environment; a resident in a city with high levels of air pollution). The model is based on the premises that "health" is a highly valued concern or goal for most individuals and that "cues to action" are widely prevalent; where these conditions are not satisfied, the model may not be useful in, or relevant to, predicting behavior.

THEORY OF PLANNED BEHAVIOR

The prediction of behavioral intentions, as the direct antecedent to behavior itself, is at the heart of Ajzen's Theory of Planned Behavior (TPB) (Ajzen, 1991; Ajzen, 2011) and its predecessor, the Theory of Reasoned Action (TRA) (Ajzen & Fishbein, 1980). Predictors of behavioral intention, according to these models, are: (1) an individual's *attitudes* toward the behavior, which are influenced, in turn, by his or her beliefs about the (a) likelihood and (b) desirability of outcomes resulting from the behavior; and (2) the *subjective norm* toward that behavior as perceived by the individual, determined by (a) what an individual perceives as the expectations of important others about the behavior, as well as (b) how motivated he or she is to comply with the beliefs of these significant others. The relative influence of these two components—attitude and subjective norms—on intention depends on the nature of the behavioral goal. For some behaviors, the attitudinal component will be the major determinant of intention, while for others, the more the individual believes that significant others are in favor of the behavior, the stronger will be his or her intention to perform it. A recent refinement of the model by its creator was the addition of "descriptive norms" as part of the "normative beliefs" component (Fishbein & Aizen, 2010). "Descriptive norms" are what a person perceives as others' actual *performance* of a particular behavior (such as the perceived extent to which peers themselves practice safer sex), not just others' *views* on the behavior.

The TPB expands on the TRA with a component representing the perceived degree of control the person has over the behavior, a concept similar to Bandura's construct of self-efficacy (Ajzen, 1991). These control beliefs take into account the presence and strength of personal and external factors that influence the behavior, such as having a workable plan, skills, social support, knowledge, time, money, willpower, and opportunity. By accounting for control perceptions, TPB increases its relevance to the large number of health-related behaviors over which people have incomplete volitional control.

FIGURE 1.3 Theory of Planned Behavior Model. (From Ajzen, 2013. Copyright 2006 Icek Ajzen. Reprinted with permission)

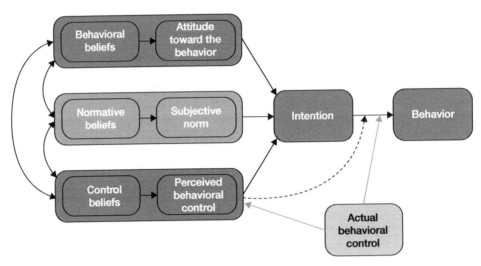

In sum, then, the TPB posits that three types of beliefs determine a person's intention to perform a particular behavior. An individual's beliefs about a behavior lead to a favorable or unfavorable *attitude* toward that behavior; his or her beliefs about how others regard the behavior determine the *subjective norm*; and beliefs about the extent to which he or she has control over the behavior determine the level of *perceived behavioral control*. Where attitudes and subjective norms are favorable, and perceived control is high, strong intention to perform the behavior should result. The ultimate execution of the behavior is not solely explained by these predictors, as actual control plays an important part as well. According to the model (Figure 1.3), perceived behavioral control can serve as a rough proxy for actual control over a behavior (perceptions of control will, of course, be more accurate in some cases than others); as such, it may contribute to the prediction of actual behavior. In other words, successful performance of the behavior will be the end result if individuals have both intention and sufficient control over the internal and external factors that influence such performance.

Operationalizing TPB components for empirical work is facilitated by the availability of a detailed guide for construction of a questionnaire measuring each of the key TPB constructs (Ajzen, 2013). The guide includes suggested formative research—such as using qualitative methods to elicit the target group's salient beliefs about behavioral outcomes, the key normative referents, and factors influencing control—as well as sample item wording. A separate document addresses the design of TPB-based behavioral interventions; for example, how to select the specific theory components to attempt to influence for a given behavior and population.

The TPB has been extensively used in health research over the last several decades and was cited over 4000 times by Google Scholar in 2010 (Ajzen, 2011). It has been applied to a wide range of health-related behaviors. A bibliography of empirical work found on the official TPB website cites TPB-based studies on such diverse behaviors as condom use, malaria prophylaxis, speeding, physical activity, use of dental floss, and cancer screening. McEachan and colleagues (McEachan, Conner, Taylor, & Lawton, 2011) performed a random-effects meta-analysis of 206 prospective studies of health behaviors using the TPB. Their analysis controlled, where possible, for the effects of past behavior on future behavior, and assessed how behavioral type (e.g., health pro-moting vs. health risk), sample characteristics, and methodological factors (e.g., length of follow-up) moderated the ability of the TPB to predict future behavior. Results of this analysis indicated that the TPB explained 19.3% of the variance in behavior and 44.3% of the variance in intention across studies, which the authors describe as being "slightly lower" than in previous meta-analytic reviews. Past behavior added 10.9% variance to the prediction of behavior and 5% to behavioral intention. In this analysis, the TPB more successfully predicted behaviors related to diet and physical activity than risk detection, safer sex, and abstinence from drugs. Behaviors in the shorter term were better predicted than behaviors in the longer term, and self-report measures of behavior were better predicted than objective measures. Notably, attitudes remained a strong predictor of intentions after controlling for past behavior, which, according to the authors, strengthens the case for trying to target attitudes as part of interventions.

In a recent article, Ajzen responds to several criticisms of the TPB (Ajzen, 2011). For example, he notes that the model has been said to ignore the affective component of decision-making, and to rely on a "rational-actor" approach to behavioral choices. He argues that both emotion and irrationality can be subsumed in the behavioral, normative, and control "beliefs" components of TPB, as these beliefs are not always formed in a rational or even accurate manner and are subject to influence by emo-tional state. Ajzen also describes attempts made by researchers to improve the pre-dictive validity of the TPB by adding components. For example, when predicting genetic testing behaviors, Wolff and colleagues (2011) added "anticipated affective outcomes" to the model's "behavioral beliefs" component; Kor and Mullan (2011) added "perceived autonomy support" to the prediction of sleep-hygiene behaviors. Ajzen cautions that for the sake of model parsimony, any new predictors proposed for addition to the model should meet strict criteria; for example, having a causal relationship with intention and action and conceptual independence from other components (Ajzen, 2011).

Research to further refine the TPB might include a greater focus on measurement context; that is, how beliefs might be activated according to mood and setting (Ajzen, 2011). Other potential areas of inquiry are the role that past behavior plays in deter-mining behavioral intention, the role of habit formation, and how stable "background factors"—for example, personality traits or demographic characteristics—might affect the relative importance of TPB components (Ajzen, 2011). Finally, MacEachen and colleagues (2011) recommend that in future tests of the TPB, researchers should consider using objective—rather than merely self-reported—measures of current behavior and of past behavior, which are currently lacking in the literature.

TRANSTHEORETICAL MODEL

The Transtheoretical Model (TTM) (Prochaska, 2009; Prochaska & Velicer, 1997), known more familiarly as the "Stages of Change" model, is one of the most prominent in health behavior research. The TTM focuses on *behavior change*, in contrast to models like the TPB that could be used equally to explain ongoing behaviors (Noar, Chabot, & Zimmerman, 2008). The TTM was the product of an effort by Prochaska and colleagues in the 1970s to identify the common elements of leading theories of psychotherapy and behavior change. The authors observed in subsequent empirical work that smokers used dif-ferent processes of change at different points in their attempts to quit, leading to the formulation of the "stage" aspect of the TTM in which behavioral change is viewed not as an event but as a six-stage process.

These stages, which represent an underlying continuum and through which movement may take place backward as well as forward, are defined as follows (Prochaska & Velicer, 1997): *precontemplation*, where people are not considering a health behavior change in the near future (usually operationalized as 6 months); *contemplation*, where people are intending to change in the next 6 months and need to be motivated to do so; *preparation*, in which people are intending to take action in the immediate future and need the skills to do so; *action*, where people are making a specific behavioral change and can be supported by intervention strategies and guidelines; *maintenance*, where a new behavior becomes more habitual and requires less ongoing effort—that is, less use of the "processes of change" described below—but where relapse prevention is still important. The final stage, somewhat theoretical in nature, is *termination*, where a behavior is permanently ingrained.

Ten *processes of change*, or activities that people use to progress through the stages, are specified by the TTM. Examples of these are counterconditioning (substituting healthy for less healthy behaviors), stimulus control (removing cues for unhealthy habits), and contingency management (e.g., a reward system). Other TTM constructs include *decisional balance* (an individual's perceived pros and cons of changing), *self-efficacy* (per social cognitive theory), and *temptation* (the intensity of urges to engage in a specific behavior when in challenging situations). The key notion of the TTM is that interventions will be more effective when they are "stage-matched"—that is, using the processes and principles of change appropriate for a given stage and a given health behavior. Thus, one way of testing the validity of the TTM is to do a "match–mismatch" experiment to assess whether stage matching enhances the intervention's effectiveness. At least one such study of a smoking cessation intervention found that participants in the "matched" condition made greater forward movement in stages (Dijkstra, Conijn, & De Vries, 2006), but another found no advantage for the stage-matched condition (Aveyard, Massey, Parsons, Manaseki, & Griffin, 2009).

Much past empirical work with the TTM has been with smoking cessation—the health behavior that gave rise to the theory—but it also has been applied to a wide range of other health-related behaviors. For example, a 2008 meta-analysis examined 48 different health behaviors which have been studied using TTM principles in 120 datasets (Hall & Rossi, 2008). This meta-analysis found consistent support across behaviors for Prochaska's so-called strong and weak principles of change, which state that for an individual to move from *precontemplation* to *action*, an individual needs to experience approximately 1 standard deviation (*SD*) increase in his or her perceived "pros" of changing, and about one-half *SD* decrease in the "cons" of changing.

A spate of recent reviews and meta-analyses demonstrate the ongoing interest in this model. These reports have examined TTM-based interventions across various behaviors: smoking cessation (Cahil, Lancaster, & Green, 2010), physical activity (Hutchison, Breckon, & Johnston, 2009), dietary change for diabetes (Salmela, Poskiparta, Kasila, Vähäsarja, & Vanhala, 2009), and diet and physical activity for weight loss (Tuah et al., 2011). Across these studies, authors noted the inconsistent and often incomplete application of the model to intervention strategies, as well as other methodological weaknesses in the studies reviewed, making it difficult to draw conclusive results about the value of the TTM for behavior-change interventions. Cahill and colleagues (2010) concluded, for example, based on 35 trials reviewed, that there does not appear to be evidence that stage-based self-help interventions and individual counseling for smoking cessation are more effective than non-stage-based equivalents. Tuah and colleagues (2011) found that TTM-based interventions for weight loss have "limited" impact in the short term, with no strong evidence for bringing about sustained weight loss.

Despite—or perhaps because of—its popularity and the appealing prospect of stage-matched interventions having the potential to produce "unprecedented impacts on entire at-risk populations" (Prochaska & Velicer, 1997), the TTM has inspired a number of critical articles describing what are viewed as the model's shortcomings. Indeed, one observer commented that the TTM has not just fame, but "notoriety" (Brug et al., 2005). Another notes that the model seems to be better accepted among practitioners than researchers (Munro et al., 2007). Examples of articles critical of the TTM are Sutton (2001), Littell and Girvin (2002), Adams and White (2005), and West (2005). Some of the common problems with the TTM described in these critiques include: weak empirical evidence for the efficacy of stage-based interventions and for the very existence of discrete stages of behavior change; implied sequencing of readiness stages; the arbitrary length of stages and the use of staging algorithms that lack validity, reliability, and consistency across studies; the difficulty of applying the model to complex behaviors like physical activity or dietary change; and a lack of evidence that moving people forward in stages ultimately results in behavior change or other health-related outcomes. Munro and colleagues (2007) also noted that stage-tailored interventions may be resource intensive and might not be appropriate when rapid behavior change is desired.

Counterpoints to these criticisms also have been made, for example, by identifying methodological shortcomings in certain studies that have not offered strong support for the model (Prochaska, Velicer, Nigg, & Prochaska, 2008) to citing empirical work that does show support for the model (Velicer, Norman, Fava, & Prochaska, 1999) to noting that in empirical work, the TTM tends to be selectively and incompletely operationalized (Hutchison et al., 2009). Suggestions for improving the application of the model also have been offered; for example, improved methods of staging individuals, and expanding the use of stage-transition strategies to include constructs from other theories/models, such as ecological models (Brug et al., 2005). Greater attention to documenting the nature and fidelity of TTM application to interventions also will contribute to a better understanding of how—and whether—the model is useful in fostering behavior change (Hutchison et al., 2009; Salmela et al., 2009).

RELAPSE PREVENTION MODEL

Relapse prevention (RP) is a cognitive-behavioral model that was developed more than three decades ago to help people who are trying to change health behaviors, particularly addictive behaviors, anticipate and cope with relapse (Marlatt & George, 1984; Hendershot, Marlatt, & George, 2009; Hendershot, Witkiewitz, George, & Marlatt, 2011). Rooted in social cognitive theory with self-regulatory efficacy playing a key role in an individual's vulnerability to relapse (Bandura, 1997), the RP model has been highly influential in practice. In fact, "relapse prevention" has become essentially a generic term describing interventions that build coping skills for dealing with situations that place individuals at high risk of relapse (Hendershot et al., 2009). Unlike the other theories and models discussed in this chapter, RP does not address initial behavior change, but rather deals with the ubiquitous challenge of maintaining the change over the long term. A major contribution of this model was its elaboration of relapse not as a failure, or end state, but rather as a transitional process which may or may not lead to previous levels of the undesired behavior. Moreover, RP provides individuals with skills and strategies to prevent a single lapse from becoming full-blown relapse (Marlatt & George, 1984).

The RP model recognizes two primary categories of factors that trigger or contribute to relapse (as described in Larimer, Palmer, & Marlatt, 1999): *immediate determinants* of relapse and *covert antecedents*. Among the *immediate determinants* are *high-risk situations*, which pose a threat to a person's sense of control over the behavior (these situations include negative emotional states like depression, interpersonal conflict, social pressure, and external cues to engage in the behavior); *coping* (that is, how the person responds to those situations; individuals who have mastered effective coping strategies are less likely to experience relapse, and success in coping also leads to greater self-efficacy to do so in the future); *outcome expectancies* for the behavior (most relevant are positive expectations; for example, relapse is more likely if a person believes that the behavior will help with short-term stress reduction); and the *abstinence violation effect* (where a person who has an initial lapse feels guilt, a lack of control, and other negative emotions, which in turn make full-blown relapse more likely).

A second category of factors (Larimer et al., 1999) consists of the broader and more subtle *covert antecedents* to relapse. These can be thought of as "lifestyle" factors that help determine the extent to which a person is confronted with high-risk situations. Successful "lifestyle balance" of obligations and pleasurable activities is seen as key for managing overall stress levels that can foster high-risk situations for relapse. The RP model specifies cognitive and behavioral intervention strategies to deal with both immediate determinants of relapse, such as skills development and cognitive restructuring, and also encourages people to achieve a healthier, more balanced lifestyle to address relapse's covert antecedents. Importantly, a recently reformulated "dynamic" version of the RP model now recognizes both "tonic" (stable personal characteristics) and "phasic" (situational or transient) influences on relapse, which interact in complex ways to determine the likelihood of relapse (see Hendershot et al., 2011, for a detailed discussion of this reformulated model).

Most empirical applications of the RP model have been to the areas of alcohol use and smoking, with some application to other addictive behaviors (Hendershot et al., 2011) and an occasional application to a nonaddictive health behavior such as physical activity maintenance (e.g., Stetson et al., 2005). Evidence for the efficacy of the RP model has been examined in systematic reviews, meta-analyses, and large RCTs, as well as in studies of specific model components such as self-efficacy and negative affect (Henderson et al., 2011). It has been noted that while the overall clinical effectiveness of the RP model and several of its components have received some empirical support, "the diffuse application of RP approaches tends to complicate efforts to define RP-based treatments and evaluate their overall efficacy" (Hendershot et al., 2011).

Both the RP model and the way it is applied to practice are continuing to evolve over time. For example, "mindfulness-based RP" refers to the addition of mindfulness techniques to the cognitive-behavioral principles used in RP (Bowen, Chawla, & Marlatt, 2011; Henderson et al., 2009; Witkiewitz, Bowen, Douglas, & Hsu, 2013). Other promising future directions that have been suggested for this model (Hendershot et al., 2011) include: using nonlinear statistical approaches to study the complex interactions proposed by the reformulated model; exploring genetic influences on relapse and relapse prevention; teasing out the mechanisms of effects in efficacious RP-based interventions; and use of functional magnetic resonance imaging to explore the neural correlates of relapse.

FUTURE DIRECTIONS IN INDIVIDUAL THEORY DEVELOPMENT

Judging from the extensive application of individual-level theories to current health behavior research—and especially the handful of popular theories described in this chapter—the value and utility of these theories would appear to be widely accepted. However, in recent years, commentators have called attention to various obstacles in the area of health behavior theory development, particularly in the realm of theory testing and of theory refinement. While ideally the field of health behavior theory would be dynamic, with the continual development of existing theories and approaches as new evidence emerges (Munro et al., 2007), some researchers see instead a state of stagnation in the field. This, in turn, has been attributed to a lack of rigorous testing and subsequent theory modification that would genuinely move the field forward (Noar & Mehrotra, 2011; Noar & Zimmerman, 2005; Weinstein & Rothman, 2005; Weinstein, 2007). Although it is beyond the scope of this chapter to describe these critiques in detail, several issues will be highlighted here, and the reader is referred to more nuanced discussions of these and other issues in the cited works.

The first is the means by which theories have traditionally been evaluated. The most common way of theory testing has been the "correlational" approach, or the "which theory explains the most variance in a particular behavior" approach. However, whether data are cross-sectional or longitudinal, associations between cognitive variables and health behaviors are inflated by the fact that the relationship between health behavior and cognitive variables is likely bidirectional. Thus, any observed cognition/behavior association may be explained, in part, by behavior's effect on cognitions; this may be particularly true in the case of ongoing or habitual behaviors (Painter et al., 2008; Weinstein, 2007). In other words, correlational approaches to theory testing assess whether given theory-based constructs are associated with a particular health behavior, when the true question of interest is whether "changes in particular theory-based constructs lead to changes in health behavior" (Noar & Mehrotra, 2011).

Noar and Mehrotra (2011) propose a "multi-methodological theory testing" framework as a way to increase the rigor of theory testing and ultimately increase the value of theory to practice. As these authors argue, any single theory-testing approach has inherent limitations, like those of the survey/correlational approach described above; while behavioral interventions based on a particular theory appear to lend support to that theory if they are proven effective, in cases where the control condition consists of minimal intervention or none at all, the specific role of the theory in intervention efficacy remains unclear. Therefore, multiple, complementary methodological tools should be used to test theory, ideally in a sequential program of research. These tools include: randomized lab experiments, randomized field experiments of theory-based interventions and mediation analysis, and meta-analysis of both lab and field experiments. Such a research program would permit greater causal inference between theory components and outcomes, and would inform theory modification that could, in turn, be used to guide more effective behavior-change interventions. Brewer and Gilkey (2012) propose "competitive hypothesis testing" as another means of increasing the value of theory testing. In this approach, researchers identify specific components of two theories that give rise to competing predictions about the nature of the relationship among particular variables; empirical data are then used to determine which theory is more accurate.

A second, broader issue regarding individual-level theories of behavior change is that a narrow focus on health decisions by individuals may downplay the importance of other levels: both the "biological underpinnings and consequences" of behavior and the social context in which it occurs (Committee on Health and Behavior: Research, Practice and Policy, Board on Neuroscience and Behavioral Health, 2001). Most of the theories discussed in this chapter incorporate interpersonal influences on attitudes, beliefs, or other antecedents of behavior; such variables also may be influenced indirectly by one's environment (e.g., workplace restrictions on smoking may factor into one's "pros and cons" of smoking cessation per the TTM).

However, Glass and McAtee (2006) write that behavioral science "has focused primarily on individual health-related behaviors ... without due consideration of the social context in which health behaviors occur and become socially patterned" (Glass & McAtee, 2006, p. 1651) and that "much of public health continues to treat behaviors such as diet, smoking, violence, drug use and sex work as if they were voluntary decisions, without regard to social constraints, inducements, or pressures" (Glass & McAtee, 2006). To better account for social and environmental context of today's pressing health behavior challenges, a "shift in emphasis, a reorientation of theories, and new methods" (Glass & McAtee, 2006, p. 1664) are all required.

Using obesity as an example, Glass and McAtee offer a detailed look at the multi-level, interacting influences on behavior using an elaborate topographic metaphor in which individual behaviors take place on the surface of a flowing stream, and are influenced by the biological levels below the water's surface; above the surface, the social, built, and natural environments all shape individual behavior as well, with the life course represented by the horizontal flow of water. They introduce the notion of "risk regulators"—factors like material conditions, social norms, and policies—as contingencies that facilitate or constrain a given behavior, and that affect biological systems within the body, which also interact with behavior. This complex, multi-dimensional way of thinking about health behavior is meant to be a framework for a "next-generation" approach to the study of behavior and health, including generating theories and organizing research (Glass & McAtee, 2006).

Finally, a brief note will be made about application of individual theories to multiple health behavior change. No existing individual-level theory explicitly considers changing multiple health behaviors (Noar et al., 2008), to the extent these may be collectively addressed in interventions. Interventions based on existing theories such as SCT and the TTM have tended to address multiple risk behaviors within communities rather than within individuals (Prochaska, Spring, & Nigg, 2008). Noar, Chabot, and Zimmerman (2008) suggest three possible approaches to using theory as it relates to multiple behaviors, each with differing implications for theory-based interventions: (a) a *"behavior change principles" approach*, wherein common principles of health behavior change can be taught to individuals, who can apply them to multiple health behaviors; (b) a *global health/behavior category approach*, which suggests using broader categories such as weight control or management of a particular illness to organize and appeal to the motives for change regarding a variety of health behaviors; and (c) a *multiple behavioral approach*, which involves intervening on multiple behaviors that may cluster together, like alcohol use and smoking. Empirical testing could reveal which of these theoretical approaches is optimal for given behaviors or circumstances. Careful study of if and how multiple health behaviors cluster is also warranted. Other, related theoretical questions that merit future exploration have to do with sequencing—that is, is it best to address multiple behaviors simultaneously or sequentially? Is there a logical hierarchy to changing behaviors (such as "gateway behaviors"), and a maximum number of behaviors to target for change? (Prochaska et al., 2008; Nigg, Allegrante, & Ory, 2002). And finally, which individual-level theories can be applied most effectively to research and to the evaluation of interventions focusing on multiple health behavior change?

CONCLUSIONS

Individual health behavior change theories have been hugely influential in shaping health behavior research and interventions over more than two decades, yet there are still many questions about the optimal use and even the validity of these theories that remain unanswered. Taking theory testing and development in new directions—including, but not limited to, those mentioned above—may help to ensure the relevance of individual-level theories in an era where a strong evidence base and multi-level, multidisciplinary approaches are viewed as critical to addressing today's biggest public health challenges.

REFERENCES

Adams, J., & White, M. (2005). Why don't stage-based activity promotion interventions work? *Health Education Research, 20*(2), 237–243.

Adih, W. K., & Alexander, C. S. (1999). Determinants of condom use to prevent HIV infection among youth in Ghana. *The Journal of Adolescent Health, 24*(1), 63–72.

Ajzen, I. (1991). The theory of planned behavior. *Organizational Behavior and Human Decision Processes, 50*(2), 179.

Ajzen, I. (2011). The theory of planned behaviour: Reactions and reflections. *Psychology & Health, 26*(9), 1113–1127.

Ajzen, I. (2013). Theory of planned behavior. In *Theory of planned behavior*. Retrieved February 4, 2013, from http://people.umass.edu/aizen/tpb.html

Ajzen, I., & Fishbein, M. (1980). *Understanding attitudes and predicting social behavior* Englewood Cliffs, NJ: Prentice-Hall.

Aveyard, P., Massey, L., Parsons, A., Manaseki, S., & Griffin, C. (2009). The effect of trans theoretical model based interventions on smoking cessation. *Social Science & Medicine (1982), 68*(3), 397–403.

Bandura, A. (1977). Self-efficacy: Toward a unifying theory of behavioral change. *Psychological Review, 84*(2), 191–215.

Bandura, A. (1980). Gauging the relationship between self-efficacy judgment and action. *Cognitive Therapy and Research, 4*(2), 263–268.

Bandura, A. (1984). Recycling misconceptions of perceived self-efficacy. *Cognitive Therapy and Research, 8*(3), 231–255.

Bandura, A. (1986). *Social foundations of thought and action: A social cognitive theory*. Englewood Cliffs, NJ: Prentice-Hall.

Bandura, A. (1997). *Self-efficacy: The exercise of control*. New York, NY: W. H. Freeman.

Bandura, A. (1999). A social cognitive theory of personality. In L. Pervin & O. John (Eds.), *Handbook of personality* (2nd ed., pp. 154–196). New York, NY: Guilford.

Bandura, A. (2001). Social cognitive theory: An agentic perspective. *Annual Review of Psychology, 52*, 1–26.

Bandura, A. (2002). Social cognitive theory in cultural context. *Journal of Applied Psychology: An International Review, 51*, 269–290.

Bandura, A. (2004). Health promotion by social cognitive means. *Health Education & Behavior, 31*(2), 143–164.

Bandura, A. (2011). Self-deception: A paradox revisited. *Behavioral and Brain Sciences, 34*(1), 16–17.

Barclay, T. R., Hinkin, C. H., Castellon, S. A., Mason, K. I., Reinhard, M. J., Marion S. D., ... Durvasula, R. S. (2007). Age-associated predictors of medication adherence in HIV-positive adults: Health beliefs, self-efficacy, and neurocognitive status. *Health Psychology, 26*(1), 40–49.

Barnard, K., Parkin, C., Young, A., & Ashraf, M. (2012). Use of an automated bolus calculator reduces fear of hypoglycemia and improves confidences in dosage accuracy in patients with type 1 diabetes mellitus treated with multiple daily insulin injections. *Journal of Diabetes Science and Technology, 6*(1), 144–149.

Becker, M. H. (1974). The health belief model and sick role behavior. *Health Education Monographs, 2*, 409–419.

Becker, M. H., Drachman, R. H., & Kirscht, J. P. (1974). A new approach to explaining sick-role behavior in low-income populations. *American Journal of Public Health, 64*, 206.

Becker, M. H., Haefner, D. P., Kasl, S. V., Kirscht, J. P., Maiman, L. A., & Rosenstock, I. M. (1977). Selected psychosocial models and correlates of individual health-related behaviors. *Medical Care, 15*(5 Suppl.), 27–46.

Benner, J. S., Glynn, R. J., Mogun, H., Neumann, P. J., Weinstein, M. C., & Avorn, J. (2002). Long-term persistence in use of statin therapy in elderly patients. *JAMA: The Journal of the American Medical Association, 288*(4), 455–461.

Bowen, C., & Marlatt, G. A. (2011). *Mindfulness-based relapse prevention for addictive behaviors: A clinician's guide*. New York, NY: Guilford Press.

Brewer, N. T., Chapman, G. B., Brownlee, S., & Leventhal, E. A. (2002). Cholesterol control, medication adherence and illness cognition. *British Journal of Health Psychology, 7*(Part 4), 433–447.

Brewer, N. T., & Gilkey, M. B. (2012). Comparing theories of health behavior using data from longitudinal studies: A comment on gerend and shepherd. *Annals of Behavioral Medicine, 44*(2), 147–148.

Bronfenbrenner, U. (1979). *The ecology of human development: Experiments by nature and design*. Cambridge, MA: Harvard University Press.

Brug, J., Conner, M., Harre, N., Kremers, S., McKellar, S., & Whitelaw, S. (2005). The transtheoretical model and stages of change: A critique: Observations by five commentators on the paper by Adams, J. & White, M. (2004). Why don't stage-based activity promotion interventions work? *Health Education Research, 20*(2), 244–258.

Burker, E. J., Evon, D. M., Galanko, J., & Egan, T. (2005). Health locus of control predicts survival after lung transplant. *Journal of Health Psychology, 10*(5), 695–704.

Cabana, M. D., Slish, K. K., Evans, D., Mellins, R. B., Brown, R. W., Lin, X., ... Clark, N. M. (2006). Impact of physician asthma care education on patient outcomes. *Pediatrics, 117*(6), 2149–2157.

Cahill, K., Lancaster, T., & Green, N. (2010). Stage-based interventions for smoking cessation. *Cochrane Database of Systematic Reviews (Online)*, (11). doi: CD004492

Cameron, L., Leventhal, E. A., & Leventhal, H. (1995). Seeking medical care in response to symptoms and life stress. *Psychosomatic Medicine, 57*(1), 37–47.

Champion, V. L., Skinner, C. S., Menon, U., Seshadri, R., Anzalone, D. C., & Rawl, S. M. (2002). Comparisons of tailored mammography interventions at two months postintervention. *Annals of Behavioral Medicine, 24*(3), 211–218.

Chen, W. W. (1995). Enhancement of health locus of control through biofeedback training. *Perceptual and Motor Skills, 80*(2), 395–398.

Clark, N. M. (1998). Management of asthma by parents and children. In H. Kotses & A. Harver (Eds.), *Self-management of asthma* (pp. 271–291). New York, NY: Marcel Dekker.

Clark, N. M. (2000). Understanding individual and collective capacity to enhance quality of life. *Health Education & Behavior, 27*(6), 699–707.

Clark, N. M., Evans, D., Zimmerman, B. J., Levison, M. J., & Mellins, R. B. (1994). Patient and family management of asthma: Theory-based techniques for the clinician. *The Journal of Asthma, 31*(6), 427–435.

Clark, N. M., & Gong, M. (2000). Management of chronic disease by practitioners and patients: Are we teaching the wrong things? *BMJ (Clinical Research Ed.), 320*(7234), 572–575.

Clark, N. M., Gong, M., & Kaciroti, N. (2001). A model of self-regulation for control of chronic disease. *Health Education & Behavior, 28*(6), 769–782.

Clark, N. M., Rakowski, W., Ostrander, L., Wheeler, J. R., Oden, S., & Keteyian, S. (1988). Development of self-management education for elderly heart patients. *The Gerontologist, 28*(4), 491–494.

Clark, N. M., & Starr-Schneidkraut, N. J. (1994). Management of asthma by patients and families. *American Journal of Respiratory and Critical Care Medicine, 149*(2, Pt. 2), S54–66; discussion S67–68.

Committee on Health and Behavior: Research, Practice and Policy, Board on Neuroscience and Behavioral Health. (2001). *Health and behavior: The interplay of biological, behavioral, and social influences*. Washington, DC: Institute of Medicine, National Academy of Sciences, National Academies Press.

Crandall, R. (1978). The measurement of self-esteem and related constructs. In J. P. Robinson & P. R. Shaver (Eds.), *Measures of social psychological attitudes* (pp. 87–94). Ann Arbor, MI: Institute of Social Research, University of Michigan.

de Wit, J. B., Vet, R., Schutten, M., & van Steenbergen, J. (2005). Social-cognitive determinants of vaccination behavior against hepatitis B: An assessment among men who have sex with men. *Preventive Medicine, 40*(6), 795–802.

Dijkstra, A., Conijn, B., & De Vries, H. (2006). A match-mismatch test of a stage model of behaviour change in tobacco smoking. *Addiction (Abingdon, England), 101*(7), 1035–1043.

DiMatteo, M. R. (2004). Social support and patient adherence to medical treatment: A meta-analysis. *Health Psychology, 23*(2), 207–218.

Eisenberg, M. E., Neumark-Sztainer, D., Story, M., & Perry, C. (2005). The role of social norms and friends' influences on unhealthy weight-control behaviors among adolescent girls. *Social Science & Medicine, 60*(6), 1165–1173.

Farquharson, L., Noble, L. M., Barker, C., & Behrens, R. H. (2004). Health beliefs and communication in the travel clinic consultation as predictors of adherence to malaria chemoprophylaxis. *British Journal of Health Psychology, 9*(Part 2), 201–217.

Fishbein, M., & Ajzen, I. (2010). *Predicting and changing behavior: The reasoned action approach*. New York, NY: Psychology Press.

Fotheringham, M. J., & Sawyer, M. G. (1995). Adherence to recommended medical regimens in childhood and adolescence. *Journal of Paediatrics and Child Health, 31*(2), 72–78.

Franklin, J., Denyer, G., Steinbeck, K. S., Caterson, I. D., & Hill, A. J. (2006). Obesity and risk of low self-esteem: A statewide survey of Australian children. *Pediatrics, 118*(6), 2481–2487.

Gallant, M. P. (2003). The influence of social support on chronic illness self-management: A review and directions for research. *Health Education & Behavior, 30*(2), 170–195.

George, J., & Shalansky, S. J. (2007). Predictors of refill non-adherence in patients with heart failure. *British Journal of Clinical Pharmacology, 63*(4), 488–493.

Glass, T. A., & McAtee, M. J. (2006). Behavioral science at the crossroads in public health: Extending horizons, envisioning the future. *Social Science & Medicine (1982), 62*(7), 1650–1671.

Gyurcsik, N. C., Estabrooks, P. A., & Frahm-Templar, M. J. (2003). Exercise-related goals and self-efficacy as correlates of aquatic exercise in individuals with arthritis. *Arthritis and Rheumatism, 49*(3), 306–313.

Hall, K. L., & Rossi, J. S. (2008). Meta-analytic examination of the strong and weak principles across 48 health behaviors. *Preventive Medicine, 46*(3), 266–274.

Hallam, J. S., & Petosa, R. (2004). The long-term impact of a four-session work-site intervention on selected social cognitive theory variables linked to adult exercise adherence. *Health Education & Behavior, 31*(1), 88–100.

Halm, E. A., Mora, P., & Leventhal, H. (2006). No symptoms, no asthma: The acute episodic disease belief is associated with poor self-management among inner-city adults with persistent asthma. *Chest, 129*(3), 573–580.

Hendershot, C., Marlatt, G. A., & George, W. (2009). Relapse prevention and the maintenance of optimal health. In S. Shumaker, J. Ockene, & K. Riekert (Eds.), *The handbook of health behavior change* (3rd ed.) (pp. 127–144). New York, NY: Springer.

Hendershot, C. S., Witkiewitz, K., George, W. H., & Marlatt, G. A. (2011). Relapse prevention for addictive behaviors. *Substance Abuse Treatment, Prevention, and Policy, 6*(1), 17.

Hong, T. B., Oddone, E. Z., Dudley, T. K., & Bosworth, H. B. (2006). Medication barriers and anti-hypertensive medication adherence: The moderating role of locus of control. *Psychology, Health & Medicine, 11*(1), 20–28.

Holt, C. L., Roberts, C., Scarinci, I., Wiley, S. R., Eloubeidi, M., Crowther, M., … Coughlin, S. S. (2009). Development of a spiritually based educational program to increase colorectal cancer screening among African American men and women. *Health Communication, 24*(5), 400–412.

Holt, C. L., Shipp, M., Eloubeidi, M., Clay, K. S., Smith-Janas, M. A., Janas, M. J., … Fouad, M. N. (2009). Use of focus group data to develop recommendations for demographically segmented colorectal cancer educational strategies. *Health Education Research, 24*(5), 876–889.

Hounton, S. H., Carabin, H., & Henderson, N. J. (2005). Towards an understanding of barriers to condom use in rural Benin using the health belief model: A cross sectional survey. *BMC Public Health, 5*, 8.

Hutchison, A. J., Breckon, J. D., & Johnston, L. H. (2009). Physical activity behavior change interventions based on the transtheoretical model: A systematic review. *Health Education & Behavior, 36*(5), 829–845.

Iannotti, R. J., Schneider, S., Nansel, T. R., Haynie, D. L., Plotnick, L. P., Clark, L. M., … Simons-Morton, B. (2006). Self-efficacy, outcome expectations, and diabetes self-management in adolescents with type 1 diabetes. *Journal of Developmental and Behavioral Pediatrics: JDBP, 27*(2), 98–105.

Ireys, H. T., Gross, S. S., Werthamer-Larsson, L. A., & Kolodner, K. B. (1994). Self-esteem of young adults with chronic health conditions: Appraising the effects of perceived impact. *Journal of Developmental and Behavioral Pediatrics: JDBP, 15*(6), 409–415.

Janz, N. K., & Becker, M. H. (1984). The health belief model: A decade later. *Health Education Quarterly, 11*(1), 1–47.

Janz, N. K., Wren, P. A., Schottenfeld, D., & Guire, K. E. (2003). Colorectal cancer screening attitudes and behavior: A population-based study. *Preventive Medicine, 37*(6, Pt. 1), 627–634.

Johnston-Brooks, C. H., Lewis, M. A., & Garg, S. (2002). Self-efficacy impacts self-care and HbA1c in young adults with type I diabetes. *Psychosomatic Medicine, 64*(1), 43–51.

Joseph, C. L., Havstad, S. L., Johnson, D., Saltzgaber, J., Peterson, E. L., Resnicow, K., …Strecher, V. J. (2010). Factors associated with nonresponse to a computer-tailored asthma management program for urban adolescents with asthma. *Journal of Asthma, 47*(6), 667–673.

Jung, M. E., Martin Ginis, K. A., Phillips, M. A., & Lordon, C. D. (2011). Increasing calcium intake in young women through gain-framed, targeted messages: A randomized control trial. *Psychology and Health, 26*(5), 531–547.

Kimmel, S. E., Chen, Z., Price, M., Parker, C. S., Metlay, J. P., Christie, J. D., …Gross, R. (2007). The influence of patient adherence on anticoagulation control with warfarin: Results from the international normalized ratio adherence and genetics (IN-RANGE) study. *Archives of Internal Medicine, 167*(3), 229–235.

Kirk, J. K., Grzywacz, J. G., Chapman, C., Arcury, T. A., Bell, R. A., Ip, E. H., & Quandt, S. A. (2011). Blood glucose symptom recognition: Perspectives of older rural adults. *The Diabetes Educator, 37*(3), 363–369.

Kirscht, J. P. (1974). The health belief model and illness behavior. *Health Education Monographs, 2,* 387–408.

Kor, K., & Mullan, B. A. (2011). Sleep hygiene behaviours: An application of the theory of planned behaviour and the investigation of perceived autonomy support, past behaviour and response inhibition. *Psychology & Health, 26*(9), 1208–1224.

Kubzansky, L. D., Park, N., Peterson, C., Vokonas, P., & Sparrow, D. (2011). Health psychological functioning and incident coronary heart disease: The importance of self regulation. *Archives of General Psychiatry, 68*(4), 400.

Larimer, M. E., Palmer, R. S., & Marlatt, G. A. (1999). Relapse prevention: An overview of Marlatt's cognitive-behavioral model. *Alcohol Research & Health, 23*(2), 151.

Larkey, L. K., Hecht, M. L., Miller, K., & Alatorre, C. (2001). Hispanic cultural norms for health-seeking behaviors in the face of symptoms. *Health Education & Behavior, 28*(1), 65–80.

Lee, T. J., Cameron, L. D., Wunsche, B., & Steven, C. (2011). A randomized trial of computer-based communications using imagery and text information to alter representations of heart disease risk and motivate protective behavior. *British Journal of Health Psychology, 16*, 72–91.

Leventhal, E. A., Hansell, S., Diefenbach, M., Leventhal, H., & Glass, D. C. (1996). Negative affect and self-report of physical symptoms: Two longitudinal studies of older adults. *Health Psychology, 15*(3), 193–199.

Leventhal, H., Leventhal, E. A., & Contrada, L. (1998). Self-regulation, health, and behavior: A perceptual-cognitive approach. *Psychological Health, 13*(4), 717–733.

Leventhal, H., Meyer, D., & Gutmann, M. (1980).The role of theory in the study of compliance to high blood pressure regimens. In R. B. Haynes, M. E. Mattson, & T. O. Engebretson, Jr. (Eds.), *Patient compliance to prescribed antihypertensive medication regimens: A report to the National Heart, Lung and Blood Institute* (pp. 1–58). Washington, DC: Department of Health and Human Services.

Littell, J. H., & Girvin, H. (2002). Stages of change: A critique. *Behavior Modification, 26*(2), 223–273.

Maiman, L. A., & Becker, M. H. (1974). The health belief model: Origins and correlates in psychological theory. *Health Education Monographs, 2,* 336–353.

Mancuso, C. A., Rincon, M., McCulloch, C. E., & Charlson, M. E. (2001). Self-efficacy, depressive symptoms, and patients' expectations predict outcomes in asthma. *Medical Care, 39*(12), 1326–1338.

Marlatt, G. A., & George, W. H. (1984). Relapse prevention: Introduction and overview of the model. *British Journal of Addiction, 79*(3), 261.

Marks, R., Allegrante, J. P., & Lorig, K. (2005). A review and synthesis of research evidence for self-efficacy-enhancing interventions for reducing chronic disability: Implications for health education practice (part I). *Health Promotion Practice, 6*(1), 37–43.

Martin, P. D., Dutton, G. R., & Brantley, P. J. (2012). Self-efficacy as a predictor of weight change in African American women. *Obesity, 12*(4), 646–651.

McEachan, R. R. C., Conner, M., Taylor, N. J., & Lawton, R. J. (2011). Prospective prediction of health-related behaviours with the theory of planned behaviour: A meta-analysis. *Health Psychology Review, 5*(2), 97–144.

Michie, S., & Prestwich, A. (2010). Are interventions theory-based? Development of a theory coding scheme. *Health Psychology, 29*(1), 1–8.

Miller, N. E., & Dollard, J. (1941). *Social learning and imitation.* New Haven, CT: Yale University Press.

Munro, S., Lewin, S., Swart, T., & Volmink, J. (2007). A review of health behaviour theories: How useful are these for developing interventions to promote long-term medication adherence for TB and HIV/AIDS? *BMC Public Health, 7*, 104.

Nigg, C. R., Allegrante, J. P., & Ory, M. (2002). Theory-comparison and multiple-behavior research: Common themes advancing health behavior research. *Health Education Research, 17*(5), 670–679.

Noar, S. M., Chabot, M., & Zimmerman, R. S. (2008). Applying health behavior theory to multiple behavior change: Considerations and approaches. *Preventive Medicine, 46*(3), 275–280.

Noar, S. M., & Mehrotra, P. (2011). Toward a new methodological paradigm for testing theories of health behavior and health behavior change. *Patient Education and Counseling, 82*(3), 468–474.

Noar, S. M., & Zimmerman, R. S. (2005). Health behavior theory and cumulative knowledge regarding health behaviors: Are we moving in the right direction? *Health Education Research, 20*(3), 275–290.

Ockene, J. K., Benfari, R. C., Nuttall, R. L., Hurwitz, I., & Ockene, I. S. (1982). Relationship of psychosocial factors to smoking behavior change in an intervention program. *Preventive Medicne, 11*, 13–28.

Osterberg, L., & Blaschke, T. (2005). Adherence to medication. *The New England Journal of Medicine, 353*(5), 487–497.

Painter, J. E., Borba, C. P., Hynes, M., Mays, D., & Glanz, K. (2008). The use of theory in health behavior research from 2000 to 2005: A systematic review. *Annals of Behavioral Medicine, 35*(3), 358–362.

Pine, C. M., McGoldrick, P. M., Burnside, G., Curnow, M. M., Chesters, R. K., Nicholson, J., & Huntington, E. (2000). Creating a successfull intervention programme to establish regular toothbrushing: Understanding parents' beliefs and motivating children. *International Dental Journal, 50*(S6_Part 1), 312–323.

Pinto, S. L., Lively, B. T., Siganga, W., Holiday-Goodman, M., & Kamm, G. (2006). Using the health belief model to test factors affecting patient retention in diabetes-related pharmaceutical care services. *Research in Social & Administrative Pharmacy: RSAP, 2*(1), 38–58.

Pozehl, B., Duncan, K., Hertzog, M., & Norman, J. F. (2010). Heart failure exercise and training camps: Effects of a multicomponent exercise training intervention in patients with heart failure. *Heart & Lung, 39*(6S), S1–S13.

Prochaska, J. (2009). The transtheoretical model of behavior change. In S. Shumaker, J. Ockene, & K. Riekert (Eds.), *The handbook of health behavior change* (3rd ed., pp. 59–83). New York, NY: Springer.

Prochaska, J., Spring, B., & Nigg, C. R. (2008). Multiple behavior change research: An introduction and overview. *Preventive Medicine, 46*(3), 181–188.

Prochaska, J., & Velicer, W. (1997). The trans theoretical model of health behavior change. *American Journal of Health Promotion, 12*(1), 38.

Prochaska, J. J., Velicer, W., Nigg, C. R., & Prochaska, J. O. (2008). Methods of quantifiying change in multiple risk factor interventions. *Preventive Medicine, 46*(3), 260–265.

Rejeski, W. J., Mihalko, S. L., Ambrosius, W. T., Bearon, L. B., & McClelland, J. W. (2011). Weight loss and self-regulatory eating efficacy in older adults: The cooperative lifestyle intervention program. *The Journals of Gerontology: Series B, 66B*(3), 278–286.

Rosenstock, I. M. (1974). Historical origins of the health belief model. *Health Education Monographs, 2*, 328–335.

Rosenstock, I. M., Strecher, V. J., & Becker, M. H. (1988). Social learning theory and the health belief model. *Health Education Quarterly, 15*(2), 175–183.

Sackett, D. L., & Snow, J. C. (1979). The magnitude of compliance and noncompliance. In R. B. Haynes, D. W. Taylor, & D. L. Sackett (Eds.), *Compliance in health care* (pp. 11–22). Baltimore, MD: Johns Hopkins University Press.

Salmela, S., Poskiparta, M., Kasila, K., Vähäsarja, K., & Vanhala, M. (2009).Transtheoretical model-based dietary interventions in primary care: A review of the evidence in diabetes. *Health Education Research, 24*(2), 237.

Schunk, D. H., & Carbonari, J. P. (1984). Self-efficacy models. In J. D. Matarazzo, S. M. Weiss, J. A. Herd, N. E. Miller, & S. M. Weiss (Eds.), *Behavorial health: A handbook of health enhancement and disease prevention* (pp. 230–247). New York, NY: Wiley.

Sevick, M. A., Stone, R., Burke, L., Wang, Y., Zickmund, S., & Korytkowski, M. (2009). Factors associated with adherence to dietary self-monitoring. *Annals of Behavioral Medicine, 37*(1S), S146.

Sevick, M. A., Zickmund, S., Korytkowski, M., Piraino, B., Sereika, S., Mihalko, S., …Burke, L. E. (2008). Design, feasibility, and acceptability of an intervention using personal digital assistant-based self-monitoring in managing type 2 diabetes. *Contemporary Clinical Trials, 29*(3), 396–409.

Shi, Q., Ostwald, S. K., & Wang, S. (2010). Improving glycaemic control self-efficacy and glycaemic control behaviour in Chinese patients with type 2 diabetes mellitus: Randomised controlled trial. *Journal of Clinical Nursing, 19*(3), 398–404.

Short, C. E., James, E. L, & Plotnikoff, R. C. (2013). How social cognitive theory can help oncology-based health professionals promote physical activity among breast cancer survivors. *European Journal of Oncology Nursing, 17*(4), 482–489.

Stetson, B. A., Beacham, A. O., Frommelt, S. J., Boutelle, K. N., Cole, J. D., Ziegler, C. H., & Looney, S. W. (2005). Exercise slips in high-risk situations and activity patterns in long-term exercisers: An application of the relapse prevention model. *Annals of Behavioral Medicine, 30*(1), 25.

Stanton-Salazar, R. D., & Spina, S. U. (2003). Informal mentors and role models in the lives of urban Mexican-origin adolescents. *Anthropology and Education Quarterly, 34*(3), 231–254.

Strauss, R. S. (2000). Childhood obesity and self-esteem. *Pediatrics, 105*(1), e15.

Sutton, S. (2001). Back to the drawing board? A review of applications of the transtheoretical model to substance use. *Addiction, 96*(1), 175.

Tierney, S., Mamas, M., Skelton, D., Woods, S., Rutter, M. K., Gibson, M., … Deaton, C. (2011). What we learn from patients with heart failure about exercise adherence? A systematic review of qualitative papers. *Health Psychology, 30*(4), 401–410.

Torres, R., Fernandez, F., & Maceira, D. (1995). Self-esteem and value of health as correlates of adolescent health behavior. *Adolescence, 30*(118), 403–412.

Tuah, N. A., Amiel, C., Qureshi, S., Car, J., Kaur, B., & Majeed, A. (2011). Transtheoretical model for dietary and physical exercise modification in weight loss management for overweight and obese adults. *Cochrane Database of Systematic Reviews (Online),* (10), CD008066.

Unger, J. B., Kipke, M. D., De Rosa, C. J., Hyde, J., Ritt-Olson, A., & Montgomery, S. (2006). Needle-sharing among young IV drug users and their social network members: The influence of the injection partner's characteristics on HIV risk behavior. *Addictive Behaviors, 31*(9), 1607–1618.

Velicer, W. F., Norman, G. J., Fava, J. L., & Prochaska, J. O. (1999). Testing 40 predictions from the transtheoretical model. *Addictive Behaviors, 24*(4), 455–469.

Venmans, L. M. A. J., Gorter, K. J., Hak, E., Grypdonck, M. H. F., de Bruijn, O., & Rutten, G. E. H. M. (2011). Management of infections in type 2 diabetes from the patient's perspective: A qualitative approach. *Primary Care Diabetes, 5*(1), 33–37.

Venmans, L. M. A. J., Gorter, K. J., Hak, E., & Rutten, G. E. H. M. (2008). Short-term effects of an educational program on health-seeking behavior for infections in patients with type 2 diabetes. *Diabetes Care, 31*, 402–407.

Wallston, B. S., & Wallston, K. A. (1984). Social psychological models of health behavior: An examination and integration. In A. Baum, S. Taylor, & J. E. Singer (Eds.), *Handbook of psychology and health* (pp. 215–222). Hillsdale, NJ: Erlbaum.

Webb, T. L., Joseph, J., Yardley, L., & Michie, S. (2010). Using the internet to promote health behavior change: A systematic review and meta-analysis of the impact of theoretical basis, use of behavior change techniques, and mode of delivery on efficacy. *Journal of Medical Internet Research, 12*(1), e4.

Weinstein, N. D. (2007). Misleading tests of health behavior theories. *Annals of Behavioral Medicine, 33*(1), 1–10.

Weinstein, N. D., & Rothman, A. J. (2005). Commentary: Revitalizing research on health behavior theories. *Health Education Research, 20*(3), 294–297.

West, R. (2005). Time for a change: Putting the transtheoretical (stages of change) model to rest. *Addiction (Abingdon, England), 100*(8), 1036.

Witkiewitz, K., Bowen, S., Douglas, H., & Hsu, S. H. (2013). Mindfulness-based relapse prevention for substance craving. *Addictive Behaviors, 38*(2), 1563–1571.

Wolff, K., Nordin, K., Brun, W., Berglund, G., & Kvale, G. (2011). Affective and cognitive attitudes, uncertainty avoidance and intention to obtain genetic testing: An extension of the theory of planned behaviour. *Psychology & Health, 26*(9), 1143.

Ziff, M. A., Conrad, P., & Lachman, M. E. (1995).The relative effects of perceived personal control and responsibility on health and health-related behaviors in young and middle-aged adults. *Health Education Quarterly, 22*(1), 127–142.

Zimmerman, B. J. (1998). Academic studying and the development of personal skill: A self-regulatory perspective. *Educational Psychologist, 33*(2/3), 73–86.

2

Understanding Population Health From Multi-Level and Community-Based Models

MARIAN L. FITZGIBBON
ANGELA KONG
LISA TUSSING-HUMPHREYS

LEARNING OBJECTIVES

- Summarize how socio-ecological models can be used in interventions that support healthy lifestyles.
- Identify the benefits and challenges of implementing community-based participatory research (CBPR).
- Discuss how the Reach, Efficacy/Effectiveness, Adoption, Implementation, and Maintenance (RE-AIM) evaluation framework has been applied in the evaluation of health behavior change trials.

POPULATION-BASED/COMMUNITY-BASED BEHAVIOR CHANGE MODELS

Modern population health is conceptualized as three major periods best defined by the conflicts and challenges at their boundaries (Susser & Susser, 1996). The era of "sanitary statistics" dates back to the early nineteenth century when "miasma" was the prevailing paradigm used to describe the cause and spread of disease. Most physicians and public officials believed diseases were caused by foul emanations from "air, water, and places." This era left its mark in the lexicon with words like "malaria," which means bad (mal) air (aria) (Young, 2004).

In the latter part of the 19th century, "contagionists" challenged the concept of miasma. The contagionists believed that diseases were caused by organisms passed from individual to individual. The French chemist Louis Pasteur (1822–1895) proposed a "germ theory" of disease, suggesting that microorganisms are the cause of disease (Karamanou, Panayiotakopoulos, Tsoucalas, Kousoulis, & Androutsos, 2012). The contagionists eventually prevailed, as careful experimentation and observation identified more and more bacteria (germs) that apparently caused tuberculosis, diphtheria, cholera, and other diseases previously believed to be linked to the worst miasmas (Karamanou et al., 2012). In 1876, the German scientist Robert Koch (1843–1910) demonstrated the procedures for linking a specific microbe to a specific disease by identifying the cause of anthrax (Karamanou et al., 2012), and in 1884, Koch and Frederick Loeffler (1852–1915) established criteria for confirming a relationship between a causative microbe and a disease (Karamanou et al., 2012). This approach, known as Koch's Postulates, remains the gold standard for confirming the causative agents of most infectious diseases.

Thus, the "germ theory" and the modern concept of disease transmission emerged as the second era of public health during the late 19th century and first half of the 20th century (Bullough & Rosen, 1992). Germ theory led to a number of advances, including the development of vaccines and antibiotics (Young, 2004). Due to these advances, death rates from infectious diseases fell substantially in the United States, and overall life expectancy increased by the middle of the 20th century. For example, in 1900, the average life expectancy at birth was 46 years for men and 48 years for women, but by 1950 it had increased to 66 and 71 years, respectively (National Center for Health Statistics, 2006).

By the second half of the 20th century, disease patterns in more developed countries were increasingly characterized by chronic, noninfectious diseases, which made the germ theory less relevant to population health research and heralded the beginning of a third period: the era of chronic disease epidemiology (Susser & Susser, 1996). To date, this era has focused on using advances in epidemiology and biostatistics to identify, understand, and address risk factors for chronic diseases.

Currently, heart disease, cancer, and stroke are the leading causes of death in the United States, accounting for more than two thirds of all deaths (Brownson & Bright, 2004). The shift to these and other chronic diseases as major causes of premature morbidity and mortality contributed to the need to reconceptualize the most effective strategies in preventive health. Chronic diseases, in contrast to infectious diseases, are not contagious in origin, usually include a long rather than an acute period of illness, are characterized by a prolonged latency period between exposure to the risk factors and adverse health outcome, and more often than not, are precipitated by the confluence of multiple risk factors (Curry & Fitzgibbon, 2009). Ample evidence indicates that the leading causes of premature morbidity and mortality—heart disease, cancer, and stroke—can be prevented or at least delayed through behavior change (e.g., lifestyle changes) (McGinnis & Foege, 1993). Therefore, adherence to certain preventive health behaviors (e.g., consuming a healthful diet and engaging in regular physical activity) is key to promoting health and prolonging life.

Early attempts to understand and influence the prevention, development, and maintenance of chronic disease included the development of several models of *individual* behavior change—for example, the Health Belief Model (Rosenstock, 1974), the Theory of Planned Behavior (Ajzen & Fishbein, 1980), and the Transtheoretical Model (Prochaska & DiClemente, 1983)—that emphasize changes in behavior and cognition to enhance health. The majority of health promotion interventions based on these models focus on the individual as the unit of change by attempting to modify an individual's behavior (e.g., diet and exercise behaviors), but do not focus on the complexity of factors that influence these behaviors (Huang & Glass, 2008). The individual approach to behavior change, which usually targets those at increased risk, has had limited impact, as it neglects these complex influences (Maziak, Ward, & Stockton, 2008). In addition, little attention has been given to the communities in which people live and how these environments affect behavior (Cashman & Forlano, 2009). For example, increased physical activity is influenced by the presence or absence of playground equipment and similar resources that promote physical activity (Jago & Bailey, 2001); dietary intake can be influenced by the availability of larger supermarkets that stock fresher produce at lower prices (Morland, Wing, Diez Roux, & Poole, 2002).

To date, we have seen that rigorously designed and theoretically informed behavior change interventions often provide only modest changes in health behavior that have not consistently translated into lasting behavior change or had a population-level impact (Glasgow, Klesges, Dzewaltowski, Bull, & Estabrooks, 2004). A criticism of some of these interventions, for example, the Multiple Risk Factor Intervention Trial (MRFIT 1982; Stamler & Neaton, 2008) and the Enhancing Recovery in Coronary Heart Disease trial (ENRICHD) (Berkman et al., 2003), is that they are not tailored to address the contexts that influence behavior (Glass, 2000; McKinlay & Marceau, 2000; Relman & Angell, 2002).

The primary purpose of this chapter is to provide an overview of several models that consider multiple factors involved in influencing, initiating, and maintaining behaviors. Specifically, we describe socio-ecological models, community-based participatory research (CBPR), and social marketing. We also provide an overview of RE-AIM (Reach, Effectiveness, Adoption, Implementation, Maintenance), an evaluation framework designed to assist researchers and practitioners in translating multi-level research into action (Glasgow, Vogt, & Boles, 1999). Finally, we more broadly discuss the role of government, social norms, and the need for policy intervention research as it relates to health promotion and sustained behavior change. In an effort to place this chapter in a more applied context, we incorporate the current public health crisis of obesity as an example to highlight the role of multi-level models.

SOCIO-ECOLOGICAL MODELS

The word "ecology," which has its origins in the biological sciences, is concerned with the interrelations between organisms and their environment (Bronfenbrenner, 1992). Many other disciplines, such as psychology, sociology, and public health, have adapted ecological models to define frameworks for how people interact with their physical, social, and cultural environments (Stokols, 1992). Within the realm of health behavior research, socio-ecological models provide a framework for the development of multi-level interventions that can systematically address mechanisms of change at various levels of an individual's environment (Sallis, Owen, & Fisher, 2008). Socio-ecological frameworks can be viewed, in part, as a reaction to the limited explanatory power of earlier behavioral and cognitive models of behavior change (Stokols, 1992) that primarily focused on the individual as the unit of analysis and did not produce a profound or sustained change in behavior when targeted in interventions (Glanz, Rimer, & Lewis, 2002). The innovation of the socio-ecological models is their consideration of both internal and external influences on health and behavior, which range from biological to global levels, as well as the interaction among these factors (Baranowski, Cullen, Nicklas, Thompson, & Baranowski, 2003).

CHARACTERISTICS OF SOCIO-ECOLOGICAL MODELS

Socio-ecological models are based on several core assumptions (Schneider & Stokols, 2008; Stokols, 1992). The first underscores the importance of acknowledging multiple factors that influence behavior at the biological, individual, interpersonal, community, environmental, policy, and global levels (Sallis & Owen, 1997; Smedley & Syme, 2000; Stokols, 1992). This is demonstrated in the emerging conceptualization of weight management and the current obesity epidemic (Huang & Glass, 2008). Historically, managing obesity was viewed as an individual's personal responsibility (Brownell et al., 2010). However, the minimal weight loss observed in both clinical interventions and well-designed trials (Brownell, 2010) suggests that obesity is better studied in a broader context. Researchers and clinicians increasingly recognize that solutions to the obesity epidemic must come from addressing the problem on multiple levels by considering the complex interactions of biology and socio-environmental changes that coalesce to promote and/or produce excessive weight gain in both adults and children (Ogden, Carroll, Kit, & Flegal, 2012).

The second core assumption addresses the importance of understanding the complex nature of human environments (Stokols, 1992). For example, descriptions of environments are not limited to their objective (actual) physical and social attributes, but also can be extended to their subjective (perceived) qualities (Schneider & Stokols, 2008). In addition, independent components of an environment (e.g., lighting, temperature, or spatial attributes) can be combined into composite relationships (Stokols, 1987).

The third assumption is that, similar to the way environments can be described in terms of their complexity, participants in those environments also can be studied at a number of levels, ranging from the individual to small groups to larger organizations to populations (Stokols, 1992). The emphasis in this assumption is that rather than focusing exclusively on the individual or the population, socio-ecological perspectives recognize that coordinated efforts and methodologies are necessary. Again using the obesity epidemic as an example, some of the changes needed to reverse the epidemic include individual-level behavior lifestyle changes, changes that help schools and workplace environments foster healthy choices, and changes in food advertising, transportation, and urban planning (Gortmaker et al., 2011).

The fourth assumption focuses on the fact that there are elements of any individual's environment that can either facilitate or impede healthful behavior (Stokols, 1992). In other words, an individual's ability to make good choices independently can be influenced more or less by the social and environmental contexts in which that individual lives and works (Schneider & Stokols, 2008). Again, as this assumption relates to obesity, most humans gain weight when their environment offers increased opportunities to consume high-fat, high-sugar choices (Brownell et al., 2010). As an example, Pima Indians in their native Mexico live an agrarian lifestyle, eating indigenous food and being highly active (Schulz et al., 2006). Most are of normal weight, and chronic diseases are rare. However, a related group of Pimas living in Arizona suffers from extremely high rates of obesity and has the highest rate of diabetes in the world (Schulz et al., 2006). Similarly, rates of obesity and chronic diseases are higher among lower-income and underserved populations in the United States who are more apt to live in "obesogenic" environments (i.e., environments with readily available energy-dense foods and limited opportunities for activity). These examples underscore the profound impact that context can have on the choices individuals make. Ultimately, although choices must be made at the individual level, the environment often dictates the choices available (Brownell et al., 2010).

The fifth assumption recognizes that even within a given environmental context, individual behavioral responses will vary (Schneider & Stokols, 2008). Understanding individual responses can help to create more tailored interventions that may be most beneficial to specific subgroups. For example, recent research on physical activity suggests that certain genetic variations may be related to a greater predisposition to exercise (De Moor et al., 2009). However, familial norms, cultural emphasis on the priority given to being active, and access to safe locations to exercise will affect activity levels through mechanisms that have nothing to do with genetic predisposition (Diez Roux, 2011). Therefore, socio-ecological models take into account individual-level differences in combination with contextual factors to identify the most promising strategies for a given subgroup.

Finally, the socio-ecological framework acknowledges the dynamic nature of behavior. Environments do not remain constant, and behavioral choices must be made and acted on in the context of a continually changing environment. Thus, flexibility must be built into any multi-level model of behavior change.

SOCIO-ECOLOGICAL MODELS AND STRATEGIES FOR OBESITY PREVENTION

With permission, we have reproduced a figure (Huang, Drewnosksi, Kumanyika, & Glass, 2009; Kumanyika, Jeffery, Morabia, Ritenbaugh, & Antipatis, 2002;) that depicts the complex and reciprocal contexts present when addressing obesity prevention (Figure 2.1). This model depicts biological and socio-environmental influences on behaviors that affect body weight (e.g., eating and activity behaviors) and illustrates the importance of multiple levels of influences on health behavior, including those ranging from genetics to the individual, family, community, and society (Huang & Glass, 2008). This model also recognizes that several factors act on the individual, including attitudes, social influences, and cultural norms (DeVries, Glasper, & Detillion, 2003; Kumanyika, Jeffery, Morabia, Ritenbaugh, & Antipatis, 2002).

While the implementation of this approach can be complex, its essence is that in order to make effective changes, individuals must have a supportive environment that both supports healthier lifestyles and provides incentives to make those healthier choices (Ashe, Graff, & Spector, 2011). For example, many people have much easier access to food

FIGURE 2.1 Societal policies and processes with direct and indirect influences on the prevalence of obesity and undernutrition. Vertical and horizontal links will vary across different societies and populations. (From Kumanyika et al., 2002)

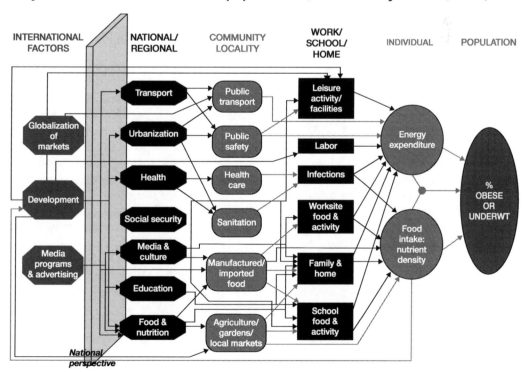

options that are high in fat and sugar rather than fruits and vegetables, and these options are typically more affordable and require little to no preparation (Walker, Keane, & Burke, 2010). This environment is not supportive of healthy dietary habits. Similarly, many neighborhoods and communities do not have safe, aesthetically pleasing facilities or built environments that support physically active lifestyles (Aboelata & Navarro, 2010).

Although this multi-level understanding of the development and prevention of obesity and other chronic diseases is useful in both theory and practice, its adoption has been slow. Note that only about 10 years ago, World Health Organization (WHO) director Dr. Gro Harlem Bundtland said in a World Health Report presentation ("Reducing Risks, Promoting Healthy Life"), "We know that most people will choose to adopt healthier behaviors, especially when they receive accurate information from authorities they trust." While this view is well intentioned, it does not take into account the challenge of modifying lifestyle behaviors. Awareness and use of multi-level models in addressing obesity and other chronic diseases have begun to erode the long held beliefs that education is the only element necessary to enable people to make the right choices and that failure to make the "right" choices is a failure to take personal responsibility (Brownell et al., 2010). Socioecological models do not obviate the role of education in promoting healthful changes, but instead underscore the need for creating an environment that makes the healthier choices feasible.

COMMUNITY-BASED PARTICIPATORY RESEARCH

Community-based participatory research (CBPR) is a collaborative research approach that uses an ecological framework to explore and address the broader context of health within a given environment (Israel, Schulz, Parker, & Becker, 1998) while enlisting the participation of the communities affected by the issue being studied. Ideally, CBPR promotes shared decision making and shared ownership of the outcomes by including representatives from community and academic organizations in all aspects of the research project (Viswanathan et al., 2004). The approach emphasizes equal involvement in an effort to create a project that truly reflects the needs of the specific community, rather than what academics and other researchers may think they need (Cornwall & Jewkes, 1995).

The complex multi-level factors present in the communities most impacted by health inequities pose tremendous challenges to any attempt to translate science into practice in these settings (Wallerstein & Duran, 2010). In the past few decades, CBPR has gained recognition as an often effective approach for addressing persistent public health disparities (Israel et al., 1998; Minkler, Blackwell, Thompson, & Tamir, 2003). As characterized by Israel and colleagues, the main aim of CBPR is "to increase knowledge and understanding of a given phenomenon and integrate the knowledge gained into interventions, policy change, and social change to improve the health and quality of life of community members" (Israel et al., 1998). This alternative research paradigm may better equip researchers to uncover and address contextual factors contributing to health disparities.

The National Institutes of Health (NIH) Office of Behavioral and Social Sciences Research (OBSSR) describes CBPR as "an applied collaborative approach that enables community residents to more actively participate in the full spectrum of research (from conception – design – conduct – analysis – interpretation – conclusions – communication of results) with a goal of influencing change in community health, systems, programs or policies" (National Institutes of Health, 2013). Whereas conventional research assumes that the academic researcher is in the best position to set the research agenda for a given community (Green & Mercer, 2001), CBPR unites researchers, community members, and relevant stakeholders to actively participate in the research process (Green & Mercer, 2001; Minkler & Wallerstein, 2008).

The partnerships formed in CBPR are dynamic, and no one set of principles is applicable to all research that includes CBPR. However, Israel and colleagues reviewed the CBPR literature and identified nine principles that serve as guides for researchers interested in using CBPR (described in detail in the latest edition of their book, *Methods for Community-Based Participatory Research for Health*, 2nd Edition) (Israel & Schulz, 2012). Of these, one of the more important is that the community is viewed as a unit of identity. For instance, community can be defined by geography (e.g., neighborhood, city, and town) or may refer to groups with a common identity (e.g., race/ethnicity, shared values, interests, culture, and goals) independent of geographic location (Israel & Schulz, 2012; Steuart, 1993). Further, compared to traditional research, scientists or academicians who use CBPR no longer hold all the power. Instead, power is shared with the community involved in the research by using strengths/resources of the community; forming equitable academic/community partnerships; fostering an exchange of skills, knowledge, and capacity building for all partners involved; using the research to benefit the community; addressing relevant concerns as identified by the community; disseminating findings to all relevant partners (e.g., community and relevant stakeholders); and making a commitment to sustainable solutions (Israel & Schulz, 2012).

A 2004 Agency for Health Research and Quality (AHRQ) report identified seven key benefits of CBPR for communities and six key benefits for researchers (Viswanathan et al., 2004). Potential benefits to the community include (1) more efficient use of existing resources, (2) better matching of research efforts to problems of interest to the community, (3) dignified approach to involving community members in the research process, (4) measures and methods that are less likely to confuse members of the target community, (5) increasing trust and bridging cultural gaps between academic/community partners, (6) findings that are a more accurate reflection of the community, and (7) community members taking pride in their accomplishment and occasionally benefiting from research-related career advancement. Potential benefits to researchers include (1) better probability of completing the research project, (2) greater likelihood of future funding if community participation yields better outcomes, (3) improved recruitment and retention due to community involvement, (4) improvements in data collected, (5) interventions/projects that are more culturally sensitive, and (6) findings that more accurately reflect the community.

While CBPR has many benefits, the approach is challenging. Minkler (2004) identified five ethical challenges researchers should consider when conducting CBPR: (1) achieving a true "community-driven" agenda; (2) insider–outsider tensions; (3) real and perceived racism; (4) the limitations of "participation"; and (5) issues involving the sharing, ownership, and use of findings for action. CBPR also has several potential methodological limitations of concern, including possible threats to external validity and scientific rigor (Wallerstein & Duran, 2010) and the potential for a lack of focus in achieving "intended" outcomes (Viswanathan et al., 2004).

Despite its challenges, CBPR continues to gain prominence in public health research due to its overwhelming value to both communities and researchers (Minkler et al., 2003). For example, the Centers for Disease Control and Prevention (CDC) established the Prevention Research Centers Program in more than 30 schools of public health or medicine to support the use of CBPR through collaborations of academic institutions and community partners in conducting research in underserved communities. In 2002, the Institute of Medicine (IOM) identified CBPR as one of eight essential content areas for emerging public health professionals (IOM, 2002). Since that time, more than a dozen institutes at the National Institutes of Health (NIH) have released funding opportunity announcements dedicated to CBPR (NIH, 2013). Along with these initiatives, experts in CBPR have developed guidelines and further refined methods to support this research approach (Minkler & Wallerstein, 2008; Israel & Schulz, 2012) in an effort to better implement and evaluate the impact of CBPR.

CBPR provides context for understanding the effects of community on behavior change (Chen, Diaz, Lucas, & Rosenthal, 2010) and may provide a foundation for developing more effective programs and interventions due to its inclusive approach and the recognition of the environmental factors that affect health. Again using the obesity epidemic as an example, CBPR recognizes that influential members of a community may be much more effective agents of change compared to outsiders who may not have intimate knowledge of key cultural and social entities within the community that affect eating and activity patterns (Cook, 2008).

CBPR EXAMPLE: OBESITY PREVENTION

Shape Up Somerville, one of the first CBPR initiatives aimed at preventing childhood obesity, tested the effectiveness of an environmental change intervention on children's weight (specifically body mass index [BMI]) (Economos et al., 2007). This non-randomized controlled trial was conducted in three culturally diverse communities in Somerville, Massachusetts, with two control communities matched on socio-demographic characteristics. Over one third of elementary school children in Somerville were either at risk for or were overweight. Researchers from Tufts University and community partners from Somerville (i.e., parents, teachers, children, school employees, and policy makers) collaborated in all stages of the research from conception through dissemination. The group determined that one of the objectives of the intervention would be to address every facet of an elementary school child's day. Accordingly, the intervention design included components that influenced environments in the home, school, and community while covering activities occurring before, during, and after school. The intervention had a modest but significant effect on BMI z score. The change in BMI z score equated to an almost 1-pound reduction over the course of 8 months for an 8-year old child. Almost 10 years after the initial study, Shape Up Somerville continues to thrive through the support of the city government and coordination by the health department and other key stakeholders.

SOCIAL MARKETING

The socio-ecological perspective maintains that individual-level behavior both impacts and is impacted by multiple levels of influence: intrapersonal, interpersonal, community, institutional, and public policy (Glanz, 1997). Since each level of influence has the potential to affect health behavior, conventional approaches that focus solely on intrapersonal factors (e.g., knowledge, beliefs, and perceptions) may limit long-term behavior change. Social marketing has been recognized as an approach that targets multiple levels of influence (e.g., social norms, barriers, and policy) to affect individual-level behavior change (Grier & Bryant, 2005). The best known social marketing approaches have been national campaigns addressing tobacco use (Farrelly et al., 2002), physical activity (Wong et al., 2004), and nutrition (Foerster et al., 1995).

One widely cited definition of *social marketing* is "the application of commercial marketing technologies to the analysis, planning, execution, and evaluation of programs designed to influence voluntary behavior of target audiences in order to improve their personal welfare and that of society" (Andreasen, 1995). As highlighted in this definition, social marketing differs from commercial marketing by its focus on influencing behavior as a means to improve the welfare of both the individual and society. While commercial marketing places a higher priority on the benefit (e.g., financial) of the organization, social marketing shifts this focus onto the target audience.

Marketing mix is a key marketing principle commonly used to guide the development of social marketing campaigns/programs. This principle is most commonly known as the four Ps: "Product," "Price," "Place," and "Promotion." We provide examples of the four P's based on the CDC's VERB™ campaign, a national mass media campaign promoting physical activity to children aged 9–13 ("tweens") (Wong et al., 2004).

In the context of social marketing, "product" refers to the desired behavioral outcome and related benefits. Defining the product of an intervention often requires formative research that gathers information on the current behaviors, perceptions, barriers, and attitudes of the target group to identify the benefits most salient to the target audience. In the VERB™ campaign, the product was promoting physical activity in "tweens" (target audience), and the related benefits included having fun and spending time with friends.

"Price" refers to the cost or barriers (e.g., financial, psychological, and social) that the target audience *perceives* to be associated with adopting the desired behavior. In commercial marketing, consumers are more prone to make a purchase if the benefits outweigh the costs. Similarly, one of the objectives of social marketing is to convince the target audience that the perceived cost–benefit ratio favors the desired behavior. In VERB™, examples of "price" or barriers included time constraints, lack of access to places to play, aversion to team sports, fear of embarrassment, and other competing interests (e.g., television, Internet, and gaming) (Asbury, Wong, Price, & Nolin, 2008). To counter these barriers, the VERB™ brand portrayed physical activity as fun rather than competitive, accessible to all children regardless of ability, and easy and appealing (Asbury et al., 2008).

"Place" is where the target audience accesses the "product" (e.g., receives information about it) or performs the behavior. The VERB™ campaign characterized "place" as any safe location for physical activity (Wong et al., 2004).

"Promotion" represents the message content, materials, and all channels or activities used to communicate the product to the target audience. Messages can be delivered through print materials, media, advertising, and other means. However, it is important to consider the target audience in selecting both the promotional messages and the form and means of delivery. In VERB™, the core content revolved around three themes: (a) physical activity is fun, (b) physical activity is an opportunity to explore and discover, and (c) physical activity is an opportunity to spend time with friends. CDC partnered with advertising and public relations agencies to develop a promotional campaign around these themes that included advertisements on television, radio (e.g., public service announcements), Internet, and billboards as well as distributing promotional items with the VERB™ logo (e.g., bracelets, tattoos, and sports equipment) (Andreasen, 1995).

Another distinct feature of social marketing is the use of audience segmentation. *Audience segmentation* is a process that identifies subgroups of a larger audience that share common characteristics. These subgroups are commonly based on demographic factors (e.g., race/ethnicity, age, or income), but a greater level of refinement is also possible with segmentation. In the context of health promotion, commonalities may be based on traits related to target behavior, risk level, or readiness to change (Forthofer & Bryant, 2000). Segmentation allows a greater understanding of the audience, which in turn allows a more tailored intervention approach. Since VERB™ was a national campaign intended to reach children across race/ethnicity, tailored strategies were developed for audience segments of specific minority ethnic groups (i.e., African American, Asian, Hispanic/Latino, and American Indian) (Huhman et al., 2008).

THE RE-AIM FRAMEWORK AND SOCIO-ECOLOGICAL APPROACHES

Multi-level socio-ecological models and community participation provide useful frameworks for addressing public health issues, such as obesity. However, much remains to be understood regarding the determinants and processes of actual population-level behavior change (Merzel & D'Affitti, 2003). Given the complexity of these models that take into account individual, social, environmental, community, and policy-level interactions, there is a need for an improved understanding of the precise way in which these interventions are operationalized, translated, and sustained in the public health domain (Merzel & D'Affitti, 2003).

Federal and private funders spend billions of dollars each year on community-based health intervention research in the United States (Fielding & Briss, 2006). However, only a small percentage of this money supports research designed to empirically evaluate the dissemination of evidence-based interventions into clinical and public health practice (Glasgow, Lichtenstein, & Marcus, 2003; Kerner, Rimer, & Emmons, 2005). Despite the best intentions of health promotion researchers, the translation of clinical community evidence-based health interventions into broader-scale dissemination and adoption is complex and often unsuccessful (Goode, Owen, Reeves, & Eakin, 2012). Unfortunately, this leaves a sizeable gap between the literature on what is possible (i.e., the evidence base) and what is actually feasible (i.e., actual public health practice) (Anderson, 1998). Glasgow and colleagues (2003) attribute this disconnect to several inter-related factors, including limited time and resources of both clinical and public health practitioners, insufficient staff training, lack of incentives to adopt evidence-based programs into practice, and inadequate infrastructure and organization at the community or systems level to support translation and maintenance of new programs. Notably, Glasgow and colleagues (2003) also place some responsibility on researchers, suggesting that the logic and assumptions behind the design of behavioral health efficacy and effectiveness trials often impede dissemination efforts.

The research paradigm historically used in community-based health intervention research stems from two influential papers published in the 1980s (Greenwald & Cullen, 1985; Flay, 1986). Both papers propose a logical progression of research beginning with hypothesis generation and ending with dissemination studies. However, this linear flow relies heavily on success at the "efficacy" and "effectiveness" stages of intervention research (Glasgow et al., 2003). Efficacy studies are designed to show that a given treatment or intervention does more good than harm (Flay, 1986). Typically, these trials are very tightly controlled and delivered in a standardized manner, by expertly trained research staff, to a highly selected target audience (Glasgow et al., 2003). This level of rigor allows the researcher to determine whether any positive or negative outcome effects can be attributed to the intervention. In contrast, an effectiveness trial examines whether the treatment or intervention produces more good than harm when conducted under "real world" conditions, by modestly trained staff, and with a more representative target audience (Flay, 1986), with the expectation that a trial of this type should produce results that are generalizable (Glasgow et al., 2003). However, the rigor of funding processes and an overemphasis on tightly controlled conditions have left the behavioral intervention research landscape with many relatively small, highly controlled efficacy studies and few successful effectiveness trials (Glasgow, Bull, Gillette, Klesges, & Dzewaltowski, 2002; Oldenburg, Ffrench, & Sallis, 2000).

Glasgow and colleagues (2003) suggest that the field has made a flawed assumption in believing that interventions proven to be successful at the efficacy stage are the best candidates for effectiveness trials. The emergence of multi-level models in public health research demonstrates why efficacy trials are poorly suited for identifying promising large-scale approaches. Specifically, at the efficacy stage of research, little emphasis is placed on external or moderating factors such as appeal to the broader target audience, adaptability to participants and stakeholders (i.e., feasibility), or variations in outcomes depending on setting or demographic or socioeconomic characteristics of the participants. In contrast, effectiveness interventions explicitly address these factors, recognizing that the interplay of complex, multi-level personal and environmental factors provides the context for success or failure (Glasgow et al., 2003). Thus, interventions focused solely on internal factors may be efficacious in a controlled setting but may not readily translate to the intended target audience in a "real world" setting (Glasgow et al., 2003). Therefore, it is important that behavioral health intervention researchers evaluate both internal and external factors across the research paradigm so that the scientific knowledge gained can be more effectively translated into broader public health use (Glasgow et al., 2003).

Researchers have developed several empirically derived intervention planning and evaluation frameworks to address the gaps between the evidence base and dissemination as well as the shift from individual health behavior change models to community and population-based paradigms (Green & Kreuter, 2005; Shediac-Rizkallah & Bone, 1998; Viswanathan et al., 2004). The Reach, Efficacy/Effectiveness, Adoption, Implementation, and Maintenance (RE-AIM) evaluation framework (Glasgow et al., 1999) emphasizes the importance of including and evaluating internal and external program elements, both individual and organizational (setting), along the research trajectory from efficacy through dissemination in an effort to improve the dissemination of evidence-based interventions into public health practice (Glasgow et al., 2003). RE-AIM can be used in the planning and evaluation of systems-level, socio-ecological, and community-based public health interventions (Glasgow et al., 1999).

Within the framework, *Reach* is an individual-level measure of participation (Glasgow et al., 1999). It represents the percentage of eligible persons in the target population who participate in an intervention and the extent to which those participants represent the target population based on socio-demographic, medical, and psychosocial characteristics (Bopp et al., 2007; Glasgow et al., 1999). If the intervention population is representative of the larger population, one can make a stronger case for generalization of the program into a community or "real world" setting (Estabrooks, 2013). Glasgow and colleagues (Estabrooks, 2013; Glasgow et al., 2003) encourage researchers to evaluate *Reach* by examining inclusion/exclusion criteria, participation rates, dropout, characteristics of participants compared to non-participants, and the use of qualitative methods to understand reach and recruitment specific to the target audience. *Efficacy* or effectiveness is an individual-level measure that assesses the extent to which the intervention has a positive effect on the hypothesized outcomes. Common measures in health interventions include biological (e.g., blood pressure and weight) and behavioral factors (e.g., dietary intake and tobacco use). Including an evaluation of unintended or negative outcomes is essential so that one can determine that harm does not outweigh benefit (Estabrooks, 2013; Glasgow et al., 1999; Glasgow et al., 2003). Researchers should also use an intent-to-treat or imputation for missing value analysis and examine moderators across subgroups as well as economic health outcomes

(Glasgow et al., 2003). *Adoption* is an organizational or setting-level factor that evaluates the percentage and representativeness of the intended setting adopting the intervention (Estabrooks, 2013; Glasgow et al., 1999; Glasgow et al., 2003). Organizations opting not to implement a given intervention also should be considered, as this may provide important information regarding barriers to adoption. Adoption is often evaluated through direct observation, surveys, and structured interviews. *Implementation* is an organizational measure that assesses the extent to which a program is delivered as intended (e.g., number of classes taught or number of pamphlets distributed) and the time and costs related to delivery (Estabrooks, 2013; Glasgow et al., 1999; Glasgow et al., 2003). Consistency of delivery by different intervention agents (i.e., fidelity) also should be evaluated. Evaluating *implementation* is crucial to determining intervention components that may be practical and effective in representative settings. *Maintenance* is an individual- and organizational-level element that assesses the extent to which an individual continues the intended outcome for 6 or more months (Estabrooks, 2013; Glasgow et al., 1999; Glasgow et al., 2003). It is also a measure of the sustainability of a program within a given setting. Researchers are encouraged to examine pushback from participants and use CBPR in the strategic planning efforts in early stages, including the efficacy state of the intervention, to improve maintenance.

The RE-AIM framework has been applied in the evaluation of many efficacy and effectiveness health intervention studies in an attempt to determine their translatability and potential for public health impact (Aittasalo, Rinne, Pasanen, Kuknen-Harjula, & Vasankari, 2012; Jenkinson, Naughton, & Benson, 2012; Toobert, Glasgow, Strycker, Barrera, & King, 2012). As an example, the RE-AIM framework was used to evaluate the Step Ahead weight gain prevention trial (Zapka et al., 2007), which used a socioecological paradigm as a means to address the social and institutional context of eating and exercise behaviors related to weight control in a hospital setting (Estabrook, Zapka, & Lemon, 2012). The 2-year intervention was conducted in six hospitals randomized to an intervention or control condition. *Reach* was evaluated by the number of participants recruited and their reported usage of the intervention components, including cafeteria signage regarding nutritional content of foods and healthy choices, use of the project website, participation in walking groups or workplace challenges, attendance at workshops, and print materials. *Effectiveness* was evaluated by assessing change in BMI and self-reported eating and activity behaviors at 12 and 24 months. Using an intent-to-treat analysis, researchers found no change in BMI at follow-up assessments (Lemon et al., 2010). Researchers also examined the impact of participation rate and differences in setting (small, medium, and large hospital) on their main outcomes. This analysis revealed that the more intervention use a person reported, the greater the decrease in BMI. Furthermore, researchers determined that a smaller hospital was associated with greater effectiveness. *Adoption* was based on upper-level management support throughout the 2-year intervention. Researchers documented meeting logs and minutes spent fostering and maintaining a relationship with administrative staff. *Implementation* was evaluated through direct observation of the hospital environments (e.g., activities and signage). The researchers found that the resarch staff exercised a high level of control over implementation of most of the intervention but that intervention components assigned to hospital food service staff were not fully implemented. Other planned components, including providing healthy lower-cost vending options, were never implemented due to vendor disinterest. Researchers found that implementation was difficult due to the lack of flexibility in scheduling for employees assigned to patient-care responsibilities. The influence of institutional size was observed at different levels, with smaller hospitals lacking a critical mass of interested participants and larger institutions contending with several competing interests. *Maintenance* was evaluated at the individual and systems levels. The program positively impacted fruit and vegetable intake at 12 months but was not maintained at 24-month follow-up. Maintenance at the institutional level was determined largely by observational environmental assessments (e.g., cafeteria signage and staff activities). Some components like cafeteria signage were maintained in the smaller hospitals, but researchers stated that lack of institutional maintenance is a likely result of the study staff implementing the majority of intervention components. The Step Ahead research team reported that assessing their study using the RE-AIM dimensions helped in understanding the strengths and weaknesses of their program and identified factors that could impede dissemination of the program into public health practice. Given the complex nature of the Step Ahead program and other population- and systems-based health interventions that intervene at both the individual and macro levels, it is essential that evaluation methods match this complexity (Glasgow et al., 1999). Researchers must go beyond assessing reach and efficacy/effectiveness, which are largely individual-level variables, by applying evaluative frameworks like RE-AIM to also examine external factors, including adoption, implementation, and maintenance, that are crucial to the wide-scale dissemination and institutionalization of evidence-based health interventions (Glasgow et al., 2003).

ENVIRONMENTAL SUPPORT AND THE ROLE OF GOVERNMENT IN OBESITY PREVENTION

Public health interventions have eliminated smallpox and polio (Young, 2004), decreased accidents due to drunk driving (Wikipedia, 2013), increased seat belt safety (National Center for Injury Prevention and Control, 2011), and helped to reduce the prevalence of smoking in the United States (Roeseler & Burns, 2010). Thus, the government clearly has an interest and a role to play in promoting the health of the population (Gearhardt et al., 2012; Novak & Brownell, 2012).

To date, a number of programs and policies have been advanced in an effort to address the obesity epidemic, including nutrition labeling on packaged foods (Nutrition Labeling Education Act, 1990), presentation of caloric information on restaurant menus (Nutrition Labeling of Standard Menu Items at Chain Restaurants, 2010), and increased availability of healthier foods for low-income populations through changes in the Special Supplemental Nutrition Program for Women, Infants, and Children (WIC) program and other initiatives (USDA, 2011). Local, regional, and national obesity campaigns have also been implemented, including the County of Los Angeles Public Health Department's program, "Improving Nutrition, Increasing Physical Activity and Reducing Obesity in LA County." This campaign stresses portion control by promoting a "Choose Less, Weigh Less" slogan (Los Angeles County Department of Public Health, 2013). This type of information has a role to play in alerting people to the benefits of choosing an appropriate portion size rather than the current standard of excessive portion sizes, and within a supportive environment, could have a more profound impact.

Interestingly, the omnipresence of the large portion sizes we see today can be traced back as far as the 1960s. David Wallerstein, a movie theater owner, wanted to increase sales by having his customers purchase more popcorn. He was not successful in getting people to purchase two servings of popcorn, but he found they were willing to purchase one serving at a larger size and slightly higher price. In Mr. Wallerstein's later position on the board of directors of the McDonald's Corporation, he convinced the company to offer a large size of fries to boost sales. Although the company's founder felt that people would buy a second order if they wanted more fries, he agreed to test the approach. The approach worked so well that today's small order of fries is the size of a large from the late 1970s, and the same is true for other menu choices. For example, the largest soda in 1955 was only 7 ounces, which is considerably smaller than the 12-ounce child size offered today (Wikipedia, 2013).

Research supports the premise that people are susceptible to environmental cues that negatively affect weight management (Wansink & Sobal, 2007). For example, a longitudinal study reported that people who live closer to fast food restaurants consume fast food more often (Boone-Heinonen et al., 2011) and that children who attend schools that serve more unhealthy foods tend to be heavier than those who attend schools that offer more healthful foods and do not allow vending machines in the school (Fox, Dodd, Wilson, & Gleason, 2009).

Recognition of the role of multiple levels of influence may have a positive effect on reducing the consumption of sugar in sweetened beverages (Han & Powell, 2013). Researchers have noted that the exposure of children to television advertising for sugar-sweetened beverages was significantly reduced from 2003 to 2009 (Powell et al., 2011; Terry-McElrath, O'Malley, & Johnston, 2012), and others have documented a significant reduction in students' access to soda in middle schools (−46%) and high schools (−37%) between 2007 and 2009 (Terry-McElrath et al., 2012). In 2009 and 2010, 11 states and 2 cities attempted to tax sugar-sweetened beverages as a means to reduce consumption. Although only one state succeeded and the bill was eventually repealed after extensive lobbying by the American Beverage Association, the willingness of individuals, communities, and policy makers to begin addressing this factor in obesity signals growing recognition that there is a need for multi-level involvement to achieve healthy lifestyle changes (American Beverage Association, 2008).

THE ENVIRONMENT, SOCIAL NORMS, AND BEHAVIOR CHANGE

Socio-ecological frameworks, CBPR, and social marketing have emerged as models in the context of obesity prevention, demonstrating the importance of social and environmental factors within the broader context of health and disease. Looking to the history of tobacco control as an example, attempts to rein in tobacco use show the value of these broader approaches to public health and underscore the need for interventions that move beyond education to include multiple levels of change (Roeseler & Burns, 2010). Just as with tobacco control efforts, this requires embracing the call for supportive environments and an altered perception of what is considered normative behavior to result in population-wide shifts in dietary and activity behaviors related to obesity. However, the recognition that changes in social norms require time is essential (Roeseler & Burns, 2010; Zhang, Cowling, & Tang, 2010). For example, cigar and pipe smoking was banned on U.S. aircraft in 1979, but it was not until 1998 that all smoking was banned on U.S. domestic flights and two more years until smoking was banned on all flights by U.S. airlines (Federal Register, 2000).

CONCLUSIONS

No single solution exists for significant public health problems such as obesity. Thus, multi-factorial approaches are our best hope for solving this type of challenge (White House Task Force on Childhood Obesity, 2010). Ultimately, individuals must take responsibility for both healthful and unhealthful choices, whether they are decisions about seat belts, driving under the influence of drugs or alcohol, food consumption, or physical inactivity. However, for obesity and other chronic diseases to be reversed on a population level, there must be dramatic shifts that make it easier for individuals to choose lifestyle behaviors aligned with healthful, active living. Unraveling the multiple contexts that have contributed to making healthful choices challenging requires a comprehensive and coordinated effort on a number of levels by individuals, communities, researchers, policy makers, and government agencies (Graff, Kappagoda, Wooten, McGowan, & Ashe, 2012).

REFERENCES

Aboelata, M. J., & Navarro, A. M. (2010). Emerging issues in improving food and physical activity environments: Strategies for addressing land use, transportation, and safety in 3 California-wide initiatives. *American Journal of Public Health, 100,* 2146–2148.

Aittasalo, M., Rinne, M., Pasanen, M., Kukkonen-Harjula, K., & Vasankari, T. (2012). Promoting walking among office employees: Evaluation of a randomized controlled intervention with pedometers and e-mail messages. *BMC Public Health, 12,* 403.

Ajzen, I., & Fishbein, M. (1980). *Understanding attitudes and predicting social behavior.* Englewood Cliffs, NJ: Prentice-Hall.

American Beverage Association. (2008). *School beverage guidelines progress report 2007–2008.* Washington, DC. Retrived from http://www.ameribev.org/files/240_SBG%20Exec%20Summary%202007-2008 .pdf. Accessed February 15, 2013.

Anderson, N. B. (1998). *After the discoveries, then what? A new approach to advancing evidence-based prevention practice* (pp. 74–75). Programs and abstracts from NIH Conference, Preventive Intervention Research at the Crossroads. Bethesda, MD.

Andreasen, A. R. (1995). *Marketing social change: Changing behavior to promote health, social development, and the environment* (1st ed.). San Francisco, CA: Jossey-Bass.

Asbury, L. D., Wong, F. L., Price, S. M., & Nolin, M. J. (2008). The VERB campaign: Applying a branding strategy in public health. *American Journal of Preventive Medicine, 34*(Suppl. 6), S183–S187.

Ashe, M., Graff, S., & Spector, C. (2011). Changing places: Policies to make a healthy choice the easy choice. *Public Health, 125,* 889–895.

Baranowski, T., Cullen, K. W., Nicklas, T., Thompson, D., & Baranowski, J. (2003). Are current health behavioral change models helpful in guiding prevention of weight gain efforts? *Obesity Research, 11*(Suppl.), 23S–43S.

Berkman, L., Blumenthal, J., Burg, M., Carney, R. M., Catellier, D., Cowan, M. J., ... Enhancing Recovery in Coronary Heart Disease Patients Investigators (ENRICHD). (2003). Effects of treating depression and low perceived social support on clinical events after myocardial infarction: The Enhancing Recovery in Coronary Heart Disease patients (ENRICHD) randomized trial. *Journal of the American Medical Association, 289,* 3106–3116.

Boone-Heinonen, J., Gordon-Larsen, P., Kiefe, C. I., Shikany, J. M., Lewis, C. E., & Popkin, B. M. (2011). Fast food restaurants and food stores: Longitudinal associations with diet in young to middle-aged adults: The CARDIA study. *Archives of Internal Medicine, 171,* 1162–1170.

Bopp, M., Wilcox, S., Laken, M., Hooker, S. P., Saunders, R., Parra-Medina, D., & McClorin, L. (2007). Using the RE-AIM framework to evaluate a physical activity intervention in churches. *Preventing Chronic Disease, 4,* A87.

Bronfenbrenner, U. (1992). Ecological systems theory. In R. Vasta (Ed.), *Six theories of child development: Revised formulations and current issues* (pp. 187–249). Philadelphia, PA: Jessica Kingsley.

Brownell, K. D. (2010). The humbling experience of treating obesity: Should we persist or desist? *Behaviour Research and Therapy, 48,* 717–719.

Brownell, K. D., Kersh, R., Ludwig, D. S., Post, R. C., Puhl, R. M., Schwartz, M. B., & Willett, W.C (2010). Personal responsibility and obesity: A constructive approach to a controversial issue. *Health Affairs (Millwood), 29,* 379–387.

Brownson, R. C., & Bright, F. S. (2004). Chronic disease control in public health practice: Looking back and moving forward. *Public Health Reports, 119,* 230–238.

Bullough, B., & Rosen, G. (1992). *Preventive medicine in the United States, 1900–1990: Trends and interpretations.* Canton, MA: Science History Publications.

Cashman, S., & Forlano, L. (2009). Collaboration between professional and mediating structures in the community: Social determinants of health and community-based participatory research. In S. A. Shumaker, J. K. Ockene, & K. A. Reikert (Eds.), *The handbook of health behavior change* (3rd ed., pp. 735–756). New York, NY: Springer.

Chen, P. G., Diaz, N., Lucas, G., & Rosenthal, M. S. (2010). Dissemination of results in community-based participatory research. *American Journal of Preventive Medicine, 39,* 372–378.

Cook, W. K. (2008). Integrating research and action: A systematic review of community-based participatory research to address health disparities in environmental and occupational health in the USA. *Journal of Epidemiology and Community Health, 62,* 668–676.

Cornwall, A., & Jewkes, R. (1995). What is participatory research? *Social Science & Medicine, 41,* 1667–1676.

Curry, S., & Fitzgibbon, M. L. (2009). Theories of prevention. In S. A. Shumaker, J. K. Ockene, & K. A. Reikert (Eds.), *The handbook of health behavior change* (3rd ed., pp. 3–18). New York, NY: Springer.

De Moor, M. H., Liu, Y. J., Boomsma, D. I., Li, J., Hamilton, J. J., Hottenga, J. J., & Deng, H. W. (2009). Genome-wide association study of exercise behavior in Dutch and American adults. *Medicine and Science in Sports and Exercise, 41,* 1887–1895.

DeVries, A. C., Glasper, E. R., & Detillion, C. E. (2003). Social modulation of stress responses. *Physiology & Behavior, 79,* 399–407.

Diez Roux, A. V. (2011). Complex systems thinking and current impasses in health disparities research. *American Journal of Public Health, 101,* 1627–1634.

Economos, C. D., Hyatt, R. R., Goldberg, J. P., Must, A., Naumova, E. N., Collins, J. J., & Nelson, M. E. (2007). A community intervention reduces BMI z-score in children: Shape Up Somerville first year results. *Obesity, 15,* 1325–1336.

Estabrook, B., Zapka, J., & Lemon, S. C. (2012). Evaluating the implementation of a hospital work-site obesity prevention intervention: Applying the RE-AIM framework. *Health Promotion Practice, 13,* 190–197.

Estabrooks, P. (2013). *Reach Effectiveness Adoption Implementation Maintenance (RE-AIM).* Virginia Tech, College of Agriculture and Life Sciences. Retrieved from http://www.re-aim.hnfe.vt.edu/index .html. Accessed February 15, 2013.

Farrelly, M. C., Healton, C. G., Davis, K. C., Messeri, P., Hersey, J. C., & Haviland, M. L. (2002). Getting to the truth: Evaluating national tobacco countermarketing campaigns. *American Journal of Public Health, 92,* 901–907.

Federal Register. The Daily Journal of the United States Government. (2000). *Smoking aboard aircraft, a rule by the Transportation Department on 06/09/2000.* Retrieved from https://www.federalregister .gov/articles/2000/06/09/00-14480/smoking-aboard-aircraft#h-8. Accessed February 18, 2013.

Fielding, J. E., & Briss, P. A. (2006). Promoting evidence-based public health policy: Can we have better evidence and more action? *Health Affairs (Millwood), 25,* 969–978.

Flay, B. R. (1986). Efficacy and effectiveness trials (and other phases of research) in the development of health promotion programs. *Preventive Medicine, 15,* 451–474.

Foerster, S. B., Kizer, K. W., Disogra, L. K., Bal, D. G., Krieg, B. F., & Bunch, K. L. (1995). California's "5 A Day–For Better Health!" campaign: An innovative population-based effort to effect large-scale dietary change. *American Journal of Preventive Medicine, 11,* 124–131.

Forthofer, M. S., & Bryant, C. A. (2000). Using audience-segmentation techniques to tailor health behavior change strategies. *American Journal of Health Behavior, 24,* 36–43.

Fox, M. K., Dodd, A. H., Wilson, A., & Gleason, P. M. (2009). Association between school food environment and practices and body mass index of U.S. public school children. *Journal of the American Dietetic Association, 109*(Suppl. 2), S108–S117.

Gearhardt, A. N., Bragg, M. A., Pearl, R. L., Schvey, N. A., Roberto, C. A., & Brownell, K. D. (2012). Obesity and public policy. *Annual Review of Clinical Psychology, 8,* 405–430.

Glanz, K., & Rimer, B. K. (1997). *Theory at a glance: A guide for health promotion practice* (NIH publication). Bethesda, MD: U.S. Department of Health and Human Services, Public Health Service, National Institutes of Health, National Cancer Institute.

Glanz, K., Rimer, B. K., & Lewis, F. M. (Eds.). (2002). *Health behavior and health education: Theory, research, and practice* (3rd ed.). San Francisco, CA: Jossey-Bass.

Glasgow, R. E., Bull, S. S., Gillette, C., Klesges, L. M., & Dzewaltowski, D. A. (2002). Behavior change intervention research in healthcare settings: A review of recent reports with emphasis on external validity. *American Journal of Preventive Medicine, 23,* 62–69.

Glasgow, R. E., Klesges, L. M., Dzewaltowski, D. A., Bull, S. S., & Estabrooks, P. (2004). The future of health behavior change research: What is needed to improve translation of research into health promotion practice? *Annals of Behavioral Medicine, 27*, 3–12.

Glasgow, R. E., Lichtenstein E., & Marcus, A. C. (2003). Why don't we see more translation of health promotion research to practice? Rethinking the efficacy-to-effectiveness transition. *American Journal of Public Health, 93*, 1261–1267.

Glasgow, R. E., Vogt, T. M., & Boles, S. M. (1999). Evaluating the public health impact of health promotion interventions: The RE-AIM framework. *American Journal of Public Health, 89*, 1322–1327.

Glass, T. A. (2000). Psychosocial interventions. In L. F. Berkman & I . Kawachi (Eds.), *Social epidemiology* (pp. 267–305). New York, NY: Oxford University Press.

Goode, A. D., Owen, N., Reeves, M. M., & Eakin, E. G. (2012). Translation from research to practice: Community dissemination of a telephone-delivered physical activity and dietary behavior change intervention. *American Journal of Health Promotion, 26*, 253–259.

Gortmaker, S. L., Swinburn, B. A., Levy, D., Carter, R., Mabry, P. L., Finegood, D. T., … Moodie, M. L. (2011). Changing the future of obesity: Science, policy, and action. *Lancet, 378*, 838–847.

Graff, S. K., Kappagoda, M., Wooten, H. M., McGowan, A. K., & Ashe, M. (2012). Policies for healthier communities: Historical, legal, and practical elements of the obesity prevention movement. *Annual Review of Public Health, 33*, 307–324.

Green, L. W., & Kreuter, M. W. (2005). *Health program planning: An educational and ecological approach* (4th ed.). New York, NY: McGraw-Hill.

Green, L. W., & Mercer, S. L. (2001). Can public health researches and agencies reconcile the push from funding bodies and the pull from communities? *American Journal of Public Health, 91*, 1926–1929.

Greenwald, P., & Cullen, J. W. (1985). The new emphasis in cancer control. *Journal of the National Cancer Institute, 74*, 543–551.

Grier, S., & Bryant, C. A. (2005). Social marketing in public health. *Annual Review of Public Health, 26*, 319–339.

Han, E., & Powell, L. M. (2013). Consumption patterns of sugar-sweetened beverages in the United States. *Journal of the Academy of Nutrition and Dietetics, 113*, 43–53.

Huang, T. T., Drewnosksi, A., Kumanyika, S., & Glass, T. A. (2009). A systems-oriented multilevel framework for addressing obesity in the 21st century. *Prevention of Chronic Disease, 6*, A82.

Huang, T. T. K., & Glass, T. A. (2008). Transforming research strategies for understanding and preventing obesity. *Journal of the American Medical Association, 300*, 1811–1813.

Huhman, M., Berkowitz, J. M., Wong, F. L., Prosper, E., Gray, M., Prince, D., & Yuen, J. (2008). The VERB campaign's strategy for reaching African-American, Hispanic, Asian, and American Indian children and parents. *American Journal of Preventive Medicine, 34*(Suppl. 6), S194–S209.

Institute of Medicine. (2002). *The future of the public's health in the 21st century*. Washington, DC: National Academies Press.

Israel, B. A., Schulz, A. J., Eng, E., & Parker, E. A. (2012). *Methods for community-based participatory research for health* (2nd ed.). San Francisco, CA: Jossey-Bass.

Israel, B. A., Schulz, A. J., Parker, E. A., & Becker, A. B. (1998). Review of community-based research: Assessing partnership approaches to improve public health. *Annual Review of Public Health, 19*, 73–202.

Jago, R., & Bailey, R. (2001). Ethics and paediatric exercise science: Issues and making a submission to a local ethics and research committee. *Journal of Sports Science, 19*, 527–535.

Jenkinson, K. A., Naughton, G., & Benson, A. C. (2012). The GLAMA (Girls! Lead! Achieve! Mentor! Activate!) physical activity and peer leadership intervention pilot project: A process evaluation using the RE-AIM framework. *BMC Public Health, 12*, 55.

Karamanou, M., Panayiotakopoulos, G., Tsoucalas, G., Kousoulis, A. A., & Androutsos, G. (2012). From miasmas to germs: A historical approach to theories of infectious disease transmission. *Infez Med, 20*, 58–62.

Kerner, J., Rimer, B., & Emmons, K. (2005). Introduction to the special section on dissemination: Dissemination research and research dissemination: How can we close the gap? *Health Psychology, 24*, 443–446.

Kumanyika, S., Jeffery, R. W., Morabia, A., Ritenbaugh, C., & Antipatis, V. J. (2002). Public Health Approaches to the Prevention of Obesity Working Group of the International Obesity Task Force (IOTF). Obesity prevention: The case for action. *International Journal of Obesity and Related Metabolic Disorders, 26*, 425–436.

Lemon, S. C., Zapka, J., Li, W., Estabrook, B., Rosal, M., Magner, R., … Hale, J. (2010). Step ahead: A worksite obesity prevention trial among hospital employees. *American Journal of Preventive Medicine, 38*, 27–38.

Los Angeles (LA) County Department of Public Health. (2013). Choose Health LA: Improving nutrition, increasing physical activity and reducing obesity in LA County. In *Choose less, weigh less*. Retrieved from http://www.choosehealthla.com/eat-healthy/portion-control/. Accessed February 15, 2013.

Maziak, W., Ward, K. D., & Stockton, M. B. (2008). Childhood obesity: Are we missing the big picture? *Obesity Review, 9*, 35–42.

McGinnis, J. M., & Foege, W. H. (1993). Actual causes of death in the United States. *Journal of the American Medical Association, 270*, 2207–2212.

McKinlay, J., & Marceau, L. (2000). Upstream healthy public policy: Lessons from the battle of tobacco. *International Journal of Health Services, 30*, 49–69.

Merzel, C., & D'Afflitti, J. (2003). Reconsidering community-based health promotion: Promise, performance, and potential. *American Journal of Public Health, 93*, 557–574.

Minkler, M. (2004). Ethical challenges for the "outside" researcher in community-based participatory research. *Health Education & Behavior, 31*, 684–697.

Minkler, M., Blackwell, A. G., Thompson, M., & Tamir, H. (2003). Community-based participatory research: Implications for public health funding. *American Journal of Public Health, 93*, 1210–1213.

Minkler, M., & Wallerstein, N. (2008). *Community-based participatory research for health: From process to outcomes* (2nd ed.). San Francisco, CA: Jossey-Bass.

Morland, K., Wing, S., Diez Roux, A., & Poole, C. (2002). Neighborhood characteristics associated with the location of food stores and food service places. *American Journal of Preventive Medicine, 22*, 23–29.

Multiple Risk Factor Intervention Trial: Risk factor changes and mortality results. (1982). *Journal of the American Medical Association, 248*, 1465–1477.

National Center for Health Statistics. (2006). *Health, United States, 2006 with chartbook on trends in the health of Americans.* Hyattsville, MD: U.S. Government Printing Office. Retrieved from http://www.cdc.gov/nchs/data/hus/hus06.pdf. Accessed February 15, 2013.

National Center for Injury Prevention and Control, Division of Unintentional Injury Prevention. (2011). *Policy impact—Seat belts.* Washington, DC: Centers for Disease Control and Prevention Retrieved from http://www.cdc.gov/MotorVehicleSafety/pdf/PolicyImpact-SeatBelts.pdf. Accessed February 15, 2013.

National Institutes of Health (NIH), Office of Behavioral and Social Sciences Research (OBSSR). (2013). *Community-based participatory research.* Retrieved from http://obssr.od.nih.gov/scientific_areas /methodology/community_based_participatory_research/index.aspx (Accessed February 15, 2013).

Novak, N. L., & Brownell, K. D. (2012). Role of policy and government in the obesity epidemic. *Circulation, 126*, 2345–2352.

Nutrition Labeling and Education Act (NLEA). (1990). Pub. L. No. 101–535, 104 Stat. 2353.

Nutrition Labeling of Standard Menu Items at Chain Restaurants. (2010). HR 3590, Sec. 4205.

Ogden, C. L., Carroll, M. D., Kit, B. K., & Flegal, K. M. (2012). Prevalence of obesity and trends in body mass index among US children and adolescents, 1999–2010. *Journal of the American Medical Association, 307*, 483–490.

Oldenburg, B. F., Ffrench, M. L., & Sallis, J. F. (2000). Health behavior research: The quality of the evidence base. *American Journal of Health Promotion, 14*, 253–257.

Powell, L. M., Schermbeck, R. M., Szczypka, G., Chaloupka, F. J., & Braunschweig, C. L. (2011). Trends in the nutritional content of television food advertisements seen by children in the United States: Analyses by age, food categories, and companies. *Archives of Pediatric and Adolescent Medicine, 165*, 1078–1086.

Prochaska, J. O., & DiClemente, C. C. (1983). Stages and processes of self-change of smoking: Toward an integrative model of change. *Journal of Consulting and Clinical Psychology, 51*, 390–395.

Relman, A. S., & Angell, M. (2002). Resolved: Psychosocial interventions can improve clinical outcomes in organic disease (con). *Psychosomatic Medicine, 64*, 558–563.

Roeseler, A., & Burns, D. (2010). The quarter that changed the world. *Tobacco Control, 19*(Suppl. 1), i3–i15.

Rosenstock, I. M. (1974). The health belief model: Origins and correlates. *Health Education Monograph, 2*, 336–353.

Sallis, J. F., & Owen, N. (1997). Ecological models. In K. Glanz, F. M. Lewis, & B. K. Rimmer (Eds.), *Health behavior and health education: Theory, research and practice* (2nd ed., pp. 403–424). San Francisco, CA: Jossey-Bass.

Sallis, J. F., Owen, N., & Fisher, E. B. (2008). Ecological models of health behavior. In K. Glanz, B. K. Rimer, & K. Viswanath (Eds.), *Health behavior and health education: Theory, research, and practice* (4th ed., pp. 465–486). San Francisco, CA: Jossey-Bass.

Schneider, M., & Stokols, D. (2008). Multilevel theories of behavior change: A social ecological framework. In S. A. Shumaker, J. K. Ockene, & K. A. Riekert (Eds.), *The handbook of health behavior change* (3rd ed., pp. 85–105). New York, NY: Springer.

Schulz, L. O., Bennett, P. H., Ravussin, E., Kidd, J. R., Kidd, K. K., Esparza, J., & Valencia, M. E. (2006). Effects of traditional and western environments on prevalence of type 2 diabetes in Pima Indians in Mexico and the U.S. *Diabetes Care, 29*, 1866–1871.

Shediac-Rizkallah, M. C., & Bone, L. R. (1998). Planning for the sustainability of community-based health programs: Conceptual frameworks and future directions for research, practice and policy. *Health Education Research, 13*, 87–108.

Smedley, B. D., & Syme, S. L., Committee on Capitalizing on Social Science and Behavioral Research to Improve the Public's Health, Division of Health Promotion and Disease Prevention. (2000). *Promoting health: Intervention strategies from social and behavioral research*. Washington, DC: National Academies Press.

Stamler, J., & Neaton, J. D. (2008). The Multiple Risk Factor Intervention Trial (MRFIT): Importance then and now. *Journal of the American Medical Association, 300*, 1343–1345.

Steuart, G. W. (1993). Social and cultural perspectives: Community intervention and mental health, 1978. *Health Education Quarterly*, (Suppl. 1), S99–S111.

Stokols, D. (1987). Conceptual strategies of environmental psychology. In D. Stokols & I. Altman, (Eds.), *Handbook of environmental psychology* (pp. 41–70). New York, NY: John Wiley & Sons.

Stokols, D. (1992). Establishing and maintaining healthy environments. Toward a social ecology of health promotion. *American Psychologist, 47*, 6–22.

Susser, M., & Susser, E. (1996). Choosing a future for epidemiology: I. Eras and paradigms. *American Journal of Public Health, 86*, 668–673.

Terry-McElrath, Y. M., O'Malley, P. M., & Johnston, L. D. (2012). Factors affecting sugar-sweetened beverage availability in competitive venues of US secondary schools. *Journal of School Health, 82*, 44–55.

Toobert, D., Glasgow, R., Strycker, L., Barrera, M., Jr., & King, D. (2012).Adapting and RE-AIMing a heart disease prevention program for older women with diabetes. *Translational Behavioral Medicine, 2*, 180–187.

United States Department of Agriculture (USDA), Food & Nutrition Service. (2011). *WIC food packages – Regulatory requirements for WIC-eligible foods*. Retrieved from http://www.fns.usda.gov/wic/benefitsandservices/foodpkgregs.HTM. Accessed February 15, 2013.

Viswanathan, M., Ammerman, A., Eng, E., Gartlehner, G., Lohr, K. N., Griffith, D., …Whitener, L. (2004). *Community-based participatory research: Assessing the evidence* (Evidence Report/Technology Assessment No. 99, Prepared by RTI–University of North Carolina Evidence-based Practice Center under Contract No. 290-02-0016). AHRQ Publication 04-E022-2. Rockville, MD: Agency for Healthcare Research and Quality.

Walker, R. E., Keane, C. R., & Burke, J. G. (2010). Disparities and access to healthy food in the United States: A review of food deserts literature. *Health & Place, 16*, 876–884.

Wallerstein, N., & Duran, B. (2010). Community-based participatory research contributions to intervention research: The intersection of science and practice to improve health equity. *American Journal of Public Health, 100*(Suppl. 1), S40–S46.

Wansink, B., & Sobal, J. (2007). Mindless eating: The 200 daily food decisions we overlook. *Environment and Behavior, 39*, 106–123.

White House Task Force on Childhood Obesity. (2010). *Let's MOVE! Solving the problem of childhood obesity within a generation* (White House Task Force on Childhood Obesity Report to the President). Retrieved from http://www.letsmove.gov/white-house-task-force-childhood-obesity-report-president. Accessed February 18, 2013.

Wikipedia. *Drunk driving in the United States*. Retrieved from http://en.wikipedia.org/wiki/Drunk_driving_in_the_United_States. Accessed February 15, 2013.

Wikipedia. *Super size me*. Retrieved from http://en.wikipedia.org/wiki/Super_Size_Me. Accessed February 15, 2013.

Wong, F., Huhman, M., Heitzler, C., Asbury, L., Bretthauer-Mueller, R., McCarthy, S., & Londe, P. (2004). VERB – A social marketing campaign to increase physical activity among youth. *Prevention of Chronic Disease, 1*, A10.

Young, T. K. (2004). *Population health, concepts and methods* (2nd ed.). New York, NY: Oxford University Press.

Zapka, J., Lemon, S. C., Estabrook, B. B., & Jolicoeur, D. G. (2007). Keeping a Step Ahead: Formative phase of a workplace intervention trial to prevent obesity. *Obesity, 15*(Suppl. 1), 27S–36S.

Zhang, X., Cowling, D. W., & Tang, H. (2010). The impact of social norm change strategies on smokers' quitting behaviours. *Tobacco Control, 19*(Suppl. 1), i51–i55.

3

Health System Models

RUSSELL E. GLASGOW
KURT C. STANGE

LEARNING OBJECTIVES

- Define and discuss the Expanded Chronic Care Model, and how it builds on the original Chronic Care Model (CCM).
- Define and describe the Practice Change Model and how it can be and has been used to facilitate health care systems/practice change.
- Describe key elements of the Reach, Efficacy/Effectiveness, Adoption, Implementation, and Maintenance (RE-AIM) model and Practical, Robust, Implementation Systems Model (PRISM), how they are related to each other, and how they help to anticipate common challenges in program implementation and dissemination.

Almost all theories of health behavior acknowledge that the behaviors of both care practitioners and the clients or patients they serve occur in a multi-level context. This chapter discusses key elements of that context and describes three widely used models of health systems as well as the research supporting these models. Twentieth-century health systems are complicated and can interact positively or negatively with the other determinants of health behaviors. The importance and many aspects of this perspective were discussed in detail in the 2012 issue of the *Journal of the National Cancer Institute* on multi-level issues in health systems (Stange, Breslau, Dietrich, & Glasgow, 2012).

The health system itself is multi-level, as illustrated in Figure 3.1. It consists of at least four overlapping but discrete levels: the team microsystem, the clinic level, the broader organization, and finally the health macrosystem consisting of both community resources and health policies. As can be seen, the persons who work together on a daily basis to serve their clients/patients are termed the *microsystem* (Wasson et al., 2006), and they reside within the larger office or practice, such as a primary care or community health clinic. Often, and especially for larger and urban settings, this practice is part of a larger network of practices that belong to a parent organization, such as a health plan, and HMO, or with the Affordable Care Act, an Accountable Care Organization (ACO). The policies, rules, norms, and culture of this larger organization often play a dominant role in influencing actions at the practice and team level. These are embedded in the broader community and the health-related resources in that community or region, such as community wellness programs, referral resources,

FIGURE 3.1 Multi-level health system.

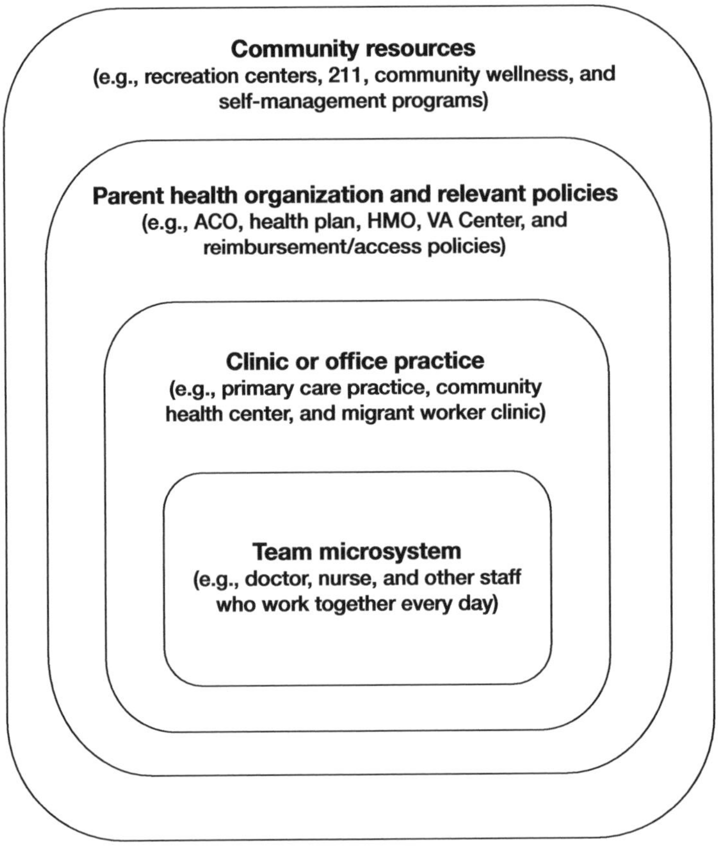

Community resources
(e.g., recreation centers, 211, community wellness, and
self-management programs)

Parent health organization and relevant policies
(e.g., ACO, health plan, HMO, VA Center, and
reimbursement/access policies)

Clinic or office practice
(e.g., primary care practice, community
health center, and migrant worker clinic)

Team microsystem
(e.g., doctor, nurse, and other staff
who work together every day)

self-management programs in community, or faith-based settings, and so on. The local, state, and national policy contexts frame all these embedded levels.

The three specific health system models in this chapter—the Chronic Care (and Extended Chronic Care) Model; the Practice Change/Complex Adaptive System Model; and the RE-AIM/PRISM Model—are technically not theories, but are frameworks that point to key aspects of health systems and/or key factors related to the success of health systems. As such, these frameworks represent important domains and interactions to pay attention to and work to understand and influence as they co-evolve together over time. They are also related to the emerging field of implementation science that is concerned with integrating research, practice, and policy (Brownson, Colditz, & Proctor, 2012; Glasgow et al., 2012).

CHRONIC CARE AND EXPANDED CHRONIC CARE MODEL

The Chronic Care Model (CCM; Bodenheimer, Wagner, & Grumbach, 2002; Wagner, Austin, Davis, Hindmarsh, & Schaefer, 2001) originated from a combination of literature review and interviews with health care systems known to produce especially high-quality chronic illness care. It was based on the developers' synthesis of the common features of successful health systems. While originally focused on chronic conditions, as the name implies, there was consideration of titling the model the "planned care

FIGURE 3.2 Chronic Care Model.

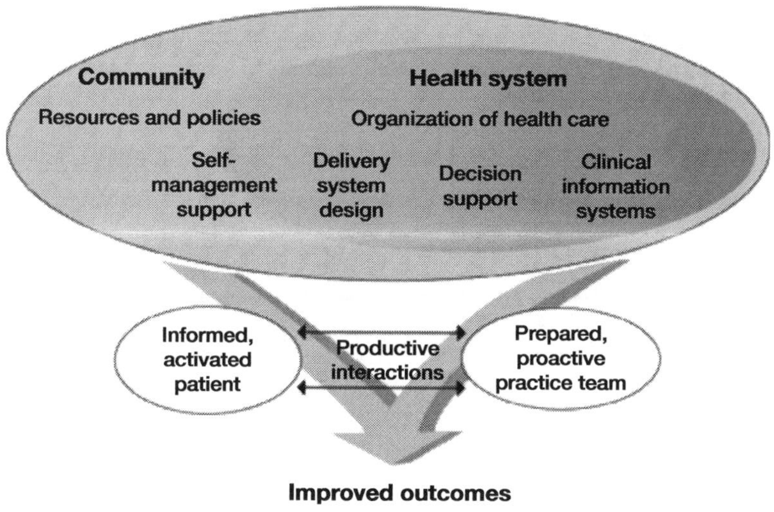

model" since, as authors later described, almost all of the same components, with slightly different emphases, are also relevant to disease prevention as well as management (Glasgow, Orleans, Wagner, Curry, & Solberg, 2001).

As can be seen in Figure 3.2, there are six core components of the CCM, all of which are hypothesized to be necessary and operating in an aligned fashion to reinforce the other components for an effective prevention or disease management health system. These components are health system support, clinical information systems, decision support, delivery system support, self-management support, and community resources.

Health care system support consists of several factors, including adequate financial and top management support, and also values and mission aligned with providing quality illness care. Clinical information systems such as electronic health records and especially disease registries are a critical and often initial focus of health systems wanting to improve their care. Knowing which patients have a given condition, and their status on key factors related to control of that condition, is a prerequisite for effective programs. A decision support system is necessary to help practitioners use the clinical information system to manage individual patients as well as their entire panel or population of patients with a condition. The decision support system often consists of guidelines or decision rules for the team microsystem to follow. Delivery system support consists of infrastructure and incentives to "make the right thing the easy thing to do."

The final two aspects of the CCM, self-management support and community resources, are both central to this volume, and also often the most challenging for health systems to implement, and in studies conducted to date are usually the elements of the model that are implemented least often (Glasgow, Davis, Funnell, & Beck, 2003). Self-management support includes listening to the patient and family or significant others; collaboratively working with the patients to identify areas to improve (ideally using decision support tools); specifying and documenting practical, achievable goals that are relevant to the patient; and collaboratively developing action plans and problem-solving strategies (Glasgow et al., 2002). Possibly the most challenging aspect of self-management support is providing consistent follow-up support once goals and an action plan are established.

For some issues, this series of activities can be implemented in the medical office, either by the clinician, or more often, by a staff member such as a nurse, educator, or behavioral specialist trained in health behavior counseling. For other self-management goals, referral to either evidence-based electronic or printed resources, or more commonly, local community resources (e.g., a stop smoking Quitline, Weight Watchers, diabetes, or chronic disease self-management support group programs) is necessary. In theory, such referral makes excellent sense; in practice, most referrals are not completed successfully due to a variety of barriers and if they are completed, the referring practice rarely receives any feedback on patient progress (Glasgow & Goldstein, 2008).

The CCM is one of the most frequently used models for health care improvement, and the most well-known application of the CCM was in collaboration with the Institute for Healthcare Improvement in the Improving Chronic Illness Care collaborative (Wagner et al., 2001). Although there have been criticisms based on the costs and selectivity of participants in such initiatives (Glasgow et al., 2003), most reviewers have concluded that these collaboratives have been successful in improving care across a variety of different chronic illness conditions and settings. In particular, the HRSA community health centers adopted the IHI Improvement model, and the CCM collaborative approach has been spread around the world (www.ihi .org/about/pages/default.aspx). Although important outcomes and successes have been reported from many of these collaboratives (Chin et al., 2007; Wagner, Glasgow, et al., 2001), there have to our knowledge been no controlled experimental studies of the collaboratives or comparisons of the use of the CCM with other approaches. Common results across different collaboratives seem to be that (a) establishment of a registry of relevant patients is a critical step to enable management of a population (or "panel") of patients, rather than treating one patient at a time; (b) "planned visits" between a motivated patient whose preferences are addressed and a prepared practice team is necessary; and (c) usually the self-management support and community resource aspects are the least well implemented of the six CCM components (Glasgow et al., 2005).

The Expanded Chronic Care Model (ECCM; Barr et al., 2003) was developed both partially in response to the results just discussed and also to insert more of a public health perspective into the CCM. The main contribution of the ECCM, and the related WHO non-communicable disease management models, is to emphasize that the health care setting (the focus of the CCM) resides within a larger environment of a community and policy/cultural context. The ECCM emphasizes the importance of also including linkages between the health care setting and community resources.

SUMMARY AND KEY LESSONS LEARNED

The CCM and the ECCM have provided the basis for several important and successful quality improvement projects for a variety of chronic conditions (Bodenheimer et al., 2002; Chin et al., 2007) and some prevention activities (Glasgow et al., 2001). Not all of these initiatives, and not all health systems participating in a given initiative or collaborative, have been uniformly successful, however. Keys to success in implementing the CCM and ECCM are summarized in this section. First, the necessary infrastructure must either exist or be established. Usually the first necessary component (in addition to necessary administrative support and resources, including time for staff to become adequately trained) is establishment of a disease or problem behavior registry. This registry is a list, usually automated to allow for data analysis, sorting, and management, of all the patients within a given practice, physician, or system having a given disease, and their relevant characteristics along a number of dimensions (e.g., severity, duration, treatments, key assessment indices, and goals).

Such a registry also provides the basis for a necessary culture shift in medical thinking and practice. This shift is from providing care to one patient in the office at that time, to providing quality care for an entire panel or "population" of patients under one's care, including those who have not been in the office recently. This fundamental change or approach, along with a parallel one in approach to self-management from telling patients what to do to listening to them and making collaborative plans that patients consider important, relevant, and achievable, is challenging for many clinicians and systems. Today, almost all practitioners self-identify as being "patient-centered" and have heard of strategies and counseling approaches such as self-management and motivational interviewing; however, observation of patient interviews reveals that implementing these practices is different from intellectual knowledge of them (Glasgow & Goldstein, 2008). Fortunately, level of resources, or how challenging one's patient population is, does not appear to be a significant determinant of success. For example, many community health centers have been equally or more successful at implementing the CCM and ECCM than health systems with vastly more resources and clinical expertise (Chin et al., 2007).

Future directions for the CCM and ECCM include the following challenges and opportunities. There is a need to both investigate and enhance the long-term results of CCM collaboratives, including both program "spread" or dissemination to all clinical teams within a setting and long-term maintenance of procedures and outcomes. Second, as described earlier, greater attention must be devoted to consistent implementation of self-management and community resource aspects of the CCM and ECCM models, and especially to establishing strong linkages between community resources and health settings (Institute of Medicine, 2012). Hopefully, developments related to the Affordable Care Act (Staff of the Washington Post, 2012), including accountable care organizations and a stronger community health worker task force, along with greatly enhanced electronic health records, will facilitate such goals. Finally, the models in which training takes places in in-person, intensive group meetings in a central location should be replaced by or supplemented with much more efficient ways to provide training and collaboration.

PRACTICE CHANGE MODEL

The Practice Change Model was born from the need to understand and facilitate the challenging process of changing clinical practice in a rapidly changing health care environment (Cohen et al., 2004). It is based on complexity theory and views medical practices and health care systems as complex adaptive systems that co-evolve with other systems. Traditional quality improvement models have been of some use, but they tend to assume a linear process of change in which inputs reliably lead to proportionate outputs. However, clinical practice—particularly primary care practice in which care is integrated, personalized, and prioritized for individuals, families, and communities—involves many non-linear processes in which small changes sometimes lead to large results in some settings and large inputs lead to limited effects in other settings. The Practice Change Model was developed from a line of investigation to understand this variation and to help guide the efforts of those trying to improve primary care practice (Crabtree et al., 2011).

This line of inquiry began with observational studies that identified the complex nature of primary care practice, and found utility from understanding primary care practice as a complex adaptive system (Miller, Crabtree, McDaniel, & Stange, 1998; Miller, 2001). In such systems, change is an emergent process that involves a complex interaction of multiple factors, including:

1. History and initial conditions, including any explicit or implicit mission and the underlying priorities for the practice.
2. Particular agents (stakeholders such as practice staff, patients, and health care system partners) and their unique styles and interests.
3. The pattern of non-linear interactions among agents.
4. The local fitness landscape (i.e., the practice's ecological niche) and its particular expectations, community values, competitive issues, and ecology.
5. Regional and global influences, such as larger health care systems, finances and regulations, and culture (Miller, 2001).

How these factors manifest and change can be understood using three complexity science principles: self-organization, co-evolution, and emergence. *Self-organization* is the development of structures and behavior in systems characterized by multiple feedback loops and non-linear dynamics. These structures are a function of the patterns of relationships among agents. Each practice seeks a niche where it can prosper and survive by interactively adapting—co-evolving—with its changing environment. As the agents of any complex adaptive system interact, novelty and surprise emerge in unpredictable ways. This emergence creates a system that is greater than the sum of its parts; it is what cannot be understood through a reductionist (one problem at a time), linear (A leads to B leads to C) examination of the practice.

The result is much (desirable and undesirable) variation between and within practices, and a perplexing set of responses to attempts to improve practice, particularly as practices co-evolve with a rapidly changing health care environment. Desirable variation occurs when practices tailor their approach to care to the unique attributes of their patients and community, and when they adapt practice improvement approaches to these attributes and those of the practice agents. Undesirable variation occurs when known helpful interventions are not taken up or adapted.

With this understanding of practices as complex adaptive systems, the Practice Change Model was developed by comparing practices that make large improvements and those that made minimal improvement in response to a practice-individualized quality improvement intervention that was successful in creating a sustained practice improvement (Goodwin et al., 2001; Stange, Goodwin, Zyzanski, & Dietrich, 2003). The sustainability of the improvement is thought to be due to having tailored the intervention to fit with the unique characteristics of each practice and practice environment (Ruhe, Carter, Litaker, & Stange, 2009). To identify the complexity science model guiding this practice change work, a multidisciplinary team evaluated data from the Study To Enhance Prevention by Understanding Practice (STEP-UP), a randomized clinical trial that was conducted to improve the delivery of evidence-based preventive services in 79 northeastern Ohio practices (Goodwin et al., 2001; Stange et al., 2003). The team conducted comparative case-study analyses of high- and low-improvement practices to identify variables that are critical to the change process and to create a conceptual model for the observed change.

The model depicts the critical elements for understanding and guiding practice change and emphasizes the importance of these elements' evolving interrelationships and how they evolve together over time. These elements are:

1. Motivation of key stakeholders to achieve the target for change;
2. Instrumental, personal, and interactive resources for change;
3. Motivators outside the practice, including the larger health care environment and community; and
4. Choices for change, that is, how key stakeholders understand the change options.

As labeled in Figure 3.3, the interaction among these factors also is important in understanding and facilitating change over time. Interventions that are based on understanding the four key elements and their interrelationships can yield sustainable quality improvements in primary care practice.

The Practice Change Model has been used to understand and to guide a number of practice improvement interventions, most recently, the National Demonstration Project (NDP) of the Patient-Centered Medical Home (Bayliss, Phillips, & Guest Editors, 2010). Using the Practice Change Model to evaluate the multiple paths by which highly motivated practices worked to make dramatic changes over a short period of time identified a relationship-centered developmental process of change (Miller, Crabtree, Nutting, Stange, & Jaen, 2010). The Practice Change Model, extended to emphasize the importance of practices' internal capabilities—their core processes, adaptive reserve, and attentiveness to the local environment—is shown in Figure 3.4. The Practice Change Model continues to be used to assess other patient-centered medical home interventions in the VA, community health centers, and integrated health care systems, and to help make sense of efforts to integrate behavioral health and primary care, such as the Advancing Care Together initiative (www.advancingcaretogether.org).

Recently, a process was articulated by which facilitators can use the Practice Change Model to assess practices and to tailor practice improvement activities to fit the needs of diverse practices and environments (Ruhe et al., 2009). A multidisciplinary team found that intervention tailoring benefits from assessment of Practice Change Model domains, that is, of key stakeholders' motivations, external influences, resources and opportunities for change, and the interactions between these factors. Using this information, intervention tailoring involves seeking and working with key stakeholders, building assets, providing options, keeping change processes flexible, offering feedback, providing exposure to scientific evidence, facilitating group processes, involving new partners, brainstorming, using stories/play acting/humor, assuming a consultant role, reframing, moving meetings off-site, and stepping back or pausing (Ruhe et al., 2009). Such a model-driven approach to guiding practice assessment enables tailored responses to the unique and emerging conditions that distinguish health care practices and influence implementation of quality improvement interventions.

The Practice Change Model provides a practical way to operationalize complexity science principles for understanding and guiding a developmental process of practice change. The model is empirically based on data showing that a practice-individualized approach can result in sustainable practice change, and subsequent experience has found the model to be useful both to those attempting to understand the process of practice change and to those working to facilitate positive change. Rather than being proscriptive, the model provides domains and interactions to pay attention to, make sense of, and act on as they develop over time. Further use and development of the model in diverse practices and their co-evolving and rapidly changing health care environments will add to the robustness of its use.

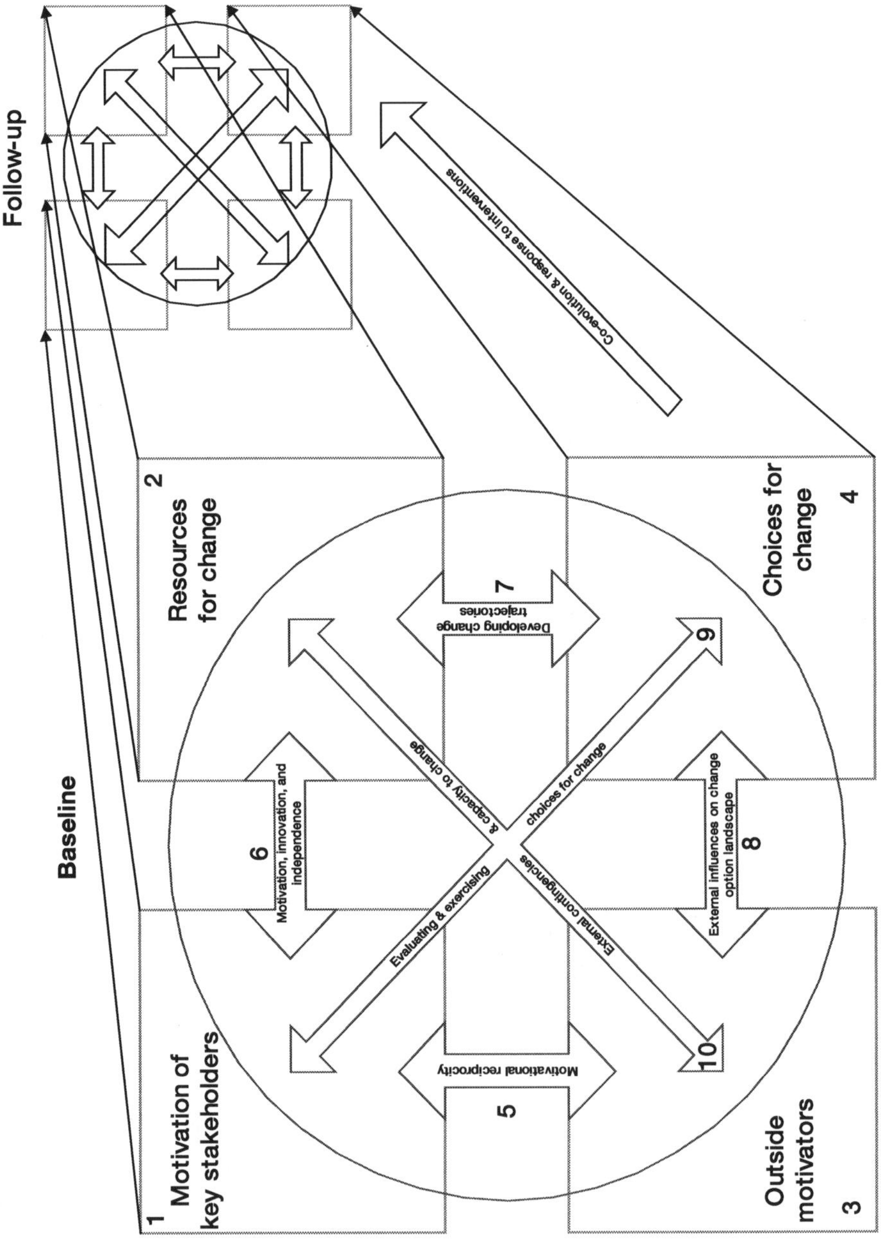

FIGURE 3.3 The Practice Change Model (Miller et al., 2010).

FIGURE 3.4 The Practice Change and Development Model (Ruhe et al., 2009).

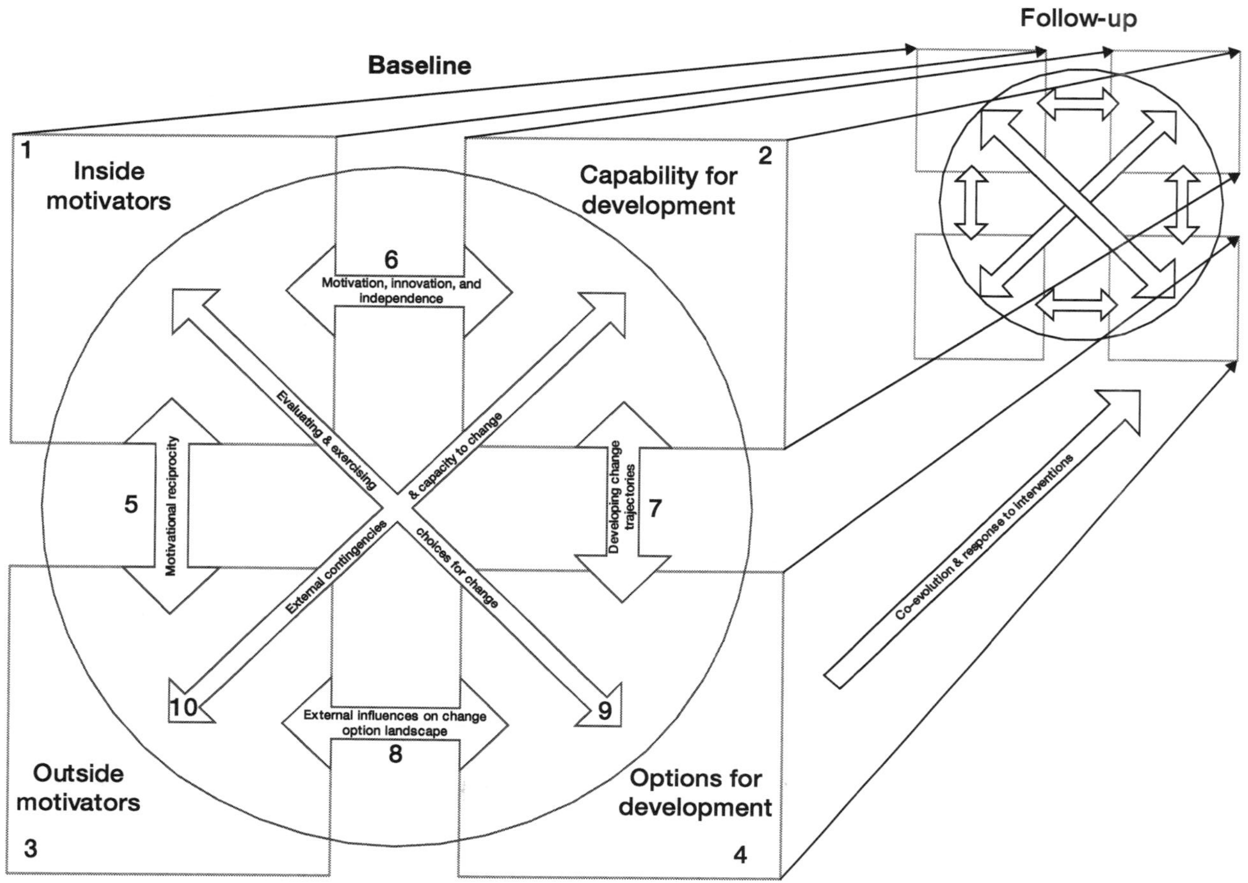

PRACTICAL, ROBUST, IMPLEMENTATION SYSTEMS MODEL (PRISM) ... AND RE-AIM

The PRISM for health system intervention planning is an adaptation of the RE-AIM (Reach, Efficacy/Effectiveness, Adoption, Implementation, and Maintenance) model. RE-AIM was developed to help address the imbalance between internal and external validity reporting in the health literature, and to provide information relevant to generalization, dissemination, and public health impact. The primary reason that practitioners give for not adopting evidence-based practices is that they do not see the research as relevant to their setting, patients, or resources (Jensen, Weersing, Hoagwood, & Goldman, 2005; Rothwell, 2005). Reporting along the RE-AIM dimensions helps to make research results more transparent and to allow potential adopters to judge the relevance of a given report to their situation. The first RE-AIM publications appeared in late 1999 and today it has become one of the most widely used evaluation models for health research grants and publications over the past 5 years, with at least 200 published studies using the framework.

CORE CONSTRUCTS

The definitions of each of the five primary RE-AIM dimensions are given in Table 3.1 and explained in more detail elsewhere (Glasgow, Nelson, Strycker, & King, 2006; Glasgow, Klesges, Dzewaltowski, Estabrooks, & Vogt, 2006). Briefly, Reach (percentage and representativeness of participants) and Effectiveness (outcomes including broad impacts on issues such as equity and quality of life and unanticipated consequences) are assessed at the individual level. Adoption (percentage and representativeness of *settings and staff* participation), Implementation (consistency and adaptations of delivery of the original protocol and costs), and Maintenance (if a program or policy is continued, adapted, or discontinued after the research or introduction period) are assessed at the setting/organizational and community levels.

Several issues that are commonly misinterpreted about RE-AIM are emphasized here:

1. Consistency (or lack of consistency) of results is important at each level. Thus, RE-AIM is concerned not only with overall mean results, but also with impacts on subgroups related to health disparities, by different implementation staff, in different settings, etc. RE-AIM requires that robustness or generalizability across these and other key dimensions be demonstrated and reported, not just assumed.

2. Cost is important in the RE-AIM model (Glasgow, Nelson, Strycker, & King, 2006; Glasgow, Klesges, Dzewaltowski, Estabrooks, & Vogt, 2006; Glasgow & Linnan, 2008). It is considered under the Implementation factor, as cost is one of the key questions decision makers have when considering practical issues such as who can implement a program, what resources it requires, etc.

3. RE-AIM is congruent with, and not opposed to, efficacy research. It simply asks that researchers report transparently (for example, using *TREND*—Transparent Reporting of Evaluations with Non-randomized Designs or *PRECIS*—Pragmatic-Explanatory Continuum Indicator Summary) on the procedures used, and detail both inclusions and exclusions made at the contextual levels of settings and staff, as well as at the patient level.

Another focus of RE-AIM has been on the multiple levels of participants (patients or end users; citizens), providers, or staff; and settings (workplaces, schools, and communities). The issues of selections, exclusions, participation rates, and representativeness at the setting and staff levels are just as important as at the individual participant level— but receive much less research attention.

TABLE 3.1 RE-AIM Guidelines for Developing, Selecting, and Evaluating Programs and Policies Intended to Have a Public Health Impact

RE-AIM ELEMENT	GUIDELINES AND QUESTIONS TO ASK
Reach Percentage and representativeness of participants	Can the program attract large and representative percentage of target population? Can the program reach those most in need and most often left out (i.e., the poor, low literacy and numeracy, complex patients)?
Effectiveness Impact on key outcomes, quality of life, unanticipated outcomes, and subgroups	Does the program produce robust effects across subpopulations? Does the program produce minimal negative side effects and increase quality of life or broader outcomes (i.e., social capital)?
Adoption Percentage and representativeness of settings and staff that participate	Is the program feasible for majority of real-world settings (costs, expertise, time, resources, etc.)? Can low-resource settings and typical staff serving high-risk populations adopt it?
Implementation Consistency and cost of delivering programs and adaptations made	Can the program be consistently implemented across program elements, different staff, time, etc.? Are the costs—personnel, up front, marginal, scale up, equipment costs—reasonable to match effectiveness?
Maintenance Long-term effects at individual and setting levels, modifications made	Does the program include principles to enhance long-term improvements (i.e., follow-up contact, community resources, peer support, ongoing feedback)? Can the settings sustain the program over time without added resources and leadership?

See www.re-aim.org or www.center-trt.org/index.cfm?fa=webtraining.reaim for more information.

PRISM

The Practical Robust Implementation and Sustainability Model (Feldstein & Glasgow, 2008) uses RE-AIM to evaluate results, but adds organizational and systems components to the model to identify key organizational issues that should be addressed in program planning. Figure 3.5 illustrates the key aspects of PRISM, which includes organizational and patient/family perspectives of the intervention and characteristics of both participants and the implementing organization. When considering the organization or health system, PRISM calls out three levels of personnel: top leadership; mid-level managers, including those leading improvement efforts; and frontline staff (clinicians and support personnel). The Feldstein and Glasgow article provides a series of key questions for health systems considering implementation of a practice, policy, or guideline, and these are reprinted in Table 3.2. PRISM has been used to design two system-wide interventions for cancer screening—one for mammography (Feldstein & Glasgow, 2008) and the other for colorectal cancer screening (Feldstein et al., 2012).

FIGURE 3.5 The Practical Robust Implementation and Sustainability Model (PRISM) (Feldstein & Glasgow, 2008).

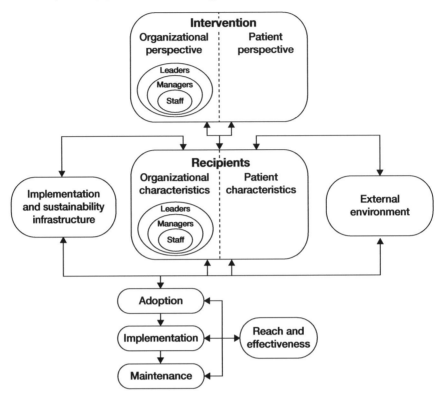

The model considers how the program or intervention design, the external environment, the implementation and sustainability infrastructure, and the recipients influence program adoption, implementation, and maintenance.

In summary, RE-AIM and PRISM have been useful in focusing attention on issues in research planning, reporting, and reviewing that have been largely neglected but are critical to external validity, translation, and stakeholders. Attention to these multi-level issues—including adoption, consistency of implementation, and sustainability—has helped to increase both the transparency and relevance of health research to those who must make decisions to adopt, implement, or fund such programs.

RE-AIM is now often used to evaluate and report on health programs. PRISM, being a decade newer, has not been used as often, but has potential to help focus attention on key organizational issues and, as Rogers addressed 20 years ago, on the fit between a given program and the organizational context into which it is being introduced (2003). Both PRISM and RE-AIM could be used more consistently in the planning phases of research. Use of tools such as the RE-AIM Self-Quiz (www.re-aim.org/resources _and_tools/self_rating_screener_and_feedback/quiz.html) to help with "evaluability assessments," as discussed by Leviton et al. (2010), could help estimate the likely success of programs and policies before millions of dollars and decades of time are invested in an endeavor that has little chance of ever being adopted, successfully implemented, or sustained in typical settings. Other opportunities include creation of more online training (such as www.centertrt.org/?p=training_webtrainings) and application to still new areas of prevention and health care.

TABLE 3.2 Key Questions and Suggestions to Enhance Implementation and Sustainability for Each PRISM Component (Feldstein & Glasgow, 2008).

PRISM COMPONENT	KEY QUESTIONS	SUGGESTIONS
Program (Intervention) from organizational perspective	• Are key staff ready to conduct intervention?	– Consider readiness of top leadership, middle management, and frontline staff before selecting intervention.
	• How much cross-departmental coordination will be necessary?	– Capitalize on need for coordination to deepen support.
	• Is the program complex and burdensome?	– Can the program be simplified while maintaining essential elements?
	• Does the clinical target area have a strong evidence base and can decision support be embedded in workflow?	– Embed tools to support evidence base in workflow whenever possible.
	• Will the program be usable and modifiable without threatening essential elements?	– Assess the usability and adaptability of the program.
	• Can staff try the program and easily stop it if needed?	– Trialability and reversibility to help convince staff to adopt new programs.
	• Will key staff be able to observe results?	– Design monitoring so results can be seen early.
Intervention from patient perspective	• Does the program address important patient barriers to response?	– Evaluate and address at least one to two important barriers with program.
	• Is the program patient-centered?	– Provide opportunities for patients to make positive steps regardless of stage of change.
	• Does the patient get the "run around" when trying to follow advice?	– Assess patient usability of program and address service issues.
	• Is the program complex and/or costly for patients?	– Simplify program and reduce patient out-of-pocket cost as much as possible.
	• Do the patients understand when they have done well?	– Integrate patient feedback into programs.

(continued)

TABLE 3.2 Key Questions and Suggestions to Enhance Implementation and Sustainability for Each PRISM Component (Feldstein & Glasgow, 2008). (continued)

PRISM COMPONENT	KEY QUESTIONS	SUGGESTIONS
Characteristics of organizational recipients	• Has the program received support of key managers? • Will financial and cultural health be barriers to success? • Does the organization have one or more clinical opinion leaders in target area? • Are systems available to support data gathering and provision of decision support? • Will staffing levels and training allow for use of existing staff? • Do staff incentives relate to target area? • Do key staff expect program to be sustainable? • How do staff at all levels perceive net benefit of program?	– Work with all levels of management to earn and communicate program support. – Assess organizational health and culture, tailor program as needed. – Engage clinical leaders from planning through implementation and maintenance stages. – Assess how and who will gather performance data. – Encourage system improvement to enhance clinical decision support whenever possible. – Use existing staff during early stages to ease implementation. – Highlight how program helps staff meet organizational expectations. – Assess factors that facilitate sustainable programs. – Encourage key managers to expect and communicate expectation of sustainability. – Assess and provide education in modifiable areas, e.g., knowledge and beliefs, and perceived risk of inaction.
Characteristics of patient recipients	• Are the prevailing characteristics and barriers of patient participants known? • Are disease burden and competing demands of target patient group understood?	– Assess target group characteristics and barriers prior to program implementation. – Assess disease burden and pattern of care to better design program.

External environment	• What are common knowledge, belief, and perceived risk patterns?	– Assess modifiable factors regarding patient perceived net benefit to address in program.
	• Have performance gaps led to patient or group payor dissatisfaction? Is this a public measure and has the competition had better performance?	– Highlight gaps in satisfaction to build support. – Use examples of improved performance elsewhere as "benchmarking" to motivate staff.
	• Have gaps in performance put the organization at legal or regulatory risk?	– Highlight these factors, as they are the most powerful in this domain.
	• Do reimbursement or coverage issues impact patient or staff behavior?	– Assess impact on staff and patients. – Work with policy and decision makers to alleviate burden or provide incentives when possible.
	• Are there community resources that can enhance program?	– Assess availability and quality of community resources and integrate when possible.
Implementation and sustainability infrastructure	• Is there an existing infrastructure that can take on key implementation tasks?	– Use existing structures as much as possible but enhance as needed to ensure completion of key tasks.
	• Should the sustainability infrastructure be the same as that used for implementation?	– Identify key tasks after start-up is over and determine who will complete them.
	• Can implementation and sustainability tasks be part of key staff job descriptions?	– Whenever possible, avoid long-term nonsustainable add-on tasks for staff—plan for sustainability.
Overall	• Can a "bridge" researcher facilitate implementation of a proven practice?	– Utilize individuals who participate in research, evaluation, and implementation.
	• Can I activate at least three or the four PRISM domains and identify at least one to two factors in each domain to capitalize upon?	– Select an intervention and implementation infrastructure that utilizes at least one important success or "leverage" factor in three to four PRISM domains.

SUMMARY AND FUTURE DIRECTIONS

A systems perspective, as employed in different ways in the CCM, the Practice Change Model, and RE-AIM (and their modifications) is essential for understanding health behavior and health systems change. These three models have been applied relatively widely, and primarily over the past decade. They have already helped direct attention to shortcomings of more traditional linear perspectives and to issues frequently neglected by much health care research. With this said, it is important to keep in mind, as George Box said, "all models (including these) are wrong; some are helpful" (1987). We hope that these models will prove helpful in both understanding and leading to the design of programs and evaluations that will advance the field and translate more consistently and rapidly into improvements in health and health care.

In contrast to the majority of models in this edition, these models focus primarily beyond the individual level, and especially at the health setting, staff, and systems level. These models imply that to produce individual change, and especially to sustain it, it is necessary to change the environment around the person. This perspective is shared with ecological theory and models such as those of Frieden (Frieden, 2010) and public health thinkers (McLeroy, Bibeau, Steckler, & Glanz, 1988). This does not mean that individual action, cognitions, emotions, and behaviors are not important, and many health system models have increasingly focused on enhanced levels of patient engagement and self-management as keys to success (Cohen et al., 2004; Crabtree et al., 2011). The models do consistently emphasize a systems approach, and predict that focusing on or assuming that only an individual (patient) can produce substantial and lasting health behavior changes in the absence of health systems and other broader ecologic levels of support is unlikely (Fisher et al., 2005; McLeroy et al., 1988).

There are limitations to all of these models, including (from a traditional perspective) the lack of direct comparisons of these models to other models or theories of health systems. In particular, studies are recommended to identify the most efficient and cost-effective ways to best implement these models (e.g., the CCM has been implemented primarily via expensive in-person intensive meetings and the Practice Change Model through trained practice consultants who may not be widely available). With the modest exception of recent RE-AIM articles (Glasgow et al., 2013), none explicitly deal with health care cost or health equity issues, which are some of the most pressing issues facing our country. Future research could use the IOM six key criteria of timeliness, equity, efficiency, effectiveness, patient-centeredness, and safety to evaluate these and other models of health systems (Glasgow, Brownson, & Kessler, 2012; Institute of Medicine, 2003; Proctor et al., 2011). None of the models described in this chapter, with the exception of complexity theory which underlies the Practice Change Model, are formal theories with postulates, falsifiable hypotheses, and related characteristics. Rather, they are frameworks or heuristic models that point to important issues to consider when designing, evaluating, or seeking to understand health systems change programs. Some key commonalities across the models are that they each imply that multiple efforts, at multiple levels, often are needed to produce health systems change. These efforts must be aligned (Stange et al., 2012) and reinforce each other, rather than compete for time and resources. All three models also point to the importance of context, and tailoring improvements to the local context. The Practice Change and RE-AIM/PRISM models both emphasize the importance of thinking broadly and assessing unanticipated consequences of actions.

CONCLUSIONS

Although the three models discussed in this chapter and their offshoots have been widely applied with reasonable success, they can each be improved. As they are applied to more and different situations and problems, we expect and hope that they will continue to evolve. For example, recent increased emphasis on the RE-AIM model of qualitative factors, adaptation of interventions, and inclusion of cost issues are seen as improvements that reflect lessons learned over time, as is the extension of the original CCM to include greater emphasis on community and contextual factors. With the advent of comparative effectiveness research (Selby, Beal, & Frank, 2012; Glasgow & Steiner, 2012), there is a need for comparison of both the models themselves to alternatives; for example, to directly test whether focusing on the multiple levels discussed in these models produces outcomes superior to those achieved with to a sole focus on individual-level behavior change. There is also a need to study and identify the most effective and efficient strategies to implement these models in different health care settings. Furthermore, there are opportunities for research on and identification of better, more practical, and more consistently used measures of these systems factors, especially clinical context (Stange & Glasgow, 2012).

These models seem especially relevant given the recent activities and initiatives in health care reform and innovation that are taking place, such as the Affordable Care Act (ACA) implementation with its Accountable Care Organizations, the Patient-Centered Medical Home projects, recent concerted attention to enhancement and "meaningful use" of electronic health records, the Patient-Centered Outcomes Research Institute (PCORI), and related focus on patient-centered prevention and disease. We hope that these activities, along with funding opportunities from the newly reissued NIH Program Announcement on Dissemination and Implementation Research (PAR 10-038), the Veteran's Health Administration Quality Enhancement Research Initiative (QUERI, and especially the eHealth QUERI—www .queri.research.va.gov), will provide opportunities for use and advancement of these models.

In closing, one particular set of opportunities for the near future concerns ways to strengthen the linkage of formal health care with public health systems and community resources. The models in this chapter should help provide suggestions and frame evaluations of efforts to accomplish this important and ambitious goal as articulated in the recent Institute of Medicine report (2012). Potentially supported by funding opportunities noted earlier, the anticipated expansion of the number of trained community health workers as part of the ACA, and the unprecedented "big data" systems never before available, progress on health care–community linkages seems more possible than ever before. By grounding innovations, quality improvement, and research in the theories discussed in this chapter, which suggest specific ways to "broaden our vision" and enhance and make transparent reporting on successes and failures at implementing change in real-world situations, we think the future is bright.

REFERENCES

Barr, V. J., Robinson, S., Marin-Link, B., Underhill, L., Dotts, A., Ravensdale, D., ... Salivaras, S. (2003). The expanded Chronic Care Model: An integration of concepts and strategies from population health promotion and the Chronic Care Model. *Hospital Quarterly, 7*, 73–82.

Bayliss, E. A., Phillips, W. R., & Guest Editors (2010). Evaluation of the American Academy of Family Physicians' Patient-centered Medical Home National Demonstration Project. *Annals of Family Medicine, 8*, S1–S92.

Bodenheimer, T., Wagner, E. H., & Grumbach, K. (2002). Improving primary care for patients with chronic illness. *Journal of the American Medical Association, 288,* 1775–1779.

Box, G. E. P., & Draper, N. R. (1987). *Empirical model-building and response surfaces* (1st ed.). New York, NY: John Wiley & Sons.

Brownson, R. C., Colditz, G. A., & Proctor, E. K. (2012). *Dissemination and implementation research in health: Translating science to practice* (1st ed.). New York, NY: Oxford University Press.

Chin, M. H., Drum, M. L., Guillen, M., Rimington, A., Levie, J. R., Kirchhoff, A. C., ... Schaefer, C. T. (2007). Improving and sustaining diabetes care in community health centers with the health disparities collaboratives. *Medical Care, 45,* 1135–1143.

Cohen, D., McDaniel, R. R., Jr., Crabtree, B. F., Ruhe, M. C., Weyer, S. M., Tallia, A., ... Stange, K. C. (2004). A practice change model for quality improvement in primary care practice. *Journal of Healthcare Management, 49,* 155–168.

Crabtree, B. F., Nutting, P. A., Miller, W. L., McDaniel, R. R., Stange, K. C., Jaen, C. R., & Stewart, E. (2011). Primary care practice transformation is hard work: Insights from a 15-year developmental program of research. *Medical Care, 49,* S28–S35.

Feldstein, A. C., & Glasgow, R. E. (2008). A practical, robust implementation and sustainability model (PRISM) for integrating research findings into practice. *Joint Commission Journal on Quality and Patient Safety, 34,* 228–243.

Feldstein, A. C., Perrin, N., Liles, E. G., Smith, D. H., Rosales, A. G., Schneider, J. L., ... Glasgow, R. E. (2012). Primary care colorectal cancer screening recommendation patterns: Associated factors and screening outcomes. *Medical Decision Making, 32*(1), 198–208.

Fisher, E. B., Brownson, C. A., O'Toole, M. L., Shetty, G., Anwuri, V. V., & Glasgow, R. E. (2005). Ecological approaches to self-management: The case of diabetes. *American Journal of Public Health, 95,* 1523–1535.

Frieden, T. R. (2010). A framework for public health action: The health impact pyramid. *American Journal of Public Health, 100,* 590–595.

Glasgow, R. E., Askew, S., Purcell, P., Levine, E., Stange, K. C., Colditz, G. A., & Bennett, G. G. (2013). Use of RE-AIM to address health inequities: Application in a low-income community health center-based weight loss and hypertension self-management program. *Translational Behavioral Medicine, 3*(2), 200–210.

Glasgow, R. E., Brownson, R. C., & Kessler, R. E. (2012). Thinking about health-related outcomes: What do we need evidence about? Submitted for publication.

Glasgow, R. E., Davis, C. L., Funnell, M. M., & Beck, A. (2003). Implementing practical interventions to support chronic illness self-management. *Joint Commission Journal on Quality and Patient Safety, 29,* 563–574.

Glasgow, R. E., Funnell, M. M., Bonomi, A. E., Davis, C., Beckham, V., & Wagner, E. H. (2002). Self-management aspects of the improving chronic illness care breakthrough series: Implementation with diabetes and heart failure teams. *Annals of Behavioral Medicine, 24,* 80–87.

Glasgow, R. E., & Goldstein, M. G. (2008). Introduction to and principles of health behavior change. In S. H. Woolf, S. Jonas, & R. S. Lawrence (Eds.), *Health promotion and disease prevention in clinical practice* (2nd ed., pp. 129–147). Philadelphia, PA: Lippincott, Williams & Wilkin.

Glasgow, R. E., Klesges, L. M., Dzewaltowski, D. A., Estabrooks, P. A., & Vogt, T. M. (2006). Evaluating the overall impact of health promotion programs: Using the RE-AIM framework to form summary measures for decision making involving complex issues. *Health Education Research, 21,* 688–694.

Glasgow, R. E., & Linnan, L. A. (2008). Evaluation of theory-based interventions. In K. Glanz, B. K. Rimer, & K. Viswanathan (Eds.), *Health behavior and health education: Theory, research, and practice* (4th ed., pp. 487–508). San Francisco, CA: Jossey-Bass.

Glasgow, R. E., Nelson, C. C., Strycker, L. A., & King, D. K. (2006). Using RE-AIM metrics to evaluate diabetes self-management support interventions. *American Journal of Preventive Medicine, 30,* 67–73.

Glasgow, R. E., Orleans, C. T., Wagner, E. H., Curry, S. J., & Solberg, L. I. (2001). Does the Chronic Care Model serve also as a template for improving prevention? *Milbank Quarterly, 79,* 579–612.

Glasgow, R. E., & Steiner, J. F. (2012). Comparative effectiveness research to accelerate translation: Recommendations for an emerging field of science. In R. C. Brownson, G. Colditz, & E. Proctor (Eds.), *Dissemination and implementation research in health: Translating science and practice* (pp. 72–93). New York, NY: Oxford University Press.

Glasgow, R. E., Vinson, C., Chambers, D., Khoury, M. J., Kaplan, R. M., & Hunter, C. (2012). National Institutes of Health approaches to dissemination and implementation science: Current and future directions. *American Journal of Public Health, 102,* 1274–1281.

Glasgow, R. E., Wagner, E., Schaefer, J., Mahoney, L., Reid, R., & Greene, S. (2005). Development and validation of the Patient Assessment of Chronic Illness Care (PACIC). *Medical Care, 43*, 436–444.

Goodwin, M. A., Zyzanski, S. J., Zronek, S., Ruhe, M., Weyer, S. M., Konrad, N., ... Stange, K. C. (2001). A clinical trial of tailored office systems for preventive service delivery: The Study to Enhance Prevention by Understanding Practice (STEP-UP). *American Journal of Preventive Medicine, 21*, 20–28.

Institute of Medicine. (2003). *Crossing the quality chasm: A new health system for the 21st century.* Washington, DC: National Academies Press.

Institute of Medicine. (2012). *Primary care and public health: Exploring integration to improve population health.* Retrieved from http://www.iom.edu/Reports/2012/Primary-Care-and-Public-Health .aspx. Accessed January 14, 2012.

Jensen, P. S., Weersing, R., Hoagwood, K. E., & Goldman, E. (2005). What is the evidence for evidence-based treatments? A hard look at our soft underbelly. *Mental Health Services Research, 7*, 53–74.

Leviton, L. C., Khan, L. K., Rog, D., Dawkins, N., & Cotton, D. (2010). Evaluability assessment to improve public health policies, programs, and practices. *Annual Review of Public Health, 31*, 213–233.

McLeroy, K. R., Bibeau, D., Steckler, A., & Glanz, K. (1988). An ecological perspective on health promotion programs. *Health Education Quarterly, 15*, 351–377.

Miller, W. I. (2001). Understanding change in primary care practice using complexity science. *Journal of Family Practice, 50*, 872–878.

Miller, W. L., Crabtree, B. F., McDaniel, R., & Stange, K. C. (1998). Understanding change in primary care practice using complexity theory. *Journal of Family Practice, 46*, 1–8.

Miller, W. L., Crabtree, B. F., Nutting, P. A., Stange, K. C., & Jaen, C. R. (2010). Primary care practice development: A relationship-centered approach. *Annals of Family Medicine, 8*(Suppl. 1), S68–S79.

Proctor, E., Silmere, H., Raghavan, R., Hovmand, P., Aarons, G., Bunger, A., ... Hensley, M. (2011). Outcomes for implementation research: Conceptual distinctions, measurement challenges, and research agenda. *Administration and Policy in Mental Health, 38*, 65–76.

Rogers, E. M. (2003). *Diffusion of innovations* (5th ed.). New York, NY: Free Press.

Rothwell, P. M. (2005). External validity of randomised controlled trials: To whom do the results of this trial apply? *Lancet, 365*, 82–93.

Ruhe, M. C., Carter, C., Litaker, D., & Stange, K. C. (2009). A systematic approach to practice assessment and quality improvement intervention tailoring. *Quality Management in Healthcare, 18*, 268–277.

Selby, J. V., Beal, A. C., & Frank, L. (2012). The Patient-Centered Outcomes Research Institute (PCORI) national priorities for research and initial research agenda. *Journal of the American Medical Association, 307*, 1583–1584.

Staff of the Washington Post. (2012). *The inside story of America's new health care law and what it means for us all.* Philadelphia, PA: Perseus Books Group.

Stange, K. C., Breslau, E. S., Dietrich, A. J., & Glasgow, R. E. (2012). State-of-the-art and future directions in multilevel interventions across the cancer control continuum. *Journal of the National Cancer Institute Monograph, 2012*, 20–31.

Stange, K. C., & Glasgow, R. E. (2012). Considering and reporting important contextual factors. In Agency for Health Care Research and Quality, *Methods brief for the AHRQ initiative in Patient-Centered Medical Home (PCMH)* (pp. 1–5). Rockville, MD: AHRQ.

Stange, K. C., Goodwin, M. A., Zyzanski, S. J., & Dietrich, A. J. (2003). Sustainability of a practice-individualized preventive service delivery intervention. *American Journal of Preventive Medicine, 25*, 296–300.

Wagner, E. H., Austin, B. T., Davis, C., Hindmarsh, M., & Schaefer, J. (2001). Improving chronic illness care: Translating evidence into action. *Health Affairs, 20*, 64–78.

Wagner, E. H., Glasgow, R. E., Davis, C., Bonomi, A. E., Provost, L., McCulloch, D., & Sixta, C. (2001). Quality improvement in chronic illness care: A collaborative approach. *Joint Commission Journal on Quality Improvement, 27*, 63–80.

Wasson, J. H., Ahles, T., Johnson, D., Kabcenell, A., Lewis, A., & Godfrey, M. M. (2006). Resource planning for patient-centered, collaborative care. *Journal of Ambulatory Care Management, 29*, 207–214.

II

Barriers to and Facilitators of Lifestyle Change and Disease Management

Many factors influence one's ability to effectively make and maintain health behavior changes and adhere to disease management strategies. It is critical to understand these factors and take them into account when designing approaches to assist individuals in making healthy lifestyle changes. The chapters in Section II delve into a wide range of barriers to and facilitators of behavior change, including psychosocial, developmental, and cultural influences, with the authors making recommendations to help researchers and clinicians integrate an understanding of these factors into their work.

In Chapter 4, "Psychosocial Predictors of Behavior Change," Williams, Haskard-Zolnierek, and DiMatteo explore such barriers to and facilitators of behavior change and disease management as qualities of the regimen itself, individual factors, demographic characteristics, and social and interpersonal factors. Regimen-related factors to be considered when designing behavior change interventions include the complexity of the regimen, clarity of instructions provided, and degree to which the behavior change affects the individual's daily routine and is compatible with his or her current lifestyle. A number of individual factors affect success in making behavior changes and adhering to disease management protocols, and should be taken into account. These include mental health, which often is not adequately assessed and can pose additional challenges to behavior change; health literacy, which has been associated with many health outcomes and nonadherence; confidence in one's ability to engage in the behavior change; coping styles; and personality or characteristic traits such as hostility, conscientiousness, and motivation. Demographic characteristics such as gender, socioeconomic status (SES), and age can be strong predictors of health behavior change, but are likely immutable. Finally, interpersonal factors such as social support play a pivotal role in making and maintaining healthy behaviors, and interventions designed to increase social support have been found to be effective in improving behavior change success. The authors recommend that health care providers focus on improving those factors that are most amenable to change and intervention, and caution awareness of the potential for nonadherence due to factors that are not changeable.

Lim, Schneider, and Janicke delve into the important influence of developmental characteristics in health behavior change in Chapter 5, "Developmental Influences on Behavior Change: Children, Adolescents, and the Elderly." These influences include an individual's functioning in four areas: physiological, physical, cognitive, and social–emotional. The authors point out that developmental changes in one area of functioning often impact other areas, and that developmental changes in these different areas often intersect and are reciprocal—an important consideration when designing behavior change interventions. Developmental transitions (e.g., starting school, initiation of adolescence, and beginning retirement) present a particular challenge, as they may add stress and affect the ability to engage in health behaviors. The developmental milestones and transitions experienced by children, adolescents, and the elderly are described, and prevention and intervention programs for health behavior change designed for each of these populations are examined with key illustrative examples presented. The authors recommend that researchers be aware of approaches used to address similar health issues across the various age groups, given that some health issues such as obesity affect individuals across the developmental spectrum. Another recommendation is to apply prevention and intervention efforts before health behaviors are solidified, and to include long-term follow-up in these populations to better assess how development affects outcomes. Finally, Lim, Schneider, and Janicke note the importance of understanding social norms and cohorts and how these impact innovations. For example, video games may be innovative ways to teach children and adolescents health behaviors, but may not be applicable to the elderly, who may benefit more from the use of technology with which they are familiar.

This section concludes with Chapter 6, "Culture, Behavior, and Health," in which Rosal, Wang, and Bodenlos describe the growing cultural diversity of the United States and pervasive disparities across health behaviors and outcomes by such characteristics as race/ethnicity, SES, and sexual orientation. They set the stage by clearly defining culture and culture-related terms for the reader, then present empirical evidence demonstrating cultural influences on a multitude of health-related behaviors, including health screening behavior, preventive behavior, illness perception, and disease management. This is followed by an excellent, in-depth discussion of the application of key theoretical frameworks to culture and health behavior that can be applied by researchers and practitioners to design culturally appropriate interventions. Finally, Rosal, Wang, and Bodenlos present methodologies that can be used to incorporate culture into research and, ultimately, health care. These include the use of qualitative methodologies to better understand individual and population-level cultural factors associated with disparities, community-based participatory research strategies to engage community members and organizations, adaptation of measurement instruments, and training cultural competency in health care providers. Recommendations include developing interventions and evaluations that are compatible with the cultural needs and traditions of diverse populations; using well-studied models for program planning, implementation, and evaluation; and developing new models for application with diverse populations. The authors conclude by emphasizing the need to understand cultural differences and their impact on health behaviors and health to ensure that programs and policies are culturally tailored and/or sensitive, and that public health and medical professionals are trained to be culturally competent to best serve an increasingly diverse population.

4

Psychosocial Predictors of Behavior Change

SUMMER L. WILLIAMS
KELLY B. HASKARD-ZOLNIEREK
M. ROBIN DIMATTEO

LEARNING OBJECTIVES

- Recognize and understand the complex regimen-related factors that affect behavior change.
- Be familiar with individual and demographic factors of the patient which may affect behavior change.
- Comprehend the various social and interpersonal factors related to behavior change.

Decades of research have investigated which psychosocial factors can help to explain how and why some individuals are able to achieve lasting changes to their health behaviors and adhere to their prescribed medical treatments. Possible predictors of an individual's success at implementing a behavior change regimen or adhering to medical advice include: (1) factors related to the regimen itself, such as complexity, burden on lifestyle, side effects, and immediacy of symptom relief; (2) factors related to the individual, such as mental health, level of health literacy, personality, coping style, self-efficacy, outcome expectancies, personal motivation, and level of cognitive impairment; (3) demographic characteristics of the individual, such as his or her gender and socio-economic status (SES); and (4) interpersonal factors, such as the availability of social support, the level of family conflict, and the patient's communication and relationship with the health care provider (see Figure 4.1). All of these predictors of behavior change success offer direction and avenues for improvement, so that health care professionals can guide and support their patients in achieving the goals of health behavior change.

MODELS PREDICTING BEHAVIOR CHANGE

Before exploring each of these four categories of predictors of behavior change, it is helpful to review models of behavior change as they relate to these predictors. One of the most extensively researched models of behavior change is the Health Belief Model

FIGURE 4.1 Predictors of behavior change and treatment adherence.

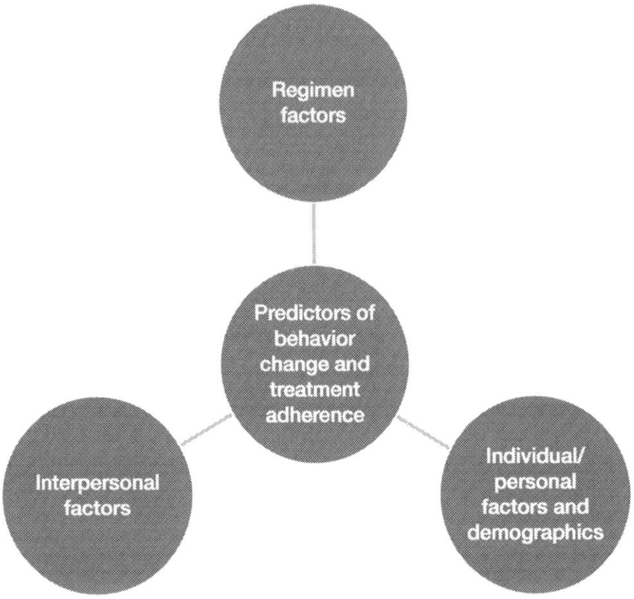

(Rosenstock, 1974). A primary goal of this model is to explain individuals' reasons for failing to take preventive measures toward overall health (such as screenings for early detection of disease) and failing to follow up on noticed symptoms and to adhere to prescribed medical regimens. The model is psychosocial in its approach to understanding an individual's motivations for change, in that it places emphasis on individuals' beliefs about severity of a condition and their susceptibility to it and attitudes toward the benefits of and barriers to change. Another widely researched model of behavior change relevant to psychosocial predictors is the Theory of Planned Behavior. In this model, an individual's intention for change as well as perceived control over that change play important roles in the success of implementation of and adherence to behavior change (Ajzen & Driver, 1991). A more integrative model, and perhaps one that best describes an individual's behavior change as a process, is the Transtheoretical Model, which emphasizes stages of individual change that occur over time, and are sometimes self-initiated, guided, and motivated, and are sometimes physician initiated or recommended. Generally, it appears that individuals moving through the five stages of change—precontemplation, contemplation, preparation, action, and maintenance—often do so in a non-linear fashion, skipping stages or repeating stages as they are progressing through change (DiClemente et al., 1991). These models are beneficial in giving a practical framework for looking at applications of behavior change in clinical practice and in overall understanding of how individuals may respond to psychosocial factors related to behavior change.

REGIMEN-RELATED FACTORS AFFECTING BEHAVIOR CHANGE

In the realm of individual behavior change and adherence to treatment, one important area of influence involves factors related to the individual's regimen. For instance, a complicated dietary regimen may be more difficult to integrate into one's life than making simple dietary changes with straightforward recipes using easy-to-find ingredients. For example, an intervention study for low-literacy patients with type 2 diabetes compared a traditional dietary change approach involving portion sizes, a food exchange system, and focus on weight loss to a simpler approach emphasizing healthy food selection and de-emphasis on weight loss (Ziemer et al., 2003). Findings revealed that the methods were both effective in changing behavior and health outcomes, and the researchers suggested that a simpler method may be more useful for a low-literacy population. An intervention currently being conducted compares (1) guiding patients with metabolic syndrome to eat a high-fiber diet with (2) guiding patients to make several dietary changes as recommended by the 2006 American Heart Association guidelines (Merriam et al., 2009, 2012). The researchers expect the findings to show that the simpler message and accompanying dietary changes of the first approach will result in better weight loss, adherence, and other health outcomes.

A prominent factor predicting an individual's success with behavior change and/or adherence to a regimen is the degree to which the change affects the individual's daily routine and habits of living. When treatment regimens require major lifestyle change and/or are complex, nonadherence can be as high as 70% (Chesney, 2000; Li et al., 2000). It may not be difficult for patients to become accustomed to taking two pills per day, but changing dietary habits or behavioral patterns (e.g., amount and type of daily exercise and poor habits such as smoking) may be more difficult for patients to maintain. Data from the Medical Outcomes Study revealed average adherence rates of 19% to exercise regimens (Kravitz et al., 1993). Those who are sedentary may struggle to make the time commitment to exercise regularly. Often the outcomes of and symptom relief for longer-term lifestyle and behavioral changes are not immediate and patients may not feel the positive effects (biologically, physically, or psychologically) for quite some time (Chesney, 2000). Patients may try to follow their regimens and may even do so in the short term; however, as in the case of regimens involving physical therapy (Sluijs, Kok, & van der Zee, 1993), or long-term lifestyle change, new habits can prove to be too difficult and/or may include negative side effects that keep patients from long-term successful adherence (Catz, Kelly, Bogart, Benotsch, & McAuliffe, 2000; Christensen, Moran, & Wiebe, 1999). Simpler medication regimens have been shown to be associated with improved adherence. For instance, a meta-analysis of studies of hypertensive patients indicated that improvements in adherence can be realized with once-daily dosing, making it easier for patients to remember their medication and integrate it into their daily routines (Iskedjian et al., 2002). Another meta-analysis of patients in treatment for *Helicobacter pylori* demonstrated that more frequent and complex dosing schedules are significantly associated with reduced medication adherence (Buring, Winner, Hatton, & Doering, 1999).

Regimen factors related to successful adherence and behavior change also revolve around the instructions patients are given when initiating a new regimen. When patients are not given clear instructions, in their native language, and with opportunity to ask questions, they may not understand the reasons, procedures, and dosing of their regimens. One study found that when prescribing new medication, physicians explained how many pills to take just 55% of the time and explained dosing frequency only 58% of the time (Tarn et al., 2006). Physicians' lack of assessment of patients' recall of new information has been associated with poorer health outcomes for diabetic patients (Schillinger et al., 2003). Likewise, with nonmedication-related lifestyle and behavior change (e.g., exercise and weight loss), patients may be given vague or broad instructions such as "lose weight," "eat better," and "exercise more." Some obese patients may not even be told by their physicians that they need to lose weight (Galuska, Will, Serdula, & Ford, 1999). One study of exercise, nutrition, and weight loss counseling revealed that physicians infrequently offered assistance with health behavior change or plans for follow-up care (Flocke, Clark, Schlessman, & Pomiecko, 2005). In one study, researchers randomly assigned HIV-positive patients to either standard care or an intervention to increase or promote adherence (i.e., included tailored information about the importance of adherence and setting realistic goals, as well as strategies for self-monitoring). Patients in the adherence-promotion intervention group showed an increase in adherence at post-intervention and follow-up, whereas the standard care group had decreased adherence (de Bruin et al., 2010). Guidelines for improving patient understanding and ultimately patient adherence must involve a regimen and behavioral lifestyle plan that is personalized and tailored to the patient's cultural background (Cooper et al., 2003).

The disease condition itself may be a factor affecting a patient's adherence and lifestyle change. Meta-analysis shows that when compared with more healthy patients, patients who are less healthy are more adherent, but only when their disease conditions are less serious. Patients whose conditions are more serious, and are in worse health, are less likely to be adherent, likely due to the nature of their illnesses (physical and psychological limitations) and their health beliefs (e.g., personal control, causes, prognosis, and consequences) (DiMatteo, Haskard, & Williams, 2007). Disease condition or seriousness of disease state may be a moderating variable in the relationship between complexity of regimen and success at adherence; it may thus be too simplistic to consider only the complexity of the regimen when determining how successful a patient may be in adhering to the regimen.

Lifestyle change regimens, as opposed to simple medication regimens, can be a challenge for many patients because such changes can affect the individual's lifestyle and established behavior patterns. For example, a systematic review of weight loss regimens indicated that those combining a reduced energy/caloric eating plan with exercise were associated with modest weight loss at 6-month follow-up compared to other types of interventions, such as advice to lose weight alone (Franz et al., 2007). It appears that a restricted diet and an exercise regimen are more difficult for patients to follow than just dietary change by itself. An additional systematic review looking at the effects of lifestyle interventions and long-term weight loss on patient lipid outcomes in obese patients recognized that weight loss alone is not the only factor that leads to beneficial lipid changes; more complex lifestyle changes are needed to sustain effective lipid-level changes (Aucott, Gray, Rothnie, Thapa, & Waweru, 2011).

INDIVIDUAL FACTORS PREDICTING BEHAVIOR CHANGE

Much of the research addressing psychosocial predictors of health behavior change focuses on the multitude of individual patient-related factors explaining success (or lack thereof) at behavior change. These individual factors can include poor mental health such as depression, low patient health literacy, personality, coping style, self-efficacy or self-confidence, self-expectancies related to health outcomes, motivation, and cognitive impairment.

MENTAL HEALTH ISSUES

Mental health problems represent one established predictor of nonadherence and difficulty with lifestyle change. A relevant issue is lack of appropriate diagnosis and recognition of mental health problems by health care providers. For instance, primary care physicians and health care professionals face many challenges to recognizing and setting treatment plans for depression in their patients (Katon, Unutzer, & Simon, 2004;

Neumeyer-Gromen, Lampert, Stark, & Kallischnigg, 2004; Schulberg, Katon, Simon, & Rush, 1999). Failure to recognize depression is a common occurrence when patients present with comorbid conditions. The primary concern of the health care professional may be the diagnosis and care of the biological aspect of the disease or illness, and the psychosocial elements associated with the disease may not be at the forefront of discussion (Badger et al., 1994; Carney & Freedland, 2003). To complicate this lack of recognition, research shows that cultural background and SES may dictate the reporting of depression by patients who are the most vulnerable (i.e., economically, socially, physically, and psychologically) (Borowsky et al., 2000; Croghan et al., 2003).

Even when recognized and diagnosed appropriately, poor mental health can be challenging to any medication regimen or behavior change plan, across many diseases. Several meta-analyses have demonstrated poorer adherence in patients with depression. One meta-analysis of 12 studies reported 3 times greater odds of nonadherence in depressed patients compared with those who were not depressed (DiMatteo, Lepper, & Croghan, 2000). Another meta-analysis of 31 studies supported these findings, reporting 1.76 times greater odds of nonadherence in medical patients with depression (Grenard et al., 2011). Patients with depression may be less likely to adhere due to cognitive difficulties (e.g., forgetting to take medication) or lack of motivation related to their health. Numerous studies across diseases provide support for the correlation between depression and nonadherence. In a meta-analysis of 95 studies, depressed patients with HIV were more likely to be nonadherent to their HIV medication regimen (Gonzalez, Batchelder, Psaros, & Safren, 2011). Two other reviews demonstrated that depression was strongly associated with nonadherence in HIV (Ammassari et al., 2002; Starace et al., 2002). A relationship between depression and poor adherence in asthma patients has also been demonstrated (Smith et al., 2006). Similar findings have been noted in patients with depression and cardiovascular disease, who are less likely to adhere to a preventive aspirin regimen, medication and health behavior change (e.g., low-fat diet and physical activity), and less likely to complete their prescribed cardiac rehabilitation or to have appropriate attendance rates (Carney, Freedland, Eisen, Rich, & Jaffe, 1995; Swardfager et al., 2011; Ziegelstein et al., 2000). The findings of a relationship between depression and poor adherence to medication or behavior change (dietary and exercise recommendations) are echoed in studies of diabetes patients as well (Ciechanowski, Katon, & Russo, 2000; Lin et al., 2004). Less clear is the connection between anxiety and nonadherence, with meta-analytic findings failing to show a significant association (DiMatteo et al., 2000; Gonzalez et al., 2004; Johnson, Heckman, Hansen, Kochman, & Sikkema, 2009). However, several more recent individual studies in cardiac patients have shown a positive, significant relationship between anxiety and nonadherence (Kuhl, Fauerbach, Bush, & Ziegelstein, 2009; McGrady, McGinnis, Badenhop, Bentle, & Rajput, 2009). The majority of research evidence seems to suggest that mental distress of varying forms reduces adherence to treatment and likelihood of successful health behavior change.

HEALTH LITERACY

Adherence and health behavior change require that patients have adequate levels of health literacy, so that they understand instructions from their physicians and follow through with those directions and recommendations (DiMatteo & DiNicola, 1982; Shumaker, Schron, & Ockene, 1998; DiMatteo, 1994; Dunbar-Jacob & Sereika, 2001). For example, in a sample of Mexican American women receiving dialysis treatment, nonadherence with phosphate restriction may have been related to participants' lack of knowledge about the consequences of elevated phosphate levels and beliefs about efficacy of the treatment (Tijerina, 2006). Some studies have demonstrated a relationship between low health literacy and nonadherence to treatment in diseases such as HIV (Kalichman, Ramachandran, & Catz, 1999) and cardiovascular disease (Gazmararian et al., 2006), although meta-analysis is needed in this area due to conflicting findings (Pignone & DeWalt, 2006). The difficulty of managing a chronic illness may be challenging for patients with low health literacy, due to the need for problem solving and active collaboration with the physician. Regarding health behaviors, findings illustrate a relationship between being sedentary and low health literacy (Wolf, Gazmararian, & Baker, 2007). There is strong evidence for a relationship between health literacy and many health outcomes; low health literacy is correlated with increased mortality (Baker, Wolf, Feinglass, & Thompson, 2008; Sudore et al., 2006b). Individuals with low health literacy use preventive services less often than those with greater health literacy (Scott, Gazmararian, Williams, & Baker, 2002), and they have more preventable hospitalizations and emergency room visits (Baker et al., 2002; Hardie, Kyanko, Busch, Losasso, & Levin, 2011). Patients with low health literacy also have worse health status and poorer clinical outcomes within a number of various chronic and severe illness categories (Dewalt, Berkman, Sheridan, Lohr, & Pignone, 2004; Schillinger, Handley, Wang, & Hammer, 2009; Schillinger et al., 2002, 2003, 2006).

Low income and education interface with health literacy issues such that low health literacy is a factor for nonadherence, poor health behavior, and poor outcomes. Studies have shown that low patient health literacy is related to poor physician–patient communication, depression, and how patients talk to their physicians (Kalichman et al., 1999; Schillinger et al., 2003). Additionally, poor health literacy can exacerbate chronic disease and lead to poor management or failure to take preventive health measures, as seen in studies with adherence to HIV regimens (Wolf et al., 2007) and glaucoma medication refill (Muir et al., 2006). The relationship between adherence and health literacy, and particularly the moderators of this relationship, are not yet clear, suggesting the importance of meta-analytic work (Fang, Machtinger, Wang, & Schillinger, 2006; Gazmararian et al., 2006; Paasch-Orlow et al., 2006).

SELF-EFFICACY

Self-efficacy may also determine an individual's ability to follow through with recommendations or make behavior change a permanent feature of his or her life. Carrying out necessary changes and maintaining those changes can be difficult, if not impossible, if individuals do not believe in their own ability to do so (e.g., resist being sedentary when tired and resist smoking when others around them are) (Catz et al., 2000; Senecal, Nouwen, & White, 2000; DiMatteo, 1994). Self-efficacy has been found to be related to adherence and lifestyle change in patients with rheumatoid arthritis (Brus, van de Laar, Taal, Rasker, & Wiegman, 1999), multiple sclerosis (Fraser, Morgante, Hadjimichael, & Vollmer, 2004), and diabetes (Kavanagh, Gooley, & Wilson, 1993). Self-efficacy has also been found to be related to adherence among patients on exercise regimens (McAuley, Courneya, Rudolph, & Lox, 1994) and those following preventive screening recommendations (Friedman, Webb, Bruce, Weinberg, & Cooper, 1995).

Humanistic theory posits that people are most likely to change in the presence of a person who accepts them as they are, which can be the key to motivating a patient to change. The patient has to feel accepted first, and then change can occur. In order to specifically target a patient's motivation for change, a humanistic patient-centered approach such as motivational interviewing can be effective (Miller & Rollnick, 2002).

INCENTIVES AND REWARDS FOR BEHAVIOR CHANGE

Another motivating factor for patients to adhere to behavior change plans is for health care providers to offer incentives or rewards for following medical recommendations. These incentives can be contingent upon a behavior contract that the patient and the health professional work on together, complete with attainable goals (Bosch-Capblanch, Abba, Prictor, & Garner, 2007; DiNicola & DiMatteo, 1984; Macharia, Leon, Rowe, Stephenson, & Haynes, 1992). Research on using financial incentives to encourage smoking cessation (Volpp et al., 2006), weight loss (Volpp & John et al., 2008), and adherence to warfarin therapy (Volpp therapy & Loewenstein et al., 2008) has demonstrated improvements in health behavior and change in response to incentives, particularly in the short term and throughout the length of the study. However, the potential for relapse once the incentives are no longer available is very real, suggesting that the change may not have been intrinsically motivated.

INDIVIDUAL HEALTH BELIEFS

Patients' health perceptions, although subjective, reflect feelings, attitudes, health beliefs about their health status, and so on, and can influence patients' participation in all aspects of their lives as well as health care, health decisions, and health behavior (Sewitch, Leffondre, & Dobkin, 2004). Patients with poor health perceptions often have negative emotional states, which can lead to decreased adherence (Olfson, Gilbert, Weissman, Blacklow, & Broadhead, 1995; Sherbourne, Hays, Ordway, DiMatteo, & Kravitz, 1992). If patients believe that nonadherence will be harmful, they are more likely to be adherent than those who believe that costs are less severe, as is reflected in the "necessity concerns framework" (Harrison, Mullen, & Green, 1992; Horne & Weinman, 1999). For example, a meta-analysis of breast cancer screening demonstrated that considering the consequences of not screening motivated greater likelihood of engaging in screening (Hay, McCaul, & Magnan, 2006). When physicians understand their patient's health perceptions, this can have a positive impact on many health outcomes, particularly adherence (Chesney, Brown, Poe, & Gary, 1983; Stewart, McWhinney, & Buck, 1979; Starfield et al., 1981).

Despite efforts by health care professionals, patients' attitudes can still often present barriers to their willingness to change and/or adhere to a behavior change regimen despite recommendations from physicians. One study examined potential impediments to asthma patients' adherence to a regimen of inhaled steroids and found that a better attitude by patients (i.e., less fear of adverse effects and stronger beliefs in benefits of the regimen) was significantly associated with better adherence (Apter et al., 2003). Meta-analytic findings demonstrate that patients' beliefs about the benefits of treatment and their certainty that barriers to adherence can be surmounted are also important in predicting motivation to adhere (Munro et al., 2007). Other research shows that transplant patients may develop a false sense of security due to improved immunosuppressive drugs; thus, they may not follow through with post-transplant recommendations because they believe that they are already getting better or that the medication will take care of it all (in particular, kidney transplant) (Rodriguez, Diaz, Colon, & Santiago-Delpin, 1991). It appears that when a behavior change regimen is primarily physician-directed, it can be harder for patients to accept and implement lifestyle change.

INDIVIDUAL COPING STYLES

Coping style also factors into how an individual will respond or adhere to medication and lifestyle change regimens. Research indicates that people with constructive problem solving styles will be more likely to adhere than those with avoidant or destructive coping styles (Johnson, Elliott, Neilands, Morin, & Chesney, 2006; Mo & Mak, 2009). How much control a patient is given in his or her treatment regimen or behavior change can also have differential effects on the patient's adherence. If a patient has a coping style that corresponds to need for control (i.e., active, internally focused coping), he or she will adhere better when behavior change treatment matches that style and allows the patient to be more in control. Conversely, patients with avoidant coping styles prefer not to have control, and may adhere better when the relationship with the health care professional follows a more active–passive model (i.e., physician dominating the decision-making process and patient is a passive recipient of care) (Christensen & Ehlers, 2002). An interesting study of hemodialysis patients revealed that when patients desired active involvement in their care, their preference was for at-home dialysis, and they generally adhered better to the dietary control and fluid-intake recommendations versus being in a more controlled setting in which dialysis is done in the hospital or outpatient setting with monitoring by health care staff (Christensen, 2000). Overall, instrumental coping and active coping are effective strategies for improving adherence because by their very nature these strategies involve seeking information, calling on others for support, and utilizing more approach-centered strategies focused on changing the problem or challenge the individual is facing. In this manner, individuals are preparing for and anticipating any problems or barriers that may occur in the process of medical care and adhering to the medical regimen (Weaver et al., 2005; Heckman, Catz, Heckman, Miller, & Kalichman, 2004).

PERSONALITY

Finally, personality and/or a person's characteristic traits may also influence adherence and behavior change. Hostile individuals generally tend to have poor adherence, whereas those who are conscientious are more likely to adhere (Christensen et al., 1999). Additionally, conscientiousness has been found to predict adherence to cholesterol-lowering medication regimens, but other Big Five personality factors such as extroversion, neuroticism, openness, and agreeableness do not (Stilley, Sereika, Muldoon, Ryan, & Dunbar-Jacob, 2004). Likewise, longitudinal studies of health and longevity point toward compelling evidence that conscientious individuals pay closer attention to their bodies, get more routine care, and take more preventive measures related to health (Friedman & Martin, 2011). Aside from medication adherence, adherence to exercise regimens seems to also be related to extroversion (Courneya, Friedenreich, Sela, Quinney, & Rhodes, 2002).

Paramount to this area is research indicating that there may be a difference in an individual's motivation for and success at behavior change dependent upon whether or not change is initiated by the individual or the health care provider. For example, there is a relationship between readiness to change diet, quit smoking, and become physically active and health professional recommendation to change those behaviors (O'Connor, Rush, Prochaska, Pronk, & Boyle, 2001). Another study found that more than two-thirds of discussions about health behavior change were initiated by physicians, and that patients were more likely to accept behavior change counseling if they were ready to change (Flocke, Kelly, & Highland, 2009).

DEMOGRAPHIC CHARACTERISTICS

In general, health behavior differs across populations of individuals, with SES serving as a particularly strong predictor of health behavior differences (Lantz et al., 1998). Distal factors related to the individual, such as poverty, can drive the more proximal factors affecting adherence, such as smoking and eating habits. Poor health behaviors and outcomes such as obesity, smoking, and sedentary lifestyles are more prevalent in lower SES populations as well as in racial and ethnic minority populations (Crespo, Smit, Andersen, Carter-Pokras, & Ainsworth, 2000; Ribisl, Winkleby, Fortmann, & Flora, 1998). Physicians may not talk as much about behavior change with patients who are of lower SES, even though these patients may want to be counseled about behavior change and may even be more likely to adhere to lifestyle change recommendations (Komaromy, Lurie, & Bindman, 1995; Taira, Safran, Seto, Rogers, & Tarlov, 1997). Likewise, ethnicity of patients may also tie into their SES, as the two constructs may be interrelated and ethnicity may be a factor affecting the type of communication a patient receives about lifestyle change or counseling (Cooper-Patrick et al., 1999; Johnson et al., 1995; Whitfield, Weidner, Clark, & Anderson, 2002). A study of racial concordance and counseling about weight loss revealed that Black overweight patients were counseled less often by White physicians than were White patients (Bleich, Simon, & Cooper, 2012). Often, lack of resources can constitute a significant impediment to behavior change despite patients' best intentions (DiMatteo & Martin, 2002). Low-income patients may not make recommended changes to their behavior and/or medication regimen because of financial concerns or challenge in fitting the change into their lifestyle (Hill-Briggs et al., 2005; Tucker et al., 2004). Patients in poverty tend to be less adherent than those who are not in poverty (Tijerina, 2006). A qualitative study of low-income women requiring follow-up after an abnormal mammogram suggested that women did not adhere for numerous economic reasons, including stress of caretaking relationships and other responsibilities, other health issues, and inability to miss work (Shelton, Goldman, Emmons, Sorensen, & Allen, 2011). Individuals who do not change or adhere due to lifestyle or socioeconomic factors may fail to take all of their medication, fail to refill prescriptions (due to limited financial resources), miss scheduled appointments with health care providers, or choose not to see their physician for matters that they deem more pressing (i.e., current daily hassles and demands). They may also feel stressed or uncomfortable during their medical visits (Martin et al., 2010). In one nationwide study, patients with serious chronic illnesses such as diabetes, hypertension, and heart disease were not refilling their prescriptions due to cost and those in the study with less than a high school education were less likely to tell their doctors of their plans to discontinue use of their medications (Piette, Heisler, & Wagner, 2004). Care by social workers may help disadvantaged patients by understanding the context of patients' illness behaviors, particularly when problems in patient adherence reflect poverty, family dynamics, and psychological stressors (Tijerina, 2006).

AGE

An individual's age can significantly influence adherence and maintenance of a behavior change regimen. Older patients generally show higher rates of adherence, perhaps because younger patients think of themselves as invulnerable to disease and/or poor health (Mo & Mak, 2009; Sherbourne et al., 1992). Younger patients may not believe in the importance of preventive or routine care if they feel healthy and are asymptomatic. Despite the higher rates of adherence in older patients, the research literature has clearly demonstrated that older patients are at increased risk for depression. Depression can put them at increased risk for nonadherence and poor behavior change outcomes (DiMatteo et al., 2000). In addition, physicians' lack of awareness of their elder patients' depression can further undermine their rapport with their patients, creating an environment void of trust and potentially leading to patient dissatisfaction and nonadherence (Hall et al., 1988; Jahng, Martin, Golin, & DiMatteo, 2005).

SOCIAL AND INTERPERSONAL FACTORS IN HEALTH BEHAVIOR CHANGE

SOCIAL SUPPORT

A patient's ability to be successful at adherence and behavior change depends heavily on his or her interpersonal relationship with important others (i.e., family, spouse, and health care professionals) and support received. Social support is typically referred to as the individual's perception or experience that he or she is loved and cared for by others, esteemed and valued, and included in a social network of mutual assistance (DiMatteo & Martin, 2002). Dimensions of support can include informational support (i.e., explaining and showing), instrumental/tangible support (i.e., money and car rides), and emotional support (i.e., advice and listening) (DiMatteo & Martin, 2002).

There are numerous studies indicating that when support is present, patients with diseases such as cancer, tuberculosis, and diabetes all experience better outcomes with their medical regimens (Classen, Koopman, Angell, & Spiegel, 1996; Barnhoorn & Adriaanse, 1992; Sherbourne et al., 1992). Meta-analysis has found that adherence to medical regimens is higher if patients have tangible support, emotional support, are married or living with someone, and have a close and cohesive family (DiMatteo, 2004). In fact, interpersonal and spousal supports appear to be vital in a patient's ability to adhere to medical recommendations. Social support leads to increased adherence, with patients who have cohesive families having 1.74 times higher adherence than those patients with family conflict (DiMatteo, 2004; Gonzalez et al., 2004; Weaver et al., 2005). Studies indicate that social support plays a vital role in patients' ability to make health-related behavior changes such as diet, physical activity, and smoking cessation. Recently poor social support has gained increased attention in diseases such as cardiovascular disease, as it is a risk factor for patients' successful health behaviors in diet and exercise regimen changes (Moyer & U.S. Preventative Services Task Force, 2012). Another recent study indicated that in cancer survivors, social support plays a vital role in patients' abilities to not only stop smoking but also maintain that health behavior, as those with perceived low social support are more likely to continue smoking (Yang et al., 2013). Studies have demonstrated the benefits of social support in maintaining an exercise program for 1 year (Litt, Kleppinger, & Judge, 2002), and a review of weight management interventions emphasizing social support demonstrated generally positive results of social support-based interventions on achievement of healthy weight (Verheijden, Bakx, van Weel, Koelen, & van Staveren, 2005). A review of social support interventions for improving self-care in diabetes patients demonstrated effectiveness of forms of support such as group health care visits and Internet peer support groups in changing lifestyle and promoting physical activity (van Dam et al., 2005).

PHYSICIAN–PATIENT COMMUNICATION

Whether or not patients willingly follow a physician's recommendations depends largely on the established rapport between the patient and the physician, and whether the patient trusts the physician. Physician communication goes a long way in the establishment of good rapport with patients, which in turn predicts how patients will adhere. When physicians are warm and invite patients to express their concerns and opinions, this encourages open communication with patients. When patients feel that their emotional needs as well their physical needs are being attended to by their physicians and that they are active participants in the decision-making process, they feel more respected in the interchange; this, in turn, makes patients more satisfied and more likely to follow recommendations (Beach et al., 2005; DiNicola & DiMatteo, 1984;

Dunbar-Jacob, Burke, & Puczynski, 1995). However, physicians may see discussion about health behavior change with patients as disappointing and/or futile (Butler, Rollnick, & Stott, 1996; Levinson, Cohen, Brady, & Duffy, 2001). A recent meta-analysis of more than 100 studies indicated that physicians' communication skill was significantly correlated with patient adherence. Findings indicated a 19% greater risk of nonadherence among patients whose physicians did not communicate well compared with those whose physicians did communicate well (Haskard-Zolnierek & DiMatteo, 2009). Physicians who are empathetic and have good bedside manners are more likely to bring about change in their patients by asking questions that are productive yet convey respect, while also remaining patient-focused, essentially helping patients in addressing barriers to change and/or any obstacles preventing them from proceeding with success (O'Connell, 2003).

CONCLUSIONS

It is evident from a plethora of research that behavior change and patient adherence are affected by a myriad of factors related to the psychosocial nature of implementing behavior change. Among these factors are the complexity, burden, and side effects of the medical regimen or the incompatibility of the behavior change plan with a patient's lifestyle; individual factors, such as poor mental health, low health literacy, personality traits, coping styles, perceived self-efficacy, motivation, and outcome expectancies of patients; demographic characteristics inherent to the patient that may be immutable, such as gender, SES, and age; and social and interpersonal factors, such as social support and socio-emotional relationships, family conflict, and trust in the health care provider. Although it may be challenging for health care professionals to consider all of these factors, the goal is to focus on those most amenable to change and intervention (see Table 4.1). While personality may present stable features resistant to change, it is clear that working on a patient's motivation and self-efficacy can clear the way for better adherence and lifestyle change outcomes. Likewise, improved recognition of poor affective states such as depression can allow a more biopsychosocial approach to the care and treatment planning of an individual. Though the links between patient health literacy and behavior change are still unclear, it may behoove health professionals to

TABLE 4.1 Provider/Clinician Strategies to Address Common Psychosocial Barriers to Health Behavior Change and Adherence

Simplify regimen or plan
Adjust change to fit individual's lifestyle
Provide clear, simple instructions
Be aware of undiagnosed, untreated mental health issues
Encourage self-efficacy
Uncover health beliefs and attitudes
Promote active, problem-focused coping
Identify resources to support low-SES individuals
Endorse the receipt of social support
Communicate openly and collaboratively

consider their patients' full understanding of regimens and prior knowledge of health and medicine, as well as health beliefs that may be inherent to the patient's culture. As more is being learned about the psychosocial factors that predict adherence and lifestyle change, research suggests the importance of making the distinction between things that can be changed and improved, and immutable factors that cannot. Efforts should be focused on influencing factors that can be improved, and the dangers of non-adherence due to factors that are not changeable should be recognized.

REFERENCES

Ajzen, I., & Driver, B. L. (1991). Prediction of leisure participation from behavioral, normative, and control beliefs: An application of the theory of planned behavior. *Leisure Sciences, 13,* 184–204.

Ammassari, A., Trotta, M. P., Murri, R., Castelli, F., Narciso, P., Noto, P., … AdICoNA Study Group. (2002). Correlates and predictors of adherence to highly active antiretroviral therapy: Overview of published literature. *Journal of Acquired Immune Deficiency Syndromes, 31*(Suppl. 3), S123–S127.

Apter, A. J., Boston, R. C., George, M., Norfleet, A. L., Tenhave, T., Coyne, J. C., … Feldman, H. I. (2003). Modifiable barriers to adherence to inhaled steroids among adults with asthma: It's not just black and white. *Journal of Allergy and Clinical Immunology, 111*(6), 1219–1226.

Aucott, L., Gray, D., Rothnie, H., Thapa, M., & Waweru, C. (2011). Effects of lifestyle interventions and long-term weight loss on lipid outcomes: A systematic review. *Obesity Reviews, 12*(5), e412–e425.

Badger, L. W., DeFruy, F. V., Hartman, J., Plant, M. A., Leeper, J., Anderson, R., … Rand, E. (1994). Patient presentation, interview, consent, and the detection of depression by primary care physicians. *Psychosomatic Medicine, 56,* 128–135.

Baker, D. W., Gazmararian, J. A., Williams, M. V., Scott, T., Parker, R. M., Green, D., … Peel, J. (2002). Functional health literacy and the risk of hospital admission among Medicare managed care enrollees. *American Journal of Public Health, 92*(8), 1278–1283.

Baker, D. W., Wolf, M. S., Feinglass, J., & Thompson, J. A. (2008). Health literacy, cognitive abilities, and mortality among elderly persons. *Journal of General Internal Medicine, 23*(6), 723–726.

Barnhoorn, F., & Adriaanse, H. (1992). In search of factors responsible for noncompliance among tuberculosis patients in Wardha District, India. *Social Science & Medicine, 34*(3), 291–306.

Beach, M. C., Sugarman, J., Johnson, R. L., Arbelaez, J. J., Duggan, P. S., & Cooper, L. A. (2005). Do patients treated with dignity report higher satisfaction, adherence, and receipt of preventive care? *Annals of Family Medicine, 3*(4), 331–338.

Bleich, S. N., Simon, A. E., & Cooper, L. A. (2012). Impact of patient-doctor race concordance on rates of weight-related counseling in visits by black and white obese individuals. *Obesity (Silver Spring), 20*(3), 562–570.

Borowsky, S. J., Rubenstein, L. V., Meredith, L. S., Camp, P., Jackson-Triche, M., & Wells, K. B. (2000). Who is at risk of nondetection of mental health problems in primary care? *Journal of General Internal Medicine, 15*(6), 381–388.

Bosch-Capblanch, X., Abba, K., Prictor, M., & Garner, P. (2007). Contracts between patients and health-care practitioners for improving patients' adherence to treatment, prevention and health promotion activities. *Cochrane Database of Systematic Reviews, 18*(2), CD004808.

Brus, H., van de Laar, M., Taal, E., Rasker, J., & Wiegman, O. (1999). Determinants of compliance with medication in patients with rheumatoid arthritis: The importance of self-efficacy expectations. *Patient Education and Counseling, 36*(1), 57–64.

Buring, S. M., Winner, L. H., Hatton, R. C., & Doering, P. L. (1999). Discontinuation rates of Helicobacter pylori treatment regimens: A meta-analysis. *Pharmacotherapy, 19*(3), 324–332.

Butler, C., Rollnick, S., & Stott, N. (1996). The practitioner, the patient and resistance to change: Recent ideas on compliance. *Canadian Medical Association Journal, 154*(9), 1357–1362.

Carney, R. M., & Freedland, K. E. (2003). Depression, mortality, and medical morbidity in patients with coronary heart disease. *Biological Psychiatry, 54*(3), 241–247.

Carney, R. M., Freedland, K. E., Eisen, S. A., Rich, M. W., & Jaffe, A. S. (1995). Major depression and medication adherence in elderly patients with coronary artery disease. *Health Psychology, 14*(1), 88–90.

Catz, S. L., Kelly, J. A., Bogart, L. M., Benotsch, E. G., & McAuliffe, T. L. (2000). Patterns, correlates, and barriers to medication adherence among persons prescribed new treatments for HIV disease. *Health Psychology, 19*(2), 124–133.

Chesney, A. P., Brown, K. A., Poe, C. W., & Gary, H. E., Jr. (1983). Physician-patient agreement on symptoms as a predictor of retention in outpatient care. *Hospital & Community Psychiatry, 34*(8), 737–739.

Chesney, M. A. (2000). Factors affecting adherence to antiretroviral therapy. *Clinical Infectious Diseases, 30*(Suppl. 2), S171–S176.

Christensen, A. J. (2000). Patient-by-treatment context interaction in chronic disease: A conceptual framework for the study of patient adherence. *Psychosomatic Medicine, 62*(3), 435–443.

Christensen, A. J., & Ehlers, S. L. (2002). Psychological factors in end-stage renal disease: An emerging context for behavioral medicine research. *Journal of Consulting and Clinical Psychology, 70*, 712–724.

Christensen, A. J., Moran, P. J., & Wiebe, J. S. (1999). Assessment of irrational health beliefs: Relation to health practices and medical regimen adherence. *Health Psychology, 18*(2), 169–176.

Ciechanowski, P. S., Katon, W. J., & Russo, J. E. (2000). Depression and diabetes: Impact of depressive symptoms on adherence, function, and costs. *Archives of Internal Medicine, 160*(21), 3278–3285.

Classen, C., Koopman, C., Angell, K., & Spiegel, D. (1996). Coping styles associated with psychological adjustment to advanced breast cancer. *Health Psychology, 15*(6), 434–437.

Cooper, L. A., Roter, D. L., Johnson, R. L., Ford, D. E., Steinwachs, D. M., & Powe, N. R. (2003). Patient-centered communication, ratings of care, and concordance of patient and physician race. *Annals of Internal Medicine, 139*(11), 907–915.

Cooper-Patrick, L., Gallo, J. J., Gonzales, J. J., Vu, H. T., Powe, N. R., Nelson, C., & Ford, D. E. (1999). Race, gender, and partnership in the patient-physician relationship. *Journal of the American Medical Association, 282*(6), 583–589.

Courneya, K. S., Friedenreich, C. M., Sela, R. A., Quinney, H. A., & Rhodes, R. E. (2002). Correlates of adherence and contamination in a randomized controlled trial of exercise in cancer survivors: An application of the theory of planned behavior and the five factor model of personality. *Annals of Behavioral Medicine, 24*(4), 257–268.

Crespo, C. J., Smit, E., Andersen, R. E., Carter-Pokras, O., & Ainsworth, B. E. (2000). Race/ethnicity, social class and their relation to physical inactivity during leisure time: Results from the Third National Health and Nutrition Examination Survey, 1988–1994. *American Journal of Preventive Medicine, 18*(1), 46–53.

Croghan, T. W., Tomlin, M., Pescosolido, B. A., Schnittker, J., Martin, J., Lubell, K., & Swindle, R. (2003). American attitudes toward and willingness to use psychiatric medications. *Journal of Nervous and Mental Disease, 191*(3), 166–174.

de Bruin, M., Hospers, H. J., van Breukelen, G. J., Kok, G., Koevoets, W. M., & Prins, J. M. (2010). Electronic monitoring-based counseling to enhance adherence among HIV-infected patients: A randomized controlled trial. *Health Psychology, 29*(4), 421–428.

Dewalt, D. A., Berkman, N. D., Sheridan, S., Lohr, K. N., & Pignone, M. P. (2004). Literacy and health outcomes: A systematic review of the literature. *Journal of General Internal Medicine, 19*(12), 1228–1239.

DiClemente, C. C., Prochaska, J. O., Fairhurst, S. K., Velicer, W. F., Velasquez, M. M., & Rossi, J. S. (1991). The process of smoking cessation: An analysis of precontemplation, contemplation, and preparation stages of change. *Journal of Consulting and Clinical Psychology, 59*(2), 295–304.

DiMatteo, M. R. (1994). Enhancing patient adherence to medical recommendations. *Journal of the American Medical Association, 271*(1), 79, 83.

DiMatteo, M. R. (2004). Social support and patient adherence to medical treatment: A meta-analysis. *Health Psychology, 23*(2), 207–218.

DiMatteo, M. R., & DiNicola, D. D. (1982). *Achieving patient compliance: The psychology of the medical practitioner's role.* Elmsford, NY: Pergamon Press.

DiMatteo, M. R., Haskard, K. B., & Williams, S. L. (2007). Health beliefs, disease severity, and patient adherence: A meta-analysis. *Medical Care, 45*(6), 521–528.

DiMatteo, M. R., Lepper, H. S., & Croghan, T. W. (2000). Depression is a risk factor for noncompliance with medical treatment: Meta-analysis of the effects of anxiety and depression on patient adherence. *Archives of Internal Medicine, 160*(14), 2101–2107.

DiMatteo, M. R., & Martin, L. R. (2002). *Health psychology.* Boston, MA: Allyn and Bacon.

DiNicola, D. D., & DiMatteo, M. R. (1984). *Practitioners, patients, and compliance with medical regimens: A social psychological perspective* (Vol. 4). Hillsdale, NJ: Erlbaum.

Dunbar-Jacob, J., Burke, L. E., & Puczynski, S. (1995). Clinical assessment and management of adherence to medical regimens. In P. M. Nicassio & T. M. Smith (Eds.), *Managing chronic illness: A biopsychosocial perspective* (pp. 313–349). Washington, DC: American Psychological Association.

Dunbar-Jacob, J., & Sereika, S. M. (2001). Conceptual and methodological problems. In L. E. Burke & I. S. Ockene (Eds.), *Compliance in healthcare and research* (pp. 93–104). Armonk, NY: Futura.

Fang, M. C., Machtinger, E. L., Wang, F., & Schillinger, D. (2006). Health literacy and anticoagulation-related outcomes among patients taking warfarin. *Journal of General Internal Medicine, 21*(8), 841–846.

Flocke, S. A., Clark, A., Schlessman, K., & Pomiecko, G. (2005). Exercise, diet, and weight loss advice in the family medicine outpatient setting. *Family Medicine, 37*(6), 415–421.

Flocke, S. A., Kelly, R., & Highland, J. (2009). Initiation of health behavior discussions during primary care outpatient visits. *Patient Education and Counseling, 75*(2), 214–219.

Franz, M. J., VanWormer, J. J., Crain, A. L., Boucher, J. L., Histon, T., Caplan, W., … Pronk, N. P. (2007). Weight-loss outcomes: A systematic review and meta-analysis of weight-loss clinical trials with a minimum 1-year follow-up. *Journal of the American Dietetic Association, 107*(10), 1755–1767.

Fraser, C., Morgante, L., Hadjimichael, O., & Vollmer, T. (2004). A prospective study of adherence to glatiramer acetate in individuals with multiple sclerosis. *Journal of Neuroscience Nursing, 36*(3), 120–129.

Friedman, H. S., & Martin, L. R. (2011). *The Longevity Project: Surprising discoveries for health and long life from the landmark eight-decade study.* New York, NY: Hudson Street Press.

Friedman, L. C., Webb, J. A., Bruce, S., Weinberg, A. D., & Cooper, H. P. (1995). Skin cancer prevention and early detection intentions and behavior. *American Journal of Preventive Medicine, 11*(1), 59–65.

Galuska, D. A., Will, J. C., Serdula, M. K., & Ford, E. S. (1999). Are health care professionals advising obese patients to lose weight? *Journal of the American Medical Association, 282*(16), 1576–1578.

Gazmararian, J. A., Kripalani, S., Miller, M. J., Echt, K. V., Ren, J., & Rask, K. (2006). Factors associated with medication refill adherence in cardiovascular-related diseases: A focus on health literacy. *Journal of General Internal Medicine, 21*(12), 1215–1221.

Gonzalez, J. S., Batchelder, A. W., Psaros, C., & Safren, S. A. (2011). Depression and HIV/AIDS treatment nonadherence: A review and meta-analysis. *Journal of Acquired Immune Deficiency Syndromes, 58*(2), 181–187.

Gonzalez, J. S., Penedo, F. J., Antoni, M. H., Duran, R. E., McPherson-Baker, S., Ironson, G., …. Fletcher, M. A. (2004). Social support, positive states of mind, and HIV treatment adherence in men and women living with HIV/AIDS. *Health Psychology, 23*(4), 413–418.

Grenard, J. L., Munjas, B. A., Adams, J. L., Suttorp, M., Maglione, M., McGlynn, E. A., & Gellad, W. F. (2011). Depression and medication adherence in the treatment of chronic diseases in the United States: A meta-analysis. *Journal of General Internal Medicine, 26*(10), 1175–1182.

Hardie, N. A., Kyanko, K., Busch, S., Losasso, A. T., & Levin, R. A. (2011). Health literacy and health care spending and utilization in a consumer-driven health plan. *Journal of Health Communication, 16*(Suppl. 3), 308–321.

Harrison, J. A., Mullen, P. D., & Green, L. W. (1992). A meta-analysis of studies of the Health Belief Model with adults. *Health Education Research, 7*(1), 107–116.

Haskard-Zolnierek, K. B., & DiMatteo, M. R. (2009). Physician communication and patient adherence to treatment: A meta-analysis. *Medical Care, 47*(8), 826–834.

Hay, J. L., McCaul, K. D., & Magnan, R. E. (2006). Does worry about breast cancer predict screening behaviors? A meta-analysis of the prospective evidence. *Preventive Medicine, 42*(6), 401–408.

Heckman, B. D., Catz, S. L., Heckman, T. G., Miller, J. G., & Kalichman, S. C. (2004). Adherence to antiretroviral therapy in rural persons living with HIV disease in the United States. *AIDS Care, 16*(2), 219–230.

Hill-Briggs, F., Gary, T. L., Bone, L. R., Hill, M. N., Levine, D. M., & Brancati, F. L. (2005). Medication adherence and diabetes control in urban African Americans with type 2 diabetes. *Health Psychology, 24*(4), 349–357.

Horne, R., & Weinman, J. (1999). Patients' beliefs about prescribed medicines and their role in adherence to treatment in chronic physical illness. *Journal of Psychosomatic Research, 47*(6), 555–567.

Iskedjian, M., Einarson, T. R., MacKeigan, L. D., Shear, N., Addis, A., Mittmann, N., & Ilersich, A. L. (2002). Relationship between daily dose frequency and adherence to antihypertensive pharmacotherapy: Evidence from a meta-analysis. *Clinical Therapeutics, 24*(2), 302–316.

Jahng, K. H., Martin, L. R., Golin, C. E., & DiMatteo, M. R. (2005). Preferences for medical collaboration: Patient-physician congruence and patient outcomes. *Patient Education and Counselling, 57*(3), 308–314.

Johnson, C. J., Heckman, T. G., Hansen, N. B., Kochman, A., & Sikkema, K. J. (2009). Adherence to antiretroviral medication in older adults living with HIV/AIDS: A comparison of alternative models. *AIDS Care, 21*(5), 541–551.

Johnson, K. W., Anderson, N. B., Bastida, E., Kramer, B. J., Williams, D., & Wong, M. (1995). Macrosocial and environmental influences on minority health. *Health Psychology, 14*(7), 601–612.

Johnson, M. O., Elliott, T. R., Neilands, T. B., Morin, S. F., & Chesney, M. A. (2006). A social problem-solving model of adherence to HIV medications. *Health Psychology, 25*(3), 355–363.

Kalichman, S. C., Ramachandran, B., & Catz, S. (1999). Adherence to combination antiretroviral therapies in HIV patients of low health literacy. *Journal of General Internal Medicine, 14*(5), 267–273.

Katon, W. J., Unutzer, J., & Simon, G. (2004). Treatment of depression in primary care: Where we are, where we can go. *Medical Care, 42*(12), 1153–1157.

Kavanagh, D. J., Gooley, S., & Wilson, P. H. (1993). Prediction of adherence and control in diabetes. *Journal of Behavioral Medicine, 16*(5), 509–522.

Komaromy, M., Lurie, N., & Bindman, A. B. (1995). California physicians' willingness to care for the poor. *Western Journal of Medicine, 162*(2), 127–132.

Kravitz, R. L., Hays, R. D., Sherbourne, C. D., DiMatteo, M. R., Rogers, W. H., Ordway, L., & Greenfield, S. (1993). Recall of recommendations and adherence to advice among patients with chronic medical conditions. *Archives of Internal Medicine, 153*(16), 1869–1878.

Kuhl, E. A., Fauerbach, J. A., Bush, D. E., & Ziegelstein, R. C. (2009). Relation of anxiety and adherence to risk-reducing recommendations following myocardial infarction. *American Journal of Cardiology, 103*(12), 1629–1634.

Lantz, P. M., House, J. S., Lepkowski, J. M., Williams, D. R., Mero, R. P., & Chen, J. (1998). Socioeconomic factors, health behaviors, and mortality: Results from a nationally representative prospective study of US adults. *Journal of the American Medical Association, 279*(21), 1703–1708.

Levinson, W., Cohen, M. S., Brady, D., & Duffy, F. D. (2001). To change or not to change: "Sounds like you have a dilemma." *Annals of Internal Medicine, 135*(5), 386–391.

Li, B. D., Brown, W. A., Ampil, F. L., Burton, G. V., Yu, H., & McDonald, J. C. (2000). Patient compliance is critical for equivalent clinical outcomes for breast cancer treated by breast-conservation therapy. *Annals of Surgery, 231*(6), 883–889.

Lin, E. H., Katon, W., Von Korff, M., Rutter, C., Simon, G. E., Oliver, M., … Young, B. (2004). Relationship of depression and diabetes self-care, medication adherence, and preventive care. *Diabetes Care, 27*(9), 2154–2160.

Litt, M. D., Kleppinger, A., & Judge, J. O. (2002). Initiation and maintenance of exercise behavior in older women: Predictors from the social learning model. *Journal of Behavioral Medicine, 25*(1), 83–97.

Macharia, W. M., Leon, G., Rowe, B. H., Stephenson, B. J., & Haynes, R. B. (1992). An overview of interventions to improve compliance with appointment keeping for medical services. *Journal of the American Medical Association, 267*(13), 1813–1817.

Martin, M. Y., Kohler, C., Kim, Y. I., Kratt, P., Schoenberger, Y. M., Litaker, M. S., … Pisu, M. (2010). Taking less than prescribed: Medication nonadherence and provider-patient relationships in lower-income, rural minority adults with hypertension. *Journal of Clinical Hypertension (Greenwich, Conn.), 12*(9), 706–713.

McAuley, E., Courneya, K. S., Rudolph, D. L., & Lox, C. L. (1994). Enhancing exercise adherence in middle-aged males and females. *Preventive Medicine, 23*(4), 498–506.

McGrady, A., McGinnis, R., Badenhop, D., Bentle, M., & Rajput, M. (2009). Effects of depression and anxiety on adherence to cardiac rehabilitation. *Journal of Cardiopulmonary Rehabilitation and Prevention, 29*(6), 358–364.

Merriam, P. A., Ma, Y., Olendzki, B. C., Schneider, K. L., Li, W., Ockene, I. S., & Pagoto, S. L. (2009). Design and methods for testing a simple dietary message to improve weight loss and dietary quality. *BMC Medical Research Methodology, 9*, 87.

Merriam, P. A., Persuitte, G., Olendzki, B. C., Schneider, K., Pagoto, S. L., Palken, J. L., & Ma, Y. (2012). Dietary intervention targeting increased fiber consumption for metabolic syndrome. *Journal of the Academy of Nutrition and Dietetics, 112*(5), 621–623.

Miller, W. R., & Rollnick, S. (2002). *Motivational interviewing: Preparing people for change* (2nd ed.). New York, NY: Guilford Press.

Mo, P. K., & Mak, W. W. (2009). Help-seeking for mental health problems among Chinese: The application and extension of the theory of planned behavior. *Social Psychiatry and Psychiatric Epidemiology, 44*(8), 675–684.

Moyer, V. A., & U.S. Preventive Services Task Force. (2012). Behavioral counseling interventions to promote a healthful diet and physical activity for cardiovascular disease prevention in adults: U.S. Preventive Services Task Force recommendation statement. *Annals of Internal Medicine, 157*(5), 367–371.

Muir, K. W., Santiago-Turla, C., Stinnett, S. S., Herndon, L. W., Allingham, R. R., Challa, P., & Lee, P. P. (2006). Health literacy and adherence to glaucoma therapy. *American Journal of Ophthalmology, 142*(2), 223–226.

Munro, S. A., Lewin, S. A., Smith, H. J., Engel, M. E., Fretheim, A., & Volmink, J. (2007). Patient adherence to tuberculosis treatment: A systematic review of qualitative research. *PLoS Medicine, 4*(7), e238.

Neumeyer-Gromen, A., Lampert, T., Stark, K., & Kallischnigg, G. (2004). Disease management programs for depression: A systematic review and meta-analysis of randomized controlled trials. *Medical Care, 42*(12), 1211–1221.

O'Connell, D. (2003). Behavior change. In M. D. Feldman & J. F. Christensen (Eds.), *Behavioral medicine in primary care* (2nd ed., pp. 135–149). New York, NY: Lange/McGraw-Hill.

O'Connor, P. J., Rush, W. A., Prochaska, J. O., Pronk, N. P., & Boyle, R. G. (2001). Professional advice and readiness to change behavioral risk factors among members of a managed care organization. *American Journal of Managed Care, 7*(2), 125–130.

Olfson, M., Gilbert, T., Weissman, M., Blacklow, R. S., & Broadhead, W. E. (1995). Recognition of emotional distress in physically healthy primary care patients who perceive poor physical health. *General Hospital Psychiatry, 17*(3), 173–180.

Piette, J. D., Heisler, M., & Wagner, T. H. (2004). Cost-related medication underuse: Do patients with chronic illnesses tell their doctors? *Archives of Internal Medicine, 164*(16), 1749–1755.

Pignone, M. P., & DeWalt, D. A. (2006). Literacy and health outcomes: Is adherence the missing link? *Journal of General Internal Medicine, 21*(8), 896–897.

Ribisl, K. M., Winkleby, M. A., Fortmann, S. P., & Flora, J. A. (1998). The interplay of socioeconomic status and ethnicity on Hispanic and white men's cardiovascular disease risk and health communication patterns. *Health Education Research, 13*(3), 407–417.

Rodriguez, A., Diaz, M., Colon, A., & Santiago-Delpin, E. A. (1991). Psychosocial profile of noncompliant transplant patients. *Transplantation Proceedings, 23*(2), 1807–1809.

Rosenstock, I. M. (1974). Historical origins of the health belief model. *Health Education Monographs, 2*, 328–335.

Schillinger, D., Grumbach, K., Piette, J., Wang, F., Osmond, D., Daher, C., … Bindman, A. B. (2002). Association of health literacy with diabetes outcomes. *Journal of the American Medical Association, 288*(4), 475–482.

Schillinger, D., Handley, M., Wang, F., & Hammer, H. (2009). Effects of self-management support on structure, process, and outcomes among vulnerable patients with diabetes: A three-arm practical clinical trial. *Diabetes Care, 32*(4), 559–566.

Schillinger, D., Machtinger, E. L., Wang, F., Palacios, J., Rodriguez, M., & Bindman, A. (2006). Language, literacy, and communication regarding medication in an anticoagulation clinic: A comparison of verbal vs. visual assessment. *Journal of Health Communication, 11*(7), 651–664.

Schillinger, D., Piette, J., Grumbach, K., Wang, F., Wilson, C., Daher, C., … Bindman, A. B. (2003). Closing the loop: Physician communication with diabetic patients who have low health literacy. *Archives of Internal Medicine, 163*(1), 83–90.

Schulberg, H. C., Katon, W. J., Simon, G. E., & Rush, A. J. (1999). Best clinical practice: Guidelines for managing major depression in primary medical care. *Journal of Clinical Psychiatry, 60*(Suppl. 7), 19–26; discussion 27–18.

Scott, T. L., Gazmararian, J. A., Williams, M. V., & Baker, D. W. (2002). Health literacy and preventive health care use among Medicare enrollees in a managed care organization. *Medical Care, 40*(5), 395–404.

Senecal, C., Nouwen, A., & White, D. (2000). Motivation and dietary self-care in adults with diabetes: Are self-efficacy and autonomous self-regulation complementary or competing constructs? *Health Psychology, 19*(5), 452–457.

Sewitch, M. J., Leffondre, K., & Dobkin, P. L. (2004). Clustering patients according to health perceptions: Relationships to psychosocial characteristics and medication nonadherence. *Journal of Psychosomatic Research, 56*(3), 323–332.

Shelton, R. C., Goldman, R. E., Emmons, K. M., Sorensen, G., & Allen, J. D. (2011). An investigation into the social context of low-income, urban Black and Latina women: Implications for adherence to recommended health behaviors. *Health Education & Behavior, 38*(5), 471–481.

Sherbourne, C. D., Hays, R. D., Ordway, L., DiMatteo, M. R., & Kravitz, R. L. (1992). Antecedents of adherence to medical recommendations: Results from the Medical Outcomes Study. *Journal of Behavioral Medicine, 15*(5), 447–468.

Shumaker, S. A., Schron, E. B., & Ockene, J. K. (1998). *The handbook of health behavior change* (2nd ed.). New York, NY: Springer.

Sluijs, E. M., Kok, G. J., & van der Zee, J. (1993). Correlates of exercise compliance in physical therapy. *Physical Therapy, 73*(11), 771–782; discussion 783–776.

Smith, A., Krishnan, J. A., Bilderback, A., Riekert, K. A., Rand, C. S., & Bartlett, S. J. (2006). Depressive symptoms and adherence to asthma therapy after hospital discharge. *Chest, 130*(4), 1034–1038.

Starace, F., Ammassari, A., Trotta, M. P., Murri, R., De Longis, P., Izzo, C., … AdICoNA Study Group, NeuroICoNA Study Group. (2002). Depression is a risk factor for suboptimal adherence to highly active antiretroviral therapy. *Journal of Acquired Immune Deficiency Syndromes, 31*(Suppl. 3), S136–S139.

Starfield, B., Wray, C., Hess, K., Gross, R., Birk, P. S., & D'Lugoff, B. C. (1981). The influence of patient-practitioner agreement on outcome of care. *American Journal of Public Health, 71*(2), 127–131.

Stewart, M. A., McWhinney, I. R., & Buck, C. W. (1979). The doctor/patient relationship and its effect upon outcome. *Journal of the Royal College of General Practitioners, 29*(199), 77–81.

Stilley, C. S., Sereika, S., Muldoon, M. F., Ryan, C. M., & Dunbar-Jacob, J. (2004). Psychological and cognitive function: Predictors of adherence with cholesterol lowering treatment. *Annals of Behavioral Medicine, 27*(2), 117–124.

Sudore, R. L., Yaffe, K., Satterfield, S., Harris, T. B., Mehta, K. M., Simonsick, E. M., … Schillinger, D. (2006). Limited literacy and mortality in the elderly: The health, aging, and body composition study. *Journal of General Internal Medicine, 21*(8), 806–812.

Swardfager, W., Herrmann, N., Marzolini, S., Saleem, M., Farber, S. B., Kiss, A., … Lanctôt, K. L. (2011). Major depressive disorder predicts completion, adherence, and outcomes in cardiac rehabilitation: A prospective cohort study of 195 patients with coronary artery disease. *Journal of Clinical Psychiatry, 72*(9), 1181–1188.

Taira, D. A., Safran, D. G., Seto, T. B., Rogers, W. H., & Tarlov, A. R. (1997). The relationship between patient income and physician discussion of health risk behaviors. *Journal of the American Medical Association, 278*(17), 1412–1417.

Tarn, D. M., Heritage, J., Paterniti, D. A., Hays, R. D., Kravitz, R. L., & Wenger, N. S. (2006). Physician communication when prescribing new medications. *Archives of Internal Medicine, 166*(17), 1855–1862.

Tijerina, M. S. (2006). Psychosocial factors influencing Mexican-American women's adherence with hemodialysis treatment. *Social Work in Health Care, 43*(1), 57–74.

Tucker, J. S., Orlando, M., Burnam, M. A., Sherbourne, C. D., Kung, F. Y., & Gifford, A. L. (2004). Psychosocial mediators of antiretroviral nonadherence in HIV-positive adults with substance use and mental health problems. *Health Psychology, 23*(4), 363–370.

van Dam, H. A., van der Horst, F. G., Knoops, L., Ryckman, R. M., Crebolder, H. F., & van den Borne, B. H. (2005). Social support in diabetes: A systematic review of controlled intervention studies. *Patient Education and Counseling, 59*(1), 1–12.

Verheijden, M. W., Bakx, J. C., van Weel, C., Koelen, M. A., & van Staveren, W. A. (2005). Role of social support in lifestyle-focused weight management interventions. *European Journal of Clinical Nutrition, 59*(Suppl. 1), S179–S186.

Volpp, K. G., Gurmankin Levy, A., Asch, D. A., Berlin, J. A., Murphy, J. J., Gomez, A., … Lerman, C. (2006). A randomized controlled trial of financial incentives for smoking cessation. *Cancer Epidemiology, Biomarkers and Prevention, 15*(1), 12–18.

Volpp, K. G., John, L. K., Troxel, A. B., Norton, L., Fassbender, J., & Loewenstein, G. (2008). Financial incentive-based approaches for weight loss: A randomized trial. *Journal of the American Medical Association, 300*(22), 2631–2637.

Volpp, K. G., Loewenstein, G., Troxel, A. B., Doshi, J., Price, M., Laskin, M., & Kimmel, S. E. (2008). A test of financial incentives to improve warfarin adherence. *BMC Health Services Research, 8*, 272.

Weaver, K. E., Llabre, M. M., Duran, R. E., Antoni, M. H., Ironson, G., Penedo, F. J., & Schneiderman, N. (2005). A stress and coping model of medication adherence and viral load in HIV-positive men and women on highly active antiretroviral therapy (HAART). *Health Psychology, 24*(4), 385–392.

Whitfield, K. E., Weidner, G., Clark, R., & Anderson, N. B. (2002). Sociodemographic diversity and behavioral medicine. *Journal of Consulting and Clinical Psychology, 70*(3), 463–481.

Wolf, M. S., Davis, T. C., Osborn, C. Y., Skripkauskas, S., Bennett, C. L., & Makoul, G. (2007). Literacy, self-efficacy, and HIV medication adherence. *Patient Education and Counseling, 65*(2), 253–260.

Wolf, M. S., Gazmararian, J. A., & Baker, D. W. (2007). Health literacy and health risk behaviors among older adults. *American Journal of Preventive Medicine, 32*(1), 19–24.

Yang, H. K., Shin, D. W., Park, J. H., Kim, S. Y., Eom, C. S., Kam, S., … Seo, H. G. (2013). The association between perceived social support and continued smoking in cancer survivors. *Japanese Journal of Clinical Oncology, 43*(1), 45–54.

Ziegelstein, R. C., Fauerbach, J. A., Stevens, S. S., Romanelli, J., Richter, D. P., & Bush, D. E. (2000). Patients with depression are less likely to follow recommendations to reduce cardiac risk during recovery from a myocardial infarction. *Archives of Internal Medicine, 160*(12), 1818–1823.

Ziemer, D. C., Berkowitz, K. J., Panayioto, R. M., El-Kebbi, I. M., Musey, V. C., Anderson, L. A., … Phillips, L. S. (2003). A simple meal plan emphasizing healthy food choices is as effective as an exchange-based meal plan for urban African Americans with type 2 diabetes. *Diabetes Care, 26*(6), 1719–1724.

5

Developmental Influences on Behavior Change: Children, Adolescents, and the Elderly

CRYSTAL S. LIM
ELIZABETH SCHNEIDER
DAVID M. JANICKE

LEARNING OBJECTIVES

- Describe important developmental issues occurring in childhood, adolescence, and old age.
- Identify aspects of health behavior change interventions that take developmental issues into consideration.
- Summarize directions for future research and clinical work focused on developmental influences to encourage health behavior change.

Facilitating health behavior change is a complex task for clinicians and researchers. A multitude of factors impact health behavior change, such as the complexity of the health behavior or condition (La Greca & Mackey, 2009) and race/ethnicity of the patient or family (Dariotis, Sifakis, Pleck, Astone, & Sonenstein, 2011; Taber et al., 2011). However, one important influence that has often been overlooked is the developmental characteristics of the targeted patient population. Development, which is often indicated by age, represents a person's functioning in a variety of domains, specifically physiological, physical, cognitive, and socio-emotional, all of which may impact health-related behavior and the course and management of disease (La Greca & Mackey, 2009). Developmental changes occur in successive, systematic, and organized ways throughout the lifespan in numerous areas (Lerner, Theokas, & Bobek, 2005). Many stage theories of development have been proposed, such as Freud's psychosexual stages (Freud, 1991), Erikson's psychosocial stages (Erikson, 1959), and more recently life-course theory (Elder, 1994). Others, such as Bronfenbrenner (1977), have emphasized ecological systems that impact development throughout the lifespan. However, developmental changes in one domain often have direct impacts on another domain and direct or indirect influences on behavior. For example, weight gain in females associated with growth spurt and sexual maturation has an impact on socio-emotional functioning, resulting in increases in body dissatisfaction (Stice & Whitenton, 2002), which is in turn associated with disordered eating practices (Bearman, Presnell, Martinez, & Stice, 2006; O'Dea & Abraham, 1999). Thus, though developmental changes are frequently viewed in their respective physical, cognitive, and socio-emotional domains, in actuality these changes intersect, are often reciprocal in nature, and are best characterized as multidimensional.

Developmental changes, milestones, and transitions are important for health behavior change researchers and clinicians to consider. The timing of developmental milestones is especially important for infants and young children, as reaching milestones at a delayed age may indicate whether early interventions are needed. For example, if a child does not walk independently by two years of age, physical therapy may be recommended to help facilitate the development of gross motor skills. As children and adults age, there is less emphasis on milestones and increased focus on transitions. Developmental transitions, such as starting school, initiation of adolescence, or beginning retirement, may create added stress and affect an individual's ability to engage in certain health behaviors, as well as effectively modify these behaviors (Drotar, 2006). Developmental milestones and transitions also may determine the focus of prevention and intervention efforts and who is the most appropriate target. For example, when working with preschool-age children, parents are often considered the targeted agent of health behavior change, as they are primarily responsible for controlling children's health behaviors. The developmental appropriateness of prevention and intervention efforts is important in facilitating successful health behavior change throughout life.

The purpose of this chapter is to review developmental influences related to health behavior change as they specifically apply to children, adolescents, and the elderly, which are all times of significant developmental changes and transitions. We will first review important developmental milestones and transitions experienced at these life stages. Second, we will examine prevention and intervention programs designed for children, adolescents, and the elderly to illustrate how development influences the facilitation of health behavior change. Last, we will discuss implications for future research, prevention, and intervention efforts related to the impact of development on health behavior change and the implementation of developmentally appropriate programs focused on modifying health behaviors.

CHILDREN

Development during infancy in physical, cognitive, and socio-emotional areas is rapid. For example, at 2 months an infant should hold its head up and begin to push up when lying on the stomach, pay attention to faces, make gurgling and cooing sounds, and begin to smile at others (CDC, 2012b). In contrast, at 1 year children may stand alone and take a few steps without help, copy gestures and use objects correctly (e.g., drinking from a cup), may say "mama" and "dada," and play games like peek-a-boo (CDC, 2012b). Other developmental milestones throughout childhood include becoming potty trained and beginning, as well as progressing through, school. Important developmental issues that arise in early childhood (0 to 5 years) and middle childhood (6–12 years) that should be considered for the relevance, design, acceptability, and effectiveness of health behavior interventions are detailed in Tables 5.1 and 5.2. One consistent characteristic throughout early and middle childhood that influences health behavior change is the role of parents.

TABLE 5.1 Developmental Influences in Early Childhood (Years 0 to 5)

DOMAIN	AREA	CONSIDERATIONS FOR HEALTH BEHAVIOR CHANGE INTERVENTIONS
Physical	Growth	Skeletal growth continues; begin to lose primary teeth
	Motor Skills	Development of gross (e.g., walking) and fine (e.g., grasping) motor skills; improvements in posture, balance, and gait; able to dress and eat independently, as well as draw and paint
	Eating/Appetite	Transition to eating solid foods and developing preference for certain foods/drinks
	Physical Activity	Increasingly more active
	Sleep	As children age, require less sleep; time spent in rapid eye movement (REM) sleep decreases
	Sensory	Touch, hearing, taste, and smell are fully developed
	Potty Training	Should be able to use the bathroom alone at the end of early childhood
Cognitive	Brain Development	Dramatic increase in brain weight; rapid cell growth in frontal lobe
	Language	Development and improvements in language skills (increased vocabulary, grammar, ability to hold conversations)
	Thought Processes	Gains in mental representations, imagination, and creativity; egocentric (cannot distinguish own views from those of others); can distinguish between real and make-believe
	Handedness	Becomes solidified in early childhood
	Academic Skills	Begins to learn counting, writing letters, and reading
Socio-Emotional	Peer Relationships	Plays and shares toys with friends during informal activities; friends change frequently during this period; begins to want to please and be like friends
	Morals	Begins to understand and agree with social rules
	Self-Awareness	Increases along with self-concept as children progress through early childhood
	Self-Esteem	Increase in self-consciousness
	Emotion Regulation	Emotional understanding and self-regulation improve; sometimes demanding and sometimes cooperative; develop shame, guilt, and empathy
	Gender	Stereotypes become more rigid

Note: This table was adapted from information from the following sources: CDC (2012); Lamb (2005); Lightfoot, Cole, and Cole (2009).

TABLE 5.2 Developmental Influences in Middle Childhood (Years 6 to 12)

DOMAIN	AREA	CONSIDERATIONS FOR HEALTH BEHAVIOR CHANGE INTERVENTIONS
Physical	Growth	Slower than in early childhood but steady with some growth spurts; body changes may indicate approaching puberty; adult teeth develop
	Motor Skills	Improvements in gross and fine motor coordination and control; girls better at fine motor skills and boys better at gross motor skills
	Eating/Appetite	Eating may fluctuate with physical activity
	Physical Activity	Difficult to balance highly active and quiet activities; vigorous activity may result in tiredness
	Sleep	Need about 10 hours of sleep per night
	Sensory	Vision fully matured
Cognitive	Thought Processes	Become more logical, flexible, and organized (concrete operational)
	Academic Skills	Continued improvements in reading and writing; become proficient at sequencing and ordering
	Memory	Increased memory capacity; increased metacognition (understanding of mental activities) and use of memory strategies
	Attention	Attention span gets increasingly longer; increased ability to focus, plan, and sustain attention
	Learning	Learn best when able to be active, able to focus more on completion of tasks
	Problem Solving	May have to talk through problems; can develop a plan to solve a problem or meet a goal
Socio-Emotional	Peer Relationships	Friends are usually the same gender, have about five best friends; nurturing and helpful with younger children and follow older children; personal qualities and trust become increasingly important
	Increased Independence	May begin to rebel to test growing knowledge and establish independence
	Morals	Rules become more flexible and intentions considered
	Self-Focused	Self-conscious and may feel small differences are noticed by others; increase in self-evaluation
	Perspective Taking	Begin understanding others' points of view
	Emotion Regulation	Fewer anger outbursts; increased ability to endure frustration though mood swings may increase; feelings may still get hurt easily
	Self-Image	Views of self are determined by appearance, possessions, and activities; value winning, being first, or leading; can describe their personality
	Role Models	Often attached to adults other than parents who they admire, engage in activities to get the attention of or to please these individuals
	Gender	Understand differences between boys and girls; increased flexibility in what boys and girls can do; boys begin to identify with masculine traits and girls with feminine traits

Note: This table was adapted from information from the following sources: CDC (2012); Lamb (2005); Lightfoot, Cole, and Cole (2009).

During infancy and childhood, parents (or caregivers) are responsible for meeting the basic physical, cognitive, social, and emotional needs of children. They also significantly influence health behaviors, such as attending well-child pediatrician visits to managing medications for a chronic illness. In addition to the role that parents play in meeting the basic needs of children, they also have important impacts on child development. In fact, according to ecological theory, the relationship between children and parents is interactional and bidirectional (Bronfenbrenner, 1977). Parenting is also considered dynamic because it varies depending on the developmental stage of the child (Lamb & Lewis, 2005). For example, in infancy the attachment between the parent and child is essential to ensure that basic needs are met, whereas in middle childhood parents are more responsible for providing guidance and emotional support. Besides the parent–child relationship, the overall functioning of the family is also important in the context of child development and behavior change. Child well-being is associated with family flexibility, effective communication, a supportive network, clear family boundaries, active coping, balancing family needs and responsibilities, and positive characteristics (Kazak, Rourke, & Navsaria, 2009). However, poor family functioning results in poorer child behavioral and health outcomes. Thus, for appropriate prevention and treatment efforts the role and influences of parents and the family are important to consider. They are likely the most appropriate target of health behavior prevention and interventions, due to children's limited cognitive abilities, independence, and control of environments that impact health behaviors and related changes.

EXAMPLES OF BEHAVIOR CHANGE INTERVENTIONS FOR CHILDREN

Important health issues in childhood include immunizations, unintentional injury and accidents, and obesity. The importance of these health issues in children will be reviewed and descriptions of interventions that address these health concerns will follow. The reviewed interventions provide examples for tailoring health behavior change interventions for children using a variety of designs.

Immunizations

From birth to 6 years of age, the Centers for Disease Control and Prevention (CDC) recommends that healthy children receive more than 28 immunizations to prevent the development of chronic diseases and even death (CDC, 2012a). Despite the recognized importance of immunizations in childhood, more than 1 in 4 children in the United States 19 to 35 months of age do not receive the recommended vaccinations (Luman, Shaw, & Stokley, 2008). Parent-identified reasons for late immunizations include a fear of side effects, having a sick child, lack of knowledge about immunization timing, and forgetting (Taylor et al., 2002; Thomas, Kohli, & King, 2004). To help increase immunization rates in young children, many prevention and intervention efforts have been utilized at a national level (George et al., 2007), which have resulted in increased immunization rates. However, underimmunization continues to be an issue for some families, especially ethnic minority families living in urban areas.

STEPPED INTERVENTION

Hambidge and colleagues (2009) developed a *Stepped Intervention* to increase immunization in infants from birth to 15 months of age in a primarily Latino and socially disadvantaged sample of families (Hambidge, Phibbs, Chandramouli, Fairclough, & Steiner, 2009). This intervention consisted of three steps, each increasingly targeted to a smaller number of families. First, all families were sent reminder postcards 10 days before each infant's well-care visit. Second, identified high-risk families received a reminder telephone call prior to the well-care visit. When infants were 10 and 21 days overdue for immunizations, additional postcards were mailed and telephone calls were placed. Step three involved extensive outreach and home visitation when immunizations were 30 days overdue. During home visits, individual family barriers related to access to medical care were assessed and addressed, as well as other nonmedical issues (e.g., transportation, insurance problems, etc.). Descriptive analyses revealed that 7% of families did not require phone calls (step one), 56% of families were contacted through postcards and telephone calls in step two, and 37% of families required at least one home visit (step 3). Results comparing families participating in the stepped intervention ($N = 408$) to those in a control group ($N = 399$) demonstrated that days infants were underimmunized were reduced 43% during the 15 months. The intervention utilized community workers and intervened with families in their community, which likely decreased the burden placed on families and increased the acceptability of the intervention for parents. The information provided about the timing of the immunizations was individualized for each family, which addressed an identified barrier and improved applicability for each family. This stepped intervention highlights the need for health behavior change interventions for young children to specifically target parents, due to the role they play in seeking out and providing access to medical care.

Unintentional Injury and Accidents

Unintentional injuries and accidents are the leading cause of death and injury in children (CDC, 2009, 2010; Jemal, Ward, Hao, & Thun, 2005). Developmental influences are important to consider when examining the patterns of injuries throughout childhood. Falls from furniture are the leading cause of injuries in infants 6 to 8 months old, whereas pedestrian injury is the leading cause of injury in children 36 to 47 months of age (Agran et al., 2003). Injury and accident prevention efforts must account for the timing of physical and motor developmental milestones and transitions (Agran et al., 2003; Morrongiello & Schwebel, 2008). Passive and active prevention efforts have been designed to reduce the rates of unintentional injury and accidents in children (Brown Kirschman, Mayes, & Perciful, 2009).

THE GREAT ESCAPE

As fires and burns are a leading cause of unintentional injury in children under 14, Morrongiello and colleagues (Morrongiello, Schwebel, Bell, Stewart, & Davis, 2012) examined the effectiveness of a fire safety computer game, *The Great Escape*, in preschoolers 3 to 6 years of age. The computer game was interactive, did not require reading, and had children help an animal character escape from various fire hazard scenarios. Throughout the game, children were provided with corrective feedback related to fire safety. Specific fire safety topics covered included lighter and basic fire knowledge, home escape plans, how to handle clothes catching fire, and how to escape a bedroom safely when fire is outside the room. Participating children ($N = 76$) were randomized to receive the fire safety computer program or a computer program about dog safety. Results from fire safety specific play and photo assessment tasks revealed that children in the fire safety group had significant increases in fire safety scores compared to the control group after the intervention. Parents of participating children also provided positive ratings about the fire safety computer program. The effectiveness of the intervention and positive feedback from parents were likely influenced by the developmental issues that were considered in the creation of *The Great Escape*. These considerations included making the animal character playful and colorful, which likely helped young children stay attentive and engaged in the program; a high level of positive feedback and encouragement that helped children feel good about their performance and improved their enjoyment; and a decreased emphasis on reading and parent supervision that likely helped preschoolers feel more independent and increased families' use of the program. This intervention demonstrates that if young children are directly targeted for behavior change, a format that is engaging, developmentally appropriate, and involves short periods of time (children played for an average of 45 minutes over a 3-week period) may be an effective way to teach preventive health behaviors to reduce the risk of unintentional injuries and accidents.

Obesity

Obesity continues to be an urgent public health issue. In infants and toddlers, the rates of obesity are almost 10% (Ogden, Carroll, Kit, & Flegal, 2012). The prevalence of overweight and obesity in children 2 to 19 years of age is almost 32%, with almost half of these children considered obese (Ogden et al., 2012). Overweight and obesity in childhood increases the risk for a variety of physical and emotional health problems (Daniels, 2006). In addition, being overweight or obese in childhood increases the risk of obesity in adulthood (Guo, Wu, Chumlea, & Roche, 2002). The high prevalence and short- and long-term negative health implications of obesity place an extensive cost burden on the U.S. health care system (Wang, Beydoun, Liang, Caballero, & Kumanyika, 2008). For these reasons, there has been an increase in the development of obesity prevention and intervention programs targeting children. Many programs developed to address weight concerns in children focus on improving healthy lifestyle habits, specifically improving dietary intake and increasing physical activity. Parents and families play an extensive role in the foods and physical activities available to children. Many prevention and intervention efforts are family-based treatments, with parent involvement associated with better child weight outcomes (Kitzmann et al., 2010). However, the level of parental and family involvement should depend on the age and developmental level of the child targeted for weight management.

Project STORY

In *Project STORY (Sensible Treatment of Obesity in Rural Youth)*, Janicke and colleagues (Janicke et al., 2008) compared the effectiveness of two weight management interventions, a behavioral family intervention and a behavioral parent-only intervention, to a waitlist control group in children 8 to 14 years of age and their parents from underserved rural counties. The behavioral family and behavioral parent-only interventions met for 12 group sessions over a 4-month period. Both children and parents were asked to work together to monitor their dietary intake through food logs and physical activity via pedometers. Changes to dietary intake were encouraged based on the Stoplight Diet, with an emphasis on decreasing high-fat/high-calorie Red foods and increasing consumption of fruits and vegetables (Green foods). Dietary and physical activity goals were individualized for each family. In the behavioral family intervention, children and parents attended simultaneous but separate groups and at the end of each session met together to develop family goals for action in between sessions. Parent group activities consisted of reviewing success and barriers since the last group and focusing on knowledge and skills training involving nutrition, physical activity, and child behavior management. The child group activities involved review of progress, engagement in physical activity, and preparation of a healthy snack. For the behavioral parent-only intervention, only parents attended group meetings. The groups were similar to the parent group in the behavioral family intervention; however, teaching parents to work with their children to set healthy lifestyle goals was emphasized.

Evaluation after treatment (month 4) revealed significant group differences in child BMI z-score, with children in the behavioral parent-only intervention demonstrating a greater decrease compared to the waitlist group. However, no group differences in child BMI z-score were found between children in the behavioral family intervention and the waitlist groups. However, 6 months after treatment completion, children in both the behavioral family and behavioral parent-only interventions exhibited significantly greater decreases in BMI z-score relative to the waitlist group. There was no group difference between BMI z-scores for the two behavioral intervention groups. There were no significant between-group changes in parent BMI or child caloric intake .

An additional strength of Project STORY was the examination of differential treatment outcomes by age. These exploratory analyses revealed that younger children (8–10 years) in the behavioral parent-only intervention exhibited decreases in BMI z-score compared to younger children in the behavioral family intervention. However, children 11 years and older in the behavioral family intervention exhibited improvement in weight status relative to their same-aged peers in the behavioral parent-only intervention. Older school-age children may benefit more from being actively engaged in a weight management intervention, due to their increased cognitive and emotional capabilities, as well as their increased independence in various settings (e.g., home, school, etc.).

ADOLESCENTS

Undoubtedly, adolescence is a period marked by rapid and significant developments in the physical, cognitive, and socio-emotional domains. As a result of these changes, perhaps more than at any other time across the lifespan, development in one domain greatly influences development in the others. Hence, first key developmental influences in each domain will be reviewed, followed by a review of behavior change interventions that have been tailored specifically for adolescents and account for intersecting developmental influences across domains.

The most significant biological development in adolescence is puberty, leading to physical growth and sexual maturation. Early adolescence (11–14 years of age) is the period in which the most rapid physical change is observed (Geithner et al., 2004; Lightfoot, Cole, & Cole, 2009), which sets the stage for the numerous cognitive and socio-emotional changes that follow. The timing of puberty has important implications, with late maturing girls and early maturing boys having the most positive outcomes overall (Graber, Seeley, Brooks-Gunn, & Lewinsohn, 2004; Mendle, Turkheimer, & Emery, 2007), such as reduction in high-risk behaviors, though individual differences exist.

Throughout adolescence, the frontal lobe continues to develop, leading to progressive improvements in memory, attention, self-regulation and inhibition, decision making, processing speed, and metacognition. Because of these rapid changes in brain development, it is believed that the adolescent is particularly vulnerable to the effects of substances such as drugs and alcohol (Lubman, Yücel, & Hall, 2007), as well as increased sensitivity to excitatory neurotransmitter messages, which is associated with heightened preferences for novelty and pleasure and intensified reactions to stress. Advances in abstract thought and scientific reasoning are also characteristic of adolescence. However, adolescents are also more self-conscious and self-focusing as a result of their ability to reflect on their own thoughts and increased perspective taking, allowing them to reflect on the thoughts of others. The increase in egocentric orientation during adolescence is likely due to the common adolescent belief that they are the focus of attention and others are not able to understand their unique thoughts and feelings.

Adolescence serves as the transitional period between childhood and adulthood, posing unique socio-emotional challenges, such as an increased desire for autonomy and identity development; gravitation toward peers and increased intimacy needs; a strong desire for social acceptability; and an egocentric orientation. Other developmental influences to consider for health behavior change interventions with adolescents are highlighted in Table 5.3.

EXAMPLES OF BEHAVIOR CHANGE INTERVENTIONS FOR ADOLESCENTS

Identifying and prioritizing intervention needs specific to adolescents and accounting for unique developmental features that contribute to designing interventions that are engaging, relevant, and effective are essential. Important health issues specific to adolescents include reducing the risks of sexually transmitted infections (STIs) and improving adherence to treatments for chronic medical conditions, such as diabetes and cancer. These health concerns will be reviewed along with interventions that provide exemplars for tailoring behavior change interventions to adolescents and use diverse formats.

Sexually Transmitted Infections (STIs)

During adolescence, increases in sexual activity are observed. A substantial number of young people are sexually active by age 14 or 15, with males tending to have first intercourse earlier than females. Approximately 25% of adolescents aged 14 to 19 years have one or more STIs, with rates for ethnic minorities being even more pronounced (CDC, 2011). Reports of low prevalence of consistent contraceptive use are implicated as one factor in STI risk (CDC, 2011). Morbidity and mortality in adolescence increase about 200% compared to childhood, as a result of unprotected sex as well as increased engagement in risky behavior, including experimentation with drugs and alcohol (Dahl, 2004). Various prevention efforts have been created to help reduce the risks of STIs in this developmental group. The following example is a brief intervention designed with developmental influences in mind.

SISTERS SAVING SISTERS
Jemmott, Jemmott, Braverman, and Fong (2005) report on a randomized-controlled trial of a small group skill-based intervention, *Sisters Saving Sisters*, targeting STI risk. The intervention is particularly relevant because it targeted sexually active Latina and African American females, populations known to be at increased risk for STIs. The authors report on a sample of 682 adolescents ranging in age from 12 to 19, with participants randomly assigned to one of three conditions: treatment group receiving the target intervention; treatment group receiving an information session on STI risk without skill-building activities; or a general health promotion control group.

The *Sisters Saving Sisters* intervention consisted of a single, 250-minute duration session conducted in a community clinic utilizing role plays, videotapes, group discussions, and a variety of exercises. Facilitators were all female and the intervention was designed to be delivered as interactive and participatory by engaging teens and relating to their life circumstances within a supportive environment. In addition to providing accurate education information on STIs, pregnancy, and prevention strategies, a core component of the intervention targeted four types of behavioral outcomes or

TABLE 5.3 Developmental Influences in Adolescence

DOMAIN	AREA	CONSIDERATIONS FOR HEALTH BEHAVIOR CHANGE INTERVENTIONS
Physical	Sexual Maturity	Increased sexual activity; limited use of contraceptives; increased risk of teen pregnancy and STIs
	Sleep	Require 8–10 hours of sleep; sleep deprivation common partially due to changes in sleep–wake cycle
	Growth Spurt	Increase in caloric needs—diet is typically energy dense (especially without nutrition education and parental monitoring); muscle mass increases more in males, while fat mass increases more in females; changes in body image and increase in body dissatisfaction
	Pubertal Timing	Gender differences, with males and females no longer being well-matched physically; females experience a significant decline in physical activity and sport participation; differences in pubertal timing associated with a range of outcomes—more positive outcomes linked to female late bloomers and male early bloomers
Cognitive	Frontal Cortex	Continued development; improvements in memory, attention, self-regulation, and inhibition; decision making, processing speed, and metacognition increase
	Neurotransmitters	Increase in sensitivity to excitatory messages which in part intensifies reactions to stress, pleasure, and novelty
	Operational Thought	Systematic and logical thinking; critical of hypocrisies; increase in abstract ideas
	Perspective Taking	Increased ability to consider others' perspectives, which leads to a new form of egocentrism focused on others' thoughts that increases self-scrutiny
Socio-Emotional	Parent–Adolescent Relationships	Increased desire for autonomy, with negotiation common between parents and adolescents; psychological and physical distancing from parent is common; parent–adolescent conflict increases in frequency and intensity but is usually over trivial matters
	Morality	Shift from "good-child" morality to "law-and-order" morality; greater focus on the individual in relation to the social group
	Identity Development	Struggles to form a unified sense of identity are common; focus on identity exploration and commitment; issues with the concept of multiple identities that may be contradictory; development of ethnic and sexual identity continues
	Peer Influence	Peers become a major focal point—adolescents spend more time than ever with peers; peer activities are more likely to be unsupervised; peer groups increase in number while close relationships (such as with romantic partners) increase in intensity; preference for peers who are similar physically
	Emotional Disturbance	Mood fluctuations, emotional intensity, and sensation seeking are common (which are associated with hormonal changes); socio-emotional problems increase, with internalizing problems more common in females and externalizing problems more common in males; rates of suicide attempts also increase
	Increased Risk Taking	Experimentation with substances increases, though only a minority transition to substance abuse; unintentional injuries, including motor vehicle accidents, are a leading cause of mortality, with alcohol a major contributing factor

Note: This table was adapted from information from the following sources: Berk (2010); Lightfoot, Cole, and Cole (2009).

outcome expectancies. For example, the intervention challenged the "Partner Reaction Belief," characterized as the belief that a partner would not approve of contraceptive use or react negatively to the proposition of their use. Negotiation, problem solving, and condom-use skills, as well as a focus on building self-efficacy in negotiating the use of protection, were also a focus of the intervention. At 12-month follow-up, participants in the intervention group reported significantly fewer days of unprotected sex during the previous 3 months, as well as significantly fewer sexual partners. In addition, adolescents were less likely to test positive for STIs.

This intervention is commendable for considering an array of developmental influences. First, it targeted an issue of significance with an at-risk, vulnerable population, with the recognition that STIs and pregnancy risk increase dramatically during adolescence and is especially pronounced for ethnic minorities. Second, it accounted for gender differences by targeting only females, as well as incorporating the use of female-only facilitators. In terms of socio-emotional considerations, the intervention strove to maintain a caring and supportive environment while also challenging participants to think more systematically and logically about the consequences of unprotected sexual activity by providing them with knowledge, basic education, and practical skills needed to navigate challenging situations. Moreover, this was done in an engaging, interactive, community-based clinic and in one session, which may be more convenient and efficient than recurring sessions in a different setting.

Adherence to Chronic Medical Conditions

Estimates of adherence rates to the management of pediatric chronic medical conditions (e.g., medication, treatment, etc.) are between 50% to 55% (Rapoff, 2010). However, adolescents with chronic medical conditions have lower rates of adherence to disease management compared to younger children (Rapoff, 2010), which may be due to adolescents having increased responsibility for their disease regimen, more desire to be accepted and fit in with peers, and biological changes associated with development (La Greca & Mackey, 2009). Diabetes is one pediatric chronic medical condition in which adherence interventions have been developed with adolescents in mind.

BEHAVIORAL FAMILY SYSTEMS THERAPY FOR DIABETES (BFST-D)

Wysocki et al. (2006) integrated diabetes-specific behavioral components into a Behavioral Family Systems Therapy (BFST) framework, resulting in the BFST for Diabetes (BFST-D) treatment for adolescents with type 1 diabetes mellitus (T1DM) or type 2 diabetes mellitus (T2DM) managed with insulin. The intervention targeted communication and problem solving at the family level in a sample of adolescents ($N = 104$) ranging in age from 11 to 16 years with poor diabetic control. Families were randomized to either a standard care condition, an educational support group, or 12 sessions of BFST-D treatment over 6 months.

Core components of the BFST-D included problem solving, communication, cognitive restructuring, and functional-structural family therapy. Moreover, each family targeted specific barriers to diabetes management; engaged in behavioral contracting; and received education on using blood glucose values to guide insulin, diet, and exercise. The intervention had parents simulate living with diabetes for one week, which included multiple daily injections, blood glucose checks, monitoring of carbohydrate intake, and a mock hypoglycemic event. Families were also given the option of extending the intervention to other social networks (through involvement of siblings, teachers, and/or peers) by conducting sessions in alternate locations.

Study results demonstrated significant improvements in adherence in regard to important facets of diabetes management—specifically, blood glucose testing, insulin administration, management of hypoglycemia, and diet and exercise regimens—in the active intervention compared to standard care or the educational support group, as well as lower levels of family conflict and reduced HbA1C levels. Moreover at 6-, 12-, and 18-month follow-up, relative to the standard care and educational support conditions, the BFST-D led to improvements in communication between adolescents and mothers, family interaction quality, and family communication and problem solving (Wysocki et al., 2008).

The BFST-D intervention accounted for both cognitive and socio-developmental influences in adolescence, with the implicit understanding that cognitive development in this period is uneven, and socio-emotional needs of adolescents call for increased autonomy within a supportive context. Even though many adolescents, particularly those in middle adolescence (15–17 years of age), are capable of systematic problem solving and perspective taking, these skills have to be fostered and developed, particularly in their generalization to a chronic condition like diabetes. The BFST-D intervention accomplished this through implementation of core components addressing problem solving and communication, and even tailored the intervention to specific barriers identified by both the adolescent and the family. It also addressed the rising parent–child conflict seen in adolescence through the use of family therapy. The intervention accommodated the widening and multiple systems of the adolescent, as influences of peer groups and school become ever increasingly important in adolescence, by providing the opportunity to extend the intervention across settings. Lastly, the integration of a simulated "diabetic week" for parents emphasized addressing the egocentric thought characteristic of adolescents, and the common adolescent sentiment that parents cannot possibly understand the adolescent's unique situation. Overall, BFST-D stands as an example of an intervention that targets physical health through behavioral changes, while accounting for important cognitive and socio-emotional influences that impact adolescents.

THE ELDERLY

In the United States, the average life expectancy in 2009 was 78.5 years, with women living 4 to 5 years longer than men (National Center for Health Statistics, 2012). The number of elderly in our nation has risen dramatically. This population requires a tailored approach to behavior change: one that considers the physical and cognitive declines that are observed, but also takes a lifespan approach to development.

Though individual differences exist, late adulthood is characterized by physical decline across all sensory systems. In terms of eyesight, dark adaptation becomes more difficult, depth perception less reliable, and visual acuity worsens (Fozard, 2001). The declines in sensory systems are thought to not only be associated with decreases in quality of life and decreased participation in leisure activities, but also pose safety risks (such as reducing the likelihood of smelling fumes from a fire). Yet, most Americans aged 65 to 75 are capable of living independent lives. After age 75, approximately 9% of the population struggles with carrying out basic self-care tasks, with that number increasing to approximately 17% for instrumental activities of daily living, such as paying bills (Berk, 2010). These numbers rise sharply as individuals progress through late adulthood.

Other physical changes of late adulthood include decreases in cardiovascular functioning (with vital lung capacity cut in half, and reduced blood flow); immune functioning (with increased susceptibility to infectious and autoimmune diseases); and a decreased need for sleep, associated with an earlier bedtime and rising time, but also more general sleep difficulties (such as insomnia and sleep apnea; Berk, 2010). Rates of illness, injuries, and disabilities also increase during late adulthood, with rates of arthritis, cancer, type 2 diabetes, and heart disease being significantly concerning. Exercise and proper nutrition act as protective factors against physical decline, but the degree of protection offered is typically greater for continued, stable exercise regimens and nutritious diets. Memory impairments and a decline in cognitive functioning are also associated with increased age (Hoyer & Verhaeghen, 2006), as are difficulties in language processing. Though memory and language impairments are observed in late adulthood, engagement in mental activities (e.g., continued education), leisure activities, and social participation are associated with a reduction in such declines.

Though many of the changes of late adulthood are framed as impairments or deficiencies, the elderly can also be a source of wisdom, reflecting their high degree of practical knowledge through years of life experience, confronting adversity, and altruistic tendencies (Berk, 2010; Brugman, 2006). Despite physical and cognitive decline, elders tend to focus on the present, and this temporal orientation is accompanied by an increase in optimism, tempered by an overall decrease in satisfaction (which may be associated with realism about death; Lennings, 2000). Despite these strengths, research has shown that the stereotype of the elderly as warm but incompetent is quite pervasive and leads to them being viewed with pity and admiration (Cuddy & Fiske, 2002). As a result of this warm–incompetent perspective, elders tend to be exposed to both helping and exclusionary behaviors from others (Cuddy, Norton, & Fiske, 2005). Table 5.4 reviews important developmental issues for the elderly that should be considered when designing health behavior interventions.

EXAMPLES OF BEHAVIORAL CHANGE INTERVENTIONS FOR THE ELDERLY

Prevention and intervention programs that empower elders, respect their years of accumulated experience, and understand their need for control within a supportive context are likely to be the most acceptable and beneficial. Important health issues faced by the elderly include non-adherence to medication regimens, unintentional injuries, and obesity. The following descriptions of interventions integrate novel components to account for the developmental issues that affect health behavior change in the elderly.

Non-Adherence to Medications

The elderly are the largest consumers of both prescription and non-prescription medication (Murdaugh, 1998). They are at risk for non-adherence to pharmacological regimens because of a variety of both drug- and patient-specific factors, as well as an associated increase in morbidity (Gellad, Grenard, & Marcum, 2011). Because of the problematic nature of non-adherence in the elderly, interventions have and continue to be developed to address potential barriers to adherence.

AUTOMATED REMINDING AND TAILORED COMPUTER-BASED INTERVENTION
Studies providing automated reminders to take medications, as well as studies using patient-specific tailored medication information delivered via computers, have demonstrated improvements in medication adherence (Cutrona et al., 2010; Haynes, Ackloo, Sahota, McDonald, & Yao, 2008; Piette, Weinberger, & McPhee, 2000). However, the majority of studies have utilized several strategies for increasing adherence in combination,

TABLE 5.4 Developmental Influences in the Elderly

DOMAIN	AREA	CONSIDERATIONS FOR HEALTH BEHAVIOR CHANGE INTERVENTIONS
Physical	Life Expectancy	Gains in life expectancy in industrialized countries, with elderly being the fastest growing segment of the U.S. population; women tend to live longer than men; life expectancy varies with SES, ethnicity, and nationality
	Activities of Daily Living	After age 75, increased difficulties carrying out activities of daily living, but even more prominent difficulties carrying out instrumental activities of daily living (such as paying bills); with age prevalence of these difficulties rises
	Nervous System	Loss of brain weight and neurons accelerates after age 60; autonomic nervous system becomes less efficient
	Sensory Systems	Decline in all five sensory systems, associated with functional impairments, increased hazard risk (such as falls), and decreases in social or leisure activities; examples: dark adaptation more difficult; reduced depth perception and visual acuity; hearing impairments at high frequency and loss of speech perception, affect more men than women; reduced sensitivity to all four basic tastes; olfactory and touch receptors decrease, resulting in declines in odor and touch sensitivity
	Cardiovascular System	Heartbeat less forceful, results in slower heart rate and decreased blood flow; vital lung capacity cut by half—less oxygen to tissues
	Immune System	Effectiveness of immune system declines; more infections and autoimmune diseases and stress-related susceptibility
	Sleep	Need less sleep, earlier bedtime and rise time, but sleep difficulties more common
	Appearance and Mobility	Skin thinner, wrinkled, and spotted; ears, nose, teeth, and hair change; lose height and weight after age 60; muscle strength and bone strength decline; less flexibility
	Nutrition and Exercise	Increased need for nutrients to protect bones and support immune functioning; barriers to nutrition increase; importance of continued exercise—benefits include improved physical capacities, brain function, and self-esteem
	Illness and Injury	Increase in medical conditions; accidents and unintentional injury rates increase (associated with sensory and cognitive declines)
	Long-Term Care	More needs with advanced age, severe disorders, and loss of support network, but vary by SES and ethnic group

(continued)

100

TABLE 5.4 Developmental Influences in the Elderly (continued)

DOMAIN	AREA	CONSIDERATIONS FOR HEALTH BEHAVIOR CHANGE INTERVENTIONS
Cognitive	Memory	Memory impairments surface, making recall more difficult; implicit memory better than deliberate memory; dementia more common with increased age
	Language Processing	Comprehension changes little, but have problems retrieving specific words and planning what to say; common compensatory techniques include use of simpler grammar, more sentences, and providing a "gist"
	Problem Solving	Tend to focus on family relations and management of daily activities; tend to extend use of strategies from middle adulthood; often consult with others and try to avoid interpersonal conflicts
	Wisdom	Depth and breadth of practical knowledge and application of knowledge to improving life developed by some elders
	Cognitive Declines	Mentally active life predictive of better cognitive functioning; health, retirement, and distance to death also have associations
Socio-Emotional	Identity	Response to sense of mortality important, including whether individuals view their lives as whole or satisfactory (leading to ego integrity) or lacking resolution (leading to despair)
	Affect and Resilience	Maximize positive and dampen negative emotions, contributes to resilience; most older adults sustain a sense of optimism and good psychological well-being; emotional perceptiveness associated with increased use of emotion-centered coping strategies
	Personality	Secure, multi-faceted self-concept; shifts in some characteristics: more agreeable, less sociable, greater acceptance of change
	Spirituality and Religion	Some may become more religious or spiritual with age, while others become less religious; more than half attend weekly services; increased spirituality associated with physical and psychological benefits and promotes social engagement
	Control/Dependency	Social context important for whether assistance supports or undermines well-being; excessive dependency should be avoided
	Psychological Health	Physical illness, including disability, is a strong risk factor of depression and suicide
	Social Support	Number of social partners decreases; choose friends similar to self; friendships are important in providing companionship, helping to cope with loss, and as link to community
	Widowhood	Most stressful event for many: experienced by 1/3 of elderly—significantly more women than men; few remarry and most live alone

Note: This table was adapted from information from the following sources: Berk (2010); Fozard and Gordon-Salant (2001); Lightfoot, Cole, and Cole (2009).

making it difficult to tease apart the individual efficacy of such strategies. To fill this gap in the literature, Ownby, Hertzog, and Czaja (2012) compared the efficacy of automated reminders versus tailored information delivery in a small sample of elders (N = 27 and mean age = 79.9 years) recruited from a memory disorder clinic. Participants were randomized to either the automated reminding, tailored information, or control conditions. Automated reminding participants received automated daily phone calls, which played a pre-recorded message reminding them to take their medication. The tailored information condition provided participants with information about their specific medications and required them to complete a survey to assess what information they would like to receive about memory disorders, as well as their language preference, health literacy, and desire for additional health information. The information from the survey was entered into a computer program that provided a personalized medication and treatment information handout tailored to their responses. Medication adherence was evaluated with the use of an electronic pill bottle, and the impact of having a caregiver involved was also examined.

Results revealed significant benefits from both interventions compared to the control group, and the presence of a caregiver was associated with higher levels of adherence. Additionally, though general cognitive status was not a significant predictor of adherence, verbal memory was. Overall, these results highlight the potential benefit of automated or computer-based interventions as a low-cost route for adherence intervention. The fact that caregivers were significantly associated with improved adherence may also highlight the important role of support for daily living activities for the elderly, and potentially, the role of social support in general. Despite the small sample of this study, both interventions present potential benefits unique to this population. For instance, the automated reminders offer a practical, low-cost intervention providing daily reminders to elders, which may be important considering their declining cognitive functioning (including memory impairments). The tailored intervention inherently demonstrated a respect for the elders' perspective on what is important to them and potentially empowering them to learn more regarding their conditions. Both interventions placed little burden on participants, which is critical in this population. However, more research examining the effectiveness of these interventions with elders is needed.

Unintentional Injuries

More than 35% to 40% of elders over age 65 suffer a fall each year, with falls being associated with significant morbidity and mortality (Cesari et al., 2002). Due to both physical and cognitive declines (such as vision problems, slowed reaction times, and balance and strength problems), unintentional injuries are also a major focus of intervention during late adulthood. Multi-component interventions have been shown to have the greatest success at reducing fall rates (Day et al., 2002) and typically target physical activity, risk prevention, and/or hazard management in the home. In addition, particularly for elders who have experienced a fall, there is an increase in fear of falling associated with decreased functional ability and quality of life, as well as activity restriction (Li, Fisher, Harmer, McAuley, & Wilson, 2003).

STEPPING ON

A multi-faceted fall prevention program, known as *Stepping On*, has been evaluated with community-residing elders aged 70 and older (N = 310) who either had a history of a fall within the past 12 months or were concerned about the possibility of falling (Clemson et al., 2004). Using a small-group format, participants were provided seven weekly sessions targeting different aspects of fall risk (e.g., risk appraisal, strength/balance exercises, home hazard management, safe footwear/clothing, the role of poor vision, use of hip protectors, and benefits of calcium and vitamin D). A follow-up home visit, to review strategies and assist with any required home modifications, and a 3-month booster session were also incorporated. Using a randomized trial, results demonstrated a fall rate reduction of 31% for the intervention group in comparison to the control group. In addition, the intervention was found to be particularly effective for men, with a fall rate reduction of approximately 66%. This study incorporated multiple components to address fall risk in the elderly and accounted for not only physical declines, but also a focus on education and empowerment. The inclusion of these components accounted for the socio-emotional need for control and challenged the common stereotype of elders as passive or incompetent. Preventing or decreasing fear of fall risk by empowering elders may help boost self-confidence and prevent further social isolation, which may be more common as a result of increased activity restriction (Li et al., 2003). In addition, the intervention provided an in-home session; considering the physical decline experienced by elders, providing logistical support to complete any home modification was likely also critical.

Obesity

More than 70% of adults over 60 years of age are considered overweight or obese (Ogden, Flegal, Carroll, & Johnson, 2002). However, after about age 60, body weight begins to decline for the majority of elders (Chen & Wittert, 2006). Despite this decrease in body weight, the proportion of intra-abdominal fat increases, which is problematic due to its association with increased morbidity and mortality (Elia, 2012). Several factors have been implicated in regard to unhealthy weight in elders and the increase in intra-abdominal body fat, including a decrease in physical activity, reduction in muscle mass, a decrease in basal metabolic rate, and poor nutrition. Lifestyle intervention programs may help to decrease morbidity and mortality associated with health conditions such as diabetes and vascular conditions (Kennedy, Chokkalingham, & Srinivasan, 2004).

TREATMENT OF OBESITY IN UNDERSERVED RURAL SETTINGS (TOURS)

Perri et al. (2008) targeted obese women ($N = 234$) in medically underserved, rural communities and examined the effectiveness of an extended care, problem-solving counseling intervention in comparison to an education control group. Participants initially participated in a standard 6-month group-based lifestyle intervention aimed at producing weight loss and incorporating consumption of a low-calorie diet, increased physical activity, goal setting, and self-monitoring. In the extended care phase, participants were randomized to an education control group, a face-to-face counseling condition, or a telephone counseling condition. Both counseling conditions received 26 biweekly sessions focused on problem solving and addressing barriers to healthy eating and physical activity for sustaining weight loss, with face-to-face sessions lasting 60 minutes in duration and telephone sessions lasting 20 minutes. The problem-solving model (Perri et al., 2001, 2008) consisted of developing an appropriate coping framework; defining the specific problem, as well as target behaviors; generating alterative solutions; anticipating the outcomes of the different proposed solutions; and implementing a plan and monitoring the effectiveness of that plan. Results revealed that both extended care counseling conditions significantly improved the maintenance of weight loss in participants in comparison to the control condition, with the authors highlighting the cost-effectiveness of the telephone condition in particular.

Overall, this study demonstrated that providing extended care counseling to elders may help to improve maintenance of healthy lifestyle changes and as a result improve the maintenance of weight loss. Focusing on engaging elders in counseling specific to eating and physical activity behaviors was likely helpful as a result of improvements in problem solving and adherence to treatment, which have been associated with weight loss (Murawski et al., 2009). The relatively large number of sessions (26 delivered biweekly) was likely helpful in terms of being able to practice these strategies repeatedly and address a range of different barriers. Establishing those skills within participants likely contributed to a greater sense of self-efficacy. In addition, using telephone counseling was just as effective as the longer, and more burdensome, face-to-face sessions, which indicates it may be a more acceptable and sustainable intervention for elders.

CONCLUSIONS

This chapter demonstrates the important influence development has on health behavior change. Previous research with children, adolescents, and the elderly provides rich examples of behavioral health issues and interventions designed to promote change while taking development into account. However, there continues to be a need for the design of developmentally appropriate interventions that encourage behavioral change. The following are recommendations for future clinical and research endeavors that take developmental influences into account.

First, it is essential to recognize that some health issues impact individuals across the developmental spectrum. For example, while in this chapter obesity is identified as affecting preschool-age children and the elderly, obesity is a challenge across all developmental stages. The same is true for adherence, which is an issue affecting infant immunizations, medical regimens, and medication use across the lifespan. It is important for researchers and clinicians to be aware of what is being done to address the same health issue across age groups, as it is likely that interventions designed for one developmental group could help inform those created for other developmental groups. In general, increased dissemination of findings to different specialty groups (e.g., pediatrics and geriatrics) is necessary for this to occur.

Second, due to lifelong behavioral health concerns, there is a pressing need for early prevention and intervention efforts. Health behaviors are often solidified at young ages and changes to these behaviors should be implemented as early as feasible. This issue is most noticeable in the increased number of obesity interventions and federal funding designed specifically for young children. Addressing weight management at an early age may lead to decreased weight gain trajectories and prevent children from developing serious medical conditions associated with obesity (e.g., type 2 diabetes) and help reduce health care costs.

Third, there is a need for longer follow-up periods in research focusing on children, adolescents, and the elderly. Longitudinal assessments and treatments will provide more information about how development impacts and interacts with outcomes of prevention and intervention efforts. Researchers should also consider developmental trajectories in the development of prevention and intervention programs and interpretation of research results. For example, an area of increasing interest in pediatric psychology is the transition of adolescents with pediatric chronic illnesses to adult medical care facilities. As there have been extensive medical developments that allow children with pediatric chronic illnesses, such as cystic fibrosis (Quittner, Barker, Marciel, & Grimley, 2009), to live longer lives, the need for developmentally appropriate transitions to adult care centers becomes increasingly important. Yet, this is a prime example of how developmental transitions could impact health behavior, and it is unknown whether health behavior changes positively or negatively during and after this transition. More research is needed focusing on specific transition periods to determine what health behavior change interventions may be the most acceptable and the most effective.

Fourth, for interventions to be innovative and engaging throughout the lifespan, understanding social norms and cohort impacts is vital. For example, video games are an innovative way to teach children and adolescents health behaviors and can lead to behavioral change. However, this type of intervention may not be applicable for the elderly, due to their limited exposure to video games; other aspects of technology (e.g., telephones) may be more appropriate. One area for future investigation would be developing interventions using new social media platforms, such as various applications (apps), Twitter, and Tumblr. To encourage change throughout life, researchers and clinicians should increase awareness of aspects of technology that could be integrated into health behavior change interventions.

Lastly, social and cultural influences impact development. For example, research suggests that industrialization, socioeconomic status, and race and ethnicity affect pubertal timing (Biro, Khoury, & Morrison, 2005; Kaplowitz, Slora, Wasserman, Pedlow, & Herman-Giddens, 2001). Social and cultural influences shape engagement in health behaviors throughout development and interact with behavioral change processes. Developmentally appropriate interventions should also take social and cultural issues into account in order to be considered relevant, acceptable, and effective.

In conclusion, developmental issues are important to consider when working with children, adolescents, and the elderly. However, development in physical, cognitive, and socio-emotional domains should be considered when working with any population, especially those related to milestones and transitions. As demonstrated, development impacts and interacts with health behaviors in numerous ways and should be acknowledged in order to encourage lasting health behavior change in clinical and research settings.

REFERENCES

Agran, P. F., Anderson, C., Winn, D., Trent, R., Walton-Haynes, L., & Thayer, S. (2003). Rates of pediatric injuries by 3-month intervals for children 0 to 3 years of age. *Pediatrics, 111,* e683–e692.

Bearman, S. K., Presnell, K., Martinez, E., & Stice, E. (2006). The skinny on body dissatisfaction: A longitudinal study of adolescent girls and boys. *Journal of Youth and Adolescence, 35,* 217–229.

Berk, L. E. (2010). *Development through the lifespan* (5th ed.). Boston, MA: Allyn & Bacon.

Biro, F. M., Khoury, P., & Morrison, J. A. (2005). Influence of obesity on timing of puberty. *International Journal of Andrology, 29,* 272–277.

Bronfenbrenner, U. (1977). Toward an experimental ecology of human development. *American Psychologist, 32,* 513–531.

Brown Kirschman, K. J., Mayes, S., & Perciful, M. S. (2009). Prevention of unintentional injury in children and adolescents. In M. C. Roberts & R. G. Steele (Eds.), *Handbook of pediatric psychology* (4th ed., pp. 286–602). New York, NY: Guilford Press.

Brugman, G. M. (2006). Wisdom and aging. In J. E. Birren & K. W. Schaie (Eds.), *The handbook of the psychology of aging* (6th ed., pp. 445–476). San Diego, CA: Academic Press.

Centers for Disease Control and Prevention (CDC). (2009). 10 leading causes of death by age group, United States – 2009. Atlanta, GA: Author.

CDC. (2010). National estimates of the 10 leading causes of nonfatal injuries treated in hospital emergency departments, United States – 2010. Atlanta, GA: Author.

CDC. (2011). *Sexually transmitted disease surveillance 2010.* Atlanta, GA: Author.

CDC. (2012a). *2012 recommended immunizations for children from birth through 6 years old.* Atlanta, GA: Author.

CDC. (2012b). *Learn the signs: Act early.* Atlanta, GA: Author.

Cesari, M., Landi, F., Torre, S., Onder, G., Lattanzio, F., & Bernabei, R. (2002). Prevalence and risk factors for falls in an older community-dwelling population. *Journals of Gerontology Series A: Biological Sciences and Medical Sciences, 57,* M722–M726.

Chen, R. Y. T., & Wittert, G. A. (2006). Obesity in the elderly. In M. S. J. Pathy, A. J. Sinclair, & J. E. Morley (Eds.), *Principles and practice of geriatric medicine* (Vol. 2) (4th ed., pp. 347–353). John Wiley & Sons Ltd., Chichester, West Sussex, England.

Clemson, L., Cumming, R. G., Kendig, H., Swann, M., Heard, R., & Taylor, K. (2004). The effectiveness of a community-based program for reducing the incidence of falls in the elderly: A randomized trial. *Journal of the American Geriatrics Society, 52,* 1487–1494.

Cuddy, A. J. C., & Fiske, S. T. (2002). Doddering but dear: Process, content, and function in stereotyping of older persons. In T. D. Nelson (Ed.), *Ageism: Stereotyping and prejudice against older persons* (pp. 3–26). Cambridge, MA: MIT Press.

Cuddy, A. J. C., Norton, M. I., & Fiske, S. T. (2005). This old stereotype: The pervasiveness and persistence of the elderly stereotype. *Journal of Social Issues, 61,* 267–285.

Cutrona, S. L., Choudhry, N. K., Fischer, M. A., Servi, A., Liberman, J. N., Brennan, T., et al. (2010). Modes of delivery for interventions to improve cardiovascular medication adherence: Review. *American Journal of Managed Care, 16,* 929.

Dahl, R. E. (2004). Adolescent brain development: A period of vulnerabilities and opportunities. Keynote address. *Annals of the New York Academy of Sciences, 1021,* 1–22.

Daniels, S. R. (2006). The consequences of childhood overweight and obesity. *Future Child, 16,* 47–67.

Dariotis, J. K., Sifakis, F., Pleck, J. H., Astone, N. M., & Sonenstein, F. L. (2011). Racial and ethnic disparities in sexual risk behaviors and STDs during young men's transition to adulthood. *Perspectives on Sexual and Reproductive Health, 43,* 51–59.

Day, L., Fildes, B., Gordon, I., Fitzharris, M., Flamer, H., & Lord, S. (2002). Randomised factorial trial of falls prevention among older people living in their own homes. *BMJ: British Medical Journal, 325,* 128.

Drotar, D. (2006). *Psychological interventions in childhood chronic illness.* Washington, DC: American Psychological Association.

Elder, G. H., Jr. (1994). Time, human agency, and social change: Perspectives on the life course. *Social Psychology Quarterly, 57,* 4–15.

Elia, M. (2012). Obesity in the elderly. *Obesity Research, 9,* 244S–248S.

Erikson, E. H. (1959). Identity and the life cycle. *Psychological Issues, 1,* 18–164.

Fozard, J. L., & Gordon-Salant, S. (2001). Changes in vision and hearing with aging. In J. E. Birren & K. W. Schaie (Eds.), *The handbook of the psychology of aging* (5th ed., pp. 241–266). San Diego, CA: Academic Press.

Freud, S. (1991). *On sexuality.* London, England: Penguin Books.

Geithner, C. A., Thomis, M. A., Vanden Eynde, B., Maes, H. H., Loos, R. J., Peeters, M., et al. (2004). Growth in peak aerobic power during adolescence. *Medicine & Science in Sports & Exercise, 36,* 1616–1624.

Gellad, W. F., Grenard, J. L., & Marcum, Z. A. (2011). A systematic review of barriers to medication adherence in the elderly: Looking beyond cost and regimen complexity. *American Journal of Geriatric Pharmacotherapy, 9,* 11–23.

George, T., Shefer, A. M., Rickert, D., David, F., Stevenson, J. M., & Fishbein, D. B. (2007). A status report from 1996–2004: Are more effective immunization interventions being used in the women, infants, and children (WIC) program? *Maternal and Child Health Journal, 11,* 327–333.

Graber, J. A., Seeley, J. R., Brooks-Gunn, J., & Lewinsohn, P. M. (2004). Is pubertal timing associated with psychopathology in young adulthood? *Journal of the American Academy of Child & Adolescent Psychiatry, 43,* 718–726.

Guo, S. S., Wu, W., Chumlea, W. C., & Roche, A. F. (2002). Predicting overweight and obesity in adulthood from body mass index values in childhood and adolescence. *American Journal of Clinical Nutrition, 76,* 653–658.

Hambidge, S. J., Phibbs, S. L., Chandramouli, V., Fairclough, D., & Steiner, J. F. (2009). A stepped intervention increases well-child care and immunization rates in a disadvantaged population. *Pediatrics, 124,* 455–464.

Haynes, R. B., Ackloo, E., Sahota, N., McDonald, H. P., & Yao, X. (2008). Interventions for enhancing medication adherence. *Cochrane Database of System Reviews, 2.*

Hoyer, W. J., & Verhaeghen, P. (2006). Memory aging. In J. E. Birren & K. W. Schaie (Eds.), *The handbook of the psychology of aging* (6th ed., pp. 209–232). San Diego, CA: Academic Press.

Janicke, D. M., Sallinen, B. J., Perri, M. G., Lutes, L. D., Huerta, M., Silverstein, J. H., et al. (2008). Comparison of parent-only vs. family-based interventions for overweight children in underserved rural settings: Outcomes from Project STORY. *Archives of Pediatrics and Adolescent Medicine, 162,* 1119–1125.

Jemal, A., Ward, E., Hao, Y., & Thun, M. (2005). Trends in the leading causes of death in the United States, 1970–2002. *Journal of the American Medical Association, 294,* 1255–1259.

Jemmott III, J. B., Jemmott, L. S., Braverman, P. K., & Fong, G. T. (2005). HIV/STD risk reduction interventions for African American and Latino adolescent girls at an adolescent medicine clinic: A randomized controlled trial. *Archives of Pediatrics & Adolescent Medicine, 159,* 440.

Kaplowitz, P. B., Slora, E. J., Wasserman, R. C., Pedlow, S. E., & Herman-Giddens, M. E. (2001). Earlier onset of puberty in girls: Relation to increased body mass index and race. *Pediatrics, 108,* 347–353.

Kazak, A. E., Rourke, M. T., & Navsaria, N. (2009). Families and other systems in pediatric psychology. In M. C. Roberts & R. G. Steele (Eds.), *Handbook of pediatric psychology* (4th ed., pp. 656–671). New York, NY: Guilford Press.

Kennedy, R. L., Chokkalingham, K., & Srinivasan, R. (2004). Obesity in the elderly: Who should we be treating, and why, and how? *Current Opinion in Clinical Nutrition & Metabolic Care, 7,* 3–9.

Kitzmann, K. M., Dalton, W. T., 3rd, Stanley, C. M., Beech, B. M., Reeves, T. P., Buscemi, J., et al. (2010). Lifestyle interventions for youth who are overweight: A meta-analytic review. *Health Psychology, 29,* 91–101.

La Greca, A. M., & Mackey, E. R. (2009). Adherence to pediatric treatment regimens. In M. C. Roberts & R. G. Steele (Eds.), *Handbook of pediatric psychology* (4th ed., pp. 130–152). New York, NY: Guilford Press.

Lamb, M. E., & Lewis, C. (2005). The role of parent-child relationships in child development. In M. H. Bornstein & M. E. Lamb (Eds.), *Developmental science: An advanced textbook* (5th ed., pp. 429–468). Mahwah, NJ: Lawrence Erlbaum.

Lennings, C. J. (2000). Optimism, satisfaction and time perspective in the elderly. *International Journal of Aging and Human Development, 51,* 167–182.

Lerner, R. M., Theokas, C., & Bobek, D. L. (2005). Concepts and theories of human development: Historical and contemporary dimensions. In M. H. Bornstein & M. E. Lamb (Eds.), *Developmental science: An advanced textbook* (5th ed., pp. 3–43). Mahwah, NJ: Lawrence Erlbaum Associates.

Li, F., Fisher, K. J., Harmer, P., McAuley, E., & Wilson, N. L. (2003). Fear of falling in elderly persons: Association with falls, functional ability, and quality of life. *Journals of Gerontology Series B: Psychological Sciences and Social Sciences, 58,* P283–P290.

Lightfoot, C., Cole, M., & Cole, S. R. (2009). *The development of children.* New York, NY: Worth.

Lubman, D. I., Yücel, M., & Hall, W. D. (2007). Substance use and the adolescent brain: A toxic combination? *Journal of Psychopharmacology, 21,* 792–794.

Luman, E. T., Shaw, K. M., & Stokley, S. K. (2008). Compliance with vaccination recommendations for U.S. children. [Research Support, U.S. Gov't, P.H.S.]. *American Journal of Preventative Medicine, 34,* 463–470.

Mendle, J., Turkheimer, E., & Emery, R. E. (2007). Detrimental psychological outcomes associated with early pubertal timing in adolescent girls. *Developmental Review, 27,* 151–171.

Morrongiello, B. A., & Schwebel, D. C. (2008). Gaps in childhood injury research and prevention: What can developmental scientists contribute? *Child Development Perspectives, 2,* 78–84.

Morrongiello, B. A., Schwebel, D. C., Bell, M., Stewart, J., & Davis, A. L. (2012). An evaluation of The Great Escape: Can an interactive computer game improve young children's fire safety knowledge and behaviors? *Health Psychology, 31,* 496–502.

Murawski, M. E., Milsom, V. A., Ross, K. M., Rickel, K. A., DeBraganza, N., Gibbons, L. M., et al. (2009). Problem solving, treatment adherence, and weight-loss outcome among women participating in lifestyle treatment for obesity. *Eating Behaviors, 10,* 146–151.

Murdaugh, C. L. (1998). Problems with adherence in the elderly. In E. B. Schron, S. A. Shumaker, J. K. Ockene, & W. McBee (Eds.), *The handbook of health behavior change* (2nd ed., pp. 357–376). New York, NY: Springer.

National Center for Health Statistics. (2012). *Health, United States 2011: With special feature on socioeconomic status and health.* Retrieved from http://www.cdc.gov/nchs/data/hus/hus11.pdf#022

O'Dea, J. A., & Abraham, S. (1999). Onset of disordered eating attitudes and behaviors in early adolescence: Interplay of pubertal status, gender, weight, and age. *Adolescence, 34,* 671–680.

Ogden, C. L., Carroll, M. D., Kit, B. K., & Flegal, K. M. (2012). Prevalence of obesity and trends in body mass index among US children and adolescents, 1999–2010. *Journal of the American Medical Association, 307*, 483–490.

Ogden, C. L., Flegal, K. M., Carroll, M. D., & Johnson, C. L. (2002). Prevalence and trends in overweight among US children and adolescents, 1999–2000. *Journal of the American Medical Association, 288*, 1728–1732.

Ownby, R. L., Hertzog, C., & Czaja, S. J. (2012). Tailored information and automated reminding to improve medication adherence in Spanish- and English-speaking elders treated for memory impairment. *Clinical Gerontologist, 35*, 221–238.

Perri, M. G., Limacher, M. C., Durning, P. E., Janicke, D. M., Lutes, L. D., Bobroff, L. B., et al. (2008). Extended-care programs for weight management in rural communities: The treatment of obesity in underserved rural settings (TOURS) randomized trial. *Archives of Internal Medicine, 168*, 2347.

Perri, M. G., Nezu, A. M., McKelvey, W. F., Shermer, R. L., Renjilian, D. A., & Viegener, B. J. (2001). Relapse prevention training and problem-solving therapy in the long-term management of obesity. *Journal of Consulting and Clinical Psychology, 69*, 722.

Piette, J. D., Weinberger, M., & McPhee, S. J. (2000). The effect of automated calls with telephone nurse follow-up on patient-centered outcomes of diabetes care: A randomized, controlled trial. *Medical Care, 38*, 218–230.

Quittner, A. L., Barker, D. H., Marciel, K. K., & Grimley, M. E. (2009). Cystic fibrosis: A model for drug discovery and patient care. In M. C. Roberts & R. G. Steele (Eds.), *Handbook of pediatric psychology* (4th ed., pp. 271–286). New York, NY: Guilford Press.

Rapoff, M. A. (2010). *Adherence to pediatric medical regimens* (2nd ed.). New York, NY: Springer.

Stice, E., & Whitenton, K. (2002). Risk factors for body dissatisfaction in adolescent girls: A longitudinal investigation. *Developmental Psychology, 38*, 669.

Taber, D. R., Stevens, J., Evenson, K. R., Ward, D. S., Poole, C., Maciejewski, M. L., et al. (2011). State policies targeting junk food in schools: Racial/ethnic differences in the effect of policy change on soda consumption. *American Journal of Public Health, 101*, 1769–1775.

Taylor, J. A., Darden, P. M., Brooks, D. A., Hendricks, J. W., Wasserman, R. C., Bocian, A. B., et al. (2002). Association between parents' preferences and perceptions of barriers to vaccination and the immunization status of their children: A study from Pediatric Research in Office Settings and the National Medical Association. *Pediatrics, 110*, 1110–1116.

Thomas, M., Kohli, V., & King, D. (2004). Barriers to childhood immunization: Findings from a needs assessment study. *Home Health Care Services Quarterly, 23*, 19–39.

Wang, Y., Beydoun, M. A., Liang, L., Caballero, B., & Kumanyika, S. K. (2008). Will all Americans become overweight or obese? Estimating the progression and cost of the US obesity epidemic. *Obesity (Silver Spring), 16*, 2323–2330.

Wysocki, T., Harris, M. A., Buckloh, L. M., Mertlich, D., Lochrie, A. S., Taylor, A., ... White, N. H. (2006). Effects of Behavioral Family Systems Therapy for Diabetes on adolescents' family relationships, treatment adherence, and metabolic control. *Journal of Pediatric Psychology, 31*, 928–938.

Wysocki, T., Harris, M. A., Buckloh, L. M., Mertlich, D., Lochrie, A. S., Taylor, A., & White, N. H. (2008). Randomized, controlled trial of behavioral family systems therapy for diabetes: Maintenance and generalization of effects on parent-adolescent communication. *Behavior Therapy, 39*, 33–46.

6

Culture, Behavior, and Health

MILAGROS C. ROSAL
MONICA L. WANG
JAMIE S. BODENLOS

LEARNING OBJECTIVES

- Understand cultural concepts and various mechanisms through which culture influences health and health behavior.
- Apply major health behavior theories to culture and health.
- Determine strategies to incorporate culture in reseach and health care.

Culture, broadly defined as what is learned, shared, transmitted intergenerationally, and reflected in a group's values, beliefs, norms, behaviors, communication, and social roles, can affect health-related behaviors both directly and indirectly (Kreuter & Haughton, 2006), and thus is highly relevant to disease prevention and management as well as health promotion. Current literature on culture, health, and health behaviors is very limited, however, and much is left to understand regarding how best to assess and intervene with diverse populations in a culturally appropriate manner. Interest in the role of culture on health continues to increase due to the growing cultural diversity of the U.S. population, as well as the pervasive disparities observed across numerous health behaviors and outcomes by characteristics such as race/ethnicity, socioeconomic status (SES), and sexual orientation.

Data from the 2010 Census indicated that, overall, the United States is increasing in diversity in numerous areas. From 2000 to 2010, both the Hispanic population (50.5 million in 2010) and the Asian population (14.7 million in 2010) grew by about 43% (Humes, Jones, & Ramirez, 2011); these growths are due in part to relatively higher levels of immigration. (Note: For this chapter, we use the term "Hispanic" to describe individuals and populations of Hispanic or Latino ethnicity.) Multiracial individuals also constitute another fast-growing subgroup. The number and proportion of individuals who speak a language other than English at home also have increased steadily over the past three decades. Over half (62%) of the 55.4 million people who spoke a language other than English at home spoke Spanish, followed by other Indo-European languages (19%), Asian and Pacific Island languages (15%), and other languages (4%) (Shin & Kominski, 2010). The 2010 American Community Survey (ACS) estimated that 13% of the U.S. population was foreign-born, with 53% of the foreign-born population migrating from Latin America (Grieco et al., 2012). Among unmarried couple house-holds, the proportion of same-sex unmarried couples has doubled from 0.3% in 2000 to 0.6% in 2010 (Lofquist, Lugaila, O'Connell, & Feliz, 2012). However, these percentages do not capture other same-sex sexual orientation individuals, including youth who iden-tify as lesbian, gay, bisexual, or transgender (LGBT), LGBT adults who did not report being part of a same-sex couple household, and same-sex couples who are legally mar-ried. Overall, these population patterns emphasize the increasing need to understand cultural differences and their impact on health behaviors and health; to develop and implement programs and policies that are culturally tailored and/or sensitive; and to train culturally competent public health and medical professionals to better serve a population that continues to increase in diversity.

In this chapter, we approach the topic of culture from an empirical and a theoretical perspective, and discuss the importance of conducting theory-based research to enhance our understanding of cultural influences on behavior. This chapter begins with a review of commonly used culture-related concepts and definitions and subsequently presents empirical evidence of the influence of culture on health-related perceptions, screening and preventive behaviors, and disease management behaviors. It also summarizes frequently cited theoretical models of behavior which can be useful in accounting for the effect of culture on behavior, and discusses key methodological recommendations to incorporate cultural considerations in clinical and population research, health care, and public health.

CULTURE-RELATED DEFINITIONS

CULTURAL INFLUENCE

Cultural influence refers to the degree to which the values, beliefs, norms, and traditions common to a particular group influence behaviors of individual members within the group. Culture can influence what is acceptable, appropriate, and desirable behavior, including behaviors related to health (Haviland, 1999).

CULTURAL CHANGE

Although there is a certain degree of permanency in cultures, changes in culture can occur to various degrees and at varying rates. Aspects of a culture may change and affect other aspects of that culture. For example, the learning of a new language, an important cultural symbol, by a group can bring on the adoption of other behaviors (e.g., greater engagement in the health care system) among members of that group. Cultural changes such as changes in beliefs and behaviors can also occur as a result of "lived experiences"—that is, experiences that individuals and populations go through as they live their lives (Garro, 2000). At the individual level, these lived experiences can include, but are not limited to, acquisition of education or migration to a new country, county, or region. Recent examples of lived experiences at the population level include disasters that affect regions (e.g., Hurricane Katrina's effects on the Gulf Coast and the effects of 9/11 on New York City and the United States).

SOCIETY

Society is a group of people who have a common homeland, are dependent on each other for survival, and share a common culture commonly referred to as "mainstream" culture (Haviland, 1999). However, no two members of a society experience the same exact culture; culture shared by members of a society is not uniform and multiple sub-cultures coexist within a single society. One aspect of the mainstream American culture (or society) that affects Americans from all subcultures is food environment. Neighbor-hood-level studies indicate that living in areas with a high density of fast food chains and decreased availability and accessibility of supermarkets is associated with higher rates of overweight and obesity (Fraser & Edwards, 2010; Morland & Evenson, 2009) and that the "obesogenic" culture of the United States has contributed significantly to the current obesity epidemic (Sallis & Glanz, 2006).

SUBCULTURES

Individuals can belong to many different cultures and subcultures (Haviland, 1999). *Subcultures* are defined as groups within a society, each functioning by its own distinc-tive standards of values, norms, and behaviors, while at the same time sharing certain standards with the overarching culture (Haviland, 1999). For example, although mem-bers of a society may share a common homeland and language, multiple subcultures exist within that society and can be characterized by gender, race/ethnicity, age group, religion, sexual orientation, SES, urbanicity of residence (i.e., urban, suburban, and rural) and regional location. The definitions of race and ethnicity warrant detailed attention, as the definitions of these terms have changed over time. The modern concept of race emphasizes social origins rather than a biological basis. *Race* refers to the group that a person belongs to as a result of physical features (i.e., skin color and hair texture), which also reflect ancestry and geographical origins (Bhopal, 2004). *Ethnicity*, derived from the Greek word *ethnos*, meaning "nation," refers to a group to which people belong or are perceived to belong as a result of certain shared characteristics, including geo-graphical and ancestral origins, cultural traditions, and languages (Bhopal, 2004). Race and ethnicity are distinct concepts but overlap in their definitions; thus, the two terms are often used interchangeably or used in conjunction ("race/ethnicity"), a practice becoming increasingly common in the United States.

As culture may overlap with race/ethnicity (e.g., both culture and ethnicity are par-tially defined by sharing of geographical origins and cultural traditions and languages), race/ethnicity is often assumed to be a proxy for culture. However, it is important to note that there is great subgroup variation in cultural identity, cultural practices, SES, and other characteristics within each racial/ethnic group. For instance, regional and SES differences between groups may be more important in determining behavior that contributes to health disparities than racial/ethnic differences (Coughlin et al., 2006; Foster, 2006; McGory, Zingmond, Sekeris, Bastani, & Ko, 2006; Parikh-Patel, Bates, & Campleman, 2006); for example, there are significant differences in health-related behav-iors within Hispanic populations based on country of origin and SES. Overall, culture is a multidimensional concept that captures aspects of the dynamic experience of iden-tifying with certain characteristics or belonging to various groups (e.g., gender, race/ethnicity, and SES) and cannot be isolated from those characteristics when examining how culture impacts health behaviors and outcomes.

HEALTH DISPARITIES AND INTRA-GROUP DIVERSITY

Health disparities refer to preventable and unjust health differences between groups of people that are closely linked with social, economic, and/or environmental disadvan-tage (U.S. Department of Health and Human Services, 2010). For this chapter, we focus on racial/ethnic-specific cultural differences that contribute to health disparities, as it is well established that compared to Whites, individuals from minority racial/ethnic backgrounds have higher rates of and poorer health outcomes in numerous preventable and treatable conditions, including cardiovascular disease and stroke, type 2 diabetes mellitus, asthma, HIV/AIDS, some cancers, and obesity (U.S. Department of Health and Human Services & Agency for Healthcare Research and Quality, 2011). However, significant heterogeneity exists within racial/ethnic groups, and failure to recognize and understand these differences can lead to inappropriate and/or inaccurate conclusions. For example, there is much diversity in the ancestry, biological characteristics, cultural traditions, belief systems, and behaviors within all major racial/ethnic categories (i.e., White, Hispanic, Black/African American, and Asian) (Bhopal & Donaldson, 1998). (Note: We use the term "Black/African American" to refer to individuals who are of African descent and/or those who identify as Black. For the remainder of the chapter, we use the term "Black" to be inclusive of individuals who may identify as Black but who are not of African descent, e.g., Haitian). Combining smaller subgroups into a larger subgroup, as is often done for statistical analysis purposes, can mask important heterogeneity of health behaviors and outcomes. For example, Hawaiian/Pacific Islanders have a high prevalence of obesity but are often included as part of the Asian category, which on average has lower rates of obesity compared to other racial/ethnic groups. Consequently, it is critical to consider the heterogeneity of health-related characteristics, behaviors, and outcomes within groups and to avoid making generalizations and assumptions based on data that do not capture intra-group diversity.

It is also important to recognize the importance and intricacies of individual-level demographics (i.e., SES, race/ethnicity, and culture) that operate within various contexts and settings. It is well established in the literature that SES influences health and contributes to health disparities through mechanisms such as ability to afford health insurance, purchase or engage in healthy behaviors, and live in healthier and safer neighborhoods. In 2009, the majority (85%) of adults in the United States reported having at least a high school degree and over a quarter (28%) reported having a bachelor's degree or higher; however, educational attainment for non-Hispanic Whites and Asians was higher than for Blacks and Hispanics (Ryan & Siebens, 2012). Black and Hispanic workers earned less at nearly all educational attainment levels than non-Hispanic Whites, and men earned more than women at each level of educational attainment. These patterns suggest that individuals' SES potential and experience are strongly correlated and intertwined with race/ethnicity and gender. Thus, it is important to consider these intricacies in understanding health behavior, conducting research and interpreting findings related to health disparities, and working with diverse populations.

CULTURE TRANSMISSION

Transmission of culture is the process by which specific aspects of a culture (e.g., language, beliefs, rituals, and normative behavior) are passed down from one generation to the next; this process is shaped by multiple spheres of influence, including family members, peers, schools, work groups, geography, politics, the physical environment, and mass media. Transmission of a culture begins soon after a child is born, through enculturation and socialization (Berry, Poortinga, Segall, & Dasen, 1992). Early in life, the most important role models and transmitters of culture are a child's caregivers and other family members. As the child matures and begins to spend more time outside the home, other spheres of influence, such as peers and the school environment, become important. These include "social acceptance," which rewards adherence to cultural standards and can become especially important during adolescence. Transmission of culture also occurs via various media channels. Given the growing ubiquity of the Internet, the media has grown exponentially in its power to shape the views, attitudes, and behaviors of individuals from early ages within and across societies worldwide (Wilson, Gutierrez, & Chao, 2003).

ACCULTURATION

Transmission of a new culture can also occur later in life, after one has already become rooted in a different culture; this usually occurs when an individual changes geographic location and has to adapt to new cultural sanctions. *Acculturation* is the degree to which cultural elements of a mainstream culture are adopted by another group (Carter-Pokras & Bethune, 2009; Sam, 2010). Individuals may have varying levels of acculturation to a mainstream culture. Degree of acculturation has been measured by the language spoken at home, number of years resident in country of immigration, citizenship status, and place of birth, as well as by various psychosocial measurements (Carter-Pokras & Bethune, 2009). The impact of acculturation on health and health-related behaviors has been extensively documented among several populations (Borrayo & Guarnaccia, 2000; Elder et al., 1991; Goel et al., 2003; Gonzalez, Haan, & Hinton, 2001; Lara, Gamboa, Kahramanian, Morales, & Bautista, 2005). Qualitative, observational, and systematic review studies indicate that a higher degree of acculturation to Western or American culture (e.g., longer residence in the United States and language acculturation) is associated with adverse health-related behaviors and outcomes. Among Hispanics who immigrate to the United States, acculturation is associated with increased sedentary behaviors (Banna, Kaiser, Drake, & Townsend, 2012), poorer quality of dietary intake (Perez-Escamilla, 2011), and increased stress (Tovar et al., 2013). Other studies found acculturation to be a risk factor for weight gain and obesity among U.S. immigrants (Fuentes-Afflick & Hessol, 2008; Oza-Frank & Cunningham, 2010). As the United States continues to increase in racial/ethnic and ethnic–immigrant diversity, acculturation will be an increasingly important process to examine in health care settings and research.

ETHNOCENTRISM

Transmission of culture from one generation to the next depends to some extent on how individuals feel about their culture. *Ethnocentrism*, the belief that one's own culture is superior to all others, is adaptive for transmission of a culture or preserving key aspects of a particular culture (Sumner, 1906). However, ethnocentrism can also become a barrier when a need exists to understand or gain information about another culture (Thiederman, 1986 [Sutherland, 2002]). This is relevant to developing health promotion or disease management interventions that meet the needs of individuals of a particular culture. In order to gain an unbiased view of someone else's culture and thus understand individuals in their own cultural terms, researchers and health care providers must be able to recognize their own cultural biases and minimize judgment on culture-related practices of targeted individuals or groups as much as possible; this process is referred to as *cultural relativism* (Haviland, 1999).

CULTURAL COMPETENCE

Cultural competence is having the capacity to function effectively as an individual or an organization within the context of the cultural beliefs, behaviors, and needs presented by a particular group or community (U.S. Department of Health and Human Services & Office of Minority Health, 2001). It involves: (1) awareness of one's own cultural values and biases, (2) knowledge of others' views and perspectives, and (3) having the skills to design and effectively deliver culturally appropriate interventions (Harris-Davis & Haughton, 2000).

CULTURAL SENSITIVITY

Cultural sensitivity refers to the extent to which ethnic and cultural aspects of a target population, as well as relevant historical, political, environmental, and social forces, are incorporated in the design, delivery, and evaluation of targeted interventions, materials, and programs (Resnicow, Baranowski, Ahluwalia, & Braithwaite, 1999). There are two types of cultural sensitivity: (1) *surface culture*, which refers to observable characteristics and includes language, dress, and music; and (2) *deep cultural structure*, which relates to nonobservable characteristics such as common values and ideology that shape health-related decisions (Kreuter, Lukwago, Bucholtz, Clark, & Sanders-Thompson, 2003; Resnicow et al., 1999; Torres, Marquez, Carbone, Stacciarini, & Foster, 2008). Strategies to develop culturally sensitive interventions are discussed later in this chapter.

EMPIRICAL EVIDENCE OF CULTURAL INFLUENCES ON HEALTH-RELATED BEHAVIORS

In this section, we review empirical evidence indicating how elements of culture influence health behaviors and outcomes ultimately contributing to health disparities, particularly racial/ethnic health disparities.

CULTURE AND HEALTH SCREENING BEHAVIOR

Health screenings are an important component of preventive care, yet adherence to health screening guidelines is suboptimal among certain groups and contributes to health disparities (Ata et al., 2006; Boltri, Okosun, Davis-Smith, & Vogel, 2005; Finney, Tumiel-Berhalter, Fox, & Jaen, 2006; Neal, Magwood, Jenkins, & Hossler, 2006). The proportion of Asian American women who receive mammograms and cervical cancer screenings and who are adherent to cancer screening guidelines are the lowest among any of the racial/ethnic groups in the United States (MacLean, 2004), and Asian Americans are the only racial/ethnic group in the United States to experience cancer as the leading cause of death (Centers for Disease Control, 2007). The cancer burden that affects this group may be significantly reduced by increasing earlier detection. Cultural beliefs can heavily influence health screening practices. For instance, Buddhism, Taoism, and Confucianism focus on acceptance of the natural order of life (Allinson, 1989; Graham, 1990) and present disease and illness as a part of the life cycle. In the Chinese culture, life events, such as health and illness, are often explained in terms of luck, fortune, or fate (Allinson, 1989); these culturally influenced perceptions are likely to contribute to the low participation in screening behaviors among Asian Americans (Kwok & Sullivan, 2006).

CULTURE AND PREVENTIVE BEHAVIOR

Several prevalent and costly diseases can be prevented, or their onset delayed, through preventive interventions and policies that promote healthy behaviors and decrease disease risk factors (Knowler et al., 2002; Turnbull, 2003). Thus, behavioral adherence to these types of interventions may be key to prolonging health and quality of life (QoL).

In the United States, Blacks comprised 44% of all new HIV infections in 2009 and face the most severe burden of HIV, including higher mortality rates, compared to all other racial/ethnic groups (Centers for Disease Control (CDC), 2011), despite significant advances in the treatment of HIV/AIDS. Cultural factors influencing safe-sex behaviors may partially contribute to these disparities. Black and Hispanic communities often have conspiracy beliefs about HIV/AIDS, such as that HIV is manmade by the government and planted in Black communities, cures exist and are withheld from the poor, people who take new HIV medications are guinea pigs for the government, much information about AIDS is being withheld from the public, and medicines used to treat HIV actually cause AIDS (Bogart & Bird, 2003; Bogart & Thorburn, 2005; Herek & Capitanio, 1994; Herek & Glunt, 1991; Klonoff & Landrine, 1999; Neff, 2006). These conspiracy beliefs have been associated with negative attitudes toward condoms and participation in risky sexual behaviors, such as inconsistent condom use, among Blacks, thus minimizing the effectiveness of HIV prevention programs (Herek & Capitanio, 1994).

Cultural influences may also positively impact health behaviors such as prevention and screening. With the exception of Asian Americans, Hispanics have lower rates of smoking (12.5%) than most other racial/ethnic groups in the United States (Centers for Disease Control and Prevention, 2011). Hispanics who currently smoke also consume fewer cigarettes per day than White and Black current smokers (Hassmiller, Warner, Mendez, Levy, & Romano, 2003; Reitzel et al., 2009; Zhu, Pulvers, Zhuang, & Baezconde-Garbanati, 2007). The Hispanic culture may in part explain lower rates and frequency of smoking compared to Whites, as Hispanics are more likely to cite family and interpersonal relationships as important reasons to quit smoking. Likewise, lack of family approval has been shown to prevent many young Hispanics from initiating smoking (Foraker, Patten, Lopez, Croghan, & Thomas, 2005). These examples highlight the influence of interdependence and importance of the family (*familialismo*) characteristic of the Hispanic culture.

CULTURE, ILLNESS PERCEPTION, AND DISEASE MANAGEMENT

Individuals from different cultures may have different attitudes, beliefs, or interpretations of bodily symptoms, what constitutes a disease, and what interventions and treatments are acceptable (Betancourt, 2006; Surbone, 2006; Waite, 2006; Ward, 2007). Cultural syndromes are a clear example of this issue. The *Diagnostic and statistical manual of mental disorders* (4th ed.; *DSM-IV*; American Psychiatric Association, 2000) defined culture-bound syndromes as "recurrent, locality-specific patterns of aberrant behavior and troubling experience that may or may not be linked to a particular *DSM-IV* diagnostic category" (American Psychiatric Association, 2000). In the recently released *DSM-5*, cultural syndromes are described as "clusters of symptoms and attributions that tend to co-occur among individuals in specific cultural groups, communities, or contexts and that are recognized locally as coherent patterns of experience" (American Psychiatric Association, 2013). Many culture-bound syndromes are considered indigenously to be "illnesses" or at least afflictions, and most have local names. One example specific to Latin American and Hispanic populations is "*susto*," a syndrome usually associated with a broad array of symptoms including nervousness, anorexia, insomnia, listlessness, despondency, involuntary muscle tics, and diarrhea. Within these cultures, the causes of *susto* are attributed to fright that can result in a loss of soul from the body and from natural or supernatural events. For instance, *susto* may occur after a near miss or accident or after witnessing a supernatural phenomenon such as a ghost. Among Mexican immigrants, *susto* is widely believed to be the cause of type 2 diabetes (Mendenhall, Fernandez, Adler, & Jacobs, 2012; Poss & Jezewski, 2002). The symptoms associated with *susto* are often misinterpreted by health care providers and often diagnosed as tuberculosis in the United States (Kemp, 2004).

Symptom reporting, pain perception, and coping among various cultural groups may also affect providers' response to patients and the interventions and treatments prescribed. A review of culture and pain among adults (Calvillo & Flaskerud, 1991) found that White Americans of Northern European origin tend to react to pain more stoically; this type of response to pain has become the cultural norm in the United States and is expected by health care providers. Findings from this review indicated that the ethnicity and culture of the patient influenced the extent of the difference between the patients' pain perception and the nurses' assessment of the patients' level of pain.

Treatment preferences for common medical conditions are also influenced by culture. An example of this is the considerable ethnic variation in the choice of knee replacement as the treatment of knee osteoarthritis, the most common procedure among hospital discharges in the United States. Joint replacements are elective procedures that provide substantial benefits in pain relief and QoL (Callahan, Drake, Heck, & Dittus, 1995). However, despite these benefits, Hispanic and Black patients are half as likely as White patients to undergo surgery, even after controlling for income and access to care (Ibrahim, Siminoff, Burant, & Kwoh, 2002a, 2002b). Black patients were least likely to consider surgery despite reporting more severe symptoms, even when significant physician counseling has been provided (Ibrahim et al., 2002a, 2002b). Willingness to undergo surgery is related to beliefs about the efficacy of the procedure, expectations of post-surgical pain and functional difficulties, and knowing individuals in their close social environment who have undergone the procedure (Ibrahim et al., 2002a, 2002b; Suarez-Almazor et al., 2005). Additionally, the perception of prayer has been shown to influence treatment preferences for arthritis, with Black patients more likely to perceive prayer as a helpful coping mechanism for arthritis than White patients, and the perception of the helpfulness of prayer shown to be a mediator between ethnicity and consideration of arthroplasty (Ang, Ibrahim, Burant, Siminoff, & Kwoh, 2002).

Assessing various perspectives related to culture, illness, and care is one way to view and explain disparities in mental health treatment among individuals with different cultural views on medicine (Kleinman, Eisenberg, & Good, 1978). In this model, both the physician and the patient operate under two different explanations of the symptoms. Health care providers of Western medicine who prescribe antidepressant medications for treatment of depressive symptoms tend to operate under the belief system that depression is a disease that may be treated with medication and psychotherapy, whereas patients may be operating under a different set of beliefs regarding the labeling, cause, and treatment of their symptoms (Kleinman et al., 1978). In Chinese cultural settings, mental health issues such as depression are highly stigmatized, and depressive symptoms are often attributed to a physiological humoral imbalance (i.e., lack of blood flow and reduced vital breath) rather than a mental illness (Kleinman et al., 1978; Kuo & Kavanagh, 1994; Ryder & Chentsova-Dutton, 2012). Findings from qualitative research suggest that cultural beliefs, including spiritual and religious attitudes, as well as stigma related to mental illness, may explain the lack of acceptability of and low adherence to antidepressant medication (Cooper-Patrick et al., 1997). For example, compared to Whites, Hispanics prefer counseling over antidepressant medication (Cooper et al., 2003). These cultural differences are likely to lead to noncompliance, strained patient–provider relations, and untreated symptoms.

APPLYING THEORETICAL FRAMEWORKS TO CULTURE AND HEALTH BEHAVIOR

In this section, we review major theoretical frameworks used in preventive and behavioral medicine and public health research that identify various mechanisms through which culture influences behavior. Table 6.1 summarizes key information of theoretical

TABLE 6.1 Major Theories Applied in Examining the Role of Culture on Health and Health Behavior

THEORY	ORIGINS	ASSUMPTIONS	CONSTRUCTS	STRENGTHS*	WEAKNESSES*
		Individual-Level Theories			
Folk/Cultural Model	Developed by Shore in 1996; roots in cognitive anthropology.	Members of a group or society share cultural models, which are not fixed but malleable through the individual's personal experiences.	Cultural models	– Can be directly applied to the role of culture on various health outcomes and behaviors. – Can explain differences within a subgroup. – Allows for individual variation in cultural models.	– May be difficult to measure cultural models. – Not explicit in addressing how dominant themes in cultural models may change across generations, or how multiple cultures may interact with one another.
Prototype Theory	Developed by Eleanor Rosch and colleagues in the 1970s. Influenced by cognitive theory.	All concepts are organized around a prototype; individuals develop categorization systems in order to understand the environment and deal with the overwhelming stimuli in it (Rosch et al., 1976).	Prototypes (basic level and informative categories)	– Useful in understanding biases that affect perceptions and behaviors of patients and providers alike.	– Certain prototypes (e.g., normative forms of exercise) may not be consistent across cultures. – Provides limited mechanisms through which health behavior change can be achieved.
Health Belief Model (HBM)	An expectancy value theory developed in the 1950s by social psychologists (Rosenstock, 1966). Influenced by stimulus–response theory and cognitive theory.	Individuals are rational actors who value health, want to avoid illness, and believe that a specific health action will prevent illness.	– Perceived illness susceptibility – Perceived illness severity – Perceived benefits of change – Perceived barriers – Cues to action (eventually dropped from model) – Self-efficacy (later added to the model)	– Considers cultural issues that translate into notions of barriers and susceptibility. – Takes individual's perceptions and beliefs into account rather relying on global measures.	– Assumptions may not be valid for all populations (e.g., good health may not be a high priority or hold high value, or may not be believed to be under an individual's control, i.e., "God's will").

(continued)

TABLE 6.1 Major Theories Applied in Examining the Role of Culture on Health and Health Behavior (continued)

THEORY	ORIGINS	ASSUMPTIONS	CONSTRUCTS	STRENGTHS*	WEAKNESSES*
Theory of Reasoned Action/Theory of Planned Behavior (TRA/TPB)	TRA developed by Azjen and Fishbein in the 1960s; Azjen added perceived behavioral control to form TPB in 1986. TRA/TPB are expectancy value theories with roots in social psychology.	Individuals are rational actors. Intention directly precedes and predicts behavior.	– Behavioral intention – Attitudes (behavioral beliefs weighted by evaluation of behavioral outcomes) – Subjective norm (normative beliefs weighted by motivation to comply) – Perceived behavioral control (control beliefs weighted by perceived power)	– Cultural context partially addressed through attitudes. – Call for formative research on target populations prior to developing instruments and interventions allows for cross-cultural applicability of this theory.	– Assumptions may not be valid for the population of interest (e.g., behavioral intent may not be a strong predictor of behavior change due to other barriers).
Integrated Behavioral Model (IBM)	An extension of the TRA/TPB that includes major constructs from other theories (Montano & Kasprzyk, 2008).	Intention directly precedes and predicts behavior.	– Behavioral intention – Attitudes (experiential and instrumental attitudes) – Perceived norm (injunctive and descriptive norms) – Personal agency (perceived control and self-efficacy) – Knowledge and skills to perform the behavior – Salience of behavior – Environmental constraints – Habit intention	– Allows the relative importance of various constructs to vary in determining behavioral intention for different behaviors and populations. – Surveys assessing this model's constructs can be designed to consider cultural issues.	– Relatively new theory that has not been extensively tested among interventions targeting culturally and/or linguistically diverse populations.

Interpersonal-Level Theories

Operant Theory	Initially proposed by BF Skinner in late 1950s–1960s. Roots in psychology and informed by laboratory behavioral studies.	Behavioral antecedents and consequences regulate behavior (Glenn, Ellis, & Greenspoon, 1992; Skinner, 1969, 1983). – Contingencies/consequences – Positive and negative reinforcement – Positive and negative punishment – Antecedents (also known as discriminant stimuli)	– Considers the role of culture in determining what events become antecedents or discriminative stimuli for a particular behavior. – Considers how culturally dominant values may affect the reinforcing or punishing value of a contingency. – Can be used to understand how population-level behavior is shaped through cultural transmission (Skinner, 1969).	– Assumes that behaviors are largely shaped by immediate antecedents and consequences, with less emphasis on the effect of intermediate and long-term consequences. – Discounts the influence of cognitive factors.
Social Cognitive Theory (SCT)	Developed by Albert Bandura in 1986; influenced by cognitive models and Operant Theory.	Individuals are able to symbolize behavior, learn through observation, anticipate outcomes of behavior, be confident in performing behavior, reflect on and analyze experiences, and self-regulate behavior (Baranowski, Cullen, Nicklas, Thompson, & Baranowski, 2002). – Reciprocal determinism – Observational learning/modeling – Self-efficacy – Outcome expectancies – Reinforcements – Emotional coping responses – Behavioral capability – Self-regulation/control – Environment	– Useful to guide understanding of how cultural beliefs can influence behavior via reciprocal determinism and outcome expectancies. – Modeling construct provides opportunities to develop interventions that are culturally specific.	– Lacks specificity regarding the mechanism by which culture influences theoretical constructs and ultimately health behaviors.

(continued)

TABLE 6.1 Major Theories Applied in Examining the Role of Culture on Health and Health Behavior (continued)

THEORY	ORIGINS	ASSUMPTIONS	CONSTRUCTS	STRENGTHS*	WEAKNESSES*
		Community-Level Theories			
Communication/ Persuasion Model	Developed by McGuire in the late 1970s and 1980s. Primarily used in advertising.	Communication output steps must be completed in chronological order before a desired behavior change can be achieved. Individuals are rational actors.	– Input communication factors (source, message, channel, receiver, destination) – Output communication factors/steps (tuning in, attending, liking, comprehending, generating related cognitions, acquiring appropriate skills, agreeing, storing, retrieving, decision-acting, acting, post-action integration, converting)	– Model provides opportunity for "diversity and culture to be considered at each of the decision points when developing campaigns that target culturally diverse population subgroups" (Kreuter & McClure, 2004).	– Interventions focusing solely on communicating messages on health without addressing actual barriers may increase health disparities (Corcoran, 2007).
		Ecological Models			
Social Ecological Model	An ecologic model derived from the work of Bronfenbrenner (1986) to investigate complex, multi-level influences contributing to health and health behaviors.	Health is influenced by multiple aspects of physical and social environments. Environments are multidimensional. Human–environment interactions can be described at varying levels of organization. Individuals may influence various levels of the environments in which they live.	– Levels of influence (intrapersonal factors, interpersonal influences, behavioral settings, sectors of influence, overarching sociocultural and political context) – Reciprocal causation	– The "expression of cultural pathways in terms of everyday practices and routines" is explicitly identified and included in this model, which can inform the design of health promotion interventions (Weisner, 2002).	– Does not explicitly consider the interplay of multiple cultural influences and how they impact the inner levels.
Ecosocial Theory	A population theory of disease distribution (Krieger, 1994). Builds on the theory of the social production of disease.	Populations are greater than the sum of individuals. Diseases are caused by our biological incorporation of the social and material conditions of the environments in which we live across the life course.	– Embodiment – Pathways of embodiment – Cumulative interplay between susceptibility, exposure, and resistance – Accountability and agency	– Comprehensive nature (socio-cultural, biological, historical). – Includes agency and accountability in examining health disparities.	– Researchers can only test a small portion of the complex relationship of causes and levels.

*Refers specifically to strengths and weaknesses of the theories/models in their application to culture and health.

frameworks or models that have been useful in understanding cultural influences on health and health behaviors, including strengths and weaknesses of each theory or model with respect to understanding cultural influences on health, followed by application of these theories to health behavior change and research. Several well-known theories emphasize the role of cognition on human behavior, including the Folk Model (otherwise known as the Cultural Model) (Shore, 1996), Prototype Theory (Rosch, Mervis, Gray, Johnson, & Bayes-Braem, 1976), the Health Belief Model (HBM) (Becker, 1974; Janz & Becker, 1984), and the Theory of Reasoned Action/Theory of Planned Behavior (TRA/TPB). Others, such as the Social Cognitive (Bandura, 1986) and Operant (Skinner, 1953, 1969, 1983) theories, explicitly emphasize dynamic interactions between the individual and the environment in shaping the development of behavior. Over the past decade, there has been greater recognition of the need to expand current theoretical frameworks and models to identify various levels of the social and physical environment that allow us to better understand and predict health-related behavior (Matson-Koffman, Brownstein, Neiner, & Greaney, 2005), and intervene to change behaviors with the ultimate purpose of improving health (i.e., Social Ecological Models). Many of these theories and models are discussed in more depth in the chapters in Section 1 of this book.

THE FOLK/CULTURAL MODEL

The Folk Model proposes that behavior is influenced by "cultural models," thought of as loose, interpretative frameworks or cognitive categories used by people to understand the world and human behavior. These models may be transmitted consciously and unconsciously, and/or overtly or subtly, between members of a group. The Folk Model (Holy & Stuchlik, 1981; Shore, 1996) can be useful in explaining phenomena such as low mammogram screening rates among Asian Americans (described previously), as dominant cultural beliefs related to health (e.g., illness is part of the life cycle) can affect participation in preventive health behaviors among this group. These models and resulting behaviors may be shaped overtly through verbal statements regarding health or health behaviors or by watching how people deal with illness, treatment, diagnoses, and the health care system. The Folk Model can also explain individual differences in behaviors within a subgroup. Since cultural models are not fixed but malleable, individual experiences can either reinforce or challenge the current model (Shore, 1996). In the example of screening behaviors among Asian American women, personal experiences (e.g., interactions with a co-worker who was diagnosed with breast cancer in early stage through mammography) can modify these cultural models and thus influence that individual's behavior.

PROTOTYPE THEORY

Prototype theory proposes that given the complexity of the stimuli in our world, individuals develop categorization systems in order to understand the environment and deal with the overwhelming stimuli in it (Rosch et al., 1976). An individual then bases his or her judgments and decisions regarding a behavior, person, or object on the similarity between its features and the prototype (Cantor & Mischel, 1979). The types of prototypes that one has are likely to differ depending on one's culture. For instance, an individual's prototype of a healthy diet is likely to differ depending on: (1) who the individual is and what that individual has learned through his or her own culture about what constitutes a healthy diet, and (2) what the individual's personal experience has been with respect to exposure to foods or diets that are considered "healthy." Another type of prototype is "exemplary" examples for different categories (Lakoff, 1982). In the clinical setting, physicians may first recommend jogging outside or joining a gym in discussing exercise with a patient, which may not be normative or applicable forms of exercise to that patient. Additional levels of complexities around prototypes include individuals' own perceptions of prototypes regarding objects, cultures, and social and behavioral patterns associated with those objects or cultures. For example, a physician may hold a prototype about Hispanic individuals being less likely to engage in exercise, which may prevent that physician from encouraging or discussing physical activity during the clinical visit. Alternatively, a patient may hold a prototype about a food diary (i.e., calorie counting and food monitoring are only done by people who have eating disorders or body image issues), which in turn inhibits willingness to be open to self-monitoring diet for weight loss.

HEALTH BELIEF MODEL (HBM)

The HBM (Becker, 1974; Janz & Becker, 1984) is a expectancy-value theory. According to HBM, people will take action to prevent, screen for, or control their health conditions if they believe they are susceptible to disease (perceived susceptibility), the disease will have serious consequences (perceived severity), there are benefits to engaging in the behavior (perceived benefits), and there are few barriers that prevent this behavior (perceived barriers). Thus, an individual will weigh perceived susceptibility and severity of the disease against the balance of benefits and barriers to making those changes. HBM can be useful in our understanding of the influence of culturally based beliefs on health-related behaviors described in previous sections. For example, the HBM has been used to develop interventions that promote mammography screening and that target risky sexual behaviors among adults in various ethnic groups (Champion et al., 2006; Wight, Abraham, & Scott, 1998).

THEORY OF REASONED ACTION/THEORY OF PLANNED BEHAVIOR (TRA/TPB) AND INTEGRATED BEHAVIORAL MODEL (IBM)

TRA/TPB is one of the few theories that explicitly calls for formative research on target populations, and thus is very useful for understanding cultural influences that may drive differences in behavior across various racial/ethnic and cultural groups. TPB posits that individuals' behavioral attitudes, subjective norm, and perceived behavioral control influence individuals' behavioral intention (perceived likelihood of engaging in the behavior), which is thought to predict and directly precede behavior change. TRA/TPB has been applied to a variety of health behaviors (exercise, smoking, drug use, risky sexual behaviors, mammography, and oral hygiene). The Integrated Behavioral Model (IBM) is an extension of the TRA/TPB and incorporates important constructs from other major theories of health behavior, such as knowledge and skills to perform a behavior and self-efficacy. Similar to TRA/TPB, the IBM has cross-cultural applicability to various health behaviors, outcomes, and target populations, as surveys assessing IBM's constructs can be designed to consider cultural issues. One example of how this relatively new theory has been used within the context of culture and health behavior is the application of the IBM to HIV prevention among rural residents in Zimbabwe (Montano & Kasprzyk, 2008). Guided by the IBM constructs, formative research was conducted to identify behavioral, normative, and efficacy beliefs related to behavioral intention of using condoms with steady partners.

OPERANT THEORY

Operant Theory proposes that behavioral antecedents and consequences regulate behavior (Glenn, Ellis, & Greenspoon, 1992; Skinner, 1969, 1983). The same general principles of discriminative stimuli, reinforcers, and punishers used to explain individual behavior in accordance with Operant Theory are applied to understand the behavior of groups and entire cultures, and have been applied to acculturation (Landrine & Klonoff, 2004). *Antecedents* are any feature of the context or environment that signal whether and what contingencies will follow a behavior, whereas *consequences* are events that occur contingent upon the behavior of interest which either increase (though reinforcement) or decrease (through punishment) the probability of occurrence of that behavior (Skinner, 1953, 1969, 1983). Culture determines what events become antecedents or discriminative stimuli for the occurrence of a particular behavior. For example, antecedent factors may play a role in increased drinking among acculturated Hispanic women. The social acceptance in the United States of higher amounts of alcohol consumption by women, as well as a variety of environmental cues for drinking (e.g., media promoting drinking), may partially contribute to higher rates of drinking among highly acculturated Hispanic women, regardless of country of origin (Black & Markides, 1993; Lara et al., 2005; Marks, Garcia, & Solis, 1990), than less acculturated Hispanic women. With regard to consequences or contingencies, the culturally dominant values of the individual culture affect, at least partly, the reinforcing or punishing value of a contingency. Contingencies that explain how behavior at the population level is shaped (relevant to cultural transmission) are known as *meta-contingencies* or *cultural contingencies* (Skinner, 1969).

SOCIAL COGNITIVE THEORY (SCT)

SCT is one of the most commonly used theoretical frameworks in behavioral science (Bandura, 1986). The theory posits that human behavior is the result of a triadic, dynamic, and reciprocal interaction of personal factors, behavior, and the environment, and mediated by cognitive processes. This model has had great applicability in understanding individual behavior and has potential for use in understanding culturally based group behavior. For instance, the low rates of breast cancer screening among Asian and Black populations (described previously) can be explained by weak outcome expectations regarding screening mammograms. Likewise, cultural beliefs leading to lack of trust in the health care system within the Black community can affect beliefs that they will adhere to a prescribed medication regimen (self-efficacy) and that taking a prescribed medication (e.g., antihypertensives) will reduce their risk of stroke (outcome expectation). Another important feature of the SCT relevant to the study of culture, cultural transmission, and acculturation is the construct of modeling. Observation of others' behavior and their consequences plays a role in transfer of culture among individuals by communicating what behaviors will be rewarded or punished in what contexts (Iversen & Lattal, 1991). SCT has been used to guide interventions targeting numerous behaviors and used among both child and adult populations. For example, SCT has been applied in conjunction with other theories to guide culturally tailored interventions to reduce obesity and to enhance diabetes control among low-income Hispanic populations (Drieling, Ma, & Stafford, 2011; Merriam et al., 2009; Rosal et al., 2009).

COMMUNICATION/PERSUASION MODEL

The Communication/Persuasion Model emphasizes the importance of sources, message content, channels, target audience, and effects when communicating messages.

Within the context of culture and health, this model provides valuable opportunities for health providers, researchers, and other health professionals to tailor the delivery, receptiveness, and effectiveness of health communication strategies in order to target knowledge, attitudes, and behaviors related to health. The Communication/Persuasion Model has been applied extensively to the development of health-communication-based interventions across diverse populations by specifically focusing on the source, message, and channel factors of the model (Kreuter & McClure, 2004). The North Carolina Native American Cervical Cancer Prevention Project trained local Native American women to deliver a cervical cancer educational intervention to other tribal women (thus matching the source of the message to the target population) (Messler, Steckler, & Dignan, 1999). Results indicated that the intervention was well received and was associated with increased self-reported rates of receiving a Pap test compared to a control group. Another example is the incorporation of cultural values, such as racial pride and spirituality, in health-related messages in a magazine-based intervention promoting fruit and vegetable consumption and mammography among African American women (Kreuter et al., 2004).

THE SOCIAL ECOLOGICAL MODEL

Ecological models focus on the interactions of people with their physical and socio-cultural environments and the impact that these interactions have on the individual's behavior. Levels of influence include intrapersonal, interpersonal, organizational, environmental, and socio-cultural. Interactions between levels of influence may shape health-related behaviors that in turn affect health outcomes. The Social Ecological Model explicitly acknowledges the role of culture on health-related behavior (Stokols, 1992, 1996). Cultural norms, values, and traditions around health-related behaviors, such as eating, physical activity, sexual practices, health screening, and drug use, can heavily influence patterns in health behaviors and outcomes between cultural groups (Sorensen et al., 2003; Stokols, 1996). Previous studies have utilized the Social Ecological Model to develop culturally sensitive health behavior interventions targeting cancer prevention, fruit and vegetable consumption, and tobacco cessation (Sorensen, Barbeau, Hunt, & Emmons, 2004; Sorensen et al., 2003; Sorensen et al., 2007). Multi-level modeling can be used to isolate the unique contribution of higher-level factors, such as the built physical and socio-cultural environment, in influencing health behaviors and outcomes while adjusting for individual-level characteristics and behaviors. An adaptation of the Social Ecological Model by the Institute of Medicine (IOM) (Koplan, Liverman, & Kraak, 2005) specific to childhood obesity prevention efforts restructured the Social Ecological Model by specifying particular behavioral settings (i.e., home, school, worksites, and communities) and sectors of influence (i.e., government, public health, health care, education, media, and transportation). The identification of the culturally influenced and culture-influencing sectors, such as the media industry, and the consideration of cultural factors that may differ across behavioral settings (e.g., cultural norms and practices in the home may be different from those in the school and work settings), may be helpful in considering the multitude of ways in which culture may impact a wide range of health behaviors and outcomes.

ECOSOCIAL THEORY

According to Ecosocial Theory (Krieger, 1994), there are numerous pathways of how individuals literally embody, biologically, the material and social world around them.

For example, in examining the role of race-based discrimination on health and health disparities, higher incidence and prevalence of numerous adverse health outcomes and behaviors among racial/ethnic minority groups relative to Whites in the United States may occur via several pathways/mechanisms (Krieger, 2001). These include: (1) *economic and social deprivation* (racial/ethnic minority groups are historically poorer due in part to race-based policies around education, occupation, and housing; thus, lower socioeconomic resources limit these groups' ability to engage in certain healthy behaviors and be healthy as well as limit their ability to live in neighborhoods with access to healthy produce and physical activity facilities) (Williams, 1999); (2) *socially inflicted trauma* (perceived discrimination has been shown to be linked with higher stress and hypertension) (Din-Dzietham, Nembhard, Collins, & Davis, 2004; Roberts, Vines, Kaufman, & James, 2008; Sims et al., 2012); (3) *targeted marketing* (Blacks have been specifically targeted by tobacco companies in the United States) (Cruz, Wright, & Crawford, 2010; Henriksen, Schleicher, Dauphinee, & Fortmann, 2012; Sutton & Robinson, 2004); (4) *inadequate or reduced access to health care* (poorer detection and management of hypertension among Blacks have been shown to increase risk of untreated and uncontrolled hypertension) (Strumpf, 2011; Svetkey et al., 1996; Weech-Maldonado, Hall, Bryant, Jenkins, & Elliott, 2012); and (5) *exposure to toxic environments* (residential segregation has led to a higher percentage of minority racial/ethnic groups living in neighborhoods with higher levels of pollution, less green space, and substandard housing, which contributes to disparities in outcomes such as asthma and lead poisoning) (Jacobs, 2011; Lanphear, Weitzman, & Eberly, 1996).

INCORPORATING CULTURE INTO HEALTH CARE AND RESEARCH: METHODS AND RECOMMENDATIONS

The goals of medicine and public health are to deliver evidence-based interventions that maintain health, prevent and manage chronic disease, and decrease human suffering. However, many existing evidence-based interventions are based on randomized controlled trials conducted on predominantly White, middle-class populations. Considerable gaps exist with regard to behavioral interventions that have been shown to be effective for individuals from other racial/ethnic and SES backgrounds. Given the increasing diversity of the American population and persisting health disparities between racial/ethnic and disadvantaged groups, translating evidence-based interventions to benefit those bearing the greatest burden of disease is of utmost importance. Systematic strategies for translating evidence-based interventions to be culturally responsive, as well as the development of new approaches or interventions based on the needs of these populations, have the potential to significantly advance the field and enhance the health of all individuals (Ang et al., 2002; Escarce, Epstein, Colby, & Schwartz, 1993; Ford & Cooper, 1995; Hannan et al., 1999; Keppel, 2007; Lee, Gehlbach, Hosmer, Reti, & Baker, 1997; Shi, 1999; Smedley, Stith, & Nelson, 2003; Suarez-Almazor et al., 2005). The next section synthesizes the literature with regard to strategies to incorporate culture in clinical and population-based research and, ultimately, in health care.

QUALITATIVE METHODOLOGIES

Qualitative methodologies are an important tool in health disparity research to gain in-depth understanding about individual and population-level cultural factors associated with the disparities, in particular deep cultural structures (Kreuter et al., 2003; Resnicow, Braithwaite, & Glanz, 2002). Commonly used qualitative methods include focus groups, a facilitated small-group discussion among selected individuals on a particular topic; and in-depth interviews (also referred to as key informant interviews), which are semi-structured guided interviews that include open-ended questions. Formative research that incorporates qualitative methods gives researchers the means of uncovering deeply seated beliefs, values, and practices specific to that culture that are relevant to a particular health disparity and which can be targeted in interventions aimed at eliminating the disparity (Resnicow et al., 1999). Qualitative methods can also provide important information about preferences for intervention, such as strategies to which a particular community might be receptive. For instance, through qualitative methods, researchers have uncovered that African Americans and Hispanics share beliefs that the government facilitates the spread of HIV among their communities (Bogart & Thorburn, 2005; Essien, Meshack, & Ross, 2002), and that these groups differ from Whites in that they report being more likely to receive HIV/AIDS information from "media" compared to "professionals or government agencies" (Essien, Ross, Linares, & Osemene, 2000). Tailoring behavioral interventions to be culturally responsive is a promising strategy for addressing health disparities among diverse populations.

The following example illustrates the use of qualitative data for tailoring a self-management intervention to low-income middle-aged and elderly Hispanic patients with uncontrolled diabetes. Findings from focus groups and key informant interviews revealed that participants had difficulty remembering health messages presented in a didactic format, but enjoyed and remembered information presented in a soap opera. This knowledge was used to develop an innovative educational drama or soap opera to be used as the core component of a diabetes self-management intervention (Rosal et al., 2009). This soap opera sought to promote models for positive attitudinal change toward diabetes self-care and modeled the implementation of basic diabetes self-management principles. Additional focus groups were used to pre-test its use with the target population, which facilitated the development of a discussion guide to highlight key themes for each episode and thus maximize its effectiveness (Rosal, Ockene, et al., 2011).

Qualitative methods, in particular cognitive interviewing, are also valuable in pre-testing intervention materials for clarity, feasibility, and acceptability. Cognitive interviewing has been used to assess the cultural appropriateness of specific intervention materials for a given population. It involves eliciting the verbalization of thoughts, feelings, interpretations, and ideas that come to mind ("think aloud") while examining specific materials or survey questions (Willis, 1994). Respondents are also asked to suggest alternative wording to increase comprehension. Lessons from this process can inform the revision of materials prior to a larger-scale use. Cognitive interview techniques have been used in the development of interactive nutrition messages for low-income populations (Carbone, Campbell, & Honess-Morreale, 2002).

COMMUNITY-BASED PARTICIPATORY RESEARCH

Community-based participatory research (CBPR) is defined as research conducted as a collaborative, equal partnership between researchers or trained experts and members of a community (Minkler & Wallerstein, 2008). CBPR actively engages community members and organizations in all aspects and products of the research process (Minkler & Wallerstein, 2008), ensuring that the research question is relevant to the socio-cultural context of the community, the research design and methods are compatible with the culture, and the research outcomes are interpreted in a manner that takes all aspects of the target community into consideration. For example, CBPR was used to examine cultural factors related to Pap testing practices among Vietnamese American immigrant women (Nguyen-Truong et al., 2012). Lower perceived cultural barriers (e.g., lack of family support and use of Eastern/Asian medicine) were associated with increased adherence to recommended Pap testing practices among Vietnamese American immigrant women (Nguyen-Truong et al., 2012). Findings from this CBPR study provided valuable information on the topics and skills that needed to be addressed in interventions targeting screening for this population.

Academic–community partnerships have considerable potential to facilitate the cultural translation of evidence-based interventions to enhance health behaviors and decrease disease risk. For example, in translating the Diabetes Prevention Program (DPP) lifestyle intervention for facilitating postpartum weight loss among culturally diverse low-income postpartum women, academic researchers collaborated with leadership, staff, and clients of a Women, Infants, and Children (WIC) program in Massachusetts to adapt the intervention to the WIC population and setting (Rosal, Lemon, Nguyen, Driscoll, & DiTaranto, 2011).

CROSS-CULTURAL ADAPTATION OF MEASUREMENT INSTRUMENTS

Currently, there is a need for validated instruments that can be used across cultures to improve medical and public health research, health care delivery, and health outcomes. For example, the interpretation of QoL can vary widely based on cultural differences in the values, beliefs, norms, and behaviors practiced daily by individuals; thus, the assessment of QoL has to reflect those differences and requires rigorous qualitative and quantitative methodology to adapt existing instruments, with the end result being an equivalent, rather than a literal, translation of the original instrument (Chwalow, 1995; Gjersing, Caplehorn, & Clausen, 2010; Symon et al., 2012). Many QoL measures examining a variety of health outcomes have been adapted to reflect cultural differences in this construct. Another example relates to the measurement of dietary intake. Validated dietary measures were developed based on the inclusion of Western-based foods, portion sizes, and recipes; other ethnic foods (i.e., plantains and fried rice) are largely missing, and thus the tools cannot accurately assess the dietary patterns of diverse populations or capture the true association between diet and health outcomes. Additionally, attention to literacy level and linguistic variations is critical to the validity of measurement tools for use with diverse groups. Literal translations may not accurately capture the intended meaning of the questions or responses of surveys, and the literacy level of the original or translated versions of a measurement tool may not be appropriate for the population of interest. Utilization of cognitive interviewing strategies (described earlier) helps enhance the literacy and linguistic appropriateness of a particular assessment instrument. Cognitive interview techniques (described earlier) have been used in the development of psychosocial and behavioral measurement instruments for low-income populations (Carbone et al., 2002; Elasy et al., 2000; Rosal, Carbone, & Goins, 2003).

CULTURAL COMPETENCY OF HEALTH CARE PROVIDERS

Up to this point, we have primarily discussed culture as it relates to research on the behavior of individuals and diverse communities. However, the cultures of health care and public health providers are also of great importance in the context of developing and delivering interventions to culturally diverse populations. Research indicates that physicians' cultural biases have the potential to adversely affect patients. Several studies indicate that patients who are racially concordant with their physician are more likely to receive HIV treatment than if the provider is Caucasian and the patient is Black (King, Wong, Shapiro, Landon, & Cunningham, 2004). Stereotypical perceptions of patient adherence may account for the greater delay in HIV treatment among Blacks and Hispanics than Caucasians (Turner et al., 2000) through health care providers' beliefs regarding adherence to Highly Active Anti-Retroviral Treatment (HAART) by Blacks and Hispanics; these beliefs may influence provision and prescriptions of HIV medications to these populations (Bogart, Catz, Kelly, & Benotsch, 2001; Bogart, Kelly, Catz, & Sosman, 2000; Wong et al., 2004). Enhancing providers' cultural competence has the potential to improve health outcomes of ethnically and culturally diverse individuals (Betancourt, 2006; Betancourt, Green, Carrillo, & Ananeh-Firempong, 2003). To this end, it is essential that providers be aware of their ethnocentric tendencies, identify how personally held prototypes of certain groups may impact their interactions with the populations they serve (Harris-Davis & Haughton, 2000), and be proactive in learning about cultural differences relevant to populations they serve. In contrast, less is known about cultural factors and biases of non-physician health care providers (i.e., allied providers) and their influence on patient behavior change, indicating the need for further studies that examine this particular population of health care providers.

METHODS FOR IMPLEMENTING CULTURALLY APPROPRIATE INTERVENTIONS

A recent review of the effectiveness of culturally appropriate interventions to prevent or manage chronic disease in culturally and linguistically diverse communities (Henderson, Kendall, & See, 2011) identified five main methodologies used to implement these types of interventions: the use of community-based bilingual health workers; providing cultural-competency training for health workers; using interpreter services; using multimedia and culturally sensitive videos; and establishing community point-of-care services for people with chronic disease. Results from this review indicated that the use of trained bilingual and culturally competent community health workers was associated with greater uptake of disease prevention strategies by the communities targeted and that delivery of health programs by community members is deemed to be culturally sensitive and appropriate by the community served. However, the number of studies that have assessed the effectiveness of these types of interventions is small (24 studies fit the inclusion and exclusion criteria for this review), indicating the need for additional research to inform and disseminate interventions that are culturally, linguistically, and economically relevant to target populations.

Current literature indicates that additional research is needed to determine the most effective strategies to build cultural competence among clinical and public health providers. There is evidence that cultural-competency training (i.e., enhancing providers' communication skills, providing educational sessions on cultural awareness, sensitivity, and competence) is associated with better communication between patients and providers (Bischoff, Perneger, Bovier, Loutan, & Stalder, 2003; Majumdar, Browne, Roberts, & Carpio, 2004), and increased provider cultural awareness and understanding of cultural differences. In addition, patients of health care professionals who completed cultural-competency training have shown increased use of social resources and greater functional capacity following provider cultural-competency training (Chevannes, 2002; Henderson et al., 2011; Majumdar et al., 2004; Schim, Doorenbos, & Borse, 2006). Strategies that help providers to translate the knowledge gained from this training to practice are critical (Chevannes, 2002).

CONCLUSIONS

Cultural awareness, competence, and sensitivity can enhance the role of health care providers and researchers alike. For providers, understanding the role and impact of culture on health can improve patient–provider communication and potentially the effectiveness of the provider in facilitating behavioral change and/or addressing the underlying causes of adverse health outcomes for the patient. For researchers, cultural understanding, as outlined in the following four ways, can enhance the development of interventions and subsequent evaluations compatible with the cultural needs and traditions of diverse populations. First, understanding the function of behaviors of interest within a culture can facilitate the understanding of factors that maintain those behaviors. Second, capitalizing on elements of cultures that support adherence to desirable health behaviors can work in favor of cultural compatibility of interventions. Third, studying cultural factors relevant to specific groups can assist in the choice of variables, methodologies, and measurements. Finally, researchers' cultural competence will be crucial to recruiting representative culturally diverse individuals into research studies and retaining these individuals until study completion so that conclusive statements can be made about the generalizability of the interventions.

As the United States continues to increase its diversity, addressing health care needs of diverse populations has become a critical priority, highlighting the importance of greater cultural awareness, a comprehensive theoretical and empirical understanding of how specific cultural factors within diverse groups influence health behaviors and, ultimately, the ability to utilize limited health care resources to improve the health of our culturally diverse population. Much of our understanding of culture and its influences on behavior is theoretical and retrospective. Recommendations for future research on culture and health to advance the field include utilization of well-studied models for program planning, implementation, and evaluation; the development of new models that further expand and facilitate our understanding of culture; and exploration of models from other disciplines such as sociology and anthropology. The iterative process of research, development of cultural-competency training and culturally appropriate interventions, and evaluation of these programs is essential to better serve the health needs of a nation and of a world increasing in cultural diversity. The implementation and dissemination of effective methodologies and practices based on these findings are essential to making significant improvements in health behaviors and outcomes at the individual and population level.

REFERENCES

Allinson, R. E. (1989). *Understanding the Chinese mind.* Hong Kong: Oxford University Press.

American Psychiatric Association. (2000). *Diagnostic and statistical manual of mental disorders* (4th ed.). Washington, DC: Author.

American Psychiatric Association. (2013). *Diagnostic and statistical manual of mental disorders* (5th ed.). Washington, DC: American Psychiatric Publishing.

Ang, D. C., Ibrahim, S. A., Burant, C. J., Siminoff, L. A., & Kwoh, C. K. (2002). Ethnic differences in the perception of prayer and consideration of joint arthroplasty. *Medical Care, 40*(6), 471–476.

Ata, A., Elzey, J. D., Insaf, T. Z., Grau, A. M., Stain, S. C., & Ahmed, N. U. (2006). Colorectal cancer prevention: Adherence patterns and correlates of tests done for screening purposes within United States populations. *Cancer Detection and Prevention, 30*(2), 134–143.

Bandura, A. (1986). *Social foundation of thought and action: A social cognitive theory.* Englewood Cliffs, NJ: Prentice-Hall.

Banna, J. C., Kaiser, L. L., Drake, C., & Townsend, M. S. (2012). Acculturation, physical activity and television viewing in Hispanic women: Findings from the 2005 California Women's Health Survey. *Public Health Nutrition, 15*(2), 198–207.

Baranowski, T., Cullen, K. W., Nicklas, T., Thompson, D., & Baranowski, J. (2002). School-based obesity prevention: A blueprint for taming the epidemic. *American Journal of Health Behavior, 26*(6), 486–493.

Becker, M. H. (1974). The health belief model and personal health behavior. *Health Education Monographs, 2*, 324–473.

Berry, J. W., Poortinga, Y. H., Segall, M. H., & Dasen, P. R. (1992). *Cross-cultural psychology: Research and applications.* New York, NY: Cambridge University Press.

Betancourt, J. R. (2006). Cultural competency: Providing quality care to diverse populations. *Consultant Pharmacist, 21*(12), 988–995.

Betancourt, J. R., Green, A. R., Carrillo, J. E., & Ananeh-Firempong, O., 2nd. (2003). Defining cultural competence: A practical framework for addressing racial/ethnic disparities in health and health care. *Public Health Reports, 118*(4), 293–302.

Bhopal, R. (2004). Glossary of terms relating to ethnicity and race: For reflection and debate. *Journal of Epidemiology and Community Health, 58*(6), 441–445.

Bhopal, R., & Donaldson, L. (1998). White, European, Western, Caucasian, or what? Inappropriate labeling in research on race, ethnicity, and health. *American Journal of Public Health, 88*(9), 1303–1307.

Bischoff, A., Perneger, T. V., Bovier, P. A., Loutan, L., & Stalder, H. (2003). Improving communication between physicians and patients who speak a foreign language. *British Journal of General Practice, 53*(492), 541–546.

Black, S. A., & Markides, K. S. (1993). Acculturation and alcohol consumption in Puerto Rican, Cuban-American, and Mexican-American women in the United States. *American Journal of Public Health, 83*(6), 890–893.

Bogart, L. M., & Bird, S. T. (2003). Exploring the relationship of conspiracy beliefs about HIV/AIDS to sexual behaviors and attitudes among African-American adults. *Journal of the National Medical Association, 95*(11), 1057–1065.

Bogart, L. M., Catz, S. L., Kelly, J. A., & Benotsch, E. G. (2001). Factors influencing physicians' judgments of adherence and treatment decisions for patients with HIV disease. *Medical Decision Making, 21*(1), 28–36.

Bogart, L. M., Kelly, J. A., Catz, S. L., & Sosman, J. M. (2000). Impact of medical and nonmedical factors on physician decision making for HIV/AIDS antiretroviral treatment. *Journal of Acquired Immune Deficiency, 23*(5), 396–404.

Bogart, L. M., & Thorburn, S. (2005). Are HIV/AIDS conspiracy beliefs a barrier to HIV prevention among African Americans? *Journal of Acquired Immune Deficiency, 38*(2), 213–218.

Boltri, J. M., Okosun, I. S., Davis-Smith, M., & Vogel, R. L. (2005). Hemoglobin A1c levels in diagnosed and undiagnosed black, Hispanic, and white persons with diabetes: Results from NHANES 1999–2000. *Ethnicity & Disease, 15*(4), 562–567.

Borrayo, E. A., & Guarnaccia, C. A. (2000). Differences in Mexican-born and U.S.-born women of Mexican descent regarding factors related to breast cancer screening behaviors. *Health Care for Women International, 21*(7), 599–613.

Callahan, C. M., Drake, B. G., Heck, D. A., & Dittus, R. S. (1995). Patient outcomes following unicompartmental or bicompartmental knee arthroplasty. A meta-analysis. *Journal of Arthroplasty, 10*(2), 141–150.

Calvillo, E. R., & Flaskerud, J. H. (1991). Review of literature on culture and pain of adults with focus on Mexican-Americans. *Journal of Transcultural Nursing, 2*(2), 16–23.

Cantor, N., & Mischel, W. (1979). Prototypes in person perception. In L. Berkowitz (Ed.), *Advances in experimental social psychology* (Vol. 12, pp. 3–52). New York, NY: Academic Press.

Carbone, E. T., Campbell, M. K., & Honess-Morreale, L. (2002). Use of cognitive interview techniques in the development of nutrition surveys and interactive nutrition messages for low-income populations. *Journal of the American Dietetic Association, 102*(5), 690–696.

Carter-Pokras, O., & Bethune, L. (2009). Defining and measuring acculturation: A systematic review of public health studies with Hispanic populations in the United States. A commentary on Thomson and Hoffman-Goetz. [Comment]. *Social Science & Medicine, 69*(7), 992–995; discussion 999-1001. doi:10.1016/j.socscimed.2009.06.042

Centers for Disease Control and Prevention (CDC). (2007). Leading causes of death in females—United States, 2007. Retrieved August 6, 2012, from http://www.cdc.gov/women/lcod/index.htm#asian

CDC. (2011). Fact sheet: Prevalence of diabetes among Hispanics in six U.S. geographic locations. Retrieved September 2, 2012, from http://www.cdc.gov/diabetes/pubs/factsheets/hispanic.htm

CDC. (2011). Vital signs: Current cigarette smoking among adults aged >/=18 years–United States, 2005-2010. *MMWR. Morbidity and Mortality Weekly Report, 60*(35), 1207–1212.

Champion, V. L., Springston, J. K., Zollinger, T. W., Saywell, R. M., Jr., Monahan, P. O., Zhao, Q., & Russell, K. M. (2006). Comparison of three interventions to increase mammography screening in low income African American women. *Cancer Detection and Prevention, 30*(6), 535–544.

Chevannes, M. (2002). Issues in educating health professionals to meet the diverse needs of patients and other service users from ethnic minority groups. *Journal of Advanced Nursing, 39*(3), 290–298.

Chwalow, A. J. (1995). Cross-cultural validation of existing quality of life scales. *Patient Education and Counseling, 26*(1–3), 313–318.

Cooper, L. A., Gonzales, J. J., Gallo, J. J., Rost, K. M., Meredith, L. S., Rubenstein, L. V., & Ford, D. E. (2003). The acceptability of treatment for depression among African-American, Hispanic, and white primary care patients. *Medical Care, 41*(4), 479–489.

Cooper-Patrick, L., Powe, N. R., Jenckes, M. W., Gonzales, J. J., Levine, D. M., & Ford, D. E. (1997). Identification of patient attitudes and preferences regarding treatment of depression. *Journal of General Internal Medicine, 12*(7), 431–438.

Corcoran, N. (2007). Theories and models in communicating health messages. In N. Corcoran (Ed.), *Communicating health strategies for health promotion.* Thousand Oaks, CA: Sage.

Coughlin, S. S., Richards, T. B., Thompson, T., Miller, B. A., VanEenwyk, J., Goodman, M. T., & Sherman, R. L. (2006). Rural/nonrural differences in colorectal cancer incidence in the United States, 1998–2001. *Cancer, 107*(5 Suppl.), 1181–1188.

Cruz, T. B., Wright, L. T., & Crawford, G. (2010). The menthol marketing mix: Targeted promotions for focus communities in the United States. [Research Support, Non-U.S. Gov't]. *Nicotine & Tobacco Research, 12*(Suppl. 2), S147–153. doi:10.1093/ntr/ntq201

Din-Dzietham, R., Nembhard, W. N., Collins, R., & Davis, S. K. (2004). Perceived stress following race-based discrimination at work is associated with hypertension in African-Americans. The metro Atlanta heart disease study, 1999-2001. [Comparative Study Research Support, U.S. Gov't, P.H.S.]. *Social Science & Medicine, 58*(3), 449–461.

Drieling, R. L., Ma, J., & Stafford, R. S. (2011). Evaluating clinic and community-based lifestyle interventions for obesity reduction in a low-income Latino neighborhood: Vivamos Activos Fair Oaks Program. *BMC Public Health, 11*, 98.

Elasy, T. A., Samuel-Hodge, C. D., DeVellis, R. F., Skelly, A. H., Ammerman, A. S., & Keyserling, T. C. (2000). Development of a health status measure for older African-American women with type 2 diabetes. *Diabetes Care, 23*(3), 325–329.

Elder, J. P., Castro, F. G., de Moor, C., Mayer, J., Candelaria, J. I., Campbell, N., & Ware, L. M. (1991). Differences in cancer-risk-related behaviors in Latino and Anglo adults. *Preventive Medicine, 20*(6), 751–763.

Escarce, J. J., Epstein, K. R., Colby, D. C., & Schwartz, J. S. (1993). Racial differences in the elderly's use of medical procedures and diagnostic tests. *American Journal of Public Health, 83*(7), 948–954.

Essien, E. J., Meshack, A. F., & Ross, M. W. (2002). Misperceptions about HIV transmission among heterosexual African-American and Latino men and women. *Journal of the National Medical Association, 94*(5), 304–312.

Essien, E. J., Ross, M. W., Linares, A. C., & Osemene, N. I. (2000). Perception of reliability of human immunodeficiency virus/AIDS information sources. *Journal of the National Medical Association, 92*(6), 269–274.

Finney, M. F., Tumiel-Berhalter, L. M., Fox, C., & Jaen, C. R. (2006). Breast and cervical cancer screening for Puerto Ricans, African Americans, and non-Hispanic Whites attending inner-city family practice centers. *Ethnicity & Disease, 16*(4), 994–1000.

Foraker, R. E., Patten, C. A., Lopez, K. N., Croghan, I. T., & Thomas, J. L. (2005). Beliefs and attitudes regarding smoking among young adult Latinos: A pilot study. *Preventive Medicine, 41*(1), 126–133.

Ford, E. S., & Cooper, R. S. (1995). Racial/ethnic differences in health care utilization of cardiovascular procedures: A review of the evidence. *Health Services Research, 30*(1, Pt. 2), 237–252.

Foster, M. W. (2006). Analyzing the use of race and ethnicity in biomedical research from a local community perspective. *Journal of Law, Medicine & Ethics* (Fall), 34(3), 508–512.

Fraser, L. K., & Edwards, K. L. (2010). The association between the geography of fast food outlets and childhood obesity rates in Leeds, UK. *Health & Place, 16*(6), 1124–1128.

Fuentes-Afflick, E., & Hessol, N. A. (2008). Acculturation and body mass among Latina women. *Journal of Women's Health (2002), 17*(1), 67–73.

Garro, L. C. (2000). Remembering what one knows and the construction of the past: A comparison of cultural consensus theory and cultural schema theory. *Ethos, 3*, 275–319.

Gjersing, L., Caplehorn, J. R., & Clausen, T. (2010). Cross-cultural adaptation of research instruments: Language, setting, time and statistical considerations. *BMC Medical Research Methodology, 10*, 13.

Glenn, S. S., Ellis, J., & Greenspoon, J. (1992). On the revolutionary nature of the operant as a unit of behavioral selection. *American Psychologist, 47*(11), 1329–1336.

Goel, M. S., Wee, C. C., McCarthy, E. P., Davis, R. B., Ngo-Metzger, Q., & Phillips, R. S. (2003). Racial and ethnic disparities in cancer screening: The importance of foreign birth as a barrier to care. *Journal of General Internal Medicine, 18*(12), 1028–1035.

Gonzalez, H. M., Haan, M. N., & Hinton, L. (2001). Acculturation and the prevalence of depression in older Mexican Americans: Baseline results of the Sacramento Area Latino Study on Aging. *Journal of the American Geriatrics Society, 49*(7), 948–953.

Graham, A. C. (1990). *Studies in Chinese philosophy and philosophical literature.* Albany, NY: SUNY Press.

Grieco, E. M., Acosta, Y. D., de la Cruz, P., Gambino, C., Gyrn, T., Larsen, L. J., & Walter, N. P. (2012). The foreign-born population in the United States: 2010. *American Community Survey Reports.* Retrieved from http://www.census.gov/prod/2012pubs/acs-19.pdf

Hannan, E. L., van Ryn, M., Burke, J., Stone, D., Kumar, D., Arani, D., … DeBuono, B. A. (1999). Access to coronary artery bypass surgery by race/ethnicity and gender among patients who are appropriate for surgery. *Medical Care, 37*(1), 68–77.

Harris-Davis, E., & Haughton, B. (2000). Model for multicultural nutrition counseling competencies. *Journal of the American Dietetic Association, 100*(10), 1178–1185.

Hassmiller, K. M., Warner, K. E., Mendez, D., Levy, D. T., & Romano, E. (2003). Nondaily smokers: Who are they? [Research Support, Non-U.S. Gov't]. *American Journal of Public Health, 93*(8), 1321–1327.

Haviland, W. A. (1999). *Cultural anthropology* (9th ed.). Fort Worth, TX: Harcourt Brace College Publishers.

Henderson, S., Kendall, E., & See, L. (2011). The effectiveness of culturally appropriate interventions to manage or prevent chronic disease in culturally and linguistically diverse communities: A systematic literature review. *Health & Social Care in the Community, 19*(3), 225–249.

Henriksen, L., Schleicher, N. C., Dauphinee, A. L., & Fortmann, S. P. (2012). Targeted advertising, promotion, and price for menthol cigarettes in California high school neighborhoods. [Research Support, Non-U.S. Gov't]. *Nicotine Tobacco Research, 14*(1), 116–121. doi: 10.1093/ntr/ntr122

Herek, G. M., & Capitanio, J. P. (1994). Conspiracies, contagion, and compassion: Trust and public reactions to AIDS. *AIDS Education and Prevention, 6*(4), 365–375.

Herek, G. M., & Glunt, E. K. (1991). AIDS-related attitudes in the United States: A preliminary conceptualization. *Journal of Sex Research, 28*, 99–123.

Holy, L., & Stuchlik, M. (Eds.). (1981). *The structure of folk models.* London, UK: Academic Press.

Humes, K. R., Jones, N. A., & Ramirez, R. R. (2011). Overview of race and Hispanic origin: 2010, 2010 Census Briefs. Retrieved September 5, 2012, from http://www.census.gov/prod/cen2010/briefs/c2010br-02.pdf

Ibrahim, S. A., Siminoff, L. A., Burant, C. J., & Kwoh, C. K. (2002a). Differences in expectations of outcome mediate African American/white patient differences in "willingness" to consider joint replacement. *Arthritis and Rheumatism, 46*(9), 2429–2435.

Ibrahim, S. A., Siminoff, L. A., Burant, C. J., & Kwoh, C. K. (2002b). Understanding ethnic differences in the utilization of joint replacement for osteoarthritis: The role of patient-level factors. *Medical Care, 40*(1 Suppl.), I44–I51.

Iversen, I. H., & Lattal, K. A. (Eds.). (1991). *Experimental analysis of behavior, Part 1 and Part 2.* Amsterdam: Elsevier.

Jacobs, D. E. (2011). Environmental health disparities in housing. [Review]. *American Journal of Public Health, 101*(Suppl. 1), S115–S122. doi:10.2105/AJPH.2010.300058

Janz, N. K., & Becker, M. H. (1984). The health belief model: A decade later. *Health Education Quarterly, 11*, 1–47.

Kemp, C. R., & Rasbridge, L. A. (2004). *Refugee and immigrant health: A handbook for health professionals.* Cambridge, UK: Cambridge University Press.

Keppel, K. G. (2007). Ten largest racial and ethnic health disparities in the United States based on Healthy People 2010 objectives. *American Journal of Epidemiology, 166*(1), 97–103.

King, W. D., Wong, M. D., Shapiro, M. F., Landon, B. E., & Cunningham, W. E. (2004). Does racial concordance between HIV-positive patients and their physicians affect the time to receipt of protease inhibitors? *Journal of General Internal Medicine, 19*(11), 1146–1153.

Kleinman, A., Eisenberg, L., & Good, B. (1978). Culture, illness, and care: Clinical lessons from anthropologic and cross-cultural research. [Case Reports]. *Annals of Internal Medicine, 88*(2), 251–258.

Klonoff, E. A., & Landrine, H. (1999). Do blacks believe that HIV/AIDS is a government conspiracy against them? *Preventive Medicine, 28*(5), 451–457.

Knowler, W. C., Barrett-Connor, E., Fowler, S. E., Hamman, R. F., Lachin, J. M., Walker, E. A., & Nathan, D. M. (2002). Reduction in the incidence of type 2 diabetes with lifestyle intervention or metformin. *New England Journal of Medicine, 346*(6), 393–403.

Koplan, J. P., Liverman, C. T., & Kraak, V. I. (2005). Preventing childhood obesity: Health in the balance: Executive summary. [Review]. *Journal of the American Dietetic Association, 105*(1), 131–138. doi:10.1016/j.jada.2004.11.023

Kreuter, M. W., & Haughton, L. T. (2006). Integrating culture into health information for African American women. *American Behavioral Scientist, 49*(6), 794–811.

Kreuter, M. W., Lukwago, S. N., Bucholtz, R. D., Clark, E. M., & Sanders-Thompson, V. (2003). Achieving cultural appropriateness in health promotion programs: Targeted and tailored approaches. *Health Education & Behavior, 30*(2), 133–146.

Kreuter, M. W., & McClure, S. M. (2004). The role of culture in health communication. *Annual Review of Public Health, 25,* 439–455.

Kreuter, M. W., Skinner, C. S., Steger-May, K., Holt, C. L., Bucholtz, D. C., Clark, E. M., & Haire-Joshu, D. (2004). Responses to behaviorally vs. culturally tailored cancer communication among African American women. *American Journal of Health Behavior, 28*(3), 195–207.

Krieger, N. (1994). Epidemiology and the web of causation: Has anyone seen the spider? *Social Science & Medicine, 39*(7), 887–903.

Krieger, N. (2001). Theories for social epidemiology in the 21st century: An ecosocial perspective. [Review]. *International Journal of Epidemiology, 30*(4), 668–677.

Kuo, C. L., & Kavanagh, K. H. (1994). Chinese perspectives on culture and mental health. *Issues in Mental Health Nursing, 15*(6), 551–567.

Kwok, C., & Sullivan, G. (2006). Chinese-Australian women's beliefs about cancer: Implications for health promotion. *Cancer Nursing, 29*(5), E14–E21.

Lakoff, G. (1982). *Categories and cognitive models Series A, No. 96.* Trier: Linguistic Agency University of Trier.

Landrine, H., & Klonoff, E. A. (2004). Culture change and ethnic-minority health behavior: An operant theory of acculturation. *Journal of Behavioral Medicine, 27*(6), 527–555.

Lanphear, B. P., Weitzman, M., & Eberly, S. (1996). Racial differences in urban children's environmental exposures to lead. [Comparative Study Research Support, Non-U.S. Gov't Research Support, U.S. Gov't, Non-P.H.S. Research Support, U.S. Gov't, P.H.S.]. *American Journal of Public Health, 86*(10), 1460–1463.

Lara, M., Gamboa, C., Kahramanian, M. I., Morales, L. S., & Bautista, D. E. (2005). Acculturation and Latino health in the United States: A review of the literature and its sociopolitical context. *Annual Review of Public Health, 26,* 367–397.

Lee, A. J., Gehlbach, S., Hosmer, Reti, M., & Baker, C. S. (1997). Medicare treatment differences for blacks and whites. *Medical Care, 35*(12), 1173–1189.

Lofquist, D., Lugaila, T., O'Connell, M., & Feliz, S. (2012). Households and families: 2010. *2010 Census Briefs.* Retrieved from http://www.census.gov/prod/cen2010/briefs/c2010br-14.pdf

MacLean, J. (2004). *Breast cancer in California: A closer look.* Oakland, CA: Breast Cancer Research Program, University of California.

Majumdar, B., Browne, G., Roberts, J., & Carpio, B. (2004). Effects of cultural sensitivity training on health care provider attitudes and patient outcomes. *Journal of Nursing Scholarship, 36*(2), 161–166.

Marks, G., Garcia, M., & Solis, J. M. (1990). Health risk behaviors of Hispanics in the United States: Findings from HHANES, 1982–1984. *American Journal of Public Health, 80*(Suppl.), 20–26.

Matson-Koffman, D. M., Brownstein, J. N., Neiner, J. A., & Greaney, M. L. (2005). A site-specific literature review of policy and environmental interventions that promote physical activity and nutrition for cardiovascular health: What works? *American Journal of Health Promotion, 19*(3), 167–193.

McGory, M. L., Zingmond, D. S., Sekeris, E., Bastani, R., & Ko, C. Y. (2006). A patient's race/ethnicity does not explain the underuse of appropriate adjuvant therapy in colorectal cancer. *Diseases of the Colon and Rectum, 49*(3), 319–329.

Mendenhall, E., Fernandez, A., Adler, N., & Jacobs, E. A. (2012). Susto, coraje, and abuse: Depression and beliefs about diabetes. [Research Support, Non-U.S. Gov't]. *Culture, Medicine and Psychiatry, 36*(3), 480–492. doi:10.1007/s11013-012-9267-x

Merriam, P. A., Tellez, T. L., Rosal, M. C., Olendzki, B. C., Ma, Y., Pagoto, S. L., & Ockene, I. S. (2009). Methodology of a diabetes prevention translational research project utilizing a community-academic partnership for implementation in an underserved Latino community. *BMC Medical Research Methodology, 9*, 20.

Messler, L., Steckler, A., & Dignan, M. (1999). Early detection of cervical cancer among Native American women: A qualitative supplement to a quantitative study. *Health Education & Behavior, 26*, 547–562.

Minkler, M., & Wallerstein, N. (Eds.). (2008). *Community-based participatory research for health from process to outcomes* (2nd ed.). San Francisco, CA: John Wiley & Sons.

Montano, D. E., & Kasprzyk, D. (2008). Theory of reasoned action, theory of planned behavior, and the integrated behavioral model. In K. Glanz, B. K. Rimer, & K. Viswanath (Eds.), *Health behavior and health education: Theory, research and practice* (4th ed., pp. 67–96). San Francisco, CA: John Wiley & Sons.

Morland, K. B., & Evenson, K. R. (2009). Obesity prevalence and the local food environment. *Health & Place, 15*(2), 491–495.

Neal, D., Magwood, G., Jenkins, C., & Hossler, C. L. (2006). Racial disparity in the diagnosis of obesity among people with diabetes. *Journal of Health Care for the Poor and Underserved, 17*(2 Suppl.), 106–115.

Neff, K. (2006). The HIV/AIDS pandemic in African American MSM: Targets for intervention. *Journal of Health Disparities Research and Practice, 1*(1), 109–126.

Nguyen-Truong, C. K., Lee-Lin, F., Leo, M. C., Gedaly-Duff, V., Nail, L. M., Wang, P. R., & Tran, T. (2012). A community-based participatory research approach to understanding Pap testing adherence among Vietnamese American immigrants. *Journal of Obstetric, Gynecologic, and Neonatal Nursing: JOGNN / NAACOG, 41*(6), E26–E40.

Oza-Frank, R., & Cunningham, S. A. (2010). The weight of US residence among immigrants: A systematic review. *Obesity Reviews, 11*(4), 271–280.

Parikh-Patel, A., Bates, J. H., & Campleman, S. (2006). Colorectal cancer stage at diagnosis by socioeconomic and urban/rural status in California, 1988–2000. *Cancer, 107*(5 Suppl.), 1189–1195.

Perez-Escamilla, R. (2011). Acculturation, nutrition, and health disparities in Latinos. *American Journal of Clinical Nutrition, 93*(5), 1163S–1167S.

Poss, J., & Jezewski, M. A. (2002). The role and meaning of susto in Mexican Americans' explanatory model of type 2 diabetes. [Research Support, Non-U.S. Gov't]. *Medical Anthropology Quarterly, 16*(3), 360–377.

Reitzel, L. R., Costello, T. J., Mazas, C. A., Vidrine, J. I., Businelle, M. S., Kendzor, D. E., . . . Wetter, D. W. (2009). Low-level smoking among Spanish-speaking Latino smokers: Relationships with demographics, tobacco dependence, withdrawal, and cessation. [Research Support, N.I.H., Extramural Research Support, Non-U.S. Gov't Research Support, U.S. Gov't, P.H.S.]. *Nicotine & Tobacco Research, 11*(2), 178–184. doi:10.1093/ntr/ntn021

Resnicow, K., Baranowski, T., Ahluwalia, J. S., & Braithwaite, R. L. (1999). Cultural sensitivity in public health: Defined and demystified. *Ethnicity & Disease, 9*(1), 10–21.

Resnicow, K., Braithwaite, R. L., & Glanz, K. (2002). Applying theory to culturally diverse and unique populations. In K. Glanz, B. K. Rimer, & F. M. Lewis (Eds.), *Health behavior and health education, theory, research, and practice* (3rd ed., pp. 485–509). San Francisco, CA: Jossey-Bass.

Roberts, C. B., Vines, A. I., Kaufman, J. S., & James, S. A. (2008). Cross-sectional association between perceived discrimination and hypertension in African-American men and women: The Pitt County Study. [Research Support, N.I.H., Extramural Research Support, Non-U.S. Gov't]. *American Journal of Epidemiology, 167*(5), 624–632. doi:10.1093/aje/kwm334

Rosal, M. C., Carbone, E. T., & Goins, K. V. (2003). Use of cognitive interviewing to adapt measurement instruments for low-literate Hispanics. *Diabetes Educator, 29*(6), 1006–1017.

Rosal, M. C., Lemon, S. C., Nguyen, O. H. T., Driscoll, N. E., & DiTaranto, L. (2011). Translation of the diabetes prevention program lifestyle intervention for promoting postpartum weight loss among low-income women. *Translational Behavioral Medicine: Practice, Policy and Research, 1*(4), 530–538.

Rosal, M. C., Ockene, I. S., Restrepo, A., White, M. J., Borg, A., Olendzki, B., ... Reed, G. (2011). Randomized trial of a literacy-sensitive, culturally tailored diabetes self-management intervention for low-income Latinos: Latinos en Control. *Diabetes Care, 34*(4), 838–844.

Rosal, M. C., White, M. J., Restrepo, A., Olendzki, B., Scavron, J., Sinagra, E., ... Reed, G. (2009). Design and methods for a randomized clinical trial of a diabetes self-management intervention for low-income Latinos: Latinos en Control. *BMC Medical Research Methodology, 9*, 81.

Rosch, E., Mervis, B., Gray, W. D., Johnson, D. M., & Bayes-Braem, P. (1976). Basic objects in natural categories. *Cognitive Psychology, 8*, 382–439.

Rosenstock, I. M. (1966). Why people use health services. *Milbank Memorial Fund Quarterly, 44*(3 Suppl.), 94–127.

Ryan, C. L., & Siebens, J. (2012). Educational attainment in the United States: 2009. *Current Population Reports.* Retrieved from http://www.census.gov/prod/2012pubs/p20-566.pdf

Ryder, A. G., & Chentsova-Dutton, Y. E. (2012). Depression in cultural context: "Chinese somatization," revisited. [Case Reports Research Support, Non-U.S. Gov't Review]. *Psychiatric Clinics of North America, 35*(1), 15–36. doi:10.1016/j.psc.2011.11.006

Sallis, J. F., & Glanz, K. (2006). The role of built environments in physical activity, eating, and obesity in childhood. *Future Child, 16*(1), 89–108.

Sam, D. L., & Berry, J. W. (2010). Acculturation: When individuals and groups of different cultural backgrounds meet. *Perspectives on Psychological Science, 5*(4), 472.

Schim, S. M., Doorenbos, A. Z., & Borse, N. N. (2006). Enhancing cultural competence among hospice staff. *American Journal of Hospice & Palliative Care, 23*(5), 404–411.

Shi, L. (1999). Experience of primary care by racial and ethnic groups in the United States. *Medical Care, 37*(10), 1068–1077.

Shin, H. B., & Kominski, R. A. (2010). Language use in the United States: 2007. *American Community Survey Reports.* Retrieved from http://www.census.gov/hhes/socdemo/language/data/acs/ACS-12.pdf

Shore, B. (1996). *Culture in mind: Cognition, culture, and the problem of meaning.* Oxford, UK: Oxford University Press.

Sims, M., Diez-Roux, A. V., Dudley, A., Gebreab, S., Wyatt, S. B., Bruce, M. A., … Taylor, H. A. (2012). Perceived discrimination and hypertension among African Americans in the Jackson Heart Study. [Research Support, N.I.H., Extramural]. *American Journal of Public Health, 102*(Suppl. 2), S258–S265. doi:10.2105/AJPH.2011.300523

Skinner, B. F. (1953). *Science and human behavior.* New York, NY: Free Press.

Skinner, B. F. (1969). *Contingencies of reinforcement.* Englewood Cliffs, NJ: Prentice-Hall.

Skinner, B. F. (1983). *A matter of consequences.* New York, NY: Knopf.

Smedley, B. D., Stith, A. Y., & Nelson, A. R. (Eds.). (2003). *Unequal treatment: Confronting racial and ethnic disparities in health care.* Washington, DC: National Academies Press.

Sorensen, G., Barbeau, E., Hunt, M. K., & Emmons, K. (2004). Reducing social disparities in tobacco use: A social-contextual model for reducing tobacco use among blue-collar workers. [Research Support, Non-U.S. Gov't Research Support, U.S. Gov't, P.H.S. Review]. *American Journal of Public Health, 94*(2), 230–239.

Sorensen, G., Emmons, K., Hunt, M. K., Barbeau, E., Goldman, R., Peterson, K., . . . Berkman, L. (2003). Model for incorporating social context in health behavior interventions: Applications for cancer prevention for working-class, multiethnic populations. [Research Support, Non-U.S. Gov't Research Support, U.S. Gov't, P.H.S.]. *Preventive Medicine, 37*(3), 188–197.

Sorensen, G., Stoddard, A. M., Dubowitz, T., Barbeau, E. M., Bigby, J., Emmons, K. M., … Peterson, K. E. (2007). The influence of social context on changes in fruit and vegetable consumption: Results of the healthy directions studies. [Randomized Controlled Trial Research Support, N.I.H., Extramural Research Support, Non-U.S. Gov't]. *American Journal of Public Health, 97*(7), 1216–1227. doi:10.2105/AJPH.2006.088120

Stokols, D. (1992). Establishing and maintaining healthy environments: Toward a social ecology of health promotion. *American Psychologist, 47*, 6–22.

Stokols, D. (1996). Translating social ecological theory into guidelines for community health promotion. *American Journal of Health Promotion, 10*(4), 282–298.

Strumpf, E. C. (2011). Racial/ethnic disparities in primary care: The role of physician-patient concordance. [Research Support, N.I.H., Extramural]. *Medical Care, 49*(5), 496–503. doi: 10.1097/MLR.0b013e31820fbee4

Suarez-Almazor, M. E., Souchek, J., Kelly, P. A., O'Malley, K., Byrne, M., Richardson, M., & Pak, C. (2005). Ethnic variation in knee replacement: Patient preferences or uninformed disparity? *Archives of Internal Medicine, 165*(10), 1117–1124.

Sumner, W. (1906). *Folkways: A study of the sociological importance of usages, manners, customs, mores, and morals.* Boston, MA: Ginn.

Surbone, A. (2006). Cultural aspects of communication in cancer care. *Recent Results in Cancer Research, 168*, 91–104.

Sutherland L. L. (2002, October). Ethnocentrism in a pluralistic society: A concept analysis. *J Transcult Nurs, 13*, 274–281.

Sutton, C. D., & Robinson, R. G. (2004). The marketing of menthol cigarettes in the United States: Populations, messages, and channels. *Nicotine & Tobacco Research, 6*(Suppl. 1), S83–S91. doi: 10.1080/14622203310001649504

Svetkey, L. P., George, L. K., Tyroler, H. A., Timmons, P. Z., Burchett, B. M., & Blazer, D. G. (1996). Effects of gender and ethnic group on blood pressure control in the elderly. [Clinical Trial Research Support, U.S. Gov't, P.H.S.]. *American Journal of Hypertension, 9*(6), 529–535.

Symon, A., Nagpal, J., Maniecka-Bryla, I., Nowakowska-Glab, A., Rashidian, A., Khabiri, R., … Wu, L. (2012). Cross-cultural adaptation and translation of a quality of life tool for new mothers: A methodological and experiential account from six countries. *Journal of Advanced Nursing, 69*(4), 970–980.

Thiederman, S. B. (1986). Ethnocentrism: A barrier to effective health care. *Nurse Practitioner, 11*(8), 52, 54, 59.

Torres, M. I., Marquez, D. K., Carbone, E. T., Stacciarini, J. M. R., & Foster, J. W. (2008). Culturally responsive health promotion in Puerto Rican communities: A structuralist approach. *Health Promotion Practice, 9*(2), 149–158.

Tovar, A., Must, A., Metayer, N., Gute, D. M., Pirie, A., Hyatt, R. R., & Economos, C. D. (2013). Immigrating to the US: What Brazilian, Latin American and Haitian women have to say about changes to their lifestyle that may be associated with obesity. *Journal of Immigrant and Minority Health/Center for Minority Public Health, 15*(2), 357–364.

Turnbull, F. (2003). Effects of different blood-pressure-lowering regimens on major cardiovascular events: Results of prospectively-designed overviews of randomised trials. *Lancet, 362*(9395), 1527–1535.

Turner, B. J., Cunningham, W. E., Duan, N., Andersen, R. M., Shapiro, M. F., Bozzette, S. A., … Zierler, S. (2000). Delayed medical care after diagnosis in a US national probability sample of persons infected with human immunodeficiency virus. *Archives of Internal Medicine, 160*(17), 2614–2622.

U.S. Department of Health and Human Services. (2010). Healthy People 2020: Disparities. Retrieved from http://www.healthypeople.gov/2020/about/disparitiesAbout.aspx

U.S. Department of Health and Human Services, & Agency for Healthcare Research and Quality. (2011). National healthcare disparities report. Retrieved from http://www.ahrq.gov/qual/nhdr11/nhdr11.pdf

U.S. Department of Health and Human Services, & Office of Minority Health. (2001). National standards for culturally and linguistically appropriate services in health care: Final report. Rockville, MD: IQ Solutions, Inc.

Waite, R. L. (2006). Variations in the experiences and expressions of depression among ethnic minorities. *Journal of National Black Nurses' Association: JNBNA, 17*(1), 29–35.

Ward, E. C. (2007). Examining differential treatment effects for depression in racial and ethnic minority women: A qualitative systematic review. *Journal of the National Medical Association, 99*(3), 265–274.

Weech-Maldonado, R., Hall, A., Bryant, T., Jenkins, K. A., & Elliott, M. N. (2012). The relationship between perceived discrimination and patient experiences with health care. [Research Support, N.I.H., Extramural Research Support, Non-U.S. Gov't]. *Medical Care, 50*(9 Suppl. 2), S62–S68. doi:10.1097/MLR.0b013e31825fb235

Weisner, T. S. (2002). Ecocultural understanding of children's developmental pathways. *Human Development, 45*, 275–281.

Wight, D., Abraham, C., & Scott, S. (1998). Towards a psycho-social theoretical framework for sexual health promotion. *Health Education Research, 13*(3), 317–330.

Williams, D. R. (1999). Race, socioeconomic status, and health. The added effects of racism and discrimination. [Comparative Study Research Support, Non-U.S. Gov't Research Support, U.S. Gov't, P.H.S. Review]. *Annals of the New York Academy of Sciences, 896*, 173–188.

Willis, G. B. (1994). Cognitive interviewing and questionnaire design: A training manual. (Working Paper Series, No. 7). Hyattsville, MD: Office of Research and Methodology, National Center for Health Statistics.

Wilson, C. C., Gutierrez, F., & Chao, L. M. (2003). *Racism, sexism and the media: The rise of class communication in multicultural America* (3rd ed.). Thousand Oaks, CA: Sage.

Wong, M. D., Cunningham, W. E., Shapiro, M. F., Andersen, R. M., Cleary, P. D., Duan, N., … HCSUS Consortium. (2004). Disparities in HIV treatment and physician attitudes about delaying protease inhibitors for nonadherent patients. *Journal of General Internal Medicine, 19*(4), 366–374.

Zhu, S. H., Pulvers, K., Zhuang, Y., & Baezconde-Garbanati, L. (2007). Most Latino smokers in California are low-frequency smokers. [Research Support, N.I.H., Extramural]. *Addiction, 102*(Suppl. 2), 104–111. doi:10.1111/j.1360-0443.2007.01961.x

III
Lifestyle Change/Disease Prevention Interventions

The message is clear in medicine and public health—many acute and chronic diseases can be prevented, or at least have their impact reduced, by increased attention to the adoption and maintenance of healthy behaviors. This recognition grows out of the many epidemiologic investigations that demonstrate the existence of a strong relationship between the prevention, onset, progression, and exacerbation of disease and subsequent quality of life and alterable health-related behaviors such as smoking, diet, physical activity, alcohol, and stress management. Using the theories and models presented in Section I regarding individual, community/population-based, and system-level models, strategies can be developed to address ways to help individuals modify the noted behaviors. A chapter now included in Section III, "Building a Science for Multiple-Risk Behavior Change," and not included in previous editions of this book, is an important addition.

The chapters in Section III demonstrate that, while we have learned much in the last several decades about facilitating the modification of behaviors needed for the maintenance of a healthy life, a common theme is that when it comes to maintenance of behavior change, such endeavors are still a challenge to individuals and their health care providers as well as to researchers. Another theme running throughout the chapters in this section is the importance of implementing comprehensive multi-level approaches. Authors of each chapter beckon us to address this challenge. Authors also call attention to the need for dissemination and translation of research results to practice for any change to occur.

Thomson and Foster in "Dietary Behaviors: Promoting Healthy Eating" (Chapter 7) stress the importance of community and organizational change for facilitating nutritional and other health-related interventions and the complementarity of individual and organizational change. They emphasize the difficulty of dietary change, given that eating is necessary for survival and individuals need to make multiple dietary choices each day. The authors assert that to make wellness a reality at the population level and to achieve sustained changes, clear and specific goals and promotion of self-monitoring is required. They also address the importance of the primary care clinician in helping patients make dietary changes and the need for them to learn how to use a brief patient-centered approach to help patients make or initiate changes.

Grieco, Sheats, and Winter in Chapter 8, "Physical Activity Behavior," call for a comprehensive approach for promoting regular physical activity and address the need to "scalable" interventions to be able to effectively disseminate proven interventions in community and health care settings. "Harnessing the power of technology to accelerate and maintain changes in physical activity" also is an important focus in this chapter. The authors remind us that among other things, we need to pay attention to eliminating disparities in physical activity participation and to do this we need to understand the impact of the built environments where people live and work.

Pbert, Jolicoeur, Hayes, and Ockene in Chapter 9, "Addressing Tobacco Use and Dependence," as other authors have done, stress the importance of a multi-faceted approach to tobacco especially given its physiologically addictive nature. The authors stress the importance of health care provider delivered interventions and the need to increase widespread treatment capacity by combining counseling and individual-level treatment options with population/community-based interventions. An important strategy that the authors note is the use of technology/e-strategies for reaching millions of smokers and the importance of mass media campaigns. The authors also make special note of the emergence of new tobacco products such as electronic nicotine delivery (END) devices or e-cigarettes. The authors conclude with noting the importance of different coverage models for providing accessible treatment services to all who need them.

In Chapter 10, "Alcohol Prevention and Treatment: Interventions for Hazardous, Harmful, and Dependent Drinkers," McGovern and Kaner point out that the greatest impact for reducing alcohol-related problems can be had by just intervene with individuals who are drinking at "hazardous or harmful" levels and not the heaviest drinkers as the former is where the greatest prevalence of drinkers exist. Therefore service should be provided for the full range of alcohol-related risk and harm. This chapter covers a range of intervention types from brief interventions that has a large and robust evidence base when delivered to non-treatment-seeking individuals. For treatment-seeking individuals the chapter covers psychological and pharmacologic therapies. The authors note that the added benefits of combining the two types of therapies offers some promise but further research is needed.

Dornelas, Gallagher, and Burg in Chapter 11, "Reducing Stress to Improve Health," note the important role of stress in health and disease and modification of health-related behaviors. They describe the mechanisms by which stress affects specific diseases such as cancer. The different interventions to reduce stress are discussed including cognitive-behavioral approaches, exercise, relaxation therapies (i.e., mindfulness-based meditation, hypnosis, and yoga), patient-centered supportive approaches, and technology/e-health strategies. The authors note that these are often addressed in the context of intervention for other health-related behaviors and because stress often negatively affects making other health-related changes, a case could be made for addressing stress prior to addressing the other behaviors. Technology such as mobile phones may help stress management skills become more widespread. The authors emphasize the importance of increasing stress resilience and stress management in work and life.

Chapter 12, "Building a Science for Multiple-Risk Behavior Change" by the Prochaskas, is a new and welcome addition addressing the integration of interventions for clinicians and researchers in all disciplines who are faced each day with patients who have a clustering of disease-promoting behaviors. Health practitioners need integrated approaches that can be applied to patients, rather than a collection of single behavior interventions. The authors note the complexities of addressing multiple health behaviors and that the chapter is focused on "building a science of multiple-risk behavior change" (MRBC). They discuss the methodological, analytic, and theoretical issues related to MRBC.

7

Dietary Behaviors: Promoting Healthy Eating

CYNTHIA A. THOMSON
GARY D. FOSTER

LEARNING OBJECTIVES

- Barriers to dietary behavior change are present at the individual, social, and environmental levels. For each level, list at least two barriers commonly identified.
- Describe why the distribution of educational materials alone is unlikely to promote change in eating behaviors.
- Understand the relevance of behavioral theories and constructs in the promotion of eating behaviors.
- List three behavioral approaches used in patient-centered counseling to promote changes in eating behaviors.

Current dietary intake patterns in Americans have been well described. The recurring NHANES data (National Center for Health Statistics, 2012; www.cdc.gov/nchs/nhanes.htm) based on self-reported dietary intake suggest that Americans are, on average, consuming diets incongruent with the Dietary Guidelines for Americans (2012) (health.gov/dietaryguidelines). Specifically, intake of dietary fat, saturated fat, sodium, and sugar-sweetened beverages and not including fiber, fruits and vegetables, and omega-3 fatty acids (USDA, What we eat in America; www.ars.usda.gov/Services/docs.htm) are well above what is estimated to be optimal for health. Further, dietary components whose greater intake is thought to be important for health are consumed well below estimated requirements. The resultant dietary patterns suggest poor eating behaviors predominant in the American diet. Alarmingly, these patterns have persisted for several decades and are a major contributing factor in the current epidemic of overweight/obesity and obesity-related chronic diseases such as diabetes, cardiovascular disease, as well as several cancers (Centers for Disease Control and Prevention, 2012; www.cdc.gov/chronicdisease/index.htm). This disconnect between what we select to eat and the strong and well-substantiated risk for disease when less healthy food selections are made has led to a resurgence in interest to more thoroughly explore eating behavior. Furthermore, behavioral counseling remains a central therapy to reduce the burden of chronic disease in U.S. adults (Lin et al., 2010). Food choices are complex and represent a variety of motivational factors ranging from taste/satisfaction, to psychosocial distress, to health, thus making absolute and sustained change challenging.

Importantly, humans must eat to survive and be healthy; thus avoidance is not a sustainable approach to positive eating behavior change. Eating behaviors require multiple choices repeated on a daily if not hourly basis. Each stimulus to eat from hunger, to visual cues, to smells or taste, most commonly acts to promote greater intake of food. The increasing abundance and availability of food also have promoted greater intake over time. But beyond the abundance and repeated exposures, research has suggested that the decision to select healthier less energy dense foods is both biological and behavioral.

This chapter serves to inform approaches to dietary behavior change by briefly reviewing the biology of eating; reviewing relevant behavioral theories, constructs, and strategies that have been effectively applied for changing eating behaviors; as well as exploring modification of the environment to promote healthy eating behaviors. The content is largely focused on individual behavior change; however, increasingly there is awareness that policy and population-level change also will be necessary in order to achieve the magnitude of sustained change in eating behavior necessary to make wellness a reality at the population level.

THE BIOLOGY OF EATING BEHAVIOR

The drive to consume energy is largely driven by paracrine, endocrine, metabolic, and hormonal signaling pathways (Sam, Troke, Tan, & Bewick, 2012; Wren & Bloom, 2007). To a lesser extent, diurnal variations in hormones such as estrogen also can influence energy consumption as can thermal influences such as fever and the rise in core temperature with intense physical activity. Figure 7.1 illustrates several of the key regulatory factors within the brain, orosensory system, and gastrointestinal tract that regulate intake. While the human body has sophisticated regulatory feedbacks to optimize energy control, it is clear that behavioral factors can have a profound impact on these

FIGURE 7.1 Biology of eating behavior. (Adapted from Sam, et al. 2012)

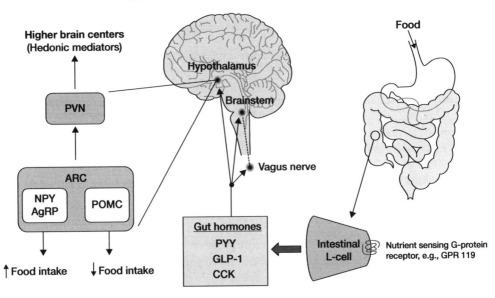

systems, particularly within the human brain and gastrointestinal tract. Further, the heterogeneity of the biological influences on eating behavior at the individual level suggests that behavioral therapy to promote changes in eating behavior will have highly variable responses as is consistently demonstrated in practice and clinical trial research.

THE BEHAVIOR OF EATING

Beyond biology, there is a significant and not fully understood role for behavior in food choices. Behavioral influences on intake include conditioned responses such as food preferences, aversions, and satiations as well as cognitive behavioral factors such as social, cultural, and esthetics. In addition, ecological influences such as relative densities and nutrient drivers also must be considered when examining the role of behavior on dietary choices. To illustrate in a more applied way, behavioral influences include a variety of factors such as stimulus response (e.g., chocolate as a "comfort food"), knowledge (e.g., consume calcium-rich dairy for bone health), social influences (e.g., mom said eat your vegetables), behavioral norms (e.g., daily lattes), role modeling (e.g., grandpa always avoided salt), aversions/attitudes (e.g., olives make me ill), and even reinforcement (e.g., coffee, beer taste wonderful).

Approaches to help individuals modify their eating behaviors, generally in an effort to support attainment of the Dietary Guidelines for Americans or some adaptation thereof, require behavioral treatment or other interventions. The distinguishing characteristics of behavioral treatment have been described by Foster and colleagues (Foster, Makris, & Bailer, 2005). Specifically effective behavioral treatment as it relates to eating and other behaviors must be goal directed, process oriented, and advocate for small rather than large change. Frequently the approach will integrate multiple components from self-monitoring to stimulus control, to cognitive restructuring.

INDIVIDUAL DIETARY BEHAVIOR CHANGE

Individual behaviors surrounding food choices may reflect personal health behavior, health-related behavior change, or health (dietary) protective behavior. Personal health behavior reflects food choices made that result in a direct effect on the individual's health. These behaviors may or may not be driven by a desire to improve one's health as food choices are more commonly the result of taste, habits, availability, beliefs, and attitudes that may indirectly alter health status despite the original or primary motivational factor driving the eating behavior. Health-related behavior change differs from personal health behavior as it captures behaviors of others that indirectly improve the target individual's health status. This would include behaviors of friends, family members, or perhaps even administrators and policymakers that affect the eating behavior of others. Health protective eating behaviors are behaviors that are undertaken with the primary, if not the sole intent, of improving a specific health indicator (e.g., serum cholesterol, blood pressure, etc.) whether it is risk for disease or control/treatment of disease.

At the individual level, changing dietary behaviors have historically relied on trained professionals (registered dietitians, medical doctors, registered nurses, etc.) who provide some specific facts or knowledge for the individual using an advice-giving mode in an attempt to elicit the desired change. While this approach in a small percentage of individuals may result in modest improvements in food choices to support health, there is a significant body of literature demonstrating that these approaches to behavior change fail in terms of magnitude of change needed as well as duration of

TABLE 7.1 Barriers to Change in Eating Behaviors to Achieve Recommended Diet Intake Patterns for Optimal Health

Individual	Lack of knowledge
	Financial/food insecurity
	Lack of or limited motivation
	Low perceived risk; insufficient benefit
	Hunger
	Taste
	Lack of awareness; mindfulness
	Habituation of food intake
Social	Cultural norms
	Holiday or religious practices
	Family composition/social isolation
	Meals consumed at home or away from home
	Shared meal environment
	Lack of social support for healthy behaviors
Environmental	Food accessibility; lack of supermarkets
	External stimulus; media
	Frequency of food exposures
	Quality of food exposures

change realized. Individuals trained in Behavioral Medicine are not surprised by these results in that these approaches often fail to engage the patient/client in the decision-making process or to ensure that the patient/client has made a conscientious effort to determine the value of specific dietary behavior changes in the context of their own risk–benefit evaluation. Yet these approaches are broadly applied even in current health care practice. A more productive client-centered approach that engages the client in developing plans and motivation for change has been demonstrated to be effective (Ockene et al., 1999). Beyond imparting knowledge and engaging the client, efforts also have been undertaken to identify barriers to making healthy food choices. Table 7.1 lists several of the more commonly reported barriers for which plans to reduce or remove the barrier may support positive changes in eating behavior. Again, reducing or removing barriers while shifting the risk–benefit ratio may or may not promote the magnitude and sustained change in eating behavior being sought.

Habituation as a Determinant of Food Intake

Epstein and colleagues have recently suggested that habituation of food intake is an important determinant of food selection and thus may be an important determinant of resistance to change in food choices (Epstein, Temple, Roemmich, & Bouton, 2009). Food intake, in this context, is the result of repeated exposure to orosensory cues that drive the decision to eat. These same cues also may drive decisions related to stoppage of eating and thus also contribute to an individual's propensity toward obesity. To dishabituate a behavior is challenging in that it requires both an awareness of the habit and cues stimulating a specific eating decision and also the capacity to alter or over-ride these habit-associated cues in an effort to make a different decision around the food behavior. To dishabituate, stimuli will need to be removed or altered. For example, food consumption is positively associated with television viewing time (Sisson, Shay, Broyles, & Leyva, 2012), particularly when combined with the availability of unhealthy snacks in the home (Pearson et al., 2012). Thus, setting a short-term goal to avoid visual stimuli from electronic sources overall and perhaps particularly during meal times will likely promote a reduction in intake. Other stimuli that should be considered include, for example, who the meal is shared with, time of day, smell of the food, visual access to the food, and related factors that may promote what has been labeled as "mindless eating" (Ogden et al., 2013; Wansink, 2010).

PROMOTION OF HEALTHY EATING BEHAVIORS

EDUCATION

There are several approaches to behavioral change. Commonly, health care providers employ one-way delivery of information, or education, in an attempt to help patients/clients change eating behavior. For example, clinicians may provide dietary handouts explaining how to reduce dietary fat, salt/sodium, or even portion sizes. Lack of information is a barrier to effective change in dietary behaviors and evidence exists to suggest that filling knowledge gaps can enhance diet change toward healthier food choices as was the case for the nutrient-rich foods consumer education program for adult primary food shoppers (Glanz et al., 2012). Many times these materials are printed in mass without formative work to determine patient understanding, interpretation, and/or ability to employ the information to change their dietary behavior. In some cases, the materials are not adapted for cultural norms or expectations or may reflect a relatively verbatim translation without modification for cultural context. Seldom is health literacy evaluated during the development of the educational handouts resulting in educational handouts that frequently include medical terminology, mathematical computations, and reading levels that are beyond the literacy level of the target population. Further, this unidirectional approach is unlikely to be effective given the complexity of eating behavior and the multiplicity of factors that contribute to the individual's risk-to-benefit assessment that can lead to significant changes in food choices. In particular, dissemination of information without application of behavioral theory is likely to ignore important psychological, social (inter- and intrapersonal), environmental, cultural, and even economic constraints. Importantly, even if the information provided through education fills a gap in the patient/client's knowledge, there is limited evidence that education alone impacts behavior change in relation to achieving complex eating goals.

BEHAVIORAL THEORIES AND CONSTRUCTS

A number of behavior change theories have been applied to dietary behavior. Commonly applied theories and constructs are described below (see Chapter 1 for a more in-depth discussion of these theories). But dietary behavior is not only complex in terms of the individual decision to eat or not eat a given food item; this decision-making process is repeated multiple times throughout a day and continuously in an individual's lifetime. Theories developed to help individuals change eating behavior must consider multiple factors at the individual, social unit, and population level that influence and inform each decision to consume or not consume food. Figure 7.2 illustrates the complexity of these interacting influences on eating behavior.

FIGURE 7.2 The Food Choice Model. (Adapted from Furst, Connors, Bisogni, Sobal, & Falk, 1996; Sobal & Bisogni, 2009)

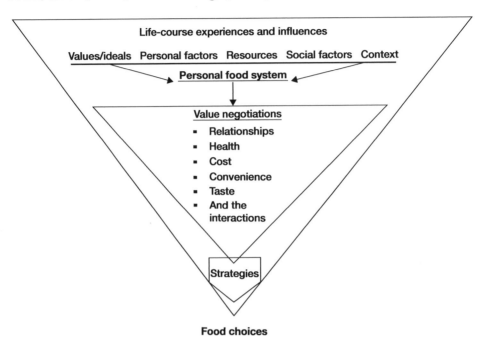

Health Belief Model

The Health Belief Model can be effectively used to promote eating behavior particularly among individuals who have true elevated risk for disease. Cues that promote eating behavior change under this model include when an individual experiences a family member or close friend diagnosed with a disease, sees a media campaign or report suggesting disease risk, or is notified by a health care provider that risk is elevated. This theory suggests that first an individual must feel personally threatened or susceptible to a disease and second the individual must believe that the benefits of taking action outweigh the risks. When promoting eating behavior change using the Health Belief Model, interventionist and health care providers should consider both how change in behavior can be incentivized to increase the benefit beyond reducing health risk alone and/or target risks of dietary behavior change along with self-empowerment strategies to build the patient/client's capacity to manage the necessary change in diet. The challenge with this theory of behavior change is that health beliefs are only one influence on eating behaviors so that perceived risk must not only be heightened above other influences it also must remain heightened over other influences (cultural, social, and personal) over time in order to sustain the behavior change. Individuals who are commonly considered appropriate for whom to employ health belief models of dietary behavior change include cancer survivors and their family members, and individuals with newly diagnosed metabolic syndrome, pre-hypertension, or perhaps premalignant lesions (adenomas, abnormal mammography, and actinic keratosis).

Social Cognitive Theory

Social Cognitive Theory builds on the interaction between personal factors and the environment suggesting that both influence each other leading to reciprocal causation in relation to eating behavior. In this model, eating behavior is thought to be a function of modeling or observed learning which is then reinforced to promote self-efficacy. Individuals learn how to make a specific dietary behavior change through observation and experiential learning (e.g., cooking demonstration, grocery store food purchasing trips, and role playing). As the individual practices the modeled behavior and increases awareness of the expected outcomes, self-efficacy is increased and eating behavior changes are effectively made. In this approach to dietary behavior change, it is important to consider significant others who play an active role in modeling the behavior of choice as well as environmental factors that may need to be considered to promote self-efficacy.

Social Determination Theory

Social Determination Theory (SDT) is an integration of other theories into a larger context and is based on the premise that reinforcement and environmental contingencies are highly effective in influencing behavior, but must remain in effect for behavior to be sustained. Both the person/personality in relation to motivations and self-regulation as well as the situation or social context motivate behavior. This theory considers four regulations for the continuum of extrinsic motivation as shown in Figure 7.3. Counseling that applies SDT will likely initiate with autonomy supportive behaviors that address the patient's current perspectives and emotions, followed by problem solving, identification of patient aspirations in relation to goal setting, and in follow-up, the integration of competence support (Deci & Ryan, 2012). For example, a patient may be entering the diet counseling session for hypertension control but be overwhelmed with a new job. This issue should be acknowledged and emotions addressed, followed by a transition to the focus of the counseling, determining the patient's aspirations and thus longer term goals for dietary health, and then problem solving perhaps around short-term goals for healthy choices in the new work environment, behavioral efforts that can then be re-evaluated to promote self-efficacy over time within future counseling sessions. SDT applied to health behavior counseling to complement behavioral change promoted through motivational interviewing (Patrick & Williams, 2012), which is a patient-centered approach to help individuals develop motivation to change a behavior (Miller & Moyers, 2007).

FIGURE 7.3 Social determination theory as it applies to healthy dietary behavior change (Patrick & Williams, 2012).

External regulation	Introjected regulation	Identified regulation	Integrated regulation
Behaving for reward or to avoid negative contingency	Behaving out of guilt, obligation, need to prove	Behaving because of the importance ascribed to the behavior	Behaving because behavior is consistent with other goals and values
Eating healthy to win a prize or stay employed	Eating healthy because food choices reflect one's character	Eating healthy because it is an important personal goal	Eating healthy because it is consistent with other health goals

Transtheoretical Model: Stages of Change

The Stages of Change Model for dietary behavior change has been employed in several dietary intervention studies. This model suggests that behavior change involves a sequence of "events" or stages that build toward sustained behavioral change. These stages include: (1) pre-contemplation during which a person is not aware, has not considered, or may be in denial about the needed behavior change, (2) contemplation wherein something happens to increase awareness and while there is some ambivalence regarding the dietary behavior change the person now has an awareness of the need for change, (3) preparation or the point at which the person actively gathers information to assess the costs and benefits of behavior change, followed by (4) action wherein the behavior is now being practiced using prior experiences, information, new skills, and motivation, and finally, (5) maintenance during which the dietary behavior is now practiced consistently and is somewhat habitual. The Stages of Change Model is sometimes applied to screen patients for eligibility in interventions or dietary change programs wherein individuals must be at the contemplation or preparation stage to be considered for program entry.

Theory of Diffusion of Innovations

While this theory is not solely applicable to dietary change, it does have a clear application in this context. This theory notes that behavior change is about the compatibility of the innovation with an individual's economic, sociocultural, and philosophical values. Several factors influence the adoption of the new behavior including the complexity, flexibility, relative advantage over current methods, cost-efficiency, and risk. Diffusion of Innovations Theory suggests that people fall into categories such that some can be described as innovators, those who develop new approaches, others are early adopters of the innovations, the majority adopt the behavior once the innovation is more diffused within the culture, and finally laggards are those who are resistant to the innovation. This theory probably has its greatest relevance to the use of e-technologies to promote dietary behavior change. Knowing an individual's "category" related to new technologies will help to determine the most appropriate plan for integrating innovations into behavior change strategies. For example, a patient/client who is resistant to writing down their daily food intake to self-monitor may be challenged and excited by the use of a smartphone application to achieve the same goal. Being aware also will ensure greater adherence. For example, if a patient is instructed to cook vegetables in the microwave and they have yet to adopt the microwave as a cooking method, they may not adapt your advice to another cooking technique and instead not eat the vegetables. In the end, they are unsuccessful in achieving the eating behavioral goal.

BEHAVIORAL APPROACHES TO PROMOTION OF DIETARY CHANGE

Goal Setting

Goal setting is an important component of dietary behavior change. Goals can not only provide the necessary clarity regarding the structure, specificity, and expected outcomes, they also support self-efficacy over time. Goal setting should include both short- and long-term goals. Short-terms goals, if achieved, should promote the eventual achievement of long-term goals as well. Short-term goals need to be specific to be effective in promoting the desired behavioral change and generally are written with the patient/client in an effort to individualize the goal to address barriers identified that may hinder a person's success in achieving a goal. For example, a short-term goal to eat vegetables every day is unlikely to be successful if the patient has reported that there are no available vegetable options to eat at work. Instead the short-term goal should be developed to address this barrier to dietary behavior change and could be revised to, "I will eat two servings of vegetables during each work day which I prepare at home and take with me to work. These will include raw carrot or celery sticks that I keep at my desk, a salad I prepare, or if not a leftover vegetable dish from dinner that I will reheat in the break area microwave at lunch time." This level of specificity promotes behavior change in a way that is achievable within the individual's "influences" on dietary decision making. Goal setting is most effective when accompanied with self-monitoring.

Self-Monitoring

Self-monitoring in the context of diet is the act of recording a specific dietary behavior on an ongoing basis. The value of self-monitoring lies in repeated awareness or cues for healthy decisions. However, the recorded information must align with the short- and long-term goals that have been set. For example, recording of all foods consumed may be relevant when energy intake goals have been set for weight loss, but may overburden patients and have less relevance when the target behavior is reduced sodium intake for blood pressure control. In this situation, having individuals record sodium content from labels of foods consumed and/or use of salt shaker/packets may have more relevance and thus be more acceptable and sustainable for self-monitoring behavior. Components of eating behavior that are frequently self-monitored for diet change include not only tracking of overall diet and specific nutrients (sodium, fiber, fat, fruit, and vegetables), but also meal spacing, location, timing, rate of eating, and stimulus control.

Self-monitoring can be challenging to initiate and matching the approach to the individual can facilitate success in this area. For example, a younger patient with a smartphone may wish to use applications (apps) to record intake and may find the immediate evaluation of outcome (sum of sodium intake throughout the day) motivating to continue self-monitoring and yet would have resisted writing down all foods consumed in a diary format. The frequency of self-monitoring also is important. General practice is to recommend that dietary monitoring be completed daily at least in the initial change period (6–12 weeks). After this point, self-monitoring frequency may be reduced without marked recidivism in behavior, but should not be eliminated as a behavior change strategy all together. Self-monitoring also should be increased in frequency and adjusted in context as new barriers to change are identified and new approaches to achieving long-term health goals are set. Self-monitoring has been consistently associated with weight loss, although there is a lack of evidence in diverse populations as well as objective measures of adherence to self-monitoring protocols or estimates of "dose" required to achieve weight loss (Burke, Wang, & Sevick, 2011). Of note, advances in electronic monitoring of eating and lifestyle behaviors suggest new electronic approaches, particularly when combined with daily feedback messages, may improve adherence to self-monitoring and thus indirectly result in greater achievement of dietary behavior change goals (Burke, Conroy et al., 2011; Burke et al., 2012).

Group Support

Support is an important factor for behavior change as well as for increased duration of change over time. Support may be in the form of groups as has been commonly employed in several long-term dietary trials requiring substantial dietary change including the Women's Health Initiative Dietary Modification trial (Anderson et al.,

2003), the PREDIMED trial (Zazpe et al., 2008), and the Look Ahead trial (Ryan et al., 2003). Attendance at group sessions also has been associated with greater adherence to dietary goals (Tinker et al., 2007). There is also evidence that group counseling may be more effective than phone-based counseling of individuals for weight control (Befort, Donnelly, Sullivan, Ellerbeck, & Perri, 2010).

Beyond group support, perceived support from clinic or study staff throughout trial participation also has been shown to promote greater change in eating behaviors mostly related to enhanced self-efficacy and to promote eating behavior change. Frequency and quality of contact as well as extended duration of contact each may have independent effects on dietary behavior change and both appear to be integral to achievement and maintenance of dietary behavioral goals (Middleton, Patidar, & Perri, 2012; Turk et al., 2009).

Additionally, Perri and colleagues have evaluated social support for healthy behaviors and identified an important role for friends and family. This work suggests that family and friend support is associated with greater success with weight loss (Kiernan et al., 2012).

Problem Solving

Behavioral approaches to dietary change generally address the issue of problem solving early in the counseling process. The important issue here is for the patient/client rather than the clinician to identify problems. This is important if there is to be ownership of the short-term goals required to address the problems as identified. Problem solving requires the use of both cognitive and behavioral techniques and not only addresses the person's perceived barriers to behavior change, but also their prior or planned approaches to overcome these barriers to promote the achievement of dietary goals. The discussion may begin with an open listing of barriers followed by a review of usual daily activities around food that may help to identify additional barriers. Developing a diagram of the behavior chain surrounding food choices can help the patient/client to identify barriers that are not as readily apparent without reviewing a typical day's activity and how these may inform eating choices. Figure 7.4 provides an example as to how a behavior chain might be developed in conversation with the patient/client.

FIGURE 7.4 Food behavior decision making: Identifying barriers to change. (Adapted from Foster et al., 2005)

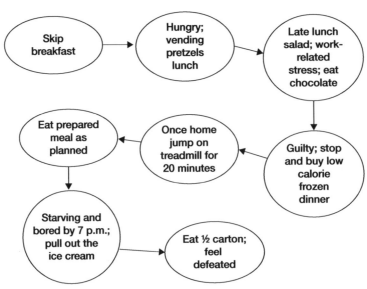

Once barriers have been identified, a discussion will commence to identify not only approaches previously employed that were successful in promoting healthy eating, but also to define and describe with specificity new strategies that the patient/client identifies as adoptable for use in meeting dietary behavioral goals. The role of the counselor is to facilitate the identification of barriers as well as change strategies. Problem solving is not a stand-alone technique but rather is generally applied within a larger behavioral plan to promote dietary change.

Motivational Interviewing

Motivational interviewing is perhaps the most commonly employed strategy to dietary behavior change. Several companies have been established in recent years to address the need for enhanced training of health care providers on this approach. It is incorrect to assume one can use motivational interviewing to effectively help patients/clients change eating behaviors without ample training on the topic. Motivational interviewing is a collaborative, person-centered form of guiding individuals to elicit and strengthen motivation for change (Miller & Moyers, 2007). Motivational interviewing helps individuals identify and resolve ambivalence with behaviors targeted for change and centers on motivational processes that facilitate the desired change. Motivational interviewing (2012) by nature is a conversation between the patient/client and the health care provider that honors autonomy and is evocative (www.motivationalinterviewing. org). An effective motivational interviewing interaction has been described to include eight tasks: openness of discussion, proficiency in client-centered counseling, identifying change and sustain talk, eliciting and strengthening change talk, reflectively hearing sustain and resistance talk, recognizing readiness toward development of a change plan, consolidating commitment, and transitioning and blending motivational interviewing techniques with other effective behavioral approaches and strategies (Miller & Moyers, 2007).

Technology and E-Strategies for Dietary Behavior Change

The wealth of new innovations, apps, and devices for dietary assessment, self-monitoring, and behavior change has presented new challenges in dietary behavior change. The theoretical model that has the most relevance here is likely the Diffusion of Innovations Theory although several studies using these methods also report use of Social Cognitive Theory, Transtheoretical Model and Precaution Adoption Process (Norman et al., 2007). Whether current health behavior models will have validity in relation to the increasingly interactive and adaptive mHealth approaches remains to be determined (Riley et al., 2011).

Overall there is limited but growing evidence as to the degree of behavioral change that can be achieved using technological approaches. Less is known about how sustainable dietary behaviors are when they are achieved with the support of e-technology. Evidence does show that significant changes in dietary behavior, including those associated with weight loss can be achieved without face-to-face contact between participants and weight loss providers (Appel et al., 2011). The lack of comprehensive evidence should not be perceived as lack of efficacy. In reality, several studies have been completed to evaluate the degree of behavior change that can be realized, although the best methods for delivery, best devices to be employed, dose, and duration have yet to be defined. A review by Norman and colleagues in 2007 identified 7 diet interventions using mHealth and 11 weight loss interventions (Norman et al., 2007). Table 7.2

TABLE 7.2 Select Studies Using e-Health Technology to Effectively Promote Dietary Behavior Change

STUDY LEAD INVESTIGATOR	TECHNOLOGY OR PLATFORM	TARGET BEHAVIOR	TARGET POPULATION
Carpenter, Finley, & Barlow, 2004	Interactive website	Healthy Eating Index score	N = 98; middle-aged, predominantly Caucasian females
Stevens, Glasgow, Toobert, Karanja, & Smith, 2003	Website	Dietary fat intake	N = 616; age 40–70 y; overweight/obese females
Nollen et al., 2013	Handheld computer program	Fruit and vegetable intake	N = 15 ; age 8–15 y; females only
Oenema, Tan, & Brug, 2005	CD-ROM	Fruits, vegetables, and fat	N = 616; middle-aged males and females, worksite-based
Baranowski, Baranowski, & Cullen, 2003	Computer games	Fruit and vegetable intake	N = 1578; children aged 8–12 y
Anderson, Winett, Wojcik, Winett, & Bowden, 2001	Grocery store kiosk	Dietary fat, fiber, fruits, and vegetables	N = 277; greater than 97% Caucasian adult females
Newman et al., 2005	Interactive telephone	Dietary fat, fruits and vegetables, and fiber	N = 3088; female breast cancer survivors
Irvine, Ary, Grove, & Gilfillan-Morton, 2004	Interactive multimedia	Fruit and vegetable and fat intake	N = 517; middle-aged, predominantly Caucasian females at worksite
Spring et al., 2012	Telephone coaching plus mobile decision support technology	Fruit and vegetable intake, saturated fat and caloric intake; sedentary time	N = 204; adults with low scores on healthy lifestyle behaviors
Block et al., 2008	e-mail lifestyle intervention	Fruits and vegetables, saturated fat, added sugars, physical activity; self-efficacy, stage of change	N = 787; age 19–65 y; 95% female; majority Caucasian

lists select dietary intervention trials that employed a variety of e-health technological approaches to effectively promote diet and/or lifestyle behavior change.

As suggested in the table, earlier studies focused primarily on the use of telephone-based counseling and CD-ROM delivery of information. More recently, efforts are ongoing to expand to smartphone applications and game-based multi-modality interventions to promote behavior change; however, there is a paucity of research providing comparative effectiveness between the methodological approaches employed. There is also the challenge of a rapidly changing technological environment in relation to available apps, devices, and delivery systems, such that by the time a study is complete and reported in the literature, new more novel and perhaps more easily implemented devices and apps may be available. Further, across cultural, gender, education, and age groups adoption of individual devices and apps can vary widely not only in relation to apps commonly used but also to the frequency of use and time to full adoption. These factors challenge the external validity of the research being done to evaluate e-technology for behavioral change.

Promoting Healthy Eating Behavior: The Clinical Setting

In addition to individual and group specific counseling efforts designed to support healthy eating choices, the clinical environment can serve as an additional reinforcement for patients and clients. First and foremost efforts by health care providers must receive adequate training on the importance of diet in health as well as effective methods to promote improvements in eating behaviors. Yet, deficiencies in current training programs continue to be identified (Vitolins et al., 2012). Providers also must develop competence in addressing eating behaviors with their patients/clients and avoid disparagement of those who report lower quality diets or who are obese, a common and generally socially acceptable prejudice in our health care system (Wolf, 2012; Teixeira, Pais-Ribeiro, & Maia, 2012). Empathy in encounters is central to meaningful interactions toward change in eating behaviors. Health care providers should ask patients their own perceptions about their weight or dietary behaviors and build from the response, affirm the difficulty in making and sustaining changes in eating behavior, and listen carefully using a patient-centered approach.

Beyond developing an empathetic initial encounter, the physical office can be modified to deliver an attitude of empathy, education, and self-empowerment. First, evaluate the clinic in relation to physical attributes (e.g., room to wait comfortably, chairs without arms, scales that are capable of weighing morbidly obese patients, examination gowns that fit all sizes, and use of large blood pressure cuffs). Second, provide access to relevant educational resources (healthy food choice/behavior pamphlets, websites, diet assessment/monitoring applications for e-health, posters on the clinic walls promoting healthy food, and even an office policy to restrict unhealthy food and beverages in the clinic setting). Third, provide clinic staff the opportunity, support, and recognition for advancing their skills in behavioral counseling to support patients who select to undertake change in eating behaviors. Consider having clinic staffs adopt dietary behavior change personally so as to gain empathy and experience with the process. Finally, understand and communicate the importance of realistic expectations.

Finally, routine integration of healthy lifestyle promotion into health services is needed if we are to succeed in improving the health of the population. Strategies should engage the health care providers, managers, researchers, and patient representatives using a socio-ecological model wherein the health care system is actively partnered, individual behavior change is supported, and educational limitations are overcome in an effort to achieve optimal dietary health (Grandes et al., 2008).

CONCLUSIONS

Changing dietary behaviors is challenging. Numerous factors contribute to every food choice including what, how much, when, and why we choose to eat. Complicating the matter more is that eating is a required behavior. Thus the decision must be repeated several times a day throughout a person's life; abstinence, employed for behavior modification of tobacco, drugs, or alcohol use, is not generally plausible except perhaps in relation to individual food omissions in the diet.

Current evidence suggests that clear and specific goals that are patient/client-identified and defined, as well as self-monitoring of the behavioral goals established, are a necessary component of any successful change in eating behavior. These goals must be complemented with clear antecedents to provide clients with the "how to" for successful eating behavior change in the context of their individual life circumstances. Additionally, relapse prevention and recovery is an essential phase in any long-term plan for sustained eating behavior change.

Promoting healthy food choices and related eating behaviors for patients/clients is critical to reducing obesity, obesity-related chronic diseases, and a variety of other clinical diagnoses. Despite the challenges, when patients are able to change eating behaviors to healthier choices there is a clear benefit that translates to numerous disease-specific outcomes.

To summarize:

- Changing dietary behavior is complex and requires long-term, dynamic approaches and strategies.
- No one behavioral theory works best; theories should be adapted for the individual intervention and/or patient/client.
- Patient-centered counseling including motivational interviewing is perhaps the most tested and effective strategy for dietary behavior change to date, but many providers lack sufficient training to effectively apply, for example, motivational interviewing in practice.
- To promote change in dietary behavior, clinicians should help clients set clear and specific goals, promote self-monitoring, recognize the role of social support and use it to enhance change in eating behavior, review the mechanisms for behavior and behavior change (antecedents), and focus on preventing relapse.
- Efforts to identify and determine "best practice" regarding behavioral theories, constructs, and strategies to help patients/clients improve dietary behaviors need to be continued.

REFERENCES

Anderson, E. S., Winett, R. A., Wojcik, J. R., Winett, S. G., & Bowden, T. (2001). A computerized social cognitive intervention for nutrition behavior: Direct and mediated effects on fat, fiber, fruits and vegetables, self-efficacy and outcome expectations among food shoppers. *Annals of Behavioral Medicine, 23*, 88–100.

Anderson, G. L., Manson, J., Wallace, R., Lund, B., Hall, D., Davis, S., ... Prentice, R. L. (2003). Implementation of the Women's Health Initiative study design. *Annals of Epidemiology, 13*(9 Suppl.), S5–S17.

Appel, L. J., Clark, J. M., Yeh, H. C., Wang, N. Y., Coughlin, J. W., Daumit, G., ... Brancati, F. L. (2011). Comparative effectiveness of weight-loss interventions in clinical practice. *New England Journal of Medicine, 365*(21), 1959–1968.

Baranowski, T., Baranowski, J., & Cullen, K. W. (2003). Squire's Quest! Dietary outcome evaluation of a multimedia game. *American Journal of Preventive Medicine, 24*, 52–61.

Befort, C. A., Donnelly, J. E., Sullivan, D. K., Ellerbeck, E. F., & Perri, M. G. (2010). Group versus individual phone-based obesity treatment for rural women. *Eating Behaviors, 11*(1), 11–7.

Block, G., Sternfeld, B., Block, C. H., Block, T. J., Norris, J., Hopkins, D., ... Clancy, H. A. (2008). Development of Alive! (A lifestyle intervention via email) and its effect on health-related quality of life presenteeism and other behavioral outcomes: Randomized controlled trial. *Journal of Medical Internet Research, 10*(4), e43.

Burke, L.E., Conroy, M.B., Sereika, S.M., Elci, O.U., Styn, M.A., Acharya, S.D., ... Glanz, K. (2011). The effect of electronic self-monitoring on weight loss and dietary intake: A randomized behavioral weight loss trial. *Obesity, 19*(2), 338–344.

Burke, L. E., Sty, M. A., Sereika, S. M., Conroy, M. B., Ye, L., Glanz, K., ... Ewing, L. J. (2012). Using mHealth technology to enhance self-monitoring for weight loss: A randomized trial. *American Journal of Preventive Medicine, 43*(1), 20–26.

Burke, L. E., Wang, J., & Sevick, M. A. (2011). Self-monitoring in weight loss: A systematic review of the literature. *Journal of the American Dietetic Association, 111*(1), 92–102.

Carpenter, R. A., Finley, C., & Barlow, C. E. (2004). Pilot test of a behavioral skill building intervention to improve overall diet quality. *Journal of Nutrition Education and Behavior, 36*, 20–26.

Centers for Disease Control and Prevention. (2012). Retrieved from http://www.cdc.gov/chronicdisease/index.htm

Deci, E. L., & Ryan, R. M. (2012). Self-determination theory in health care and its relations to motivational interviewing: A few comments. *International Journal of Behavioral Nutrition and Physical Activity, 9*, 24.

Dietary Guidelines for Americans. (2012). Retrieved from http://health.gov/dietaryguidelines

Epstein, L. H., Temple, L., Roemmich, J. N., & Bouton, M. E. (2009). Habituation as a determinant of human food intake. *Psychological Review, 116*(2), 384–407.

Foster, G. D., Makris, A. P., & Bailer, B. A. (2005). Behavioral treatment of obesity. *American Journal of Clinical Nutrition, 82*(Suppl.), 230S–235S.

Furst, T., Connors, M., Bisogni, C. A., Sobal, J., & Falk, L. W. (1996). A conceptual model of the food choice process. *Appetite, 26*(3), 247–265.

Glanz, K., Hersey, J., Cates, S., Muth, M., Creel, D., Nocholis, J., Fulgoni, V., 3rd, & Zaripheh, S. (2012). Effect of a nutrient rich foods consumer education program: Results from the nutrition advice study. *Journal of the Academy of Nutrition and Dietetics, 112*(1), 56–63.

Grandes, G., Sanchez, A., Cortada, J. M., Balague, L., Calderon, C., Arrazola, A., ... Prescribe Vida Saludable Group. (2008). Is integration of healthy lifestyle promotion into primary care feasible? Discussion and consensus sessions between clinicians and researchers. *BMC Health Services Research, 8*, 13.

Irvine, A. B., Ary, D. V., Grove, D. A., & Gilfillan-Morton, L. (2004). The effectiveness of an interactive, multimedia program to influence eating habits. *Health Education Research, 19*, 290–305.

Kiernan, M., Moore, S. D., Schoffman, D. E., Lee, K., King, A. C., Taylor, C. B., ... Perri, M. G. (2012). Social support for healthy behaviors: Scale psychometrics and prediction of weight loss among women in a behavioral program. *Obesity, 20*, 756–764.

Lin, J. S., O'Connor, E., Whitlock, E. P., Beil, T. L., Zuber, S. P., Perdue, L. A., ... Luz, K. (2010). Behavioral counseling to promote physical activity and a healthful diet to prevent cardiovascular disease in adults: Update of evidence for the U.S. Preventive Services Task Force [Internet]. Report No. 11-051490EF-1. Agency for Healthcare Research and Quality, Rockville, MD.

Middleton, K. M., Patidar, S. M., & Perri, M. G. (2012). The impact of extended care on the long-term maintenance of weight loss: A systematic review and meta-analysis. *Obesity Reviews, 13*(6), 509–517.

Miller, W. R., & Moyers, T. B. (2007). Eight stages in learning motivational interviewing. *Journal of Teaching and Addictions, 5*, 3–17.

Motivational Interviewing. (2012). Retrieved from http://motivationalinterviewing.org

National Center for Health Statistics. (2012). Retrieved from http://www.cdc.gov/nchs/nhanes.htm

Newman, V. A., Thomson, C. A., Rock, C. L., Flatt, S. W., Kealey, S., Bardwell, W. A., ... Women's Healthy Eating and Living (WHEL) Study Group. (2005). Achieving substantial changes in eating behavior among women previously treated for breast cancer – an overview of the intervention. *Journal of the American Dietetic Association, 105* (3), 382–391.

Nollen, N. L., Hutchenson, T., Carlson, S., Rapoff, M., Goggin, K., Mayfield, C., & Ellerbeck, E. (2013). Development and functionality of a handheld computer program to improve fruit and vegetable intake among low-income youth. *Health Education Research, 28*(2), 249–264. [epub ahead of print. PMID 22949499].

Norman, G. J., Zabinski, M. F., Adams, M. A., Rosenberg, D. E., Yaroch, A. L., & Atienza, A. A. (2007). A review of eHealth interventions of physical activity and dietary behavior change. *American Journal of Preventive Medicine, 33*(4), 336–345.

Ockene, I. S., Hebert, J. R., Ockene, J. K., Saperia, G. M., Stanek, E., Nicolosi, R., Merriam, P. A., & Hurley, T. G. (1999). Effect of physician-delivered nutrition counseling training and an office-support program on saturated fat intake, weight, and serum lipid measurements in a hyperlip-idemic population: Worcester-Area Trial for Counseling in Hyperlipidemia (WATCH). *Archives of Internal Medicine, 159*, 725–731.

Oenema, A., Tan, F., & Brug, J. (2005). Short-term efficacy of a web-based intervention: Main effects and mediators. *Annals of Behavioral Medicine, 29*, 54–63.

Ogden, J., Coop, N., Cousins, C., Crump, R., Field, L., Hughes, S., & Woodger, N. (2013). Distraction, the desire to eat and food intake: Towards an expanded model of mindless eating. *Appetite, 62*, 119–126. [epub ahead of print; PMID 23219989].

Patrick, H., & Williams, G.C. (2012). Self-determination theory: Its application to health behavior and complementarity with motivational interviewing. *International Journal of Behavioral Nutrition and Physical Activity, 9*, 18.

Pearson, N., Biddle, S.J., Williams, L., Worsley, A., Crawford, D., & Ball, K. (2012). Adolescent television viewing and unhealthy snack food consumption: The mediating role of home availability of unhealthy snacks. *Public Health Nutrition, 30*, 1–7.

Riley, W. T., Rivera, D. E., Atienza, A. A., Nilsen, W., Allison, S. M., & Mermelstein, R. (2011). Health behavior models in the age of mobile interventions: Are our theories up to the task? *Translational Behavioral Medicine, 1*(1), 53–71.

Ryan, D. H., Espeland, M. A., Foster, G. D., Haffner, S. M., Hubbard, V. S., Johnson, K. C., ... Look AHEAD Research Group. (2003). Look AHEAD (Action for Health in Diabetes): Design and meth-ods for a clinical trial of weight loss for the prevention of cardiovascular disease in type 2 diabetes. *Controlled Clinical Trials, 24*(5), 610–628.

Sam, A. H., Troke, R. C., Tan, T. M., & Bewick, G. A. (2012). The role of the gut/brain axis in modulating food intake. *Neuropharmacology, 63*, 46–56.

Sobal, J., & Bisogni, C. A. (2009). Constructing food choice decisions. *Annals of Behavioral Medicine, 38*(S1), S37–S46.

Spring, B., Schneider, K., McFadden, H. G., Vaughn, J., Kozak, A. T., Smith, M., ... Lloyd-Jones, D. M. (2012). Multiple behavior changes in diet and activity: A randomized controlled trial using mobile technology. *Archives of Internal Medicine, 172*(10), 789–796.

Sisson, S. B., Shay, C. M., Broyles, S. T., & Leyva, M. (2012). Television-viewing time and dietary quality among U.S. children and adults. *American Journal of Preventive Medicine, 43*(2),196–200.

Stevens, V. J., Glasgow, R. E., Toobert, D. J., Karanja, N., & Smith, K. S. (2003). One-year results from a brief, computer-assisted intervention to decrease consumption of fat and increase consumption of fruits and vegetables. *Preventive Medicine, 36*, 594–600.

Teixeira, F. V., Pais-Ribeiro, J. L., & Maia, A. R. (2012). Beliefs and practices of healthcare providers regarding obesity: A systematic review. *Revista da Associacao Medica Brasileira, 58*(2), 254–262.

Tinker, L. F., Rosal, M. C., Young, A. F., Perri, M. G., Patterson, R. E., VanHorn, L., ... Wu, L. (2007). Predictors of dietary change and maintenance in the Women's Health Initiative Dietary Modifica-tion trial. *Journal of the American Dietetic Association, 107*(7), 1155–1166.

Turk, M. W., Yang, K., Hravnak, M., Sereika, S. M., Ewing, L. J., & Burke, L. E. (2009). Randomized trials of weight loss maintenance: A review. *Journal of Cardiovascular Nursing, 24*(1), 58–80.

USDA. (2012). *What we eat in America.* Retrieved from http://www.ars.usda.gov/Services/docs.htm

Vitolins, M. Z., Crandall, S., Miller, D., Ip, E., Marion, G., & Spangler, J. G. (2012). Obesity educational interventions in U.S. medical schools: A systematic review and identified gaps. *Teaching and Learning in Medicine, 24*(3), 267–272.

Wansink, B. (2010). From mindless eating to mindlessly eating better. *Physiology & Behavior, 100*(5), 545–563.

Wolf, C. (2012). Physician assistants' attitudes about obesity and obese individuals. *Journal of Allied Health, 41*(2), e45–e48.

Wren, A. M., & Bloom, S. R. (2007). Gut hormones and appetite control. *Gastroenterology, 132*, 2116–2130.

Zazpe, I., Sanchez-Tainta, A., Estruch, R., Lamuela-Raventos, R.M., Schroder, H., Salas-Salvado, J., ... Martinez-Gonzalez, M. A. (2008). A large randomized individual and group intervention con-ducted by registered dietitians increased adherence to Mediterranean-type diets: The PREDIMED study. *Journal of the American Dietetic Association, 108*(7), 1134–1144.

8

Physical Activity Behavior

LAUREN A. GRIECO
JYLANA L. SHEATS
SANDRA J. WINTER
ABBY C. KING

LEARNING OBJECTIVES

- Describe the epidemiology and significance of physical activity behavior.
- Identify frameworks, perspectives, and technologies that can be used to broaden the targets and contexts of physical activity interventions.
- Explain individual, social, and built environment factors that contribute to physical activity behavior.
- Discuss the challenges and opportunities in the field of physical activity research.

This chapter provides an overview of the significance, challenges, intervention strategies, and future directions regarding physical activity behavior. Physical activity is defined as "any bodily movement produced by skeletal muscles that result in energy expenditure" (Caspersen, Powell, & Christenson, 1985). "Exercise," meanwhile, is typically defined as a subset of physical activity that involves "planned, structured, and repetitive bodily movements done to improve or maintain one or more components of physical fitness" (Caspersen et al., 1985). For much of the 20th century, research from exercise science focusing primarily on sport and fitness has driven the field. However, the gradual development of an increased public health focus has expanded research in this area to broader dimensions of physical activity behavior (U.S. Department of Health and Human Services [USDHHS], 2008).

EPIDEMIOLOGY AND SIGNIFICANCE

HISTORY AND DEVELOPMENT OF PHYSICAL ACTIVITY RESEARCH

Over the past 30 to 40 years, the focus of physical activity research has shifted along a continuum that began with an initial focus on vigorous-intensity physical activity, and moved to an examination of moderate-intensity physical activity to light-intensity physical activity (Powell, Paluch, & Blair, 2011). More recently, the focus has shifted to the negative effects of prolonged periods of physical inactivity, operationalized as sedentary behavior (Owen, Healy, Matthews, & Dunstan, 2010). The broad concept of "active living" recognizes that physical activity can be classified into different domains that not only include exercise, but also recreational activities, household and occupational activities, and active transportation (Sallis, Linton, & Kraft, 2005).

Research into the various domains and modes of physical activity has been facilitated by improvements in both subjective and objective physical activity assessment, as well as a growing body of literature regarding the effects of the neighborhood environment on physical activity levels. A number of population-based questionnaires now assess physical activity in more than one domain across the life course. For example, the Behavioral Risk Factor Surveillance System, the National Health and Nutrition Examination Survey (NHANES), and the Youth Risk Behavior Survey all gather data regarding leisure-time, domestic, and transportation physical activity. Additionally, there have been improvements in the objective measurement of physical activity using unobtrusive technologies that are increasingly more sophisticated, for example, accelerometers, heart rate monitors, pedometers, body temperature sensors, and motion detectors. The built environment, which includes land-use patterns, natural and constructed features, and the transportation system, also has been shown to affect physical activity and this area remains fertile ground for continued research and intervention (Gebel, Bauman, & Petticrew, 2007).

HEALTH-RELATED OUTCOMES

The potential health benefits of physical activity have long been appreciated. These include increased bone density, lower risk of hip fracture, improved sleep quality, reduced abdominal obesity, lower risk of lung and endometrial cancers, weight maintenance following weight loss, and functional health improvements in older adults (USDHHS, 2008). Evidence also exists showing reduced symptoms of anxiety and depression with regular physical activity (USDHHS, 2008). However, for a number of decades the scientific evidence base demonstrating the negative health outcomes associated with lack of physical activity has lagged behind that of other key health behaviors. Physical inactivity is now recognized as one of the three major health behaviors (in addition to tobacco use and dietary patterns) contributing to chronic diseases accountable for 50% of global mortality (Oxford Health Alliance, 2009). Chronic diseases and conditions strongly linked with inactivity are cardiovascular disease, stroke, some forms of cancer (e.g., colon and breast), type 2 diabetes, depression, loss of physical function, weight gain, cognitive decline in older adults, and all-cause mortality (USDHHS, 2008).

Health risks associated with physical inactivity generally reflect a dose–response curve, with individuals at the most inactive portion of the curve at greatest risk. While typically increasing as a function of age, health risks incurred through a physically inactive lifestyle are evident across demographic characteristics such as race/ethnicity, gender, education, income, and body size (USDHHS, 2008). Important biomarkers of chronic disease risk also have been linked with physical activity levels, including body weight, blood pressure, cholesterol, blood clotting factors, insulin sensitivity, autonomic nervous system regulation, bone and muscle strength, inflammatory processes, and brain vascularization (USDHHS, 2008; Hamer, 2007; Hamer & Chida, 2009).

PREVALENCE OF PHYSICAL ACTIVITY AND NATIONAL PHYSICAL ACTIVITY GUIDELINES

Despite the known benefits of physical activity and negative health outcomes related to inactivity, national surveillance data report that most Americans do not meet national physical activity recommendations, with 20% to 30% of adults reporting no leisure-time physical activity (Centers for Disease Control and Prevention [CDC], 2008). The prevalence of U.S. adults failing to meet recommended levels combined with the risks of being physically inactive or unfit creates a significant public health burden that is similar to, or exceeds, other major chronic disease risk factors (Haskell, Blair, & Hill, 2009).

Current national physical activity guidelines (USDHHS, 2008) make recommendations for Americans across the life course. For adults, the current physical activity recommendations are to participate in at least 150 minutes per week of moderate-intensity aerobic physical activity (i.e., sufficient to increase heart rate and breathing to some degree) or 75 minutes per week of vigorous-intensity aerobic physical activity (i.e., sufficient to increase heart rate and breathing to a noticeable extent), or a combination of the two. These guidelines also describe the recommended mode, frequency, duration, and intensity needed to achieve health benefits. See Tables 8.1 through 8.4 for a summary of the physical activity guidelines according to group: adults, older adults, children and adolescents, and for safety (USDHHS, 2008). Different types of physical activity cause different physiologic changes that result in different health outcomes (Powell et al., 2011). Physical activity health behavior change research and practice continue to be informed by an examination of how much physical activity (i.e., dose–response), of what type (aerobic, ambulatory, strength-training, and balance activities), and at what intensity (light, moderate, and vigorous) are required to achieve which kind of health benefit (e.g., improvements to metabolic or cardiorespiratory systems, or strength, functioning, and balance improvements). To achieve health benefits, current evidence suggests that physical activity can be performed in episodes of 10 minutes or more, preferably spread throughout the week (USDHHS, 2008).

TABLE 8.1 Physical Activity Guidelines for Adults (USDHHS, 2008)

- All adults should avoid inactivity. Some physical activity is better than none, and adults who participate in any amount of physical activity gain some health benefits.

- For substantial health benefits, adults should do at least 150 minutes (2 hours and 30 minutes) a week of moderate-intensity, or 75 minutes (1 hour and 15 minutes) a week of vigorous-intensity aerobic physical activity, or an equivalent combination of moderate- and vigorous-intensity aerobic activity. Aerobic activity should be performed in episodes of at least 10 minutes, and preferably, it should be spread throughout the week.

- For additional and more extensive health benefits, adults should increase their aerobic physical activity to 300 minutes (5 hours) a week of moderate-intensity, or 150 minutes a week of vigorous-intensity aerobic physical activity, or an equivalent combination of moderate- and vigorous-intensity activity. Additional health benefits are gained by engaging in physical activity beyond this amount.

- Adults should also do muscle-strengthening activities that are moderate or high intensity and involve all major muscle groups on 2 or more days a week, as these activities provide additional health benefits.

TABLE 8.2 Physical Activity Guidelines for Older Adults (USDHHS, 2008)

- When older adults cannot do 150 minutes of moderate-intensity aerobic activity a week because of chronic conditions, they should be as physically active as their abilities and conditions allow.
- Older adults should do exercises that maintain or improve balance if they are at risk of falling.
- Older adults should determine their level of effort for physical activity relative to their level of fitness.
- Older adults with chronic conditions should understand whether and how their conditions affect their ability to do regular physical activity safely.

TABLE 8.3 Physical Activity Guidelines for Children and Adolescents (USDHHS, 2008)

It is important to encourage young people to participate in physical activities that are appropriate for their age, that are enjoyable, and that offer variety. Children and adolescents should do 60 minutes (1 hour) or more of physical activity daily. These may consist of:

- **Aerobic:** Most of the 60 or more minutes a day should be either moderate- or vigorous-intensity aerobic physical activity, and should include vigorous-intensity physical activity at least 3 days a week.
- **Muscle strengthening:** As part of their 60 or more minutes of daily physical activity, children and adolescents should include muscle-strengthening physical activity on at least 3 days of the week.
- **Bone strengthening:** As part of their 60 or more minutes of daily physical activity, children and adolescents should include bone-strengthening physical activity on at least 3 days of the week.

TABLE 8.4 Guidelines for Safe Physical Activity (USDHHS, 2008)

- Understand the risks and yet be confident that physical activity is safe for almost everyone.
- Choose to do types of physical activity that are appropriate for current fitness level and health goals, because some activities are safer than others.
- Increase physical activity gradually over time whenever more activity is necessary to meet guidelines or health goals. Inactive people should "start low and go slow" by gradually increasing how often and how long activities are done.
- Protect themselves by using appropriate gear and sports equipment, looking for safe environments, following rules and policies, and making sensible choices about when, where, and how to be active.
- Be under the care of a health care provider if they have chronic conditions or symptoms. People with chronic conditions and symptoms should consult their physician.

In summary, despite the known benefits of regular, reasonably modest amounts of physical activity, the vast majority of individuals are either physically inactive or inadequately physically active. The 2008 Physical Activity Guidelines for Americans provide detailed recommendations for individuals across the lifespan. The next section will examine the various factors that contribute to whether or not an individual may be regularly physically active.

FACTORS CONTRIBUTING TO REGULAR PHYSICAL ACTIVITY

As noted above, an abundance of scientific evidence has found that regularly engaging in physical activity may result in substantial improvements in health, psychological, and cognitive well-being, overall quality of life, and lower health care costs (Lee et al., 2012; Kaplan, 2000; McAuley, Blissmer, Marquez, Jerome, Kramer, & Katula, 2000). For at least some populations, the effects of even modest levels of activity (i.e., fewer minutes per week than recommended) have been found to extend the lifespan by three years compared to individuals who are inactive (Wen et al., 2011).

Individuals of all ages have the potential to benefit from physical activity regardless of racial/ethnic background or socio-economic status (SES) (USDHHS, 2008). Utilizing a social-ecological framework (Sallis, Owen, & Fisher, 2008), this section provides an overview of individual, social, and built environment factors associated with regular physical activity. An understanding of these potential relations may provide areas for future research and assist program planners, interventionists, and policymakers in the development of individual and population-based efforts to promote and improve physical activity across the life course.

INDIVIDUAL-LEVEL FACTORS

Individuals become physically active for a variety of reasons, including weight control, to maintain or increase flexibility and balance, and to engage in social interactions or recreational or leisure pursuits. Physical activity researchers have identified genetic and evolutionary factors that may contribute to the propensity for being physically active or inactive (Bauman, Sallis, Dzewaltowski, & Owen, 2002). Similarly, prior and current participation in physical activity are positively associated with one another. Among U.S. adults, factors negatively associated with commonly investigated physical activities (e.g., leisure and aerobic activities such as brisk walking, swimming, and jogging) include, but are not limited to, advancing age, being female, having lower SES and lower perceived health status, illness, overweight and obesity, and being disabled (Bauman et al., 2002; Dowda, Ainsworth, Addy, Saunders, & Riner, 2003; Trost, Owen, Sallis, & Brown, 2002; CDC, 2007a; CDC, 2007b). Social cognitive variables such as greater levels of physical activity related self-efficacy (i.e., confidence in one's capability to be physically active) and self-regulation (i.e., skills for planning and monitoring exercise activities) have been linked with higher levels of physical activity (McAuley & Blissmer, 2000; Rovniak, Anderson, Winett, & Stephens, 2002). Furthermore, individuals' expectations for and realization of positive outcomes related to being regularly active (Neff & King, 1995; Brassington, Atienza, Perczek, DiLorenzo, & King, 2002; Carels et al., 2005; Wilcox, Castro, & King, 2006), having positive intentions to perform physical activity, and enjoyment of physical activity have been associated with increased levels of physical activity (USDHHS, 2008; Salmon, Owen, Crawford, Bauman, & Sallis, 2003).

Demographic factors such as age, race/ethnicity, and SES have been found to be associated with physical activity levels. There are consistent findings in the literature that as children mature to adolescence they often become less physically active, with girls declining at a younger age than boys (Dumith, Gigante, Domingues, & Kohl, 2011). Increasing physical activity among children and adolescents is a major public health challenge, as physical activity during childhood and adolescence may be an indicator for activity during later years of life (Taylor, Blair, Cummings, Wun, & Malina, 1999; Trudeau, Laurencelle, Tremblay, Rajic, & Shephard, 1999; Cousins, 1997). In children and adolescents, psychosocial and behavioral factors such as intention to be active, perceived barriers, perceived competence, social support (e.g., from parents and others), healthy diet, and sedentary behaviors after school and on weekends have been associated with physical activity (Sallis, Prochaska, & Taylor, 2000). Self-reported physical activity levels among White children are higher than children from racial/ethnic minority groups (Andersen, Crespo, Bartlett, Cheskin, & Pratt, 1998; Pate, Heath, Dowda, & Trost, 1996). Some additional investigations into reasons for this disparity have indicated that, among barriers and facilitators of physical activity among urban African American youth, social support was a stronger facilitator of physical activity for young men and women than other individual and socio-environmental and cultural variables being studied (Ries, Voorhees, & Gittelsohn, 2010). While such results provide useful insights, further research is needed on physical activity disparities across race and ethnicity in children.

A research agenda focused on factors influencing physical activity among older adults is a growing area of interest (Lim & Taylor, 2005; Schutzer & Graves, 2004; King, 2001). Given that older adults comprise the fastest growing age group in the United States (U.S. Census Bureau, Population Division, 2008; USDHHS, 2010) and are among the most inactive (Troiano et al., 2008; White, Wojcicki, & McAuley, 2012), the investigation of this particular population segment is particularly important (Marcus et al., 2006). Poor health (Hardy & Grogan, 2009; Moschny, Platen, Klaaßen-Mielke, Trampisch, & Hinrichs, 2011) and chronic pain (Tu, Stump, Damush, & Clark, 2004) are major factors that present unique challenges for older adults' participation in physical activities. Further barriers to older adults' engagement in physical activity include their beliefs that physical activity cannot prolong one's life, perceived lack of fitness, lack of energy (Crombie et al., 2004), minimal opportunities for sport or leisure activities (Moschny et al., 2011), lack of transport (Moschny et al., 2011), lack of access to facilities, and personal safety and security concerns (Chaudhury, Mahmood, Michael, Campo, & Hay, 2012; Hardy & Grogan, 2009).

In addition to age and race/ethnicity, SES is another demographic factor associated with levels of physical activity in both adolescents and adults (Stalsberg & Pedersen, 2010; Zambon, Lemma, Borraccino, Dalmasso, & Cavallo, 2006). Increased levels of physical activity may be due to the ability to invest in gym memberships and purchase equipment and other items that are necessary for some recreational activities (Stalsberg & Pedersen, 2010). Further, individuals with higher incomes may have more opportunities for physical activity via increased access to facilities and may live in communities that make it easier to be active (Cerin & Leslie, 2008; McNeill, Kreuter, & Subramanian, 2006). Given that personal as well as social and environmental factors may play important roles in influencing participation in physical activity, strategies for physical activity promotion should utilize a multidisciplinary approach and target all SES groups.

SOCIAL FACTORS

Positive social support from family, friends, co-workers, and other people in an individual's environment is consistently associated with increased levels of physical activity (Booth, Owen, Bauman, Clavisi, & Leslie, 2000; Eyler et al., 1998; Giles-Corti & Donovan, 2003; McNeill, Wyrwich, Brownson, Clark, & Kreuter, 2006; Smith, 1999).

For example, receiving social support from significant others, family, or friends has been associated with higher levels of physical activity across a range of adult populations (van Stralen, De Vries, Mudde, Bolman, & Lechner, 2009; Mathews et al., 2010; Bourdeaudhuij et al., 2012; Eyler et al., 1998). Among children and adolescents, Sallis, Prochaska, and Taylor (2000) found that direct parental support and sibling physical activity were positively associated with levels of physical activity. The potential influences of other sources of social support on physical activity have similarly been explored through the human–companion animal bond. This area of research suggests that pets can provide social support that promotes weight loss (Kushner, Blatner, Jewell, & Rudolff, 2012) and increased physical activity (Christian, Giles-Corti, & Knuiman, 2010). For example, a study of older adults conducted by Shibata and colleagues (Shibata et al., 2012) revealed that dog walkers engaged in more total physical activity and minutes per week of moderate-to-vigorous physical activity than non-dog walkers and non-dog owners. Social networks also have been shown to be important in facilitating physical activity and reducing the odds of obesity, particularly for older adults (Leroux, Moore, Richard, & Gauvin, 2012).

BUILT ENVIRONMENT FACTORS

The built environment includes constructed features (e.g., sidewalks), natural features (e.g., green spaces), land-use patterns, and the transportation system (Brownson, Hoehner, Day, Forsyth, & Sallis, 2009). Commonly assessed built environment variables include residential density and land-use mix (how the land is used), availability and accessibility of recreational facilities, street connectivity, sidewalk availability, amount and speed of vehicular traffic, and aesthetic characteristics of the neighborhood (e.g., scenery, foliage, and shade) (Brownson et al., 2009). Public transit and related transportation factors also comprise the built environment and are associated with walking in a variety of populations (Saelens & Handy, 2008). In addition to individual built environment factors, composite variables and indices (i.e., a combination of different environmental variables) have been developed and successfully used in capturing physical activity levels in different locales (Frank et al., 2010; King et al., 2011; Brownson et al., 2009; Friel, Chopra, & Satcher, 2007; Handy, Boarnet, Ewing, & Killingsworth, 2002).

A growing recognition exists concerning the associations between physical activity and personal, social, and physical environmental factors (Wendel Vos, Droomers, Kremers, Brug, & Van Lenthe, 2007; USDHHS, 2010; McNeill, Wyrwich, Brownson, Clark, & Kreuter, 2006; Giles-Corti & Donovan, 2003). Both perceived and objectively measured environmental elements have been linked with variations in physical activity across different types of neighborhoods. Among the positive associations that have been found between physical activity levels and perceived and objective measures of environmental variables are the availability, accessibility, and convenience of destinations and public facilities as well as neighborhood features (e.g., the presence of sidewalks and lower traffic volume) (McCormack et al., 2004). Additional perceived environment measures consistently associated with physical activity are attractive neighborhood aesthetics (e.g., gardens and foliage), absence of stray dogs, presence of intersection safety features, and social features such as the presence of other people in the community being active (King et al., 2000, 2006; Sallis, King, Sirard, & Albright, 2007). In an examination of neighborhood environments and physical activity in 11 countries, it was reported that in order to meet physical activity recommendations, multiple activity-friendly features and neighborhood attributes would need to be present (as opposed to single features or attributes) (Sallis et al., 2009).

The impact of environmental variables on the practice of health behaviors such as physical activity may be particularly pronounced for special populations such as ethnic/racial minorities and older adults. For example, living in street blocks within a neighborhood that are characterized by low SES and a high proportion of minorities has been associated with reduced access to physical activity facilities and lower levels of physical activity (Gordon-Larsen, Nelson, Page, & Popkin, 2006). A systematic review of African Americans and the built environment revealed that minimal traffic, the presence of sidewalks, and safety from crime were perceived built environment variables that were positively associated with physical activity (Casagrande, Whitt-Glover, Lancaster, Odoms-Young, & Gary, 2009). However, among African American girls it was found that perceptions of neighborhood safety and access to facilities for physical activity were not associated with physical activity levels, which leads to questions about other individual, interpersonal, environmental, and/or cultural factors that may play a role (Adkins, Sherwood, Story, & Davis, 2004). Environmental correlates of physical activity among older adults have been less examined. Programs that are in close proximity to older adults' households and factors such as the availability of open spaces, safe paths and sidewalks, and weather are potential environmental facilitators to physical activity for this population (Lim & Taylor, 2005).

In summary, there are many factors at the individual, social, and environmental levels that affect physical activity levels across the lifespan. Continued research in this field will help to further clarify the social and built environments that facilitate healthy decision making at the population level.

PHYSICAL ACTIVITY INTERVENTIONS

Acknowledgement of the influence of environmental contexts and differences across and within subgroups of the population are important in the development and implementation of successful physical activity interventions (King et al., 2000; Marcus et al., 2006). The Task Force on Community Preventive Services regularly conducts systematic intervention reviews in the physical activity field and categorizes these by approach. These include behavioral, social, informational, environmental, and policy-based approaches (Guide to Community Preventive Services, 2012). Although physical activity interventions may be categorized many different ways, this chapter will use the aforementioned groupings.

BEHAVIORAL AND SOCIAL APPROACHES

Behavioral and social interventions typically utilize a combination of cognitive and behavioral strategies that can be delivered through a range of communication channels. These channels include face-to-face (Rejeski et al., 2003), telephone programs (King, Haskell, Taylor, Kraemer, & DeBusk, 1991; Castro & King, 2002; Eakin, Lawler, Vandelanotte, & Owen, 2007), print and other mass media (Marcus et al., 2006), and communication technologies. Communication technologies may be classified into categories of Internet/web-based (Napolitano et al., 2003; Tate, Jackvony, & Wing, 2003; Verheijden, Jans, Hildebrandt, & Hopman-Rock, 2007), text message, smartphone apps (Grieco et al., 2012), hand-held computers/tablets (Bauman et al., 2012; Grieco et al., 2012; King et al., 2008), interactive voice-response "tele-health" systems (King et al., 2007), and pedometers (Bravata et al., 2007). These provide a range of possible intervention delivery modalities.

Behavioral interventions, based on social cognitive theory and its derivatives (Glanz & Bishop, 2010), typically teach individuals skills that aid in the adoption and maintenance of physical activity behaviors, and aim to enhance immediate social and environmental circumstances that support and facilitate their practice. Common components of individual-level theoretically based behavioral interventions include goal setting and self-regulation, provision of accurate information about the benefits of physical activity, and awareness enhancement (i.e., increasing awareness of opportunities to be active). Receiving reliable personalized feedback about progress, building social support for regular physical activity, and engaging in active problem solving related to barriers to physical activity are additional self-regulatory strategies shown to improve physical activity participation (Brassington et al., 2002; Carels et al., 2005; Marcus et al., 2000; Rejeski et al., 2003).

Social interventions are designed to provide individuals with strategies for receiving and giving support and encouragement to and from family, friends, co-workers, and others. Family-based social support interventions have shown increased participation around physical activity. Similarly, social support interventions in community settings that have focused on strengthening existing or new relationships and social networks for behavior change outside of the family (e.g., at worksites or in other community settings) have generally been found to be effective (Guide to Community Preventive Services, 2012). Thus, by involving others in an individual's physical activity goals, this social context can provide increased support for physical activity participation.

INFORMATIONAL APPROACHES

Informational interventions use educational strategies to target constructs related to behavior change. Specifically, knowledge, attitudes, and beliefs about the benefits of regular physical activity are key factors to target for initiating behavior change. Examples of interventional messages include notifying people of the locations of current opportunities for physical activity within their community. Other strategies include providing people with normative information regarding how and where others around them are engaging in physical activity, and instructions to help enable them to increase their regular physical activity levels.

Evidence on large-scale community-wide campaigns delivered through print, TV, and radio has shown some increases in knowledge about exercise and physical activity, as well as intention to be more physically active (Guide to Community Preventive Services, 2012). Other types of useful information include educating people on the benefits of being physically active. Such benefits include, but are not limited to, improved health, wellness and quality of life, and decreased risk of disease.

ENVIRONMENTAL AND POLICY-BASED APPROACHES

Environmental and policy-based interventions aim to alter some aspect of the physical or policy environment (Schmid, Pratt, & Howze, 1995). This is done often as a means for reducing barriers to physical activity. Incorporating environmental strategies into health promotion efforts may result in more effective community health interventions that support and sustain positive health behaviors across a wider segment of the community. Examples of specific environmental/policy approaches that may improve levels of physical activity are incorporating sidewalk and bike lanes into community design and urban planning, providing funds for hiking and walking trails as a part of highway projects, designing safe routes for walking or bicycling to school, developing "complete street" policies (i.e., increasing street aesthetics and safety though foliage, cross walks, speed bumps, traffic lights, roundabouts, etc.), and the provision of incentives for the establishment of mixed-use developments involving both residential and commercial destinations. Additional research is needed to better understand the measurement issues and impacts of environment and policy approaches to promoting regular physical activity (Story et al., 2009).

Environmental interventions have the potential for complementing informational, social, and behavioral interventions. Given their scale and scope, their population reach can be greater in addition to their potential for benefiting all individuals in a community (Glanz & Bishop, 2010; King et al., 1995; Milstein, Homer, Briss, Burton, & Pechacek, 2011; Schmid et al., 1995).

Interventions to promote physical activity in specific community settings, such as schools and worksites, also have the potential for broad impact. However, the need for better controlled, scientifically rigorous studies remains. An examination of controlled trials in their area has shown that for a number of population segments, such as adolescents, effective physical activity interventions will likely need to contain multiple program components, including school, family, and/or community involvement (van Sluijs, McMinn, & Griffin, 2007). Successful school-based physical activity interventions also have incorporated environmental and policy strategies to extend the reach of and involve others potentially influential in a child's physical activity behavior (Luepker et al., 1996; Timperio, Salmon, & Ball, 2004). A well-designed health-related physical education curriculum delivered either by teachers or physical education specialists has been shown to increase the amount of time children spend at school being physically active (Sallis et al., 1997). However, the efficacy of school-based interventions has been reported to be, at times, inconsistent (Biddle, Gorely, & Stensel, 2004; Timperio et al., 2004), and the need for further work in this area remains.

Similar to school settings for children, worksites present a potentially convenient setting for health promotion programming for working-age adults. Challenges in enacting rigorous methods in such settings notwithstanding, worksite programs have shown some favorable outcomes for increasing physical activity (Marcus et al., 2006). Effective worksite interventions have included changes in the social and physical environments to support recommended health behaviors (Carnethon et al., 2009; Osilla et al., 2012). Examples of these strategies are incorporating structured physical activity breaks during the work day, promoting the use of stairs rather than elevators, locating parking lots further away from the worksite to encourage more walking, and providing tailored motivational programs based on behavior change theory (Marcus et al., 2006). Evidence also supports the use of environmental cues and point-of-decision prompts in successfully promoting physical activity in such settings (Guide to Community Preventive Services, 2012).

In summary, a comprehensive approach that appropriately targets behavioral, informational, environmental, and policy-based interventions is required to improve and better understand the complex factors that affect physical activity behavior.

FUTURE DIRECTIONS IN PHYSICAL ACTIVITY PROMOTION

Several emerging directions in the physical activity promotion arena are summarized below. These approaches have the potential for broadening both the overall impact and population "reach" of interventions in the field.

EMERGING ROLE OF PHYSICAL INACTIVITY AND SEDENTARY BEHAVIOR AS TARGETS FOR INTERVENTION

There has been growing recognition of the negative health effects linked with prolonged sedentary behaviors (e.g., sitting, television viewing, and prolonged screen time), independent of physical activity levels (Owen, Heally, Matthews & Dunston, 2010). Among the factors associated with increased sedentary behavior are overweight and obesity, older age, lower education and income levels, unemployment, financial costs to physical activity programs, family and work commitments, feeling tired, and poor health (Bowman, 2006; CDC, 2008; Salmon et al., 2003). Television viewing also has been found to be an indicator of other sedentary behaviors among adult women, though not necessarily men (Sugiyama, Healy, Dunstan, Salmon, & Owen, 2008).

A recent article aimed to quantify the public health burden worldwide of physical inactivity resulting from major non-communicable diseases (NCDs) (Lee et al., 2012). Population-attributable fractions (the proportion of excess disease in the population attributable to physical inactivity) were used to calculate the prevalence of inactivity and the relative risk of the outcome of interest. After adjusting for confounding factors and applying meta-analytic statistical procedures, the results indicated that 6% to 10% of major NCDs worldwide were attributed to physical inactivity, and that eliminating physical inactivity could save over 5.3 million deaths and increase life expectancy by 0.68 years worldwide (Lee et al., 2012). Such analyses underscore the adverse effects of physical inactivity on the population worldwide.

The most frequently studied sedentary activity to date is television viewing. High U.S. population levels of television viewing (i.e., greater than 14 hours per week) have been associated with lower household income, increasing age, being divorced or separated, lower self-rated health, smoking, higher body mass index (BMI), fewer average minutes per week in leisure-time physical activity, more depression, lower fruit and vegetable intake, reporting unsupportive neighborhood environments for walking (e.g., crime, traffic congestion, poor lighting, and lack of aesthetics or scenery), and regularly eating dinner in front of the television (King et al., 2010). Furthermore, regularly eating dinner in front of the television was found to be the strongest single correlate of high levels of TV viewing across the U.S. population derived sample under study (King et al., 2010).

Suggested strategies to increase physical activity and decrease physical inactivity include developing a multi-level system approach to physical activity promotion, establishing a set of guiding principles that can be used by researchers and decision makers alike, making physical activity behavior an integral focus of disease prevention and health promotion modeling endeavors, and developing and implementing programs in both the private and academic sectors to this end (Kohl et al., 2012).

STEALTH INTERVENTIONS

"Stealth" health promotion interventions typically refer to interventions that are carried out for a particular non-health purpose, but have as a side effect the promotion of healthy behaviors (Robinson, 2010). Examples of health-promoting stealth interventions can be found in the field of climate change, urban planning, and altruism (Swinburn, 2008). For example, campaigns that focus on reducing the use of non-renewable energy by substituting walking and cycling in place of driving could have a positive effect on human health, not only by reducing global carbon emissions, but also by increasing physical activity (Egger, 2007). More popular in Europe than in the United States, fiscal policies that seek to reduce air and noise pollution as well as traffic congestion by charging drivers a "congestion tax" may also promote active transportation such as bicycling and walking (Roberts, 2003). Engaging community residents in fundraising events arranged by nonprofit organizations, such as fun runs or walks, while also financially supporting a worthy cause, is an increasingly popular stealth intervention that promotes physical activity (Higgins & Lauzon, 2002). Another example of a stealth physical activity intervention is the use of computer and video games that promote dance as well as other types of active play or entertainment. Preliminary evidence indicates that this type of play has the potential to increase physical activity, improve motor skills, and provide motivation for physical activity, as well as improving knowledge, skills, attitudes, and behaviors around physical activity and health more generally (Papastergiou, 2009; Biddiss & Irwin, 2010; Foley & Maddison, 2010; Chen, Hekler, & King, 2011). It is also possible that promoting physical activity may itself be a "stealth" intervention for promoting other values or goals. For example, for some individuals, sport and physical activity interventions may promote personal and social development (Sandford, 2006).

MULTIPLE BEHAVIOR CHANGE INTERVENTIONS

Heart disease, cancer, and stroke are the major causes of death and disease, not only in the United States (Kochanek, Xu, Murphy, Minino, & Kung, 2011) but worldwide (Alwan 2011), and the burden of disease is often felt more strongly by minorities and low-income individuals (Beodenheimer, Chen, & Bennert, 2009). From 1999 to 2009, the number of Americans aged 45 years and older with two or more chronic conditions increased from 16.1% to 21.0%, and this increase occurred for both men and women and across all racial and ethnic groups (Freid, Bernstein, & Bush, 2012). Individuals with multiple chronic conditions often have high health care expenditures, may be less productive workers, are more likely to develop disability, and are at increased risk of premature death (Edington, 2001). The multiple health risk behaviors associated with chronic disease include physical inactivity, poor diet, tobacco use, alcohol abuse, and chronic stress. These health behaviors are often co-occurring, and are associated with more than one chronic condition. As part of the American Heart Association's 2020 Strategic Impact Goals (Lloyd-Jones et al., 2010), a new index of optimal cardiovascular health has been developed which targets three cardiovascular health behaviors (physical activity and dietary intake consistent with current guidelines and status as a nonsmoker), and four additional health factors influenced by these health behaviors (a BMI between 18.0 kg/m^2 and 24.9 kg/m^2, untreated total cholesterol less than 200 mg/dL, untreated blood pressure less than 120/less than 80 mmHg, and fasting blood glucose less than 100 mg/dL). Fewer than 1% of 14,515 adults aged 20 years and older who participated in the National Health and Nutrition Examination Survey (NHANES) between 2003 and 2008 reported achieving all seven of these metrics (Shay et al., 2012). Other studies have found similarly low percentages of the population meeting these healthy behavior criteria (Appel, 2012).

Multiple health behavior change interventions can target several health behaviors either simultaneously (i.e., at the same time) or sequentially (i.e., by starting with one health behavior and subsequently adding others). Compared to single behavior change interventions, these types of multiple health behavior interventions have the potential to be as, or more, effective in changing health behaviors. They also can provide a better use of resources, maximize health promotion contact opportunities, have greater real-world applicability, and be more relevant for behaviors that co-occur (Nigg & Long, 2012). Successfully changing one health behavior may lead to increased confidence and self-efficacy that other health behaviors can be successfully changed, particularly if the change process for the different health behaviors is similar (Prochaska, Spring, & Nigg, 2008). It is also possible that multiple health behavior change interventions may not be as effective as single health behavior change interventions because such approaches can be overwhelming and confusing, and different behaviors may require different behavior change strategies. Single health behavior change interventions facilitate a greater focus on specific content, can be more comprehensive for a particular health behavior, and may be less cognitively demanding than combined health behavior change interventions (Nigg & Long, 2012). Further research in this field is required to better understand the potential that multiple behavior change interventions have to improve health, particularly with respect to different populations. For instance, in a study of midlife and older adults reporting greater than average stress levels, either beginning with a physical activity intervention first or simultaneously delivering physical activity and healthy diet interventions together resulted in generally improved 12-month levels of both physical activity and dietary behaviors relative to an attention-control intervention (King et al., 2013). In contrast, beginning with dietary intervention first appeared to interfere with subsequently learning how to increase physical activity (King et al., 2013).

BROADENING THE TARGETS AND CONTEXTS OF PHYSICAL ACTIVITY INTERVENTIONS

The adoption and maintenance of health-promoting physical activity are complex and warrant examination from a broad perspective. Possible approaches to consider include using a social ecological model (individual, interpersonal, organizational, environmental, and public policy), incorporating an inter-disciplinary and multi-sector approach, examining physical activity across the life course, and considering a variety of physical activity modes (frequency, intensity, time, and type) and domains (leisure, occupational, household, and transport-related activities).

Applying a Social Ecological Framework

Health behavior change can be usefully studied through applying a social ecological framework that considers not only an individual's behavior, but also the contexts in which an individual lives (Sallis, Owen & Fisher, 2008; Sallis et al., 2006). For example, an individual may set personal goals to be more physically active, but these goals may be thwarted by a lack of social support and encouragement from family and friends, an absence of wellness programs available at school or in the workplace, a lack of appropriate recreational facilities in the neighborhood, and/or by an absence of state and local policies that make travel by foot or bicycle safe and easy. Broadening the targets of physical activity research and interventions to incorporate a more holistic, social ecological perspective requires a multi-sector approach that includes professionals not only from public health and health care, but also from parks and recreation, law enforcement, education, transportation, urban planning, education, policy, and business (USDHHS, 2008). Support for the different levels that comprise such a social ecological approach can be found in the literature (Ockene et al., 2007).

Utilizing a Life-Course Perspective

The life-course approach is an alternative or complementary framework in which to consider physical activity. The 2008 Physical Activity Guidelines for Americans provide information for children and adolescents aged 6 to 17, adults aged 18 to 64, older adults aged 65 and older, and special populations such as pregnant women and people with disabilities and chronic medical conditions (USDHHS, 2008). Rarely, however, are interventions developed that target or include more than one age group or population. Doing so could potentially harness social and contextual forces shared across age groups and life stages, with broadened intervention impact a possible consequence.

CHALLENGES AND OPPORTUNITIES IN THE FIELD OF PHYSICAL ACTIVITY RESEARCH

Many factors affect the adoption and maintenance of regular physical activity during the life course, including biological and socio-cultural determinants, some of which are invariant (e.g., age and gender), and some of which are modifiable (e.g., behavioral patterns and a number of social and environmental contexts) (Seefeldt, Malina, & Clark, 2002). Similar to other health behaviors and conditions, while short-term adoption of increased physical activity can often be achieved by many individuals, longer-term maintenance of a more active lifestyle typically proves far more challenging (Marcus et al., 2000). Further research is needed regarding how best to maintain physical activity behavior over the longer term. To do this typically requires extending study periods, which necessitates a greater investment of resources (both financial and human). Currently, funding agencies do not typically support studies of a sufficient length to study maintenance strategies and relapse prevention over time.

The body of knowledge regarding health behavior change research that targets physical activity is ever increasing. One of the challenges facing researchers in this field is to determine appropriate ways of summarizing and integrating the literature. Meta-analyses are increasingly being used to combine and compare the results of different studies, but if not conducted properly, meta-analyses can result in spurious results (Sox & Goodman, 2012). Common areas of bias include inadequate identification and selection of studies (publication, search, and selection bias), integrating studies in which study methods are far from homogeneous, insufficient availability of information regarding the methods and results in the studies being combined, and using incorrect statistical techniques to analyze the integrated data (Dwan et al., 2008; Moher, Liberati, Tetzlaff, & Altman, 2009). As such, increased rigor in conducting meta-analyses is required.

THE CHALLENGE OF DISSEMINATION AND TRANSLATION OF RESULTS

Despite the growing body of knowledge regarding evidence-based interventions to promote physical activity previously discussed, less is known about how to effectively disseminate proven interventions in community and health care settings. Successful dissemination of an effective intervention typically requires a comprehensive approach that targets external validity as well as internal validity (Rabin, Brownson, Kerner, & Glasgow, 2006). Successful approaches may include (Rabin et al., 2006):

- Broadening study designs to be more representative of real-world settings;
- Measuring outcomes that include practitioner, organizational, economic, and policy change indicators and reporting of both positive and negative outcomes;
- Better documenting external validity to include measures of dissemination mediators (such as reach, adoption, and maintenance) and moderators (such as contextual factors and adopter characteristics);

- Applying tools to enhance dissemination, such as ensuring that the communication channels used are appropriate for the intervention and the target population;
- Understanding context and balancing fidelity and reinvention;
- Obtaining funding specifically for dissemination;
- Increasing organizational commitment from academic institutions and community and health care organizations;
- Encouraging research–practice partnerships; and
- Increasing organizational capacity and resources.

In addition to the many opportunities for broadening the target of physical activity interventions and research, there are additional areas within the physical activity behavior change field that also warrant further effort. These areas include eliminating disparities in physical activity participation that have been observed in the United States (Gordon-Larsen et al., 2006), increasing global collaborations, conducting a greater number of comparative effectiveness studies in identifying the most cost-effective interventions for different subgroups in the field, and expanding the use of information and assessment technologies to both promote health behavior change and disseminate interventions found to be efficacious.

Changes in the way the global population lives—through increasing globalization made possible by improved transportation and communication, increasing urbanization, and changing lifestyles that include improved access to food, decreased levels of physical activity, and the consumption of "western diets"—are contributing to increases in the prevalence and incidence of chronic diseases worldwide. Population-based strategies such as health education campaigns and fiscal and regulatory measures, in combination with behavior change initiatives that promote healthful behaviors, are urgently needed to improve health on a global scale. Practitioners and researchers in developed countries have substantial knowledge regarding physical activity behavior change accumulated over the past half century that can be shared with their counterparts in developing countries.

HARNESSING THE POWER OF INFORMATION TECHNOLOGY

The use of information and communication technologies (e.g., landline and mobile telephones, Internet, and broadband) has reached saturation levels in many developed countries and continues to increase in developing countries (International Telecomunnications Union: Measuring the Information Society, 2011). The use of these technologies to promote health is increasing—both as an intervention medium (e.g., to distribute health information or change behavior through tailored messages) and as a research focus (e.g., to gather data or reach research subjects) (Lintonen, Konu, & Seedhouse, 2008). Further, scientifically rigorous research is needed to determine the most effective components and modes of delivery of health-promoting technology interventions. Initial results suggest that health behavior change interventions are more likely to be successful if they are grounded in theory, use more rather than fewer evidence-based behavior change strategies, and combine more than one method of communication (Webb, Joseph, Yardley, & Michie, 2010). Additional research regarding the most effective ways to disseminate promising health behavior interventions in a global context is also required.

Many research studies focus on identifying the causes and correlates of diseases and their risk factors in the hopes of understanding the mechanisms associated with an existing health problem. This problem-oriented approach may have the unintended consequence of limiting hypotheses about treatment and prevention to issues that have been associated previously with the problem. A complementary approach that is future-focused, solution-oriented, and that identifies what works to address a particular problem to improve health may be more directly relevant for policy and practice (Robinson & Sirard, 2005) and, in addition, shorten the timeline to disseminate and translate research into practice. For example, Robinson and Sirard suggest that a problem-oriented approach may focus on testing the association of perceived or objective measures of neighborhood safety on physical activity, whereas a solution-oriented approach would focus on identifying and implementing practices and policies that increase perceived or objective measures of neighborhood safety and examining the effect of the intervention on physical activity. Furthermore, future directions include the need for improved measures of correlates, objective measures of physical activity, prospective designs, and advanced data modeling to assess causal determinants (Bauman et al., 2012).

CONCLUSIONS

In summary, although engaging in even modest amounts of physical activity on a regular basis has been shown to have important health benefits across the lifespan, promoting physical activity adoption and sustained maintenance remains challenging. An individual's ability to engage regularly in physical activity and reduce sedentary time is affected not only by personal characteristics but also by the social, built, and policy environments in which the individual lives, works, and plays. A comprehensive approach for promoting regular physical activity is therefore required that intervenes across the range of social ecological levels and across the life course. Adequately disseminating, translating, and scaling up successful physical activity health behavior change research and best practices continue to challenge researchers and practitioners alike. To tackle these issues, a multidisciplinary approach that incorporates a broad perspective with input from health care providers, researchers, local government, and nonprofit organizations is recommended. Finally, harnessing the power of technology to accelerate and sustain positive physical activity behavior change is an area that holds much promise for the future. Through this wide array of approaches and perspectives, the promise of creating and sustaining a physically active population may be more fully realized.

ACKNOWLEDGMENTS

Dr. King was supported by U.S. Public Health Service grants R01 HL089694, RC1 HL099340, and U01 AG022376. Drs. Grieco, Sheats, and Winter were supported by U.S. Public Health Service grant T32 HL007034 From the National Heart, Lung, and Blood Institute.

REFERENCES

Adkins, S., Sherwood, N. E., Story, M., & Davis, M. (2004). Physical activity among African-American girls: The role of parents and the home environment. *Obesity Research*, (12), 38S–45S. doi: 10.1038/oby.2004.267

Alwan, A. (2011). *Global status report on noncommunicable diseases 2010*. World Health Organization. Geneva, Switzerland

Andersen, R. E., Crespo, C. J., Bartlett, S. J., Cheskin, L. J., & Pratt, M. (1998). Relationship of physical activity and television watching with body weight and level of fatness among children. *Journal of the American Medical Association*, 279(12), 938–942.

Appel, L. J. (2012). Empirical support for cardiovascular health: The case gets even stronger. *Circulation, 125,* 973–974. doi: 10.1161/CIRCULATIONAHA.111.0088542

Bauman, A. E., Reis, R. S., Sallis, J. F., Wells, J. C., Loos, R. J., & Martin, B. W. (2012). Correlates of physical activity: Why are some people physically active and others not? *The Lancet, 380*(9838), 258–271.

Bauman, A. E., Sallis, J. F., Dzewaltowski, D. A., & Owen, N. (2002). Toward a better understanding of the influences on physical activity: The role of determinants, correlates, causal variables, mediators, moderators, and confounders. *American Journal of Preventive Medicine, 23*(2S), 5–14.

Beodenheimer, T., Chen, E., & Bennert, H. D. (2009). Confronting the growing burden of chronic disease: Can the US health care workforce do the job? *Health Affairs, 28*(1), 64–74.

Biddiss, E., & Irwin, J. (2010). Active video games to promote physical activity in children and youth: A systematic review. *Archives of Pediatrics & Adolescent Medicine, 164*(7), 664.

Biddle, S. J., Gorely, T., & Stensel, D. J. (2004). Health-enhancing physical activity and sedentary behaviour in children and adolescents. *Journal of Sports Sciences, 22,* 679–701.

Booth, M. L., Owen, N., Bauman, A., Clavisi, O., & Leslie, E. (2000). Social-cognitive and perceived environment influences associated with PA in older Australians. *Preventive Medicine, 31,* 15–22.

Bourdeaudhuij, I., Lefevre, J., Deforche, B., Wijndaele, K., Matton, L., & Philippaerts, R. (2012). Physical activity and psychosocial correlates in normal weight and overweight 11 to 19 year olds. *Obesity Research, 13*(6), 1097–1105. doi: 10.1038/oby.2005.128

Bowman, S. A. (2006). Television-viewing characteristics of adults: Correlations to eating practices and overweight and health status. *Preventing Chronic Disease, 3*(2), A38.

Brassington, G. S., Atienza, A. A., Perczek, R. E., DiLorenzo, T. M., & King, A. C. (2002). Intervention-related cognitive versus social mediators of exercise adherence in the elderly. *American Journal of Preventive Medicine, 23*(2 Suppl.), 80–86.

Brownson, R. C., Hoehner, C. M., Day, K., Forsyth, A., & Sallis, J. F. (2009). Measuring the built environment for physical activity: State of the science. *American Journal of Preventive Medicine, 36*(4 Suppl.), S99–S123.e111.

Bungum, T. J., & Vincent, M. L. (1997). Determinants of physical activity among female adolescents. *American Journal of Preventive Medicine, 13*(2), 115–122.

Carels, R. A., Darby, L. A., Rydin, S., Douglass, O. M., Cacciapaglia, H. M., & O'Brien, W. H. (2005). The relationship between self-monitoring, outcome expectancies, difficulties with eating and exercise, and physical activity and weight loss treatment outcomes. *Annals of Behavioral Medicine, 30*(3), 182–190.

Carnethon, M., Whitsel, L. P., Franklin, B. A., Kris-Etherton, P., Milani, R., Pratt, C. A., & Wagner, G. R. (2009). Worksite wellness programs for cardiovascular disease prevention. *Circulation, 120*(17), 1725–1741. doi: 10.1161/circulationaha.109.192653

Casagrande, S. S., Whitt-Glover, M. C., Lancaster, K. J., Odoms-Young, A. M., & Gary, T. L. (2009). Built environment and health behaviors among African Americans: A systematic review. *American Journal of Preventive Medicine, 36*(2), 174–181.

Caspersen, C. J., Powell, K. E., & Christenson, G. M. (1985). Physical activity, exercise, and physical fitness: Definitions and distinctions for health-related research. *Public Health Reports, 100*(2), 126.

Castro, C. M., & King, A. C. (2002). Telephone-assisted counseling for physical activity. *Exercise and Sport Sciences Reviews, 30*(2), 64–68.

Centers for Disease Control and Prevention (CDC). (1997). Monthly estimates of leisure-time physical activity—United States, 1994. *Morbidity and Mortality Weekly Report, 46,* 393–397.

CDC. (2001). Increasing physical activity: A report on recommendations of the Task Force on Community Preventive Services. *Morbidity and Mortality Weekly Report, 50*(18), 1–24.

CDC. (2007a). Physical activity among adults with a disability—United States, 2005. *Morbidity and Mortality Weekly Report, 56,* 1021–1024.

CDC. (2007b). Physical activity among adults—United States 2001 and 2005. *Morbidity and Mortality Weekly Report, 23, 56,* 1209–1212.

CDC. (2008). Physical Activity Statistics: 1988–2008 Leisure-Time Physical Activity Trend Chart. Retrieved from http://www.cdc.gov/nccdphp/dnpa/physical/stats/leisure_time.htm

Cerin, E., & Leslie, E. (2008). How socio-economic status contributes to participation in leisure-time physical activity. *Social Science & Medicine, 66,* 2596–2609.

Chaudhury, H., Mahmood, A., Michael, Y. L., Campo, M., & Hay, K. (2012). The influence of neighborhood residential density, physical and social environments on older adults' physical activity: An exploratory study in two metropolitan areas. *Journal of Aging Studies, 26*(1), 35–43.

Chatterjee, N., Blakely, D. E., & Barton, C. (2005). Perspectives on obesity and barriers to control from workers at a community center serving low-income Hispanic children and families. *Journal of Community Health Nursing, 22*(1), 23–36.

Chen, F. X., Hekler, E. B., & King, A. C. (2011). How might we change behavior through the design of physically active video games? Medicine 2.0 Annual Meeting, Stanford, CA.

Christian, H., Giles-Corti, B., & Knuiman, M. (2010). "I'm just a'-walking the dog" correlates of regular dog walking. *Family and Community Health, 33*(1), 44–52.

Cohen-Mansfield, J., Marx, M., & Guralnik, J. (2003). Motivators and barriers to exercise in an older community-dwelling population. *Journal of Aging and Physical Activity, 11*, 242–253.

Cousins, S. O. (1997). Elderly tomboys? Sources of self-efficacy for physical activity in later life. *Journal of Aging and Physical Activity, 5*, 229–243.

Crombie, I. K., Irvine, L., Williams, B., McGinnis, A. R., Slane, P. W., Alder, E. M., & McMurdo, M. E. T. (2004). Why older people do not participate in leisure time physical activity: A survey of activity levels, beliefs and deterrents. *Age and Ageing, 33*(3), 287–292. doi: 10.1093/ageing/afh089

Dowda, M., Ainsworth, B. E., Addy, C. L., Saunders, R., & Riner, W. (2003). Correlates of physical activity among U.S. young adults, 18 to 30 years of age, from NHANES III. *Annals of Behavioral Medicine, 26*(1), 15–23.

Dumith, S. C., Gigante, D. P., Domingues, M. R., & Kohl, H. W. (2011). Physical activity change during adolescence: A systematic review and a pooled analysis. *International Journal of Epidemiology, 40*(3), 685–698. doi: 10.1093/ije/dyq272

Dunn, A.L., Marcus, B.H., Kampert, J.B., Garcia, M.E., Kohl, H.W., & Blair, S.N. (1999). Comparison of lifestyle and structured interventions to increase physical activity and cardiorespiratory fitness: A randomized trial. *Journal of the American Medical Association, 281*(4), 327–34.

Dwan, K., Altman, D. G., Arnaiz, J. A., Bloom, J., Chan, A. W., Cronin, E., & Williamson, P. R. (2008). Systematic review of the empirical evidence of study publication bias and outcome reporting bias. *PLoS One, 3*(8), e3081.

Eakin, E. G., Lawler, S. P., Vandelanotte, C., & Owen, N. (2007). Telephone interventions for physical activity and dietary behavior change: A systematic review. *American Journal of Preventive Medicine, 32*(5), 419–434.

Edington, D. W. (2001). Emerging research: A view from one research center. *American Journal of Health Promotion, 15*(5), 341–349.

Egger, G. (2007). Personal carbon trading: A potential "stealth intervention" for obesity reduction? *Medical Journal of Australia, 187*(3), 185–187.

Evenson, K. R., Sarmiento, O. L., Macon, M. L., Tawney, K. W., & Ammerman, A. S. (2002). A qualitative study of physical activity determinants among Latina immigrants. *Women's Health, 36*, 43–57.

Eyler, A. A., Baker, E., Cromer, L., King, A. C., Brownson, R. C., & Donatelle, R. J. (1998). Physical activity and minority women: A qualitative study. *Health Education & Behavior, 25*, 640–652.

Foley, L., & Maddison, R. (2010). Use of active video games to increase physical activity in children: A (virtual) reality? *Pediatric Exercise Science, 22*(1), 7–20.

Frank, L. D., Sallis, J. F., Saelens, B. E., Leary, L., Cain, K., Conway, T. L., & Hess, P. M. (2010). The development of a walkability index: Application to the Neighborhood Quality of Life Study. *British Journal of Sports Medicine, 44*(13), 924–933.

Freid, V. M., Bernstein, A. B., & Bush, M. A. (2012). Multiple chronic conditions among adults aged 45 and over: Trends over the past 10 years. *Women, 45*, 64.

Friel, S., Chopra, M., & Satcher, D. (2007). Unequal weight: Equity oriented policy responses to the global obesity epidemic. *BMJ: British Medical Journal, 335*(7632), 1241.

Gebel, K., Bauman, A. E., & Petticrew, M. (2007). The physical environment and physical activity: A critical appraisal of review articles. *American Journal of Preventive Medicine, 32*, 361–369.

Giles-Corti, B., & Donovan, R. J. (2003). Relative influences of individual, social environmental, and physical environmental correlates of walking. *Journal of Information, 93*(9), 1583–1589.

Glanz, K., & Bishop, D. B. (2010). The role of behavioral science theory in development and implementation of public health interventions. *Annual Review of Public Health, 31*, 399–418.

Gordon-Larsen, P., Nelson, M. C., Page, P., & Popkin, B. M. (2006). Inequality in the built environment underlies key health disparities in physical activity and obesity. *Pediatrics, 117*(2), 417–424.

Grieco, L. A., Sheats, J. L., & Winter, S. J. (2012). *Health technology development and research in older adults: Challenges and solutions.* In section symposium at the annual meeting of the Society of Behavioral Medicine. New Orleans, LA.

Grieco, L. A., Sheats, J. L., Winter, S. J., Hekler, E. B., Buman, M. P., Cirimele, J., Chen, F. X., & King, A. C. (2012). Mobile health application development and deployment: Behavioral sciences perspectives on functional issues. *CHI 2012*, May 5–10, 2012, Austin, TX, USA.

Guide to Community Preventive Services. (2012). Promoting physical activity: Environmental and policy approaches. Retrieved from http://www.thecommunityguide.org/pa/index.html

Hamer, M. (2007). The relative influences of fitness and fatness on inflammatory factors. *Preventive Medicine, 44*(1), 3–11.

Hamer, M., & Chida, Y. (2009). Physical activity and risk of neurodegenerative disease: A systematic review of prospective evidence. *Psychological Medicine, 39*(1), 3–11.

Handy, S. L., Boarnet, M. G., Ewing, R., & Killingsworth, R. E. (2002). How the built environment affects physical activity: Views from urban planning. *American Journal of Preventive Medicine, 23*(2), 64–73.

Hardy, S., & Grogan, S. (2009). Preventing disability through exercise. *Journal of Health Psychology, 14*(7), 1036–1046. doi: 10.1177/1359105309342298

Haskell, W. L., Blair, S. N., & Hill, J. O. (2009). Physical activity: Health outcomes and importance for public health policy. *Preventive Medicine, 49*(4), 280–282.

Henderson, K. A., & Ainsworth, B. E. (2003). A synthesis of perceptions about physical activity among older African American and American Indian women. *American Journal of Public Health, 93*(2), 313–317. doi: 10.2105/ajph.93.2.313

Higgins, J., & Lauzon, L. (2002). Finding the funds in fun runs: Exploring physical activity events as fundraising tools in the nonprofit sector. *International Journal of Nonprofit and Voluntary Sector Marketing, 8*(4), 363–377.

International Telecommunication Union. Measuring the information society. (2011). Retrieved from http://www.itu.int/ITUD/ict/publications/idi/material/2011/MIS_2011_without_annex_5.pdf

Kaplan, R. M. (2000). Two pathways to prevention. *American Psychologist, 55*(4), 382–396.

King, A. C., Ahn, D. K., Oliveira, B. M., Atienza, A. A., Castro, C. M., & Gardner, C. D. (2008). Promoting physical activity through hand-held computer technology. *American Journal of Preventive Medicine, 34*(2), 138–142.

King A. C., Castro C. M., Buman M. P., Hekler E. B., Urizar G. G., Ahn D. K. (2013). Behavioral impacts of sequentially versus simultaneously delivered dietary plus physical activity interventions: The CALM trial. *Annals of Behavioral Medicine, 46*(2), 157–168. doi: 10.1007/s12160-013-9501-y

King, A. C., Castro, C., Wilcox, S., Eyler, A. A., Sallis, J. F., & Brownson, R. C. (2000). Personal and environmental factors associated with physical inactivity among different racial-ethnic groups of U.S. middle-aged and older-aged women. *Healthy Psychology, 19*(4), 354–364.

King, A. C., Friedman, R., Marcus, B., Castro, C., Napolitano, M., Ahn, D., & Baker, L. (2007). Ongoing physical activity advice by humans versus computers: The Community Health Advice by Telephone (CHAT) trial. *Health Psychology, 26*(6), 718–727.

King, A. C., Goldberg, J. H., Salmon, J., Owen, N., Dunstan, D., Weber, D., & Robinson, T. N. (2010). Identifying subgroups of US adults at risk for prolonged television viewing to inform program development. *American Journal of Preventive Medicine, 38*(1), 17–26.

King, A. C., Jeffery, R. W., Fridinger, F., Dusenbury, L., Provence, S., Hedlund, S. A., & Spangler, K. (1995). Environmental and policy approaches to cardiovascular disease prevention through physical activity: Issues and opportunities. *Health Education & Behavior, 22*(4), 499–51. doi: 10.1177/109019819502200407

King, A. C., Sallis, J. F., Frank, L. D., Saelens, B. E., Cain, K., Conway, T. L., & Kerr, J. (2011). Aging in neighborhoods differing in walkability and income: Associations with physical activity and obesity in older adults. *Social Science & Medicine, 73*(10), 1525–1533.

King, A. C., Toobert, D., Ahn, D., Resnicow, K., Coday, M., Riebe, D., & Sallis, J. F. (2006). Perceived environments as physical activity correlates and moderators of intervention in five studies. *American Journal of Health Promotion, 21*(1), 24–35.

Kochanek, K. D., Xu, J., Murphy, S. L., Minino, A. M., & Kung, H.-C. (2011). Deaths: Preliminary data for 2009. *National Vital Statistics Reports, 59*(4), 1–51.

Kohl, H. W., Craig, C. L., Lambert, E. V., Inoue, S., Alkandari, J. R., Leetongin, G., & Kahlmeier, S. (2012). The pandemic of physical inactivity: Global action for public health. *The Lancet, 380*(9838), 9–19.

Kushner, R. F., Blatner, D. J., Jewell, D. E., & Rudloff, K. (2012). The PPET Study: People and pets exercising together. *Obesity, 14*(10), 1762–1770.

Lee, I. M., Shiroma, E. J., Lobelo, F., Puska, P., Blair, S. N., & Katzmarzyk, P. T. (2012). Effect of physical inactivity on major non-communicable diseases worldwide: An analysis of burden of disease and life expectancy. *The Lancet, 380*(9838), 219–229.

Leroux, J. S., Moore, S., Richard, L., & Gauvin, L. (2012). Physical inactivity mediates the association between the perceived exercising behavior of social network members and obesity: A cross-sectional study. *PLoS One, 7*(10), e46558.

Lintonen, T., Konu, A., & Seedhouse, D. (2008). Information technology in health promotion. *Health Education Research, 23*(3), 560–566.

Lim, K., & Taylor, L. (2005). Factors associated with physical activity among older people—a poulation-based study. *Preventive Medicine, 50,* 33–40.

Lloyd-Jones, D. M., Hong, Y., Labarthe, D., Mozaffarian, D., Appel, L. J., Van Horn, L., & Rosamond, W. D. (2010). American Heart Association Strategic Planning Task Force and Statistics Committee. Defining and setting national goals for cardiovascular health promotion and disease reduction: The American Heart Association's strategic Impact Goal through 2020 and beyond. *Circulation, 121*(4), 586–613.

Luepker, R. V., Perry, C. L., McKinlay, S. M., Nader, P. R., Parcel, G. S., & Stone, E. J. (1996). Outcomes of a field trial to improve children's dietary patterns and physical activity. The Child and Adolescent Trial for Cardiovascular Health. CATCH collaborative group. *Journal of the American Medical Association, 275*(10), 768–776.

Marcus, B. H., Bock, B. C., Pinto, B. M., Forsyth, L. H., Roberts, M. B., & Traficante, R. M. (1998). Efficacy of an individualized, motivationally-tailored physical activity intervention. *Annals of Behavioral Medicine, 20,* 174–180.

Marcus, B. H., Forsyth, L. H., Stone, E. J., Dubbert, P. M., McKenzie, T. L., Dunn, A. L., & Blair, S. N. (2000). Physical activity behavior change: Issues in adoption and maintenance. *Health Psychology, 19*(1S), 32.

Marcus, B. H., Williams, D. M., Dubbert, P. M., Sallis, J. F., King, A. C., Yancey, A. K., & Claytor, R. P. (2006). Physical activity intervention studies what we know and what we need to know: A scientific statement from the American Heart Association Council on Nutrition, Physical Activity, and Metabolism (Subcommittee on Physical Activity); Council on Cardiovascular Disease in the Young; and the Interdisciplinary Working Group on Quality of Care and Outcomes Research. *Circulation, 114*(24), 2739–2752.

Mathews, A. E., Laditka, S. B., Laditka, J. N., Wilcox, S., Corwin, S. J., Liu, R., ... Logsdon, R. G. (2010). Older adults' perceived physical activity enablers and barriers: A multicultural perspective. *Journal of Aging and Physical Activity, 18*(2), 119.

McAuley, E., & Blissmer, B. (2000). Self-efficacy determinants and consequences of physical activity. *Exercise and Sport Sciences Reviews, 28,* 85–88.

McAuley, E., Blissmer, B., Marquez, D.X., Jerome, G.J., Kramer, A.F., & Katula, J. (2000). Social relations, physical activity, and well-being in older adults. *Preventive Medicine, 31*(5), 608–617.

McNeill, L., Kreuter, M., & Subramanian, S. (2006). Social environment and physical activity: A review of concepts and evidence. *Social Science & Medicine, 63,* 1011–1022.

McNeill, L., Wyrwich, K. W., Brownson, R. C., Clark, E. M., & Kreuter, M. W. (2006). Individual, social environmental and physical environmental influences on physical activity among black and white adults: A structural equation analysis. *Annals of Behavioral Medicine, 31*(1), 36–44.

McCormack, G., Giles-Corti, B., Lange, A., Smith, T., Martin, K., & Pokora, T. (2004). An update of recent evidence of the relationship between objective and self-reported measures of the physical environmental and physical activity behaviours. *Journal of Science and Medicine in Sport, 7*(1), 81–92.

Milstein, B., Homer, J., Briss, P., Burton, D., & Pechacek, T. (2011). Why behavioral and environmental interventions are needed to improve health at lower cost. *Health Affairs, 30*(5), 823–832.

Moher, D., Liberati, A., Tetzlaff, J., & Altman, D. G. (2009). Preferred reporting items for systematic reviews and meta-analyses: The PRISMA statement. *PLoS Medicine, 6*(7), e1000097.

Moschny, A., Platen, P., Klaaßen-Mielke, R., Trampisch, U., & Hinrichs, T. (2011). Barriers to physical activity in older adults in Germany: A cross-sectional study. *International Journal of Behavioral Nutrition and Physical Activity, 8*(1), 121.

Napolitano, M. A., Fotheringham, M., Tate, D., Sciamanna, C., Leslie, E., Owen, N., ... Marcus, B.(2003). Evaluation of an internet-based physical activity intervention: A preliminary investigation. *Annals of Behavioral Medicine, 25*(2), 92–99.

Napolitano, M. A., & Marcus, B. H. (2002). Targeting and tailoring physical activity information using print and information technologies. *Exercise and Sport Sciences Reviews, 30*(3), 122–128.

Neff, K. L. F., & King, A. C. (1995). Exercise program adherence in older adults: The importance of achieving one's expected benefits. *Medicine, Exercise, Nutrition, & Health, 4,* 355–362.

Neumark-Sztainer, D., Story, M., Hannan, P. J., Tharp, T., & Rex, J. (2003). Factors associated with changes in physical activity: A cohort study of inactive adolescent girls. *Archives of Pediatrics & Adolescent Medicine, 157*(8), 803–810.

Nigg, C. R., & Long, C. R. (2012). A systematic review of single health behavior change interventions vs. multiple health behavior change interventions among older adults. *Translational Behavioral Medicine, 2*(2), 163–179.

Ockene, J. K., Edgerton, E. A., Teutsch, S. M., Marion, L. N., Miller, T., Genevro, J. L., & Briss, P. A. (2007). Integrating evidence-based clinical and community strategies to improve health. *American Journal of Preventive Medicine, 32*(3), 244–252.

Osilla, K. C., Van Busum, K., Schnyer, C., Larkin, J. W., Eibner, C., & Mattke, S. (2012). Systematic Review of the impact of worksite wellness programs. *American Journal of Managed Care, 18*(2), e68–e81.

Owen, N., Healy, G. N., Matthews, C. E., & Dunstan, D. W. (2010). Too much sitting: The population health science of sedentary behavior. *Exercise and Sport Sciences Reviews, 38*(3), 105–113.

Oxford Health Alliance. Oxford Vision 2020: Community interventions for health. (2009). Oxford, UK: Oxford Health Alliance.

Papastergiou, M. (2009). Exploring the potential of computer and video games for health and physical education: A literature review. *Computers & Education, 53*(3), 603–622. doi: 10.1016/j.compedu.2009.04.001

Parks, S., Houseman, R., & Brownson, R. (2002). Differential correlates of physical activity in urban and rural adults of various socioeconomic backgrounds in the United States. *Journal of Epidemiology and Health, 57*, 29–35.

Pate, R. R., Heath, G. W., Dowda, M., & Trost, S. G. (1996). Associations between physical activity and other health behaviors in a representative sample of US adolescents. *American Journal of Public Health, 86*(11), 1577–1581.

Powell, K. E., Paluch, A. E., & Blair, S. N. (2011). Physical activity for health: What kind? How much? How intense? On top of what? *Annual Review of Public Health, 32*, 349–365. doi: 10.1146/annurev-publhealth-031210-101151

Prochaska, J. J., Spring, B., & Nigg, C. R. (2008). Multiple health behavior change research: An introduction and overview. *Preventive Medicine, 46*, 181–188.

Rabin, B., Brownson, R., Kerner, J., & Glasgow, R. (2006). Methodological challenges in disseminating evidence-based interventions to promote physical activity. *American Journal of Preventive Medicine, 31*(4s), s24–s34.

Rejeski, W. J., Brawley, L. R., Ambrosius, W. T., Brubaker, P. H., Focht, B. C., Foy, C. G., & Fox L. D. (2003). Older adults with chronic disease: Benefits of group-mediated counseling in the promotion of physically active lifestyles. *Healthy Psychology, 22*(4), 414–423.

Ries, A., Voorhees, C., & Gittelsohn, J. (2010). Environmental barriers and facilitators of physical activity among urban African-American youth. *Children, Youth and Environments, 20*(1), 26–51. Retrieved from http://www.colorado.edu/journals/cye/

Roberts, I. (2003). Congestion charging and the walking classes. *British Medical Journal, 326*(7385), 345–346.

Robinson, T. N. (2010). Save the world, prevent obesity: Piggybacking on existing social and ideological movements. *Obesity, 18*, S17–S22.

Robinson, T., & Sirard, J. (2005). Preventing childhood obesity: A solution oriented research paradigm. *American Journal of Preventive Medicine, 28*(2S2), 194–201. doi: 10.1016/j.amepre.2004.10.030.

Rovniak, L. S., Anderson, E. S., Winett, R. A., & Stephens, R. S. (2002). Social cognitive determinants of physical activity in young adults: A prospective structural equation analysis. *Annals of Behavioral Medicine, 24*(2), 149–156.

Saelens, B. E., & Handy, S. L. (2008). Built environment correlates of walking: A review. *Medicine and Science in Sports and Exercise, 40*(7 Suppl.), S550–S566.

Sallis, J. F., Bowles, H. R., Bauman, A., Ainsworth, B. E., Bull, F. C., Craig, C. L., ... Bergman, P. (2009). Neighborhood environments and physical activity among adults in 11 countries. *American Journal of Preventive Medicine, 36*(6), 484–490.

Sallis, J., Cervero, R., Ascher, W., Henderson, K. A., Kraft, M. K., & Kerr, J. (2006). An ecological approach to creating more physically active communities. *Annual Review of Public Health, 26*, 297–322.

Sallis, J. F., King, A. C., Sirard, J. R., & Albright, C. L. (2007). Perceived environmental predictors of physical activity over 6 months in adults: Activity counseling trial. *Health Psychology, 26*(6), 701–709.

Sallis, J., Linton, L., & Kraft, M. (2005). The first Active Living Research conference: Growth of a transdisciplinary field. *American Journal of Preventive Medicine, 28*(2 Suppl. 2), 93–95.

Sallis, J. F., McKenzie, T. L., Alcaraz, J. E., Kolody, B., Faucette, N., & Hovell, M. F. (1997). The effects of a 2-year physical education program (SPARK) on physical activity and fitness in elementary school students. Sports, play and active recreation for kids. *American Journal of Public Health, 87*(8), 1328–1334.

Sallis, J. F., Owen, N., & Fisher, E. (2008). Ecological models of health behavior. In K. Glanz, B. K. Rimer, & K. Viswanath (Eds.), *Health behavior and health education: Theory, research and practice* (4th ed., pp. 465–482). San Francisco, CA: Jossey-Bass.

Sallis, J., Owen, N., & Fotheringham, M. (2000). Behavioral Epidemiology: A sytematic framework to classify phases of research on health promotion and disease prevention. *Annals of Behavioral Medicine, 22*, 294–298.

Sallis, J., Prochaska, J., & Taylor, C. (2000). A review of correlates of physical activity of children and adolescents. *Medicine and Science in Sports and Exercise, 32*(5), 963–975.

Salmon, J., Owen, N., Crawford, D., Bauman, A., & Sallis, J. F. (2003). Physical activity and sedentary behavior: A population-based study of barriers, enjoyment, and preference. *Health Psychology, 22*(2), 178–188.

Sandford, R. A. (2006). Re-engaging disaffected youth through physical activity programmes. *British Educational Research Journal, 32*(2), 251–271.

Schmid, T. L., Pratt, M., & Howze, E. (1995). Policy as intervention: Environmental and policy approaches to the prevention of cardiovascular disease. *American Journal of Public Health, 85*, 1207–1211.

Schutzer, K., & Graves, S. (2004). Barriers and motivation to exercise in older adults. *Preventive Medicine, 39*, 1056–1061.

Seefeldt, V., Malina, R., & Clark, M. (2002). Factors affecting levels of physical activity in adults. *Sports Medicine, 32*(3), 143–168.

Shay, C. M., Ning, H., Allen, N. B., Carnethon, M. R., Chiuve, S. E., Greenlund, K. J., & Lloyd-Jones, D. M. (2012). Epidemiology and Prevention: Status of cardiovascular health in US adults. *Circulation, 125*, 45–56.

Shibata, A., Oka, K., Inoue, S., Christian, H., Kitabatake, Y., & Shimomitsu, T. (2012). Physical activity of Japanese older adults who own and walk dogs. *American Journal of Preventive Medicine, 43*(4), 429–433.

Smith, A. L. (1999). Perceptions of peer relationships and physical activity participation in early adolescence. *Journal of Sport & Exercise Psychology, 21*, 329–350.

Sox, H. C., & Goodman, S. N. (2012). The methods of comparative effectiveness research. *Annual Review of Public Health, 33*, 425-445.

Stalsberg, R., & Pedersen, A. V. (2010). Effects of socioeconomic status on the physical activity in adolescents: A systematic review of the evidence. *Scandinavian Journal of Medicine & Science in Sports, 20*(3), 368–383.

Story, M., Giles-Corti, B., Yaroch, A. L., Cummins, S., Frank, L. D., Huang, T. T. K., & Lewis, L. B. (2009). Work group IV: Future directions for measures of the food and physical activity environments. *American Journal of Preventive Medicine, 36*(4), 182–188.

Sugiyama, T., Healy, G.N., Dunstan, D.W., Salmon, J., & Owen N. (2008). Is television viewing time a marker of a broader pattern of sedentary behavior? *Annals of Behavioral Medicine, 35*(2), 245–50.

Swinburn, B. (2008). Obesity prevention: The role of policies, laws and regulations. *Australia New Zealand Health Policy, 5*(12), 1–6. doi: 10.1186/1743-8462-5-12

Taylor, W. C., Blair, S. N., Cummings, S. S., Wun, C. C., & Malina, R. M. (1999). Childhood and adolescent physical activity patterns and adult physical activity. *Medicine and Science in Sports and Exercise, 31*(1), 118–23.

Timperio, A., Salmon, J., & Ball, K. (2004). Evidence-based strategies to promote physical activity among children, adolescents and young adults: Review and update. *Journal of Science Medicine in Sport, 7*(1), 20–29.

Troiano, R. P., Berrigan, D., Dodd, K. W., Masse, L. C., Tilert, T., & Macdowell, M. (2008). Physical activity in the United States measured by accelerometer. *Medicine and Science in Sports and Exercise, 40*, 181–188.

Trost, S. G., Owen, N., Bauman, A. E., Sallis, J. F., & Brown, W. (2002). Correlates of adults' participation in physical activity: Review and update. *Medicine and Science in Sports and Exercise, 34*(12), 1996–2001.

Trudeau, F., Laurencelle, L., Tremblay, J., Rajic, M., & Shephard, R. J. (1999). Daily primary school physical education: Effects on physical activity during adult life. *Medicine and Science in Sports and Exercise, 31*(1), 111.

Tu, W., Stump, X. A., Damush, X. M., & Clark, D. O. (2004). The effects of health and environment on exercise class participation in older, urban women. *Journal of Aging and Physical Activity, 12*, 480–496.

U.S. Census Bureau, Population Division. (2008). Table 2. Projections of the population. 2008. Retrieved from http://www.census.gov/population/www/projections/summarytables.html

U.S. Department of Health and Human Services. (1996). Physical activity and health: A report of the Surgeon General. Atlanta, GA: U.S. Department of Health and Human Services, Centers for Disease Control and Prevention, National Center for Chronic Disease Prevention and Health Promotion.

U.S. Department of Health and Human Services. (2008). *Physical Activity Guidelines for Americans*. Retrieved from http://www.health.gov/paguidelines/guidelines/default.aspx

U.S. Department of Health and Human Services. (2010). Administration on aging. Aging statistics. Retrieved from http://www.aoa.gov/aoaroot/aging_statistics/index.aspx

Van Sluijs, E. M., McMinn, A. M., & Griffin, S. J. (2007). Effectiveness of interventions to promote physical activity in children and adolescents: Systematic review of controlled trials. *British Medical Journal, 335,* 703.

Van Stralen, M. M., De Vries, H., Mudde, A. N., Bolman, C., & Lechner, L. (2009). Determinants of initiation and maintenance of physical activity among older adults: A literature review. *Health Psychology Review, 3*(2), 147–207. doi:10.1080/17437190903229462

Verheijden, M. W., Jans, M. P., Hildebrandt, V. H., & Hopman-Rock, M. (2007). Rates and determinants of repeated participation in a web-based behavior change program for healthy body weight and healthy lifestyle. *Journal of Medical Internet Research, 9*(1), e1.

Webb, T. L., Joseph, J., Yardley, L., & Michie, S. (2010). Using the internet to promote health behaviour change: A systematic review and meta-analysis of the impact of theoretical basis, use of behaviour change techniques, and mode of delivery on efficacy. *Journal of Medical Internet Research, 12*(1), e4. doi: 10.2196/jmir.1376

Wen, C. P., Wai, J. P. M., Tsai, M. K., Yang, Y. C., Cheng, T. Y. D., Lee, M. C., & Wu, X. (2011). Minimum amount of physical activity for reduced mortality and extended life expectancy: A prospective cohort study. *The Lancet, 378*(9798), 1244–1253.

Wendel Vos, W., Droomers, M., Kremers, S., Brug, J., & Van Lenthe, F. (2007). Potential environmental determinants of physical activity in adults: A systematic review. *Obesity Reviews, 8*(5), 425–440.

White, S. M., Wójcicki, T. R., & McAuley, E. (2012). Social cognitive influences on physical activity behavior in middle-aged and older adults. *The Journals of Gerontology Series B: Psychological Sciences and Social Sciences, 67*(1), 18–26.

Wilbur, J., Chandler, P., Dancy, B., Choi, J., & Plonczynski, D. (2002). Environmental, policy, and cultural factors related to physical activity in urban, African American women. *Women & Health, 36*(2), 17–28. doi: 10.1300/J013v36n02_02

Wilcox, S., Castro, C., & King, A. C. (2006). Outcome expectations and physical activity participation in caregiving and non-caregiving women. *Journal of Health Psychology, 11*(1), 65–77.

Wilcox, S., Castro, C., King, A. C., Housemann, R., & Brownson, R. C. (2000). Determinants of leisure time physical activity in rural compared with urban older and ethnically diverse women in the United States. *Journal of Epidemiology and Community Health, 54*(9), 667–672.

Young, D., & King, A. C. (1995). Exercise adherence: Determinants of PA and applications of health behavior change theories. *Medicine Exercise Nutrition and Health, 4,* 335–348.

Young, D., & Voorhees, C. C. (2003). Personal, social, and environment correlates of physical activity in urban African-American women. *American Journal of Preventive Medicine, 25*(3Si), 38–44.

Zambon, A., Lemma, P., Borraccino, A., Dalmasso, P., & Cavallo, F. (2006). Socio-economic position and adolescents' health in Italy: The role of the quality of social relations. *European Journal of Public Health, 16*(6), 627–632.

9

Addressing Tobacco Use and Dependence

LORI PBERT
DENISE JOLICOEUR
RASHELLE B. HAYES
JUDITH K. OCKENE

LEARNING OBJECTIVES

- Understand the prevalence of tobacco use and cessation.
- Identify the biological, psychological, and social factors that influence tobacco use and dependence.
- Describe intervention approaches that can be used to help people change tobacco use behavior.

Tobacco use is multi-faceted, involving a complex interplay of biological, psychological, and social factors. This chapter begins by providing an overview of the unique challenges associated with changing tobacco use behavior due to its multi-faceted nature and the dependence it creates, describing the myriad factors involved in the creation of dependence and cessation. Next, the major components of effective individual-level treatment interventions including behavioral and pharmacologic options, as well as health care provider delivered interventions and the importance of connecting individual-level clinical treatment options with population-based interventions to increase widespread treatment capacity, are reviewed. And finally, conclusions and future directions in research and clinical practice are presented.

EPIDEMIOLOGY AND SIGNIFICANCE OF THE PROBLEM OF TOBACCO USE

Since the first Surgeon General's report in 1964 on the health effects of smoking, a wide variety of tobacco control efforts have been implemented throughout the United States. The net impact of these strategies resulted in a remarkable 50% decrease in the prevalence of smoking, from 42.4% in 1965 to 19.0% in 2011 (Centers for Disease Control and Prevention [CDC], 2012a). The magnitude of this population-level drop in tobacco use behavior within a nearly 50-year time frame is an astounding public health success. Much more work, however, needs to be done. Tobacco use unfortunately remains the single largest preventable cause of death, disease, and disability for both men and women in the United States and worldwide. Although the mortality rate attributable to smoking has declined as a result of the reduction in smoking prevalence (Rodu & Cole, 2007), tobacco use still accounts for more than 440,000 annual deaths in the United States and about 6 million deaths annually worldwide (World Health Organization [WHO], 2011). A significant proportion of these deaths are from heart disease, chronic lung and respiratory diseases, and from cancers from every body organ or system (U.S. Department of Health and Human Services [UDHHS], 2010a). Nonsmokers also are at risk for these illnesses due to the harmful exposure of secondhand smoke (UDHHS, 2010a). Indeed, every Surgeon General Report from 1964 to 2010 has reported on a strong and growing evidence-based science that concludes that "there is no safe tobacco product," and importantly, "there is no risk-free level of exposure to tobacco smoke" (UDHHS, 2010a).

Over the years the CDC, the U.S. Food and Drug Administration (FDA), and other federal agencies have worked to implement and maintain tobacco control policies and regulations as a strategy toward ending the tobacco epidemic. A recent and significant public health landmark initiative, for example, was the *Family Smoking Prevention and Tobacco Control Act* enacted in 2009. This gave the FDA explicit regulatory authority over tobacco products to protect and promote the health of the American public, which included requiring companies to reveal all ingredients in tobacco products and regulating tobacco advertising. Implementing these tobacco policies and regulations, as well as effectively disseminating efficacious tobacco dependence treatment, is essential because these measures are associated with cessation for many smokers. Policies and treatments also have changed smoking patterns. For example, relative to 50 years ago, the majority of smokers have substantially limited their daily cigarette intake. Definitions of "heavy" versus "light" smoker have changed, and the proportion of smokers who use tobacco intermittently (e.g., nondaily, intermittent smokers) versus daily is growing rapidly. Also, some smokers may choose to additionally use alternative tobacco products, like smokeless tobacco, including chew or snuff, or other tobacco products such as cigars, water pipes (e.g., hookah), bidis, or PREPS ("Potentially Reduced Exposure Products") while others may choose to switch to these tobacco products completely. These smoking behaviors and patterns may differ among subpopulations of smokers.

Becoming familiar with the epidemiology of tobacco use among various subpopulations can inform policy and treatment practices. Below, the current prevalence rates of adult tobacco use are outlined by subpopulations in the United States and important recent trends in tobacco use are highlighted. Given more available research on cigarette and smokeless tobacco use, the prevalence and smoking patterns among adults for each of these tobacco products are presented and trends in alternative tobacco products are briefly addressed in a later section. Finally, rates of cigarette smoking cessation are outlined, also by subpopulation.

ADULT CIGARETTE SMOKING RATES

Currently, nearly one in every five adults aged 18 years or older smoke (19.0% in 2011, 43.8 million people) and rates have not dramatically changed since 2005 (20.9%) (CDC, 2011b). Tobacco control policies such as excise cigarette taxes and workplace smoking bans, and the de-normalization of smoking have effected significant changes in how people smoke. For example, the percentage of adult daily smokers who smoke 30 or more cigarettes per day decreased from 12.6% in 2005 to 9.1% in 2011, while the percentage of daily smokers who smoke between 1 and 9 cigarettes per day increased from 16.4% to 22% (CDC, 2012a). Additionally, between 21% and 33% of all adult smokers now smoke nondaily or on "some days," and these patterns of smoking are expected to continue and increase (CDC, 2012a; Shiffman, 2009).

Cigarette smoking varies substantially across subpopulations. In general, the prevalence of smoking is higher among men (21.6%) than women (16.5%). Adults aged 18 to 24 (18.9%), 25 to 44 years (22.1%), and 45 to 64 years (21.4%) have similar, but higher smoking prevalence rates compared to adults 65 years and older (7.9%). Among racial/ethnic populations, American Indians/Alaska Natives have the highest prevalence (31.5%), followed by non-Hispanic Whites (20.6%) and non-Hispanic Blacks (19.4%). Hispanics (12.9%) and Asians (9.9%) have the lowest prevalence of cigarette use, but wide variability exists within ethnic subpopulations and between gender and country of origin (Caraballo, Yee, Gfroerer, & Mirza, 2008; Cokkinides, Bandi, Siegel, & Jemal, 2012). For example, among the major Hispanic subgroups, Cuban and Puerto Rican men and women have higher rates of smoking (Cuban: 20.7% and 15.1%; Puerto Rican: 19.0% and 16.6%), compared to Dominicans (6.2% for both men and women) (Cokkinides et al., 2012). Typically, Hispanics born in the United States are more likely to smoke compared to those who are foreign-born (16.8% vs. 10.7%) (Fagan, Moolchan, Lawrence, Fernander, & Ponder, 2007). For Asian Americans, smoking among men (14.7%) is significantly higher than smoking among Asian American women (4.3%) (CDC, 2012a), and rates for Southeast Asian (Cambodian, Laotian, and Vietnamese), Korean, and Filipino American men are generally much higher than other Asian American groups (Kim, Ziedonis, & Chen, 2007). Other factors that influence smoking rates are education, income, and U.S. region and state. Smoking prevalence generally decreases with increasing education (e.g., General Educational Degree [45.3%], high school graduate [23.8%], undergraduate degree [9.3%], and graduate degree [5.0%]), and is higher among adults living below the poverty level (29.0%) compared to those at or above the poverty level (17.9%). Prevalence is also highest in the Midwest (21.8%) and South (20.7%), followed by the Northeast (17.3%), and lowest in the West (15.9%). By state, smoking prevalence is lowest in Utah (9.1%) and California (12.1%) and highest in West Virginia (26.8%) and Kentucky (24.8%).

ADULT SMOKELESS TOBACCO RATES

Smokeless tobacco, also called spit or chewing tobacco, comes in two forms: snuff and chewing tobacco. Similar to cigarette smoking, it can cause adverse health consequences and nicotine addiction, and should not be considered a safe alternative to smoking cigarettes. The most recent national survey results show that smokeless tobacco prevalence rates in the United States among those aged 12 years and older were 3.4% or 8.6 million in 2009 and have remained stable since 2002 (3.3%) (Substance Abuse and Mental Health Services Administration [SAMHSA], 2005, 2009). Rates, however, have increased from 2002 to 2009 among high school students (5.9% to 6.7%) and among those between 18 and 25 (4.8% to 6.1%), while generally remaining stable among middle school students (3.6% to 2.6%) and among those older than 26 years (3.2% to 3.1%).

Of importance is that specific populations predominantly use smokeless tobacco. For example, males (6.7%) are more likely to use smokeless tobacco compared to females (0.3%). Students in high school (6.7%) and those between the ages of 18 and 25 (5.9%) are also more likely to use smokeless tobacco compared to middle school students (2.6%)

and those older than 26 years old (3.2%). With regard to racial/ethnic populations, among those 12 and older, American Indian/Alaska Natives have the highest prevalence (9.8%), followed by non-Hispanic Whites (4.5%), Hispanics (1.0%), non-Hispanic Blacks (0.9%), and Asian Americans (0.5%) (SAMHSA, 2010). Most smokeless tobacco users also smoked cigarettes at some point in their lives (85.8%), while 38.8% are dual users (use both smokeless and cigarettes) within the past month. Again, this rate of dual use is higher among those aged 18 to 25 (66.9%) and among those 12 to 17 (52.8%), compared to those 26 or older (29.3%) (King, Dube, & Tynan, 2012). Among states that have the highest cigarette smoking prevalence, many also have the highest prevalence of smokeless tobacco use including Alabama, Alaska, Arkansas, Kentucky, Mississippi, Oklahoma, and West Virginia (CDC, 2010).

ADULT CIGARETTE QUITTING INTEREST AND SUCCESS

With regard to interest in quitting, as of 2010, 68.8% of current smokers reported that they want to stop smoking completely. Interest in quitting smoking was generally higher among those aged ≤ 65 years (70.2%) than among those aged ≥ 65 years (53.8%). By race/ethnicity, interest in quitting was highest among non-Hispanic Black smokers (75.6%), followed by non-Hispanic Whites (69.1%), persons of other race/ethnicities (62.5%), and Hispanics (61.0%). Greater interest in quitting also is associated with higher education levels (some college 73.4% vs. high school degree 65.9%). Those with private insurance (70.4%) or Medicaid (71.2%) were more likely to report interest in quitting compared to those with Medicare (60.7%).

Quit attempts, defined as no smoking for ≥ 1 day in the past year, were more likely to be made among those younger in age (62.4% of those aged 18 to 24 reported a quit attempt vs. 43.5% of those ≥ 65 years), and among non-Hispanic Blacks compared to non-Hispanic Whites (59.1% vs. 50.7%). Quit attempts also were more prevalent among those with a college (55.9%) or an undergraduate degree (56.0%) compared to those with a high school diploma (46.9%). With regard to successful cessation, overall rates are 6.2%. Cessation is more likely to occur among non-Hispanic Whites (6.0%) than among non-Hispanic Blacks (3.3%). Cessation rates also increase with level of education (undergraduate degree 11.4% vs. high school degree or less 3.2%). Also, those with private health plans (7.8%) were more likely to have quit smoking than those with Medicaid (4.6%) or no health plan (3.6%) (CDC, 2011a).

UNIQUE CHALLENGES TO CHANGING TOBACCO BEHAVIOR

DEFINING DEPENDENCE

The fifth edition of the American Psychiatric Association's (APA) *Diagnostic and Statistical Manual* (*DSM-5*) (APA, 2013) has broadened the definitions of substance-related and addictive disorders, including tobacco. Tobacco use disorder includes 11 possible symptoms and is defined at three levels, Mild (2–3 symptoms), Moderate (4–5 symptoms) and Severe (6 or more symptoms). Symptoms are considered to belong to one of four groupings. Criteria related to impaired control include the inability to reduce or stop using tobacco and strong desire or craving. Experiencing cravings has been predictive of the likelihood of relapse (Killen & Fortmann, 1997; Piasecki et al., 2000), and was added to the *DSM-5*. The categories of social impairment and risky use capture continued use of tobacco despite observable negative effects on social relationships and physical harm. Tolerance and withdrawal are both considered pharmacological criteria. Withdrawal, in particular, is thought to significantly impact the ability to stop tobacco use. It includes: (1) depressed mood; (2) insomnia; (3) irritability, frustration, or anger; (4) anxiety; (5) difficulty concentrating; (6) restlessness; and (7) increased appetite (American Psychiatric Association, 2013). Withdrawal symptoms are thought to occur independent of heaviness of smoking (Piper, McCarthy, & Baker, 2006). In fact, the appearance of withdrawal symptoms may occur very early in the use of tobacco, even in the context of light and intermittent smoking (DiFranza et al., 2000; DiFranza et al., 2007; Shiffman, Ferguson, Dunbar, & Scholl, 2012). Regardless of the diagnostic category and level of tobacco dependence, the initiation and maintenance of tobacco use are influenced by a combination of biological, psychological, and sociocultural factors. The interaction of these factors is reflected in the "biopsychosocial" model, endorsed by researchers and clinicians to explain the intricate nature of dependence. Direct influence on any of the three factors of dependence can significantly impact the other two. Below, each factor is discussed in more detail.

Neurobiology of Nicotine Dependence

When a person smokes, nicotine on the tar droplets produced by cigarette smoke is carried into the lungs, then to the heart, and then to the brain within 7 to 10 seconds. Once in the brain, nicotine diffuses readily into brain tissue and binds to nicotinic acetylcholine receptors (nAChRs). The nAChR complex is composed of several subunits found in the peripheral and central nervous system, but it is the $\alpha4\beta2$ receptor subtype that is found most in the brain and believed to be the primary receptor mediating nicotine dependence.

As with many other drugs of abuse, the role of the mesolimbic system of the brain appears to be the most significant and so far the best understood in nicotine dependence. Stimulation of nAChRs by nicotine results in the release of several neurotransmitters in the brain, most importantly dopamine. The release of dopamine within the mesolimbic system, which includes the ventral tegmental area and the nucleus accumbens, is critical in drug-induced reward and the sensation of pleasure. This system and its reward pathway's primary purpose was to ensure survival by associating pleasure with natural stimulants such as food, water, sex, and nurturing, but nicotine's stimulation of this system "hijacks" this pathway when it too is associated with intense pleasure (Balfour, 2004; Dani, 2001).

Nicotine's stimulation of nAChRs also results in the release of other neurotransmitters such as norepinephrine, acetylcholine, and serotonin, which also mediate various behaviors associated with nicotine (e.g., appetite suppression and cognitive enhancement). An increase in the neurotransmitter glutamate facilitates the effect of dopamine in pleasure sensation because it is thought to contribute to the reinforcement of the pleasurable memory (Lambe, Picciotto, & Aghajanian, 2003). By contrast the inhibitory effect of GABA, whose function is to regulate the amount of available dopamine, is reduced. Thus these complementary functions serve to increase dopamine or facilitate its neurotransmission, which reinforces the pleasurable effects of nicotine (Kalivas & Volkow, 2005), leading to continued use.

Nicotine withdrawal is an essential component of nicotine addiction and a key barrier to abstinence success. It is associated with deficient dopamine release and subsequent decreased sensations of pleasure. With chronic exposure to nicotine, neuroadaptation occurs, or brain chemistry is altered. An example of neuroadaptation is an increase of nAChRs in the brain. This increase or upregulation is in response to desensitization or an unresponsiveness of the receptors to chronic nicotine administration. However, after a period of abstinence such as during sleep the receptors become responsive again, which results in withdrawal symptoms and cravings. Because these receptors are once again sensitive or responsive, when a person smokes again (e.g., in the morning) nicotine will bind to the receptors and alleviate the withdrawal symptoms. Thus, smokers may try to maintain their receptors in a desensitized state, smoking throughout the day to maintain nicotine levels to prevent the occurrence of withdrawal symptoms (Balfour, 2004; Brody et al., 2006; Dani & De Biasi, 2001; Dani & Heinemann, 1996; Wang & Sun, 2005).

The role of these neurobiological processes is significant in understanding the mechanisms of dependence and has led to the development of pharmacologic treatments beneficial in assisting with cessation (Harris & Anthenelli, 2005). For example, optimal tobacco pharmacotherapy treatments should limit the strong and positive reinforcing effects of nicotine while reducing withdrawal symptoms. Nicotine from nicotine replacement therapies (NRTs) primarily relieves withdrawal symptoms when a person stops tobacco use. However, it does not provide as strong a positive reinforcement as smoking because it is not rapidly absorbed, and thus is less likely to be abused. Pharmacotherapy also would be beneficial if it targeted or partially blocked the specific nicotinic receptor subtype $\alpha4\beta2$ that binds to nicotine. Varenicline, for example, partially blocks the nAChRs allowing only for a limited amount of dopamine neurotransmission, but some dopamine neurotransmission subsequently reduces withdrawal symptoms. Varenicline also blocks the effects of any nicotine to the system (e.g., nicotine cannot bind to the nAChRs). Over time the reinforcing effects of nicotine from cigarette smoking are reduced (Coe et al., 2005).

Psychological Aspects of Dependence

Tobacco users report a myriad of benefits from its use. Paradoxical effects such as stress reduction and relaxation to modulating their level of arousal and mood all have been reported as perceived benefits. Some smokers also report improved concentration, reaction time, and performance of certain tasks, but it is not entirely clear if these improved abilities are direct effects of tobacco use or the result of relief of withdrawal (Heishman, 2000). Nevertheless, these perceived benefits, in addition to avoiding withdrawal symptoms, contribute to the basis of nicotine dependence.

Unfortunately, all drug-taking behavior is learned and reinforced by the rewarding effects of the drug. Smokers associate the pleasurable rewards with the daily activities, emotions, and situations in which they smoke (e.g., talking on the phone, driving, and coping with anger). These associations become "triggers" for the urge to use tobacco and strongly reinforce its habitual use. Tobacco use becomes essential to daily functioning even in the absence of conscious forethought. The conditioned "trigger" thus becomes a major factor that often leads to relapse after a period of cessation and must be addressed during the cessation process, typically through behavioral and counseling support.

For individuals with psychiatric and substance use comorbidities the psychological benefits appear to be more pronounced and even more intricately linked with daily functioning. Nearly all psychiatric and other substance use disorders are associated with an increased prevalence for smoking, lower rates of cessation, and higher relapse rates (Hughes, 1995a; Hughes, 1993, 1996; Kalman, Morissette, & George, 2005). For example, from a national population survey, the prevalence of smoking among those with any mental illness (AMI) versus no mental illness was 31.6% versus 21.4%, and on average, smokers with AMI smoked 331 cigarettes per month compared to 310 cigarettes per month by those without mental illness. Likewise, cessation rates among those with AMI compared to those without was 34.7% versus 53.4% (Centers for Disease Control and Prevention, 2013; Hughes, 1995b; Hughes et al., 1996; Hughes, 1993). Smoking rates of over 85% are observed in alcoholics, opiate addicts, and poly-drug users (Fertig & Allen, 1995; Kalman et al., 2005) and because of this smoking can be considered a marker of other substance use. It is encouraging to note however that abstinence from tobacco appears to enhance recovery and reduce relapse to other substance use (Prochaska, Delucchi, & Hall, 2004). Although use of evidence-based interventions improves cessation outcomes for all tobacco users, those who have comorbidity, particularly with mental illness, and who smoke more heavily are likely to require more intensive interventions in order to become tobacco free.

Social and Cultural Factors Associated With Dependence

There are a number of important individual and population level smoker characteristics associated with differences in smoking prevalence, motivation to quit, and some cessation outcomes. Some of these factors are important to consider when reaching out to smokers in the hope of motivating them to stop smoking, and encouraging them to use the best interventions available to increase the likelihood of success and reduce the high rates of relapse after quit attempts. These factors include gender, education, income, age, and racial and ethnic background.

Women differ from men in their biological responses to nicotine (Perkins, Donny, & Caggiula, 1999); however, there is mixed data regarding whether women have more difficulty quitting than men (Killen, Fortmann, Varady, & Kraemer, 2002; Wetter et al., 1999). Concerns about weight gain, stress reduction, and the need for social support may contribute to differences between men and women smokers.

Educational attainment, income level, and age are among the strongest predictors of smoking. As mentioned earlier, rates of smoking decline with greater educational attainment (5% among those graduating with a graduate degree vs. 45.3% among those with a GED); smoking is greater in those living below poverty level (29.0%) versus those living above poverty level (17.9%), and smoking rates are similar across all age groups (range from 18.9% to 22.1% for ages 18 to 65), except those older than 65 (7.9%) (CDC, 2012a).

There is also wide variation between cultural and ethnic groups, as noted earlier, as well as within any cultural or ethnic group. For example, although the aggregate smoking rate for Asians/Pacific Islanders is relatively low (CDC, 2012a), other surveys generally report that Southeast Asian (Cambodian, Laotian, and Vietnamese), Korean, and Filipino American populations smoke at much higher rates compared to other Asian American and other ethnic groups, and rates also vary by gender and acculturation.

The between and within group differences suggest that differences in cultural history, context, attitudes, and biology of a subpopulation can influence smoking behavior. For example, there are biological group differences in metabolizing nicotine. African Americans and Chinese both metabolize nicotine at a slower rate compared to Whites (Benowitz, Perez-Stable, Herrera, & Jacob, 2002; CDC, 1998; Perez-Stable, Herrera, Jacob, & Benowitz, 1998), which may contribute to their typical relatively reduced cigarette consumption on days smoked compared to Whites.

With regard to quitting, there also are ethnic differences in quit attempts, quit success rates, use of medication for smoking cessation, and receipt of physician advice to quit smoking. While minority groups are more likely to attempt quitting compared to Caucasians, they are less likely to succeed. Overall, 50% of Caucasians have successfully quit smoking compared to 37.5% of African Americans and 42.9% of Hispanics (Giovino, 2002). This possibly may be due to differences in the use of NRT, which varies from 31% for Caucasians, and 22% each for African Americans, Hispanics, and Asians (Fu et al., 2008). Ethnic differences in quitting also may be influenced by differential receipt of physician advice to quit among Caucasians (72%) versus African Americans (61%) and Hispanics (50%) (Houston, Scarinci, Person, & Greene, 2005).

Smoking patterns among adolescents are more variable than among adults, with many adolescents smoking intermittently as opposed to daily. Sociocultural factors such as parental smoking and socioeconomic stress affect smoking rates among adolescents and the most significant predictor is peer smoking (Milton et al., 2004). Ethnic and cultural differences can be seen here as well with the highest rates of smoking among American Indian/Alaska Native teens, followed by Caucasian teens (CDC, 2006).

While few generalizations can be made regarding effective treatment strategies for subgroups, whenever possible both behavioral and pharmacologic treatment should be tailored and monitored in order to best meet the needs of the individual. Smokers who are at higher risk due to certain bio-behavioral or socioeconomic vulnerabilities may benefit from more intensive, longer, or specialized clinical interventions. The following section provides a foundation upon which effective treatment strategies at the individual and systems level are based.

INTERVENTIONS TO CHANGE TOBACCO USE BEHAVIOR

In order to effectively reduce tobacco use, a multi-pronged approach is needed including public health messages and policies such as smoke-free laws, ordinances and taxation, health care delivery systems primed to identify and treat tobacco use, and access to treatment. This is evidenced by smoking prevalence being lower than the national average (19.3%) (CDC, 2011b) in those states with strong, visible, comprehensive, and sustained antismoking programs, for example, 14.9% in California and 17.8% in Massachusetts (Institute of Medicine [IOM], 2007). Access to effective tobacco treatment resources is a key component of such comprehensive programs. The full impact of cessation interventions on the intended target population is a product of the proportion of the population reached and the efficacy and fidelity of implementation of the intervention delivered (Impact = Reach × Efficacy); see Abrams et al. (2003, 1993) for details. Thus, in addition to trying to motivate more smokers to make quit attempts, there is an enormous opportunity to further increase cessation outcomes by implementing systems-level interventions that reach more smokers and increase access to treatment. Diverse strategies that include clinical, medical, and community interventions can contribute significantly to improving the health of the public (Ockene et al., 2007). This is consistent with social ecological models described in Chapter 3.

Treatment services for nicotine dependence are recommended as an integral component of the multi-pronged approach that has contributed to the decline in smoking (USDHHS, 2012). The Clinical Practice Guideline, Treating Tobacco Use and Dependence, published by the Public Health Service has compiled the available research demonstrating that effective smoking cessation interventions exist, including behavioral and pharmacologic treatment (Fiore et al., 2008). Using evidence-based treatment significantly increases success from almost double to as much as fourfold the cessation rate of quitting on one's own. Despite the social climate that is making it more difficult to smoke (e.g., bans in worksites and higher taxes), effective cessation programs are greatly underutilized. The IOM has recommended a "comprehensive, coordinated system of care management for cessation treatment" that includes five key elements: (1) motivating tobacco users to make more frequent quit attempts, (2) educating tobacco users to use evidence-based treatments when they try to quit, (3) reducing the very high rates of relapse to tobacco use after successfully quitting, (4) ensuring that all tobacco users have access to the best care available and full insurance coverage for treatment services, and (5) structuring the system of care to provide additional levels of more intensive/specialized treatment for tobacco users who need them (IOM, 2007).

There are many intervention approaches that can be implemented to help smokers change tobacco use behavior. These include *education* of tobacco users about evidence-based treatments and approaches, *behavioral strategies* including treatment strategies at each phase of the quitting process, *pharmacologic approaches, health care provider directed interventions* including individual and systems level interventions to reach more tobacco users and increase access to effective tobacco treatment resources, *technology/e-strategies,* and *patient-centered/supportive strategies* to enhance motivation and support tobacco users in their efforts to quit. These are each described in detail below.

EDUCATION

The vast majority of smokers who make quit attempts do so without any form of assistance, and unfortunately, over 95% relapse (National Institutes of Health, 2006). Few smokers know about treatment efficacy, few use any treatments at all, and of those who do use an evidence-based program, they may not use or have access to the best programs to address their individual needs. Consequently there is a need to increase the interest and motivation of smokers to make more quit attempts, to use evidence-based interventions when quitting to improve the likelihood of cessation, and to reduce the likelihood of relapse (Orleans & Slade, 1993; Orleans, 2007; Orleans & Alper, 2003).

The simplest form of education for tobacco treatment is with self-help materials. In general, standard self-help materials increase quit rates when compared to no intervention but the effect is small. Because the effect is small, they may have limited added benefit when used in addition to other interventions such as health care provider advice or NRT. In general, when these materials are tailored to the individual (e.g., based on gender, ethnicity, level of motivation, and confidence to quit) there is a strong effect compared to no intervention and even compared to standard materials (Durkin, Brennan, & Wakefield, 2012; Durkin, Biener, & Wakefield, 2009; Lancaster & Stead, 2005). A more complex method for educating individuals is through mass media campaigns (e.g., television, radio, billboards, newspapers, and posters) where information is distributed to a large number of people. In general, when these campaigns are conducted in the context of comprehensive tobacco control programs they can reduce adult smoking prevalence. However, each campaign's reach, intensity, duration, and message type will influence effectiveness. For example, use of television continues to most effectively reach low socioeconomic smokers. Negative health effect messages or ads that are emotionally arousing or are personalized stories about the effects of smoking and quitting have been most successful in increasing knowledge, beliefs, and quitting behavior, particularly among low socioeconomic smokers.

BEHAVIORAL TREATMENT STRATEGIES

In general, the greater the intensity of treatment (duration and number of contacts and more modalities of intervention) the greater the cessation outcomes, and delivery of treatment via in-person (1:1 or group) and proactive telephone counseling is equally effective (Fiore et al., 2008). Although the following classification is an oversimplification, for many purposes treatment intensity can be classified into three categories: (1) minimal; (2) moderate; and (3) intensive. Many of the cognitive behavioral strategies described in the following sections are derived from several theories and models of individual behavior, including Social Cognitive Theory and the Health Belief Model. For an in-depth description of these and other relevant models for behavior change, see Chapter 2.

Level 1: Minimal Treatment Intensity

It is recommended by the United States Preventive Services Task Force (USPSTF, 2009) that tobacco users seen in a clinical setting should receive at least brief intervention. Therefore, all clinicians should at least deliver brief interventions of minimal intensity, consistent with the Public Health Service (PHS) recommended 5A model (Fiore et al., 2008): *Ask* about tobacco use, *Advise* tobacco users to quit, including sharing the risks of smoking and benefits of quitting, *Assess* willingness to make a quit attempt, *Assist* with cessation, and *Arrange* follow-up. Often, the most feasible brief intervention to deliver in the busy clinic setting is *Ask* and *Advise*, combined with *Referral* to more intensive treatment. This step reflects the importance of ensuring linkages to referral sources in the clinical setting and in the community. Minimal intensity interventions usually entail less than 10 minutes of counseling during contact for another issue. It may be a single occurrence or repeated in subsequent contacts. The addition of *Assess, Assist,* and *Arrange* components is consistent with moderate (level 2) and maximal service (level 3) (see below).

Level 2: Moderate Treatment Intensity

Characteristics of moderate treatment intensity include one or more sessions devoted exclusively to tobacco treatment, with more than 30 minutes of total contact time. This level includes a comprehensive assessment of tobacco use, development of a treatment plan, assistance with pharmacotherapy (typically mono-therapy), and referral to more intensive treatment as appropriate. Moderate treatment intensity is often guided by a clear, scripted protocol.

Level 3: Intensive Treatment

Intensive treatment involves four or more sessions. A comprehensive assessment of tobacco use and related issues is conducted, with the development of a highly individualized treatment plan and assistance with pharmacotherapy that may include combination therapy. Intensive treatment is typically provided to individuals with complex nicotine addiction and/or co-occurring conditions, and requires coordination of care with providers treating the co-occurring conditions.

PHASES OF QUITTING

Quitting tobacco use consists of three phases: (1) Preparation (getting ready); (2) Cessation (quitting); and (3) Maintenance (relapse prevention). Effective treatment planning must address all three phases. Below are specific behavioral treatment strategies for use in the preparation, cessation, and maintenance or relapse prevention phases of quitting (Abrams et al., 2003). Pharmacologic treatment and combined treatment are covered in a later section.

Preparation Phase

The primary objective of the *preparation phase* is to help the smoker strengthen and renew his or her motivation to quit tobacco use. Key strategies include establishing a clear target quit date, self-monitoring tobacco behavior, and development of an action plan that includes strategies to use if a lapse or relapse occurs. A thorough assessment of current and past use patterns and past relapses or return to smoking is important at this stage. This assessment includes reviewing the motivation and strategies related to past quit attempts and exploration of current use patterns including situations, moods, and routines that trigger smoking. These triggers are often identified during a period of behavioral self-monitoring that involves recording time, place, situation, mood, thoughts, and need level associated with each instance of tobacco use.

Cessation Phase

In the *cessation or quitting phase* of treatment, the period just prior to and during the quit attempt, the key objective is for the smoker to learn specific self-management skills for quitting. Skill development in specific cognitive behavioral techniques helps the tobacco user develop strategies to address identified triggers and anticipated problems. Practical skills focus on developing coping strategies such as: identifying and avoiding or removing oneself from high-risk situations; replacing tobacco use with other incompatible behaviors; using cognitive strategies and restructuring cognitions to reshape positive beliefs about smoking, counteract irrational thinking, and reduce negative moods; and developing refusal skills and other skills necessary to effectively manage triggers and urges. Examples of urge coping strategies include understanding that urges are time limited and gradually diminish in intensity after quitting; distraction; "urge-surfing" imagery (imagining oneself as a surfer, riding the urge like a wave to the peak then through its completion, when the urge diminishes in intensity then ends); and the 4Ds: delay, drink water, deep breathe, and distract.

Maintenance Phase

In the *maintenance or relapse prevention phase* the key objective is for the smoker to sustain abstinence by focusing on the use and practice of the skills noted above for the quitting phase. Focusing on these skills is critical in treatment programs as the majority of treated tobacco users will resume use of tobacco (i.e., relapse). Between 65% and 95% of quit attempts end in relapse (Pierce & Gilpin, 2003) with the greatest proportion of relapse (44%) occurring within 14 days (Garvey, Bliss, Hitchcock, Heinold, & Rosner, 1992) of a serious quit attempt. In addition, behavioral treatment programs that are extended and treat smoking as a chronic disease have demonstrated efficacy for long-term abstinence (Hall et al., 2011). However, in the study by Hall and colleagues, brief extended contact performed as well as extended behavioral treatment. Thus, it may be effective to use and develop brief contact approaches such as an Internet intervention that can have a large public health impact and help reduce relapse and improve the likelihood that people will stop again (i.e., recycle). It allows continuous recycling. In one preliminary study, there was a very strong correlation between use of chat rooms for support and successful maintenance of cessation at 3-month follow-up (Cobb, Graham, Bock, Papandonatos, & Abrams, 2005).

Taking up smoking again at any time after the quit date counts as relapse; therefore, no clear definition of a relapse prevention intervention exists distinct from extended cessation treatment (Hall et al., 2011). In general, interventions explicitly implemented to reduce relapse following successful cessation after a treatment phase or self-quit attempt is considered relapse prevention. Since the duration of the treatment phase varies, the point at which measurement of a relapse prevention effect begins is variable.

Although repeated quit attempts are common, overall results of studies encouraging repeat quit attempts (recycling) have been discouraging. Lando and colleagues (Lando, Pirie, Roski, McGovern, & Schmid, 1996) reported that a telephone support intervention significantly increased recycling but not long-term abstinence. Tonnesen and colleagues (Tonnesen et al., 1996) found that introducing nicotine replacement after one year did not appreciably increase abstinence (6% for nasal spray and 0% for patch). Relapse prevention and recycling are a huge public health opportunity but the research base to inform effective and efficient recycling/relapse prevention intervention is sparse (Brandon, Herzog, & Webb, 2003).

PHARMACOTHERAPY

The Public Health Service Guideline (Fiore et al., 2008) recommends that all patients working on cessation be offered pharmacotherapy, unless medically contraindicated or in the presence of other special situations such as pregnancy, lactation, adolescence, or smoking fewer than 10 cigarettes per day. As of this writing, there are seven first-line medications approved by the FDA for use in smoking cessation: five NRT products (transdermal patch, gum, lozenge, inhaler, and nasal spray) and two non-nicotine medications (bupropion and varenicline). The nicotine patch, gum, and lozenge are available over the counter; all other medications require a prescription. Below is a brief description of each medication. Please see Table 9.1 for specific precautions, dosing instructions, and adverse effects of each product.

Determining Appropriate Medications

In general, all seven first-line FDA-approved smoking cessation medications produce similar efficacy rates. The one exception to this may be varenicline, which has been found to have higher quit rates in three randomized control trials (Keating & Siddiqui, 2006). The effectiveness of NRT has been demonstrated even when used in the absence of counseling (West & Zhou, 2007), and it is likely that bupropion and varenicline have similar effects. However, the combination of counseling plus pharmacotherapy has been found to be superior in helping tobacco users quit, and should be utilized if available (Fiore et al., 2008).

While there are no established algorithms to guide the selection of first-line medications (Fiore et al., 2008), there are a number of factors to consider in helping individuals choose the appropriate pharmacotherapy. One is the level of nicotine dependence, especially in relation to the use of NRT products or combination therapy. A simple assessment can include time to the first cigarette and the number of cigarettes per day (less than 30 minutes and greater than 25 cigarettes indicate high dependence) which has been found to be an indicator of the level of nicotine dependence (Heatherton, Kozlowski, Frecker, & Fagerstrom, 1991). Other factors to consider in determining which type of medication a particular patient should use include patient preference, contraindications, prior experience of success or failure with a medication, cost and/or insurance coverage, patient ability to adhere to usage and dosing instructions, side effects, availability, and access. The final decision should be the patient's. For additional details on the management of pharmacotherapies for smoking cessation, see Goldstein (in Abrams et al., 2003).

TABLE 9.1 Pharmacologic Product Guide: FDA-Approved Medications for Smoking Cessation

| | NICOTINE REPLACEMENT THERAPY (NRT) FORMULATIONS | | | | | | |
	GUM	LOZENGE	TRANSDERMAL PATCH	NASAL SPRAY	ORAL INHALER	BUPROPION SR	VARENICLINE
Product	Nicorette,[1] Generic OTC 2 mg, 4 mg original, cinnamon, fruit mint, orange	Nicorette Lozenge,[1] Nicorette Mini Lozenge,[1] Generic OTC 2 mg, 4 mg cherry, mint	NicoDerm CQ,[1] Generic OTC (NicoDerm CQ, generic) Rx (generic) 7 mg, 14 mg, 21 mg (24-hour release)	Nicotrol NS[2] Rx Metered spray 0.5 mg nicotine in 50 mcL aqueous nicotine solution	Nicotrol Inhaler[2] Rx 10 mg cartridge delivers 4 mg inhaled nicotine vapor	Zyban,[1] Generic Rx 150 mg sustained-release tablet	Chantix[2] Rx 0.5 mg, 1 mg tablet
Precautions	• Recent (≤ 2 weeks) myocardial infarction • Serious underlying arrhythmias • Serious or worsening angina pectoris • Temporomandibular joint disease • Pregnancy[3] and breastfeeding • Adolescents (<18 years)	• Recent (≤ 2 weeks) myocardial infarction • Serious underlying arrhythmias • Serious or worsening angina pectoris • Pregnancy[3] and breastfeeding • Adolescents (<18 years)	• Recent (≤ 2 weeks) myocardial infarction • Serious underlying arrhythmias • Serious or worsening angina pectoris • Pregnancy[3] (Rx formulations, category D) and breastfeeding • Adolescents (<18 years)	• Recent (≤ 2 weeks) myocardial infarction • Serious underlying arrhythmias • Serious or worsening angina pectoris • Underlying chronic nasal disorders (rhinitis, nasal polyps, sinusitis) • Severe reactive airway disease • Pregnancy[3] (category D) and breastfeeding • Adolescents (<18 years)	• Recent (≤ 2 weeks) myocardial infarction • Serious underlying arrhythmias • Serious or worsening angina pectoris • Broncho spastic disease • Pregnancy[3] (category D) and breastfeeding • Adolescents (<18 years)	• Concomitant therapy with medications or medical conditions known to lower the seizure threshold • Severe hepatic cirrhosis • Pregnancy[3] (category C) and breastfeeding • Adolescents (<18 years) **Warning:** • BLACK-BOXED WARNING for neuropsychiatric symptoms[4] **Contraindications:** • Seizure disorder • Concomitant bupropion (e.g., Wellbutrin) therapy • Current or prior diagnosis of bulimia or anorexia nervosa • Simultaneous abrupt discontinuation of alcohol or sedatives/benzodiazepines • MAO inhibitor therapy in previous 14 days	• Severe renal impairment (dosage adjustment is necessary) • Pregnancy[3] (category C) and breastfeeding • Adolescents (<18 years) **Warnings:** • BLACK-BOXED WARNING for neuropsychiatric symptoms[4] • Cardiovascular adverse events in patients with existing cardiovascular disease

(continued)

TABLE 9.1 Pharmacologic Product Guide: FDA-Approved Medications for Smoking Cessation (continued)

	NICOTINE REPLACEMENT THERAPY (NRT) FORMULATIONS						
	GUM	**LOZENGE**	**TRANSDERMAL PATCH**	**NASAL SPRAY**	**ORAL INHALER**	**BUPROPION SR**	**VARENICLINE**
Dosing	*First cigarette ≤30 minutes after waking: 4 mg* *First cigarette >30 minutes after waking: 2 mg* Weeks 1–6: 1 piece q 1–2 hours Weeks 7–9: 1 piece q 2–4 hours Weeks 10–12: 1 piece q 4–8 hours • Maximum, 24 pieces/day • Chew each piece slowly • Park between cheek and gum when peppery or tingling sensation appears (~15–30 chews) • Resume chewing when tingle fades • Repeat chew/park steps until most of the nicotine is gone (tingle does not return; generally 30 min) • Park in different areas of mouth • No food or beverages 15 minutes before or during use • Duration: up to 12 weeks	*First cigarette ≤30 minutes after waking: 4 mg* *First cigarette >30 minutes after waking: 2 mg* Weeks 1–6: 1 lozenge q 1–2 hours Weeks 7–9: 1 lozenge q 2–4 hours Weeks 10–12: 1 lozenge q 1–8 hours • Maximum, 20 lozenges/day • Allow to dissolve slowly (20–30 minutes for standard; 10 minutes for mini) • Nicotine release may cause a warm, tingling sensation • Do not chew or swallow • Occasionally rotate to different areas of the mouth • No food or beverages 15 minutes before or during use • Duration: up to 12 weeks	*>10 cigarettes/day* 21 mg/day × 4 weeks (generic) 6 weeks (NicoDerm CQ) 14 mg/day × 2 weeks 7 mg/day × 2 weeks *≤10 cigarettes/day:* 14 mg/day × 6 weeks 7 mg/day × 2 weeks • May wear patch for 16 hours if patient experiences sleep disturbances (remove at bedtime) • Duration: 8–10 weeks	1–2 doses/hour (8–40 doses/day) One dose = 2 sprays (one in each nostril); each spray delivers 0.5 mg of nicotine to the nasal mucosa • Maximum – 5 doses/hour or – 40 doses/day • For best results, initially use at least 8 doses/day • Do not sniff, swallow, or inhale through the nose as the spray is being administered • Duration: 3–6 months	6–16 cartridges/day Individualize dosing; initially use 1 cartridge q 1–2 hours • Best effects with continuous puffing for 20 minutes • Initially use at least 6 cartridges/day • Nicotine in cartridge is depleted after 20 minutes of active puffing • Inhale into back of throat or puff in short breaths • Do NOT inhale into the lungs (like a cigarette) but "puff" as if lighting a pipe • Open cartridge retains potency for 24 hours • No food or beverages 15 minutes before or during use • Duration: 3–6 months	150 mg po q AM × 3 days, then 150 mg po bid • Do not exceed 300 mg/day • Begin therapy 1–2 weeks **prior** to quit date • Allow at least 8 hours between doses • Avoid bedtime dosing to minimize insomnia • Dose tapering is not necessary • Can be used safely with NRT • Duration: 7–12 weeks, with maintenance up to 6 months in selected patients	Days 1–3: 0.5 mg q AM Days 4–7: 0.5 mg po bid Weeks 2–12: 1 mg po bid • Begin therapy 1 week prior to quit date; alternatively, the patient can begin therapy and then quit smoking between days 8–35 of treatment • Take dose after eating and with a full glass of water • Dose tapering is not necessary • Dosing adjustment is necessary for patients with severe renal impairment • Duration: 12 weeks; an additional 12-weeks course may be used in selected patients

Adverse Effects						

• Mouth/jaw soreness
• Hiccups
• Dyspepsia
• Hypersalivation
• Effects associated with incorrect chewing technique:
  – Lightheadedness
  – Nausea/vomiting
  – Throat and mouth irritation
	• Nausea
	• Hiccups
	• Cough
	• Heartburn
	• Headache
	• Flatulence
	• Insomnia
		• Local skin reactions (erythema, pruritus, burning)
		• Headache
		• Sleep disturbances (insomnia, abnormal/vivid dreams); associated with nocturnal nicotine absorption
			• Nasal and/or throat irritation (hot, peppery, or burning sensation)
			• Rhinitis
			• Tearing
			• Sneezing
			• Cough
			• Headache
				• Mouth and/or throat irritation
				• Cough
				• Headache
				• Rhinitis
				• Dyspepsia
				• Hiccups
					• Insomnia
					• Dry mouth
					• Nervousness/difficulty concentrating
					• Rash
					• Constipation
					• Seizures (risk is 0.1%)
					• Neuropsychiatric symptoms (rare; see Precautions)
						• Nausea
						• Sleep disturbances (insomnia, abnormal/vivid dreams)
						• Constipation
						• Flatulence
						• Vomiting
						• Neuropsychiatric symptoms (rare; see Precautions)

Advantages						
• Might satisfy oral cravings • Might delay weight gain • Patients can titrate therapy to manage withdrawal symptoms • Variety of flavors are available	• Might satisfy oral cravings • Might delay weight gain • Easy to use and conceal • Patients can titrate therapy to manage withdrawal symptoms • Variety of flavors are available	• Provides consistent nicotine levels over 24 hours • Easy to use and conceal • Once daily dosing associated with fewer compliance problems	• Patients can titrate therapy to rapidly manage withdrawal symptoms	• Patients can titrate therapy to manage withdrawal symptoms • Mimics hand-to-mouth ritual of smoking (could also be perceived as a disadvantage)	• Easy to use; oral formulation might be associated with fewer compliance problems • Might delay weight gain • Can be used with NRT • Might be beneficial in patients with depression	• Easy to use; oral formulation might be associated with fewer compliance problems • Offers a new mechanism of action for patients who have failed other agents

(continued)

193

TABLE 9.1 Pharmacologic Product Guide: FDA-Approved Medications for Smoking Cessation (continued)

	GUM	LOZENGE	TRANSDERMAL PATCH	NASAL SPRAY	ORAL INHALER	BUPROPION SR	VARENICLINE
			NICOTINE REPLACEMENT THERAPY (NRT) FORMULATIONS				
Disadvantages	• Need for frequent dosing can compromise compliance • Might be problematic for patients with significant dental work • Patients must use proper chewing technique to minimize adverse effects • Gum chewing may not be socially acceptable	• Need for frequent dosing can compromise compliance • Gastrointestinal side effects (nausea, hiccups, heartburn) might be bothersome	• Patients cannot titrate the dose to acutely manage withdrawal symptoms • Allergic reactions to adhesive might occur • Patients with dermatologic conditions should not use the patch	• Need for frequent dosing can compromise compliance • Nasal/throat irritation may be bothersome • Patients must wait 5 minutes before driving or operating heavy machinery • Patients with chronic nasal disorders or severe reactive airway disease should not use the spray	• Need for frequent dosing can compromise compliance • Initial throat or mouth irritation can be bothersome • Cartridges should not be stored in very warm conditions or used in very cold conditions • Patients with underlying bronchospastic disease must use with caution	• Seizure risk is increased • Several contraindications and precautions preclude use in some patients (see PRECAUTIONS) • Patients should be monitored for potential neuropsychiatric symptoms[4] (see PRECAUTIONS)	• May induce nausea in up to one-third of patients • Patients should be monitored for potential neuropsychiatric symptoms[4] (see PRECAUTIONS)
Cost/Day[5]	2 mg or 4 mg: $1.89–$5.48 (9 pieces)	2 mg or 4 mg: $3.05–$4.38 (9 pieces)	$1.52–$3.40 (1 patch)	$4.12 (8 doses)	$7.35 (6 cartridges)	$2.38–$6.22 (2 tablets)	$5.96–$6.5Q (2 tablets)

[1] Marketed by GlaxoSmithKline.

[2] Marketed by Pfizer.

[3] The U.S. Clinical Practice Guideline states that pregnant smokers should be encouraged to quit without medication based on insufficient evidence of effectiveness and theoretical concerns with safety. Pregnant smokers should be offered behavioral counseling interventions that exceed minimal advice to quit.

[4] In July 2009, the FDA mandated that the prescribing information for all bupropion- and varenicline-containing products include a black-boxed warning highlighting the risk of serious neuropsychiatric symptoms, including changes in behavior, hostility, agitation, depressed mood, suicidal thoughts and behavior, and attempted suicide. Clinicians should advise patients to stop taking varenicline or bupropion SR and contact a health care provider immediately if they experience agitation, depressed mood, and any changes in behavior that are not typical of nicotine withdrawal, or if they experience suicidal thoughts or behavior. If treatment is stopped due to neuropsychiatric symptoms, patients should be monitored until the symptoms resolve.

[5] Wholesale acquisition cost from Red Book Online. Thomson Reuters, September 2012.

MAO, monoamine oxidase; NRT, nicotine replacement therapy; OTC, over-the-counter (non-prescription product); Rx, prescription product.

For complete prescribing information, please refer to the manufacturers' package inserts.

Nicotine Replacement Therapy (NRT)

The goal of NRT is to gradually wean the tobacco user by replacing the nicotine from tobacco products and blunting nicotine withdrawal symptoms. A factor that may reduce the effectiveness of NRT is that the recommended dosages of NRT deliver only about half the amount of nicotine a smoker would typically receive by smoking a pack of cigarettes under typical conditions. The rate at which nicotine is delivered also varies with the NRT product. For instance, the *transdermal nicotine patch (TNP)* delivers nicotine at a relatively steady rate over 24 hours and has few barriers to adherence. In contrast, the *nicotine nasal spray* raises nicotine levels the most rapidly of all NRT products and may be more effective in reducing acute cravings in highly dependent smokers (Pbert, Luckmann, & Ockene, 2004), but also has a greater potential for abuse and dependence. Another factor affecting the effectiveness of NRT is compliance. The patch has been found to have the highest compliance rates (Henningfield, Fant, Buchhalter, & Stitzer, 2005) and can be combined with acute therapies (gum, lozenge, inhaler, and spray) on an ad lib basis to manage breakthrough cravings in heavy smokers. *Nicotine gum (NG), nicotine lozenge, nicotine inhaler* (puffed into the mouth and absorbed through the oral mucosa), and *nicotine nasal spray* require multiple dosing regimens, require careful explanation about proper usage, and may cause irritating side effects, all of which may lessen compliance.

Non-Nicotine Medications

Sustained release bupropion (Zyban, Wellbutrin, Buproban, and Budeprion) is an antidepressant found to be effective in helping smokers manage withdrawal and cravings when quitting smoking. Bupropion potentially postpones weight gain and reduces relapse rates making it a good alternative for smokers with multiple failed quit attempts or those who fear weight gain (Hays et al., 2001). *Varenicline (Chantix)* addresses nicotine dependence by stimulating dopamine release while simultaneously blocking nicotine receptors. This serves to blunt withdrawal, reduce cravings, and reduce the rewarding effects of nicotine (Foulds, Steinberg, Williams, & Ziedonis, 2006). Because varenicline works at the nicotinic receptor sites, adjuvant use of NRT is not recommended.

Combination Therapy

Among first-line medications there is evidence for increased long-term abstinence rates compared to placebo for a number of specific combinations of therapy. This includes combining the nicotine patch long term (greater than 14 weeks) (providing a stable level of nicotine) with the NG or nicotine nasal spray (ad lib short-acting NRT), the nicotine patch with the nicotine inhaler, or the nicotine patch with bupropion SR (Fiore et al., 2008). In practice, NRT products are frequently used in combination with no evidence of nicotine toxicity or other adverse events. The combination of varenicline with any NRT medications has been associated with increased side effects and is not recommended (Fiore et al., 2008).

Using Extended Pharmacotherapy for Sustained Abstinence

Tobacco dependence medications can be used long term (e.g., up to 6 months) (Fiore et al., 2008). Extended use of pharmacotherapy can be particularly useful for smokers reporting persistent withdrawal symptoms during treatment, who have relapsed in the past after stopping medication, or who desire long-term therapy. Indeed, extended treatment with some pharmacotherapies has shown promise for sustained abstinence (Gonzales, 2010). There are no known health risks to the use of these medications for up to 6 months, and the development of dependence on the medications is uncommon. In addition, the FDA has approved the use of bupropion SR, varenicline, and some NRT medications for 6-month use.

Pharmacotherapy for Special Populations

Some evidence supports the concept that tailoring of interventions to individual smoker characteristics or targeting of intervention to group characteristics (e.g., race or ethnic background, gender, and age) improves outcomes. Using proven behavioral and pharmacologic methods may be especially important for tobacco users with comorbidity. Persons with a history of mental health or substance abuse disorders may need higher levels of medications for longer periods of time and require more monitoring (Hughes, 2008). Persons suffering from depression or a history of depression may do well with bupropion due to its antidepressant qualities. Nicotine replacement medications also appear to help patients with a past history of depression (Fiore et al., 2008). For an evidence-based guide of behavioral tools for treating smokers with comorbid psychiatric conditions, see Brown (in Abrams et al., 2003).

Behavioral strategies should be considered the preferred treatment approach for pregnant women. Use of pharmacotherapy in pregnant women is usually not recommended unless the woman and her physician agree that the risks of continuing to smoke outweigh the possible risks of using pharmacotherapy (Fiore et al., 2008). Note that all the first-line prescription medications are FDA-rated C or D, so caution is warranted. Additionally, while pharmacotherapy has been found to be safe in adolescents, studies to date have not found it to be particularly effective (Fiore et al., 2008; Grimshaw & Stanton, 2006). For smokers concerned about weight gain, bupropion SR and NRTs, particularly the 4-mg NG and 4-mg nicotine lozenge, delay but do not prevent post-cessation weight gain (Grimshaw & Stanton, 2006).

HEALTH CARE PROVIDER DIRECTED INTERVENTIONS

The national rate at which physicians provide advice and assistance to their patients who smoke has remained low (Thorndike, Regan, & Rigotti, 2007). A common rationale for this includes lack of time and resources for the physician. However, studies have demonstrated the feasibility of developing linkages between clinical settings and community level services (Bentz et al., 2006; Perry, Keller, Fraser, & Fiore, 2005) thus helping to lessen the burden for the clinician. An example of such a program is Quit-Works currently operating in Massachusetts through collaboration between the Massachusetts Tobacco Control Program and major health plans in the Commonwealth. QuitWorks coordinates clinical and community-based efforts by linking patient, clinicians, and a proactive telephone counseling quitline through the use of faxed referral forms (Warner, Land, Rodgers, & Keithly, 2012). Linking quitline services with free NRT also has proved to be an effective method for reaching large numbers of smokers. Frieden, Mostashari, and colleagues (Frieden et al., 2005) reported on the effectiveness of a large-scale distribution of free NRT patches in New York City. Using a conservative intent to treat (ITT) analysis (all non-respondents were considered to be smoking at 6-month follow-up), the cessation rate was 20%. Those who received counseling also were more likely to quit than those who did not (38% vs. 27%). A study of the Minnesota QUITPLAN Helpline before and after the availability of free NRT found that participation in counseling, use of medications, and abstinence rates all increased (An et al., 2006). Easy access to free NRT cessation medication in diverse populations can help large numbers of smokers to quit.

Implementation of comprehensive care management systems can ensure that each smoker receives continuity and the appropriate level of care based on screening and triage into a level and type of treatment that meets their needs (Abrams et al., 2003). Treatment intensity can range from minimal (e.g., over-the-counter nicotine replacement, Internet-based interventions, and brief primary care), to moderate (e.g., proactive telephone), to intense (e.g., outpatient and inpatient multi-session clinical care delivered by specialists trained to treat severe tobacco addiction). This is not to suggest a novice quitter should only have access to minimal treatment, rather that this range of treatment should be available to best meet the needs and interest of the tobacco user at the time of their quit attempt. Even a first time quitter should have access to intensive treatment if interested in order to reduce the recycling so common among tobacco users.

Generally there is broad consensus that proven tobacco dependence interventions (either behavioral or pharmacologic) will roughly double the quit rate of users versus controls. Combined behavioral and pharmacologic treatments can result in as much as a three to fourfold increase in cessation outcomes. The PHS guideline (Fiore et al., 2008) details best practice recommendations; Table 9.2 depicts a practical application of these recommendations. In addition, there are resources available to assist practitioners in developing evidence-based treatment protocols including a comprehensive handbook for the assessment and treatment of smokers that covers program planning, assessment, and a range of treatment options from brief intervention to intensive treatment for smokers with comorbid psychiatric conditions (Abrams et al., 2003) as well as several other manuals (McEwen, Hajek, McRobbie, & West, 2006; Perkins, Conklin, & Levine, 2007).

Recommendations for health care providers to treat special populations such as adolescents (Sussman & Sun, 2009), pregnant smokers (Lumley, Oliver, Chamberlain, & Oakley, 2004), and those with mental health disorders (Williams & Ziedonis, 2004) also have been published. In addition, a number of tobacco treatment specialist training programs now exist (see www.attud.org). All evidence-based treatment protocols address both pharmacologic treatment (except where contraindicated) and psychosocial components that are based upon many of the behavior change theories described elsewhere in this book (see Section I). A brief summary of the application of psychosocial and pharmacologic strategies for tobacco treatment is presented here.

The role of private payers (i.e., health plans and employers) must be considered in this discussion as well. State and local departments of health cannot be expected to bear the burden of providing accessible treatment services to all tobacco users. With the passing of the Affordable Care Act (ACA) in 2010, the opportunity for increased attention to preventive services was realized. Requirements for Medicaid programs include treatment services for pregnant women beginning immediately, and in January of 2014 tobacco cessation medications must be covered (American Lung Association, 2012). Also effective immediately was the requirement for all new employer-sponsored insurance plans to cover tobacco cessation treatment. However, coverage was not clearly defined and a review of 39 plans in 2012 found wide variations, significant ambiguity, and in some cases contradictory policies regarding cessation services (Kofman, Dunton, & Senkewicz, 2012). State Health Insurance Exchanges

TABLE 9.2 5A Tobacco Intervention

ASK ABOUT TOBACCO USE AT EVERY VISIT

✓ Implement an office system that ensures that, for every patient at every visit, tobacco-use status is queried and documented.

ADVISE ALL TOBACCO USERS TO QUIT

✓ "I strongly advise you to quit smoking and I can help you."

ASSESS READINESS TO QUIT

✓ Ask every tobacco user if s/he is willing to make a quit attempt at this time:

- If willing to quit, provide assistance (see below)
- If unwilling to quit, provide motivational intervention

ASSIST TOBACCO USERS IN QUITTING

✓ Provide brief counseling:

- Reasons to quit
- Barriers to quitting
- Lessons from past quit attempts
- Set a quit date, if ready
- Enlist social support

✓ Recommend use of combination or single pharmacotherapy (patch, gum, lozenge, nasal spray, inhaler, bupropion, or varenicline) unless contraindicated.

✓ Be aware of insurance coverage. Many health plans cover some or all medications.

✓ Provide supplementary educational material.

ARRANGE FOLLOW-UP

✓ Refer to 1-800-QUIT-NOW (1-800-784-8669).

✓ If quit:

- Congratulate success, encourage maintenance

✓ If tobacco use has occurred:

- Ask for recommitment to total abstinence
- Review circumstances that caused lapse
- Use lapse as a learning experience
- Assess pharmacotherapy use and problems

✓ Consider referral to more intensive treatment.

to be implemented in 2014 are required to cover Essential Health Benefits, although the coverage of comprehensive tobacco cessation treatment is not yet defined (American Lung Association, 2012).

TECHNOLOGY/E-STRATEGIES

The Internet has the potential to reach millions of smokers cost-effectively. Many cessation websites exist, but few have been evaluated and in a review of over 300 websites, less than 10 met criteria for having content outlined as effective in the

PHS guideline (Bock et al., 2004). In a European study, 3,501 purchasers of a nicotine patch who proactively logged on to use a free Internet program and consented to participate in a research study (76%) were randomly assigned to a tailored versus an untailored program (Strecher, Shiffman, & West, 2005). At 3-month follow-up, the tailored condition (22.8%) outperformed the untailored condition (18.1%) in 10-week continuous abstinence (ITT). A preliminary large-scale evaluation of a broadly disseminated smoking cessation website reported cessation at 3 months in the range of 7% (ITT) to 30% (responders only) (Cobb et al., 2005). It is noteworthy from a comprehensive systems perspective that approximately 30% of those surveyed indicated they had already quit smoking at registration and were using the website for relapse prevention.

More recently, research has been conducted comparing the utilization and effectiveness of a variety of treatment modalities. In a study comparing clinic, worksite, phone, and web-based treatment programs in Minnesota (An et al., 2010), results indicated that enrollment was greatest for the web-based program followed by the helpline. The helpline reached more "socially disadvantaged" smokers, and the treatment centers saw more highly nicotine-dependent smokers. In terms of abstinence rates, 30-day quit rates were highest for the helpline (29%), followed by the treatment centers (26%), then worksites (20%), and web-based program (13%). The lowest cost per quit was found in the website program ($291/quit), which also attracted younger smokers. The authors concluded that each type of program is important in assisting different populations of tobacco users in their efforts to quit. In another study comparing clinic, phone, and web-based treatment programs in Vermont through both the VT Adult Tobacco Survey and VT Cessation Services Report (Hughes, Suiter, & Marcy, 2010), the helpline was found to be used by the greatest percentage of smokers (2.8%; 56% returned for a second visit) compared to the clinic (1.8%; 82% returned for a second visit) and web program (1.2%; 26% returned for a second visit). The clinic participants were older and heavier, more dependent smokers. The authors concluded that reach and outcomes were similar for all modalities, and that clinics serve the more dependent smokers. In a randomized controlled trial, comparing basic Internet treatment to enhanced Internet treatment (including interactivity) and enhanced Internet plus proactive telephone counseling, the combined enhanced Internet with telephone intervention demonstrated the highest quit rates (Graham et al., 2011).

In addition to the Internet, there is a growing interest in the use of text support and social media to assist smokers in their efforts to quit (Abroms et al., 2012; Cobb, Graham, Byron, Niaura, & Abrams, 2011). An early review of mobile phone apps by the Cochrane Collaboration found insufficient evidence to support their efficacy (Whittaker et al., 2009). However, a more recent trial has indicated efficacy (Free et al., 2011). The use of apps is relatively new, and a recent content analysis has found that the majority of apps are not evidence-based (Abroms, Padmanabhan, Thaweethai, & Phillips, 2011). A new text support program designed for young adults by the National Cancer Institute, SmokefreeTXT, has recently been released and is currently being evaluated.

PATIENT-CENTERED/SUPPORTIVE STRATEGIES

Motivation is important for a smoker to be able to make the decision to quit and to set goals consistent with this objective, such as increasing knowledge, changing attitudes, or setting a quit date. Motivation for smoking cessation refers to both a smoker's reasons for quitting, as well as the strength of their desire to quit (Curry, Wagner, & Grothaus, 1990). Patient-centered counseling (PCC) is an intervention style that has demonstrated significant results when implemented by physicians for modification of smoking, nutrition, and alcohol use (Ockene et al., 1999; Ockene et al., 1994; Ockene et al., 1988; Ockene, Wheeler, Adams, Hurley, & Hebert, 1997). It consists of helping smokers by engaging them to focus on their own strengths, resources, and past experiences with smoking cessation that can help them to develop a plan for change (Ockene, 1992; Ockene & Ockene, 1992; Ockene et al., 1988). It is guided by the principle that people need to be actively engaged in behavior change and can develop their own plans for change using strengths and past experiences. Motivational interviewing (MI; Rollnick, Miller, & Butler, 2007) uses client or patient-centered techniques to increase motivation, primarily among substance abuse patients who are often ambivalent about stopping or decreasing their addictive behavior(s). While the body of evidence regarding the effectiveness of MI for tobacco treatment is limited (Burke, Arkowitz, & Menchola, 2003; Heckman, Egleston, & Hofmann, 2010; Lai, Cahill, Qin, & Tang, 2010; Lundahl, Kunz, Brownwell, Tollefson, & Burke, 2010), a combination of MI techniques and skill training is common practice.

Prochaska and colleagues (1983), using a Stages of Change Model (Prochaska, DiClemente, Velicer, & Rossi, 1993), have suggested that tailoring interventions to motivational level may increase smoking cessation among less motivated smokers. The Stages of Change Model (Prochaska & Velicer, 2004) lends itself to the development of interventions tailored to the smoker's motivational readiness to change. It also provides a useful roadmap for smokers in that it provides milestones (pre-contemplation, contemplation, preparation, action, and maintenance) and guidelines for processes used at every phase of the journey from smoking initiation to various patterns of use to efforts at cessation, relapse, and recycling to the ultimate success of permanent maintenance of cessation. (See Chapters 2 and 13 for more information about this model.) There is some debate over the ultimate utility of a Stages of Change Model, especially regarding its ability to accurately assess readiness to change and its prospective predictive value (Herzog & Blagg, 2007; Sutton, 2001; West, 2005). Continuous measures to assess motivation, such as the Contemplation Ladder, also have been used as an alternative to a categorical staging algorithm (Herzog & Blagg, 2007). Despite the potential limitations, outcome research has supported some components of this model when applied to written and electronic materials for smoking cessation (Becona & Vazquez, 2001; Etter & Perneger, 2001; Prochaska, Velicer, Fava, Rossi, & Tsoh, 2001).

ASSESSING MOTIVATION TO QUIT

Patient-Centered Counseling (PCC) can use techniques and an understanding of the stages of change to help the clinician assess the tobacco user's willingness and confidence in quitting. Despite the appeal of a Stages of Change Model, it should also be noted that some smokers suddenly decide to quit smoking in an unpredictable fashion that does not follow the rational and sequential flow of such a model (West & Sohal, 2006). As many as 49% of smokers may quit without any advance planning (West & Sohal, 2006).

Tobacco users vary widely in their motivation to quit and initial interventions are most effective when clinicians take the time to actively listen to their patients, and encourage them to articulate the pros/cons of tobacco use and quitting. For the tobacco user who is not ready to quit (pre-contemplation) this exploration may begin to open the door for future consideration of a cessation attempt. For those considering or preparing to quit (contemplation and preparation) this discussion will begin to uncover the facilitators and barriers to change that will be faced by the patient. As mentioned earlier, the level of self-efficacy or confidence expressed by the patient may strongly influence readiness to change. Low confidence is often a barrier and increasing confidence will be a proximal goal. The basic PCC skills of using open-ended questions and asking the smoker to identify his own strengths, challenges, and resources are essential at this stage of the process. For a more detailed discussion of the tools available to address motivation to quit, see Emmons and colleagues (in Abrams et al., 2003).

CONCLUSIONS

Despite a significant history of success in reducing tobacco use, progress has stalled and there is a need to focus attention on new methods while sustaining proven practices. Healthy People 2010 targets for smoking among adults (12%) and use of all tobacco products by adolescents (21%) were not reached and have been retained in the Healthy People 2020 objectives (USDHHS, 2010b). In 2010, the Department of Health and Human Services published a strategic plan that provided a framework for re-invigorating the comprehensive efforts required to promote a continued decline in tobacco use (USDHHS, 2010b). This framework includes four major components: (1) strengthen the implementation of evidence-based tobacco control interventions, (2) change social norms around tobacco use, (3) lead by example, and (4) advance knowledge. The first year of implementation of this strategic plan resulted in action in all areas. However continued funding and focused efforts will be required to achieve the desired reduction in tobacco use (USDHHS, 2012).

Efforts to ensure the availability of tobacco treatment resources must continue to be a component of comprehensive tobacco control programs. Smoking prevalence is lower than the national average (19.3%) in those states with strong, visible, comprehensive, and sustained antismoking programs, for example, 12.1% in California (IOM, 2007). Such comprehensive programs include components with wide reach that may produce a lower ratio of quitting and more intensive programs with less reach and higher quit results. Mass media campaigns have been shown to motivate interest in quitting as evidenced by increased calls to quitlines (CDC, 2012b). Social media promises to provide a new venue for disseminating information about the risks of tobacco use and cessation methods. This may be especially true in reaching young tobacco users. The National Cancer Institute has implemented several web and mobile phone applications tailored to specific groups such as teens, women, and Spanish-speaking populations (www.smokefree.gov). Research is under way to determine the efficacy of some novel health promotion and treatment programs (Sadasivam et al., 2011) and there is a need for continued innovation. To further improve treatment for tobacco dependence, Baker and colleagues (2011) suggest that new research needs to be focused on the phases of treatment defined as motivation, pre-cessation, cessation, and maintenance. The authors propose that understanding effective methods within each of these phases will help to increase the long-term abstinence rate among tobacco users who quit.

Although much is known about the neurobiology of tobacco addiction, still more work needs to be done. Recent research, for example, has shown specific genetic or cellular mechanisms involved in dependence, such as the role of the allelic variation in the CYP2A6 gene related to differential rates of nicotine to cotinine metabolism. Decreased metabolism rates, for example, result in higher nicotine levels over time and a lower need to redose. The opportunity to use this type of information and other basic science discoveries could lead to a better understanding of differential use and effectiveness of cessation aides and possible gender or racial differences, leading to more effective and efficient use of tailored pharmacotherapies (Lerman & Niaura, 2002). It is expected that nicotine dependence treatment can be improved and abstinence will be achievable on a broader scale (Lerman & Niaura, 2002).

The emergence of new tobacco products presents an additional challenge regarding how to implement effective treatment methods. A report by the American Lung Association calls attention to the increasing availability and use of smokeless tobacco products. The use of traditional products chew and snuff are increasing. Novel products such as Ariva (a lozenge), various dissolvable products, and Snus provide an array of products to choose from (American Lung Association, 2012). Also alternative tobacco products are increasingly available as the number of hookah bars grows in the United States (CDC, 2013). This very social form of tobacco use is especially popular among college students (Brockman, Pumper, Christakis, & Moreno, 2012). The tobacco industry is focused on developing and promoting products that help tobacco users circumvent smoke-free policies and the higher cost of cigarettes. Products such as orbs, sticks, and strips are designed to appeal to young consumers and subtly imply that they can be used to help quit smoking (American Legacy Foundation, 2012; University of Medicine & Dentistry of New Jersey, 2012). In reality, these products are likely to lead to dual use and contribute to increased dependence and more difficulty in quitting. Perhaps the most rapidly growing market among new tobacco products is for Electronic Nicotine Delivery Devices (ENDS) also known as electronic cigarettes or e-cigarettes. Consecutive surveys in the United States found that in 2009, 16.4% of respondents were aware of ENDS, doubling to 32.2% by 2010. In this same time frame, the use of ENDS increased fourfold, from 0.6% to 2.7% (Regan, Promoff, Dube, & Arrazola, 2013). There is wide variability among ENDS, no manufacturing safety regulations, and currently little information regarding health effects. However, a culture and lingo are quickly developing, which is likely a sign that this product is here to stay (Etter, 2013).

Effective treatment methods for light and nondaily smokers are not yet identified despite the recognition that this population has difficulty quitting (Kotz, Fidler, & West, 2012; Tindle & Shiffman, 2011). This is an area ripe for research and development of innovative motivational and treatment methods.

In addition, there is an enormous opportunity to further increase cessation outcomes by implementing systems level interventions that reach more smokers and increase access to treatment. Diverse strategies that include a combination of clinical, medical, and community interventions can contribute significantly to improving the health of the public (Ockene et al., 2007). There is interest in receiving counseling from health care providers to help with a quit attempt (Weber et al., 2007). Despite this, the national rate at which physicians provide advice and assistance to their patients who smoke has remained low (Thorndike et al., 2007). New tobacco cessation metrics of tobacco treatment delivery by the Joint Commission have the possibility of promoting increased interventions in hospital settings. Unfortunately these measures are currently voluntary and therefore it is a missed opportunity for hospitals to adopt policies that address the requirements. The Center for Medicare and Medicaid will be considering a review of these measures in 2014 and a requirement to implement the new measures would increase interventions (Fiore, Goplerud, & Schroeder, 2012). The Electronic Health Record (EHR) Incentive Program applies to both hospital and office settings and includes criteria related to meaningful use. Stage 2 requirements were released on August 23, 2012 and include the requirement to document screening for tobacco use and intervention with all patients 18 and older. Implementation of EHR documentation has been shown to increase interventions and motivation to quit (Lindholm et al., 2010).

Interventions that are translated from clinical to community settings to proactively reach more smokers in a cost-effective manner vary widely in outcome effectiveness. This is due to variability of factors present in real world settings such as more heterogeneous characteristics of the target groups, and differences in pro-grams, providers, delivery system, and other contextual or setting factors. Channels of intervention delivery also must be factored in, such as health care organizations and medical settings from hospitals to private practice, worksites, schools, telephone quit lines, the Internet, and other print and electronic media.

Systems level models are needed to address the diversity of channels and of popu-lations of users. Models such as stepped care, the tailoring of interventions to moti-vational readiness to quit (e.g., Stages of Change Model and MI), and the targeting of interventions to channels of delivery (e.g., primary care offices, managed care orga-nizations, worksites, schools, the Internet, and telephone quitlines) or to population groups (e.g., younger or older smokers, underserved or uninsured groups, women, and minorities) will need to be evaluated empirically to demonstrate their utility and cost-effectiveness.

It is not just state and local departments of health that should bear the costs of provid-ing treatment to tobacco users. Private payers such as health plans and employers have a role to play as well. It remains to be seen how healthcare reform efforts will help to balance the burden of providing treatment services to tobacco users. Medicare and in some states Medicaid programs are setting the example in covering pharmacologic and counseling services for its beneficiaries and private insurers are slowly increasing their coverage as well (CDC, 2006; Curry & Orleans, 2005; Curry, Orleans, Keller, & Fiore, 2006).

REFERENCES

Abrams, D., Niaura, R., Brown, R., Emmons, K. A., Goldstein, M., & Monti, P. (2003). *The tobacco dependence treatment handbook: A guide to best practices*. New York, NY: The Guilford Press.

Abrams, D. B., Orleans, C. T., Niaura, R., Goldstein, M., Velicer, W., & Prochaska, J. O. (1993). Treatment issues: Towards a stepped care model. *Tobacco Control, 2*(Suppl.), S17–S37.

Abroms, L. C., Ahuja, M., Kodl, Y., Thaweethai, L., Sims, J., Winickoff, J. P., & Windsor, R. A. (2012). Text2Quit: Results from a pilot test of a personalized, interactive mobile health smoking cessation program. *Journal of Health Communication, 17*(Suppl. 1), 44–53.

Abroms, L. C., Padmanabhan, N., Thaweethai, L., & Phillips, T. (2011). iPhone apps for smoking cessation: A content analysis. *American Journal of Preventive Medicine, 40*(3), 279–285.

American Legacy Foundation. (2012). Fact Sheets. Retrieved from http://www.legacyforhealth.org/what-we-do/tobacco-control-research/fact-sheets

American Lung Association. (2012). The emergence of new smokeless tobacco products [Electronic Version]. Retrieved from http://www.lung.org/stop-smoking/tobacco-control-advocacy/reports-resources/tobacco-policy-trend-reports/new-smokeless-tobacco-products.pdf

American Psychiatric Association. (2000). *Diagnostic and statistical manual of mental disorders* (4th ed., text rev.). Washington, DC: American Psychiatric Association.

An, L. C., Betzner, A., Schillo, B., Luxenberg, M. G., Christenson, M., Wendling, A., & Joseph, A. M. (2010). The comparative effectiveness of clinic, work-site, phone, and Web-based tobacco treatment programs. *Nicotine & Tobacco Research, 12*(10), 989–996.

An, L. C., Schillo, B. A., Kavanaugh, A. M., Lachter, R. B., Luxenberg, M. G., Wendling, A. H., & Joseph, A. M. (2006). Increased reach and effectiveness of a statewide tobacco quitline after the addition of access to free nicotine replacement therapy. *Tobacco Control, 15*(4), 286–293.

Baker, T. B., Mermelstein, R., Collins, M., Piper, M. E., Jorenby, D. E., Smith, S. S., et al. (2011, April). New methods for tobacco dependence treatment research. *Ann Behav Med, 41*(2), 192–207.

Balfour, D. J. (2004). The neurobiology of tobacco dependence: A preclinical perspective on the role of the dopamine projections to the nucleus accumbens [corrected]. *Nicotine & Tobacco Research, 6*(6), 899–912.

Becona, E., & Vazquez, F. L. (2001). Effectiveness of personalized written feedback through a mail intervention for smoking cessation: A randomized-controlled trial in Spanish smokers. *Journal of Consulting and Clinical Psychology, 69*(1), 33–40.

Benowitz, N. L., Perez-Stable, E. J., Herrera, B., & Jacob, P., 3rd. (2002). Slower metabolism and reduced intake of nicotine from cigarette smoking in Chinese-Americans. *Journal of the National Cancer Institute, 94*(2), 108–115.

Bentz, C., Bayley, K., Bonin, K., Fleming, L., Hollis, J., & McAfee, T. (2006). The feasibility of connecting physician offices to a state-level tobacco quit line. *American Journal of Preventive Medicine, 30*(1), 31–37.

Bock, B., Graham, A., Sciamanna, C., Krishnamoorthy, J., Whiteley, J., Carmona-Barros, R., … Abrams, D. (2004). Smoking cessation treatment on the Internet: Content, quality, and usability. *Nicotine & Tobacco Research, 6*(2), 207–219.

Brandon, T. H., Herzog, T. A., & Webb, M. S. (2003). It ain't over till it's over: The case for offering relapse-prevention interventions to former smokers. *American Journal of the Medical Sciences, 326*(4), 197–200.

Brockman, L. N., Pumper, M. A., Christakis, D. A., & Moreno, M. A. (2012). Hookah's new popularity among US college students: A pilot study of the characteristics of hookah smokers and their Facebook displays. *BMJ Open, 2*(6), 1–8.

Brody, A. L., Mandelkern, M. A., London, E. D., Olmstead, R. E., Farahi, J., Scheibal, D., … Mukhin, A. G. (2006). Cigarette smoking saturates brain alpha 4 beta 2 nicotinic acetylcholine receptors. *Archives of General Psychiatry, 63*(8), 907–915.

Burke, B. L., Arkowitz, H., & Menchola, M. (2003). The efficacy of motivational interviewing: A meta-analysis of controlled clinical trials. *Journal of Consulting and Clinical Psychology, 71*(5), 843–861.

Caraballo, R. S., Yee, S. L., Gfroerer, J., & Mirza, S. A. (2008). Adult tobacco use among racial and ethnic groups living in the United States, 2002–2005. *Preventing Chronic Disease, 5*(3), A78.

Centers for Disease Control and Prevention. Smoking & tobacco use – Hookahs. Retrieved from http://www.cdc.gov/tobacco/data_statistics/fact_sheets/tobacco_industry/hookahs/index.htm

Centers for Disease Control and Prevention (CDC). (1998). Tobacco use among high school students–United States, 1997. *MMWR Morbidity and Mortality Weekly Report, 47*(12), 229–233.

CDC. (2006). Racial/ethnic differences among youths in cigarette smoking and susceptibility to start smoking – United States, 2002–2004. *MMWR Morbidity and Mortality Weekly Report, 55*(47), 1275–1277.

CDC. (2010). State-specific prevalence of cigarette smoking and smokeless tobacco use among adults—United States, 2009. *MMWR Morbidity and Mortality Weekly Report, 59*(43), 1400–1406.

CDC. (2011a). Quitting smoking among adults–United States, 2001–2010. *MMWR Morbidity and Mortality Weekly Report, 60*(44), 1513.

CDC. (2011b). Vital signs: Current cigarette smoking among adults aged ≥ 18 years – United States, 2005-2010. *MMWR Morbidity and Mortality Weekly Report, 60*(33), 1207–1212.

CDC. (2012a). Current cigarette smoking among adults–United States, 2011. *MMWR Morbidity and Mortality Weekly Report, 61*(44), 889–894.

CDC. (2012b). Increases in quitline calls and smoking cessation website visitors during a national tobacco education campaign–March 19-June 10, 2012. *MMWR Morbidity and Mortality Weekly Report, 61*(34), 667-670.

CDC. (2013). Vital signs: Current cigarette smoking among adults aged ≥18 years with mental illness – United States, 2009–2011. *MMWR Morbidity and Mortality Weekly Report, 62*(5), 81–87.

Centers for Disease Control and Prevention: Morbidity and Mortality Weekly Report. (2006). State Medicaid coverage for tobacco-dependence treatments – United States, 2005. *Journal of the American Medical Association, 296*(24), 2917–2919.

Cobb, N. K., Graham, A. L., Bock, B. C., Papandonatos, G., & Abrams, D. B. (2005). Initial evaluation of a real-world Internet smoking cessation system. *Nicotine & Tobacco Research, 7*(2), 207–216.

Cobb, N. K., Graham, A. L., Byron, M. J., Niaura, R. S., & Abrams, D. B. (2011). Online social networks and smoking cessation: A scientific research agenda. *Journal of Medical Internet Research, 13*(4), e119.

Coe, J. W., Brooks, P. R., Vetelino, M. G., Wirtz, M. C., Arnold, E. P., Huang, J., … O'Neill, B. T. (2005). Varenicline: An alpha4beta2 nicotinic receptor partial agonist for smoking cessation. *Journal of Medicinal Chemistry, 48*(10), 3474–3477.

Cokkinides, V. E., Bandi, P., Siegel, R. L., & Jemal, A. (2012). Cancer-related risk factors and preventive measures in US Hispanics/Latinos. *CA: A Cancer Journal for Clinicians, 62*(6), 353–363.

Curry, S., & Orleans, C. T. (2005). Addressing tobacco treatment in managed care. *Nicotine & Tobacco Research, 7*(Suppl. 1), s5–s8.

Curry, S., Wagner, E. H., & Grothaus, L. C. (1990). Intrinsic and extrinsic motivation for smoking cessation. *Journal of Consulting and Clinical Psychology, 58*(3), 310–316.

Curry, S. J., Orleans, C. T., Keller, P., & Fiore, M. (2006). Promoting smoking cessation in the healthcare environment: 10 years later. *American Journal of Preventive Medicine, 31*(3), 269–272.

Dani, J. A. (2001). Overview of nicotinic receptors and their roles in the central nervous system. *Biological Psychiatry, 49*(3), 166–174.

Dani, J. A., & De Biasi, M. (2001). Cellular mechanisms of nicotine addiction. *Pharmacology Biochemistry and Behavior, 70*(4), 439–446.

Dani, J. A., & Heinemann, S. (1996). Molecular and cellular aspects of nicotine abuse. *Neuron, 16*(5), 905–908.

DiFranza, J. R., Rigotti, N. A., McNeill, A. D., Ockene, J. K., Savageau, J. A., St Cyr, D., & Coleman, M. (2000). Initial symptoms of nicotine dependence in adolescents. *Tobacco Control, 9*(3), 313–319.

DiFranza, J. R., Savageau, J. A., Fletcher, K., O'Loughlin, J., Pbert, L., Ockene, J. K., … Wellman, R. J. (2007). Symptoms of tobacco dependence after brief intermittent use: The development and assessment of nicotine dependence in youth-2 study. *Archives of Pediatric and Adolescent Medicine, 161*(7), 704–710.

Durkin, S., Brennan, E., & Wakefield, M. (2012). Mass media campaigns to promote smoking cessation among adults: An integrative review. *Tobacco Control, 21*(2), 127–138.

Durkin, S. J., Biener, L., & Wakefield, M. A. (2009). Effects of different types of antismoking ads on reducing disparities in smoking cessation among socioeconomic subgroups. *American Journal of Public Health, 99*(12), 2217–2223.

Etter, J. F. (2013). *The electronic cigarette: An alternative to tobacco.* CreateSpace Independent Publishing Platform.

Etter, J. F., & Perneger, T. V. (2001). Effectiveness of a computer-tailored smoking cessation program: A randomized trial. *Archives of Internal Medicine, 161*(21), 2596–2601.

Fagan, P., Moolchan, E. T., Lawrence, D., Fernander, A., & Ponder, P. K. (2007). Identifying health disparities across the tobacco continuum. *Addiction, 102*(Suppl. 2), 5–29.

Fertig, J., & Allen, J. (1995). *Alcohol and tobacco: From basic science to policy*: National Institute on Alcohol Abuse and Alcoholism Monograph.

Fiore, M. C., Goplerud, E., & Schroeder, S. A. (2012). The Joint Commission's new tobacco-cessation measures–will hospitals do the right thing? *New England Journal of Medicine, 366*(13), 1172–1174.

Fiore, M. C., Jaen, C. R., Baker, T. B., Bailey, W. C., Benowitz, N. L., Curry, S. J., …Wewers, M. E. (2008). *Treating tobacco use and dependence: 2008 update.* Rockville, MD: U.S. Department of Health and Human Services. Public Health Service.

Foulds, J., Steinberg, M. B., Williams, J. M., & Ziedonis, D. M. (2006). Developments in pharmacotherapy for tobacco dependence: Past, present and future. *Drug and Alcohol Review, 25*(1), 59–71.

Free, C., Knight, R., Robertson, S., Whittaker, R., Edwards, P., Zhou, W., … Roberts, I. (2011). Smoking cessation support delivered via mobile phone text messaging (txt2stop): A single-blind, randomised trial. *Lancet, 378*(9785), 49–55.

Frieden, T. R., Mostashari, F., Kerker, B. D., Miller, N., Hajat, A., & Frankel, M. (2005). Adult tobacco use levels after intensive tobacco control measures: New York City, 2002–2003. *American Journal of Public Health, 95*(6), 1016–1023.

Fu, S. S., Kodl, M. M., Joseph, A. M., Hatsukami, D. K., Johnson, E. O., Breslau, N., … Bierut, L. (2008). Racial/ethnic disparities in the use of nicotine replacement therapy and quit ratios in lifetime smokers ages 25 to 44 years. *Cancer Epidemiology, Biomarkers & Prevention, 17*(7), 1640–1647.

Garvey, A. J., Bliss, R. E., Hitchcock, J. L., Heinold, J. W., & Rosner, B. (1992). Predictors of smoking relapse among self-quitters: A report from the Normative Aging Study. *Addictive Behaviors, 17*(4), 367–377.

Giovino, G. A. (2002). Epidemiology of tobacco use in the United States. *Oncogene, 21*(48), 7326–7340.

Gonzales, D. (2010). Nicotine patch plus lozenge gives greatest increases in abstinence from smoking rates at 6 months compared with placebo; smaller effects seen with nicotine patch alone, bupropion or nicotine lozenges alone or combined. *Evidence Based Medicine, 15*(3), 77–78.

Graham, A. L., Cobb, N. K., Papandonatos, G. D., Moreno, J. L., Kang, H., Tinkelman, D. G., … Abrams, D. B. (2011). A randomized trial of Internet and telephone treatment for smoking cessation. *Archives of Internal Medicine, 171*(1), 46–53.

Grimshaw, G. M., & Stanton, A. (2006). Tobacco cessation interventions for young people. *Cochrane Database of Systematic Reviews* (4), CD003289.

Hall, S. M., Humfleet, G. L., Munoz, R. F., Reus, V. I., Prochaska, J. J., & Robbins, J. A. (2011). Using extended cognitive behavioral treatment and medication to treat dependent smokers. *American Journal of Public Health, 101*(12), 2349–2356.

Harris, D. S., & Anthenelli, R. M. (2005). Expanding treatment of tobacco dependence. *Current Psychiatry Reports, 7*(5), 344–351.

Hays, J. T., Hurt, R. D., Rigotti, N. A., Niaura, R., Gonzales, D., Durcan, M. J., … White J. D. (2001). Sustained-release bupropion for pharmacologic relapse prevention after smoking cessation. A randomized, controlled trial. *Annals of Internal Medicine, 135*(6), 423–433.

Heatherton, T., Kozlowski, L., Frecker, R., & Fagerstrom, K. (1991). The Fagerstrom Test for nicotine dependence: A revision of the Fagerstrom tolerance questionnaire. *British Journal of Addiction, 86*(9), 1119–1127.

Heckman, C. J., Egleston, B. L., & Hofmann, M. T. (2010). Efficacy of motivational interviewing for smoking cessation: A systematic review and meta-analysis. *Tobacco Control, 19*(5), 410–416.

Heishman, S. (2000). Cognitive and behavioral effects of nicotine. In R. Ferrence, J. Slade, R. Room, & M. Pope (Eds.), *Nicotine and Public Health* (pp. 93–113). Washington, DC: American Public Health Association.

Henningfield, J. E., Fant, R. V., Buchhalter, A. R., & Stitzer, M. L. (2005). Pharmacotherapy for nicotine dependence. *CA: A Cancer Journal for Clinicians, 55*(5), 281–299; quiz 322–283, 325.

Herzog, T. A., & Blagg, C. O. (2007). Are most precontemplators contemplating smoking cessation? Assessing the validity of the stages of change. *Health Psychology, 26*(2), 222–231.

Houston, T. K., Scarinci, I. C., Person, S. D., & Greene, P. G. (2005). Patient smoking cessation advice by health care providers: The role of ethnicity, socioeconomic status, and health. *American Journal of Public Health, 95*(6), 1056–1061.

Hughes, J. (1995a). Clinical implications of the association between smoking and alcoholism. In J. Fertig & R. Fuller (Eds.), *Alcohol and tobacco: From basic science to policy. NIAAA research monograph 30* (pp. 171–181). Washington, DC: U.S. Government Printing Office.

Hughes, J. (1995b). Treatment of nicotine dependence: Is more better? *Journal of the American Medical Association, 274*, 171–181.

Hughes, J., Fiester, S., Goldstein, M., Resnick, M., Rock, N., & Ziedonis, D. (1996). American Psychiatric Association Practice Guideline for the treatment of patients with nicotine dependence. *American Journal of Psychiatry, 153*(10 Suppl.), s1–s31.

Hughes, J. N. (2008). An algorithm for choosing among smoking cessation treatments. *Journal of Substance Abuse Treatment, 34*(4), 426–432.

Hughes, J. R. (1993). Pharmacotherapy for smoking cessation: Unvalidated assumptions, anomalies, and suggestions for future research. *Journal of Consulting and Clinical Psychology, 61*(5), 751–760.

Hughes, J. R. (1996). The future of smoking cessation therapy in the United States. *Addiction, 91*(12), 1797–1802.

Hughes, J. R., Suiter, C., & Marcy, T. (2010). Use and outcomes of a state-funded in-person counselling program. *Tobacco Control, 19*(3), 260.

Institute of Medicine (IOM). (2007). *Ending the tobacco problem: A blueprint for the nation.* Washington, DC: The National Academies Press.

Kalivas, P. W., & Volkow, N. D. (2005). The neural basis of addiction: A pathology of motivation and choice. *American Journal of Psychiatry, 162*(8), 1403–1413.

Kalman, D., Morissette, S. B., & George, T. P. (2005). Co-morbidity of smoking in patients with psychiatric and substance use disorders. *American Journal of Addictions, 14*(2), 106–123.

Keating, G. M., & Siddiqui, M. A. (2006). Varenicline: A review of its use as an aid to smoking cessation therapy. *CNS Drugs, 20*(11), 945–960.

Killen, J. D., & Fortmann, S. P. (1997). Craving is associated with smoking relapse: Findings from three prospective studies. *Experimental and Clinical Psychopharmacology, 5*(2), 137–142.

Killen, J. D., Fortmann, S. P., Varady, A., & Kraemer, H. C. (2002). Do men outperform women in smoking cessation trials? Maybe, but not by much. *Experimental and Clinical Psychopharmacology, 10*(3), 295–301.

Kim, S. S., Ziedonis, D., & Chen, K. W. (2007). Tobacco use and dependence in Asian Americans: A review of the literature. *Nicotine & Tobacco Research, 9*(2), 169–184.

King, B. A., Dube, S. R., & Tynan, M. A. (2012). Current tobacco use among adults in the United States: Findings from the National Adult Tobacco Survey. *American Journal of Public Health, 102*(11), e93–e100.

Kofman, M., Dunton, K., & Senkewicz, J. D. (2012). Implementation of tobacco cessation coverage under the Affordable Care Act: Understanding how private health insurance policies cover tobacco cessation treatments [Electronic Version]. Retrieved from http://www.tobaccofreekids.org/pressoffice/2012/georgetown/coveragereport.pdf

Kotz, D., Fidler, J., & West, R. (2012). Very low rate and light smokers: Smoking patterns and cessation-related behaviour in England, 2006-11. *Addiction, 107*(5), 995–1002.

Lai, D. T. C., Cahill, K., Qin, Y., & Tang, J. L. (2010). Motivational interviewing for smoking cessation. *Cochrane Database of Systematic Reviews Issue 1*. Art. No.: CD006936. doi: 10.1002/14561858.CD006936.pub.2

Lambe, E. K., Picciotto, M. R., & Aghajanian, G. K. (2003). Nicotine induces glutamate release from thalamocortical terminals in prefrontal cortex. *Neuropsychopharmacology, 28*(2), 216–225.

Lancaster, T., & Stead, L. F. (2005). Self-help interventions for smoking cessation. *Cochrane Database of Systematic Reviews* (3), CD001118.

Lando, H. A., Pirie, P. L., Roski, J., McGovern, P. G., & Schmid, L. A. (1996). Promoting abstinence among relapsed chronic smokers: The effect of telephone support. *American Journal of Public Health, 86*(12), 1786–1790.

Lerman, C., & Niaura, R. (2002). Applying genetic approaches to the treatment of nicotine dependence. *Oncogene, 21*(48), 7412–7420.

Lindholm, C., Adsit, R., Bain, P., Reber, P. M., Brein, T., Redmond, L., & Fiore, M. C. (2010). A demonstration project for using the electronic health record to identify and treat tobacco users. *World Medical Journal, 109*(6), 335–340.

Lumley, J., Oliver, S. S., Chamberlain, C., & Oakley, L. (2004). Interventions for promoting smoking cessation during pregnancy. *Cochrane Database of Systematic Reviews* (4), CD001055.

Lundahl, B. W., Kunz, C., Brownwell, C., Tollefson, D., & Burke, B. L. (2010). A meta-analysis of motivational interviewing: Twenty-five years of empirical studies. *Research on Social Work Practice, 22*(2), 137–160.

McEwen, A., Hajek, P., McRobbie, H., & West, R. (2006). *Manual of smoking cessation: A guide for counsellors and practitioners*. Oxford, UK: Blackwell Publishing.

Milton, B., Cook, P. A., Dugdill, L., Porcellato, L., Springett, J., & Woods, S. E. (2004). Why do primary school children smoke? A longitudinal analysis of predictors of smoking uptake during pre-adolescence. *Public Health, 118*(4), 247–255.

National Institutes of Health. (2006). State-of-the-science conference statement: Tobacco use: Prevention, cessation, and control. *Annals of Internal Medicine, 145*(11), 839–844.

Ockene, I. S., Hebert, J. R., Ockene, J. K., Saperia, G. M., Stanek, E., Nicolosi, R., ... Hurley, T. G. (1999). Effect of physician-delivered nutrition counseling training and an office-support program on saturated fat intake, weight, and serum lipid measurements in a hyperlipidemic population: Worcester Area Trial for Counseling in Hyperlipidemia (WATCH). *Archives of Internal Medicine, 159*(7), 725–731.

Ockene, J. (1992). Smoking intervention: A behavioral, educational, and pharmacologic perspective. In I. Ockene & J. Ockene (Eds.), *Prevention of coronary heart disease* (pp. 201–230). Boston, MA: Little, Brown and Company.

Ockene, J., Kristeller, J., Pbert, L., Hebert, J., Luippold, R., Goldberg, R., ... Kalan, K. (1994). The PDSIP: Can short-term interventions produce long-term effects for a general outpatient population. *Health Psychology, 13*(3), 278–281.

Ockene, J., & Ockene, I. (1992). Helping patients to reduce their risk for coronary heart disease: An overview. In I. Ockene & J. Ockene (Eds.), *Prevention of coronary heart disease* (pp. 173–199). Boston, MA: Little, Brown and Company.

Ockene, J., Quirk, M., Goldberg, R., Kristeller, J., Donnelly, G., Kalan, K., ... Williams, J., et al (1988). A residents' training program for the development of smoking intervention skills. *Archives of Internal Medicine, 148*, 1039–1045.

Ockene, J., Wheeler, E., Adams, A., Hurley, T., & Hebert, J. (1997). Provider training for patient-centered alcohol counseling in a primary care setting. *Archives of Internal Medicine, 157*, 2334–2341.

Ockene, J. K., Edgerton, E. A., Teutsch, S. M., Marion, L. N., Miller, T., Genevro, J. L., ... Briss, P. A. (2007). Integrating evidence-based clinical and community strategies to improve health. *American Journal of Preventive Medicine, 32*(3), 244–252.

Orleans, C., & Slade, J. (1993). *Nicotine addiction: Principles and management*. New York, NY: Oxford University Press.

Orleans, C. T. (2007). Increasing the demand for and use of effective smoking-cessation treatments reaping the full health benefits of tobacco-control science and policy gains–in our lifetime. *American Journal of Preventive Medicine, 33*(6 Suppl.), S340–S348.

Orleans, C. T., & Alper, J. (2003). Helping addicted smokers quit. In S. Issacs & J. Knickman (Eds.), *To improve health and health care, Vol. VI.* Princeton, New Jersey: Robert Wood Johnson Foundation.

Pbert, L., Luckmann, R., & Ockene, J. K. (2004). Smoking cessation treatment. In L. J. Haas (Ed.), *Handbook of primary care psychology* (pp. 527–549). New York, NY: Oxford University Press.

Perez-Stable, E. J., Herrera, B., Jacob, P., 3rd, & Benowitz, N. L. (1998). Nicotine metabolism and intake in black and white smokers. *Journal of the American Medical Association, 280*(2), 152–156.

Perkins, K., Conklin, C., & Levine, M. (2007). *Cognitive-behavioral therapy for smoking cessation: A practical guidebook to the most effective treatments.* New York, NY: Routledge.

Perkins, K. A., Donny, E., & Caggiula, A. R. (1999). Sex differences in nicotine effects and self-administration: Review of human and animal evidence. *Nicotine & Tobacco Research, 1*(4), 301–315.

Perry, R., Keller, P., Fraser, D., & Fiore, M. (2005). Fax to quit: A model for delivery of tobacco cessation services to Wisconsin residents. *Wisconsin Medical Journal, 104*(4), 37–44.

Piasecki, T. M., Niaura, R., Shadel, W. G., Abrams, D., Goldstein, M., Fiore, M. C., & Baker, T. B. (2000). Smoking withdrawal dynamics in unaided quitters. *Journal of Abnormal Psychology, 109*(1), 74–86.

Pierce, J. P., & Gilpin, E. A. (2003). A minimum 6-month prolonged abstinence should be required for evaluating smoking cessation trials. *Nicotine & Tobacco Research, 5*(2), 151–153.

Piper, M. E., McCarthy, D. E., & Baker, T. B. (2006). Assessing tobacco dependence: A guide to measure evaluation and selection. *Nicotine & Tobacco Research, 8*(3), 339–351.

Prochaska, J., DiClemente, C., Velicer, W., & Rossi, J. (1993). Standardized, individualized, interactive and personalized self-help programs for smoking cessation. *Health Psychology, 12,* 399–405.

Prochaska, J. J., Delucchi, K., & Hall, S. M. (2004). A meta-analysis of smoking cessation interventions with individuals in substance abuse treatment or recovery. *Journal of Consulting and Clinical Psychology, 72*(6), 1144–1156.

Prochaska, J. O., & Velicer, W. F. (2004). Integrating population smoking cessation policies and programs. *Public Health Reports, 119*(3), 244–252.

Prochaska, J. O., Velicer, W. F., Fava, J. L., Rossi, J. S., & Tsoh, J. Y. (2001). Evaluating a population-based recruitment approach and a stage-based expert system intervention for smoking cessation. *Addictive Behaviors, 26*(4), 583–602.

Regan, A. K., Promoff, G., Dube, S. R., & Arrazola, R. (2013). Electronic nicotine delivery systems: Adult use and awareness of the 'e-cigarette' in the USA. *Tobacco Control, 22*(1), 19–23.

Rodu, B., & Cole, P. (2007). Declining mortality from smoking in the United States. *Nicotine & Tobacco Research, 9*(7), 781–784.

Rollnick, S., Miller, W., & Butler, C. (2007). *Motivational interviewing in health care: Helping patients change behavior.* New York, NY: Guilford Press.

Sadasivam, R. S., Delaughter, K., Crenshaw, K., Sobko, H. J., Williams, J. H., Coley, H. L., … Houston, T. K. (2011). Development of an interactive, Web-delivered system to increase provider-patient engagement in smoking cessation. *Journal of Medical Internet Research, 13*(4), e87.

Shiffman, S. (2009). Light and intermittent smokers: Background and perspective. *Nicotine & Tobacco Research, 11*(2), 122–125.

Shiffman, S., Ferguson, S. G., Dunbar, M. S., & Scholl, S. M. (2012). Tobacco dependence among intermittent smokers. *Nicotine & Tobacco Research, 14*(11), 1372–1381.

Strecher, V. J., Shiffman, S., & West, R. (2005). Randomized controlled trial of a web-based computer-tailored smoking cessation program as a supplement to nicotine patch therapy. *Addiction, 100*(5), 682–688.

Substance Abuse and Mental Health Services Administration. (2005). *Results from the 2005 National Survey on Drug Use and Health.* Rockville, MD: Office of Applied Studies, DHHS Publication SMA 05-4061.

Substance Abuse and Mental Health Services Administration. (2009). *The NSDUH report: Smokeless tobacco use, initiation, and relationship to cigarette smoking, 2002 to 2007.* Rockville, MD.

Substance Abuse and Mental Health Services Administration. (2010). Results from the 2009 National Survey on Drug Use and Health. Volume 1, Summary of National Findings (Office of Applied Studies, NSDUH Series H-38A, HHS Publication No. SMA 10-4856 Findings). Rockville, MD.

Sussman, S., & Sun, P. (2009). Youth tobacco use cessation: 2008 update. *Tobacco Induced Diseases, 5,* 3.

Sutton, S. (2001). Back to the drawing board? A review of applications of the transtheoretical model to substance use. *Addiction, 96*(1), 175–186.

Thorndike, A. N., Regan, S., & Rigotti, N. A. (2007). The treatment of smoking by US physicians during ambulatory visits: 1994–2003. *American Journal of Public Health, 97*(10), 1878–1883.

Tindle, H. A., & Shiffman, S. (2011). Smoking cessation behavior among intermittent smokers versus daily smokers. *American Journal of Public Health, 101*(7), e1–e3.

Tobacco use among middle and high school students – United States, 2000-2009. *MMWR Morbidity and Mortality Weekly Report, 59*(33), 1063–1068.

Tonnesen, P., Mikkelsen, K., Markholst, C., Ibsen, A., Bendixen, M., Pedersen, L., … Evald, T. (1996). Nurse-conducted smoking cessation with minimal intervention in a lung clinic: A randomized controlled study. *European Respiratory Journal, 9*(11), 2351–2355.

U.S. Department of Health and Human Services. (2010). *Ending the tobacco epidemic: A tobacco control strategic action plan for the U.S. Department of Health and Human Services.* Washington, DC: Office of the Assistant Secretary for Health.

U.S. Department of Health and Human Services. (2012). *Ending the tobacco epidemic: Progress toward a healthier nation.* Washington, DC: U.S. Department of Health and Human Services, Office of the Assistant Secretary for Health. Retrieved from http://www.hhs.gov/ash/initiatives/tobacco/

U.S. Department of Health and Human Services. (2010a). *How tobacco smoke causes disease: The biology and behavioral basic for smoking attributable disease: A report of the Surgeon General.* Atlanta, GA: U.S. Department of Health and Human Services, Centers for Disease and Control and Prevention, National Center for Chronic Disease Prevention and Health Promotion, Office on Smoking and Health.

U.S. Department of Health and Human Services. (2010b). *Healthy People 2020.* Retrieved from http://www.healthypeople.gov/2020/topicsobjectives2020/objectiveslist.aspx?topicId=41

U.S. Preventive Services Task Force. (2009). *Counseling and interventions to prevent tobacco-caused disease in adults and pregnant women: Reaffirmation recommendation statement.* Retrieved from http://www.uspreventiveservicestaskforce.org/uspstf09/tobacco/tobaccors2.htm

University of Medicine & Dentistry of New Jersey. (2012). *Trinkets and trash: Artifacts of the tobacco epidemic.* Retrieved from http://www.trinketsandtrash.org/index.php

Wang, H., & Sun, X. (2005). Desensitized nicotinic receptors in brain. *Brain Research Review, 48*(3), 420–437.

Warner, D. D., Land, T. G., Rodgers, A. B., & Keithly, L. (2012). Integrating tobacco cessation quitlines into health care: Massachusetts, 2002–2011. *Preventing Chronic Disease, 9*, e133.

Weber, D., Wolff, L. S., Orleans, T., Mockenhaupt, R. E., Massett, H. A., & Vose, K. K. (2007). Smokers' attitudes and behaviors related to consumer demand for cessation counseling in the medical care setting. *Nicotine & Tobacco Research, 9*(5), 571–580.

West, R. (2005). Time for a change: Putting the Transtheoretical (Stages of Change) Model to rest. *Addiction, 100*(8), 1036–1039.

West, R., & Sohal. (2006). "Catastrophic" pathways to smoking cessation: Findings from national survey. *British Medical Journal, 332*(7539), 458–460.

West, R., & Zhou, X. (2007). Is nicotine replacement therapy for smoking cessation effective in the "real world"? Findings from a prospective multinational cohort study. *Thorax, 62*(11), 998–1002.

Wetter, D. W., Kenford, S. L., Smith, S. S., Fiore, M. C., Jorenby, D. E., & Baker, T. B. (1999). Gender differences in smoking cessation. *Journal of Consulting and Clinical Psychology, 67*(4), 555–562.

Whittaker, R., Borland, R., Bullen, C., Lin, R. B., McRobbie, H., & Rodgers, A. (2009). Mobile phone-based interventions for smoking cessation. *Cochrane Database of Systematic Reviews*, (4) CDC00611. doi: 10.1002/14561858.CD00661.pub.2

Williams, J. M., & Ziedonis, D. (2004). Addressing tobacco among individuals with a mental illness or an addiction. *Addictive Behaviors, 29*(6), 1067–1083.

World Health Organization. (2011). *WHO report on the global tobacco epidemic, 2011: Warning about the dangers of tobacco.* Retrieved from http://www.who.int/tobacco/global_report/2011/en/index.html

10

Alcohol Prevention and Treatment: Interventions for Hazardous, Harmful, and Dependent Drinkers

RUTH MCGOVERN
EILEEN KANER

LEARNING OBJECTIVES

- Describe different interventions for individuals who drink alcohol excessively.
- Understand the theoretical and practice bases of the interventions.
- Evaluate the evidence for the effectiveness of the interventions.

Alcohol consumption has been rising over recent decades in many developing countries and continues to do so in Eastern Europe. While there is significant variation in consumption levels globally, excessive drinking is a major public health concern worldwide. Contributing to over 60 types of diseases, alcohol is the second greatest disease burden in high income countries after tobacco use and third worldwide after childhood underweight and unsafe sex (World Health Organization, 2009). As well as the harm to health, 20% of deaths due to road traffic accidents, 30% of deaths caused by esophageal and liver cancer, epilepsy, and homicide, and 50% of all deaths caused by liver cirrhosis are attributable to alcohol (World Health Organization, 2009). Indeed, alcohol is responsible for 3.6% of worldwide deaths and 5% in young people (Jernigan, 2001). Moreover, in young people the adverse effects of alcohol exceeds that caused by tobacco, with accident trauma and suicide caused by the acute effects of alcohol, accounting for much of the disability and death attributed to alcohol consumption (Jernigan, 2001). The disease burden relating to alcohol consumption is costly. In the United Kingdom the most recent estimates indicated that alcohol-related problems cost the National Health Service between £2.7 ($4.3) (Health Improvement Analytical Team & Department of Health, 2008) and £3 ($4.8) billion (Balakrishnan, Allender, Scarborough, Webster, & Rayner, 2009) per annum. Furthermore, the cabinet calculated that the total cost to the UK economy is £25.1 ($40.2) billion each year (National Audit Office, 2008).

Epidemiologic data indicate that the majority of alcohol-related problems in a population are not due to the most problematic drinkers, such as individuals who are alcohol dependent, but those who are hazardous or harmful drinkers. Hazardous drinking is a repeated pattern of drinking that increases the risk of physical or psychological problems (Saunders & Lee, 2000) while harmful drinking is defined by the presence of these problems (World Health Organization, 1992). In the UK, hazardous and harmful drinkers outnumber dependent drinkers by a ratio of 7:1 and therefore represent a much larger group (Drummond et al., 2004). Collectively they contribute a large number of chronic health problems due to frequent heavy drinking, and acute health problems and social disorder resulting from intoxication. Consequently it is not sufficient to target the heaviest drinkers alone. While it is essential that specialist alcohol treatment for severely dependent drinkers is provided, the greatest impact on reduction of alcohol-related problems at a population level can be made by facilitating a decrease in alcohol consumption in hazardous and harmful drinkers. This is sometimes known as the preventive paradox (Kreitman, 1986), a term first coined by Geoffrey Rose (Rose, 1981). The preventive paradox describes a situation wherein the majority of cases of disease are found within individuals in low to moderate risk and only a minority within individuals of high risk. This seemingly contradictory situation is caused by the high risk population being much smaller than the low to moderate risk population.

Behavioral change and treatment services therefore should be provided for the full range of alcohol-related risk and harm. Interventions with personalized feedback that seek to prevent harm particularly in individuals at risk for alcohol use disorders are fundamental and can be effective in reducing harm at a population level. These interventions are known as secondary prevention. Preventive medicine is typically described in terms of primary, secondary, and tertiary levels, wherein secondary prevention involves methods to diagnose and treat existing disease during early stages. For some individuals with more intensive drinking problems, however, more in-depth treatment which focuses upon abstinence may be necessary to achieve and maintain change. This chapter will consider the robust evidence base for secondary prevention, including recent technological advances within the field, before progressing to discuss lesser evidenced psychological and pharmacologic interventions.

The moderation goal has become far more acceptable in the UK (Cox, Rosenberg, Hodgins, Macartney, & Maurer, 2004), Australia (Donovan & Healther, 1997), and other countries than it has in the United States (Cox et al., 2004), whose acceptance of moderation is largely limited to populations requiring brief alcohol intervention. Therefore, interventions such as psychological and pharmacologic therapies are likely to have varying goals ranging from harm reduction to abstinence depending upon country. The goal of an intervention is essentially a clinical decision which should be negotiated with the client. As such, it is unhelpful to specify intent of intervention at a modality level, other than to say all interventions seek to achieve improvements in the client's situation. For this reason, this chapter will be structured according to the intervention type as opposed to the intervention goal.

PREVENTION

BRIEF INTERVENTIONS

Brief intervention is a secondary preventive activity, aimed at individuals who are drinking excessively or in a drinking pattern that is likely to be harmful to their health or well-being (Kaner, Newbury-Birch, & Heather, 2009). Concerned with understanding and changing behavior, brief interventions are grounded in psychological theory and broadly based upon social learning theory (Bandura, 1997), which views behavior as a dynamic interaction between the individual, behavior, and environment. The approach assumes that both the cognitive and affective attributes of individuals impact upon behavior and the extent to which they are influenced by the external world. Moreover, all individuals have the capacity to observe and learn from the behavior of other people around them or situations they have previously encountered. Consequently, drinking behavior is influenced not only by an individual's attitudes toward alcohol, their knowledge about its risks, and perceptions of its reinforcing effects, but also by the attitudes of family members and friends toward drinking and the patterns of use within relevant groups. Thus brief intervention focuses on both personal and contextual factors related to drinking behavior. The beliefs of the individual, attitudes, self-efficacy, and normative comparison (where individuals are encouraged to consider their own drinking behavior compared to other people's drinking behavior) are emphasized within brief interventions.

Brief Intervention Structure

Brief intervention largely consists of two different approaches (National Institute for Health and Clinical Excellence, 2010): simple structured advice which seeks to raise awareness through the provision of personalized feedback following screening and practical steps on how to reduce drinking behavior and its adverse consequences; and extended brief intervention which generally involves patient-centered counseling techniques, often motivational interviewing (MI). Extended brief intervention introduces and evokes change by giving the patient the opportunity to explore their alcohol use and motivations, past experiences, and strategies for change. Both forms of brief intervention share the common aim of helping people to change drinking behavior to promote health but they vary in the precise means by which this is achieved. Motivational interviewing is a person-centered, directive approach, which seeks to resolve the conflict inherent in ambivalence, thus enhancing motivation to change (Miller & Rollnick, 1991). The approach can be characterized by the FRAMES acronym:

F—personalized *feedback*
R—promoting personal *responsibility*
A—providing *advice*
M—considering a *menu* of options
E—offering *empathy*
S—promoting *self-efficacy*

Brief interventions are not simply traditional psychotherapy delivered in a short duration of time (Babor, 1994; Miller & Rollnick, 1991). Typically they are applied to opportunistic, non-treatment seeking populations, delivered by practitioners other than addiction specialists. There is a wide variation in the duration and frequency of brief alcohol interventions; however, brief interventions are typically delivered in a single session or a series of related sessions (not exceeding five sessions), lasting between 5 and 60 minutes (Kaner et al., 2007). They can be implemented by a range of health professionals such as physicians and nurse practitioners in a wide variety of settings (Heather, 2007). Brief alcohol interventions target hazardous and harmful drinkers rather than dependent drinkers. Such individuals may not know they are experiencing alcohol-related problems. Typically, brief interventions aim to reduce alcohol consumption rather than achieve abstinence.

Brief Intervention Evidence

There is a large amount of high quality evidence that has accumulated to support the effectiveness of brief interventions with adults who have an alcohol use disorder

(Kaner et al., 2007). Indeed, the evidence base for brief interventions represents the largest, most robust body of evidence for alcohol interventions (Kaner, 2012) with other psychological and pharmacologic interventions being less well evidenced.

The most comprehensive systematic review of brief interventions was conducted by Moyer and colleagues (2002) which included 56 controlled trials conducted in a wide range of settings, with treatment seeking and non-treatment seeking patients (Moyer, Finney, Swearingen, & Vergun, 2002). The review identified 34 trials which compared brief interventions (defined as no more than four sessions) to control conditions in non-treatment seeking populations and 20 trials comparing brief interventions to more extended interventions within treatment seeking populations. Meta-analyses of the 34 trials showed brief interventions had significantly different effect sizes relating to alcohol consumption and other alcohol-related outcomes at less than 3-month, 3- to 6-month, and 6- to 12-month follow-up whereas the 20 trials comparing brief interventions to extended interventions did not find effect sizes significantly different from zero. Thus this indicates superior outcomes from brief interventions. The effects from a single session brief intervention have been found to be still present at 2 years (Ockene, Reed, & Reiff-Hekking, 2009) and 4 years follow-up after intervention (Fleming et al., 2002; Ockene et al., 2009), while in a different study no evidence was found at 10 years follow-up (Wutzke, Conigrave, Saunders, & Hall, 2002).

Most of the evidence for brief alcohol intervention in non-treatment seeking groups is within primary health care (Ballesteros, Duffy, Querejeta, Arino, & Gonzalez-Pinto, 2004; Bertholet, Daeppen, Wietlisbach, Fleming, & Burnand, 2005; Kaner et al., 2007; Littlejohn, 2006; Ockene, Adams, Hurley, Wheeler, & Hebert, 1999; Ockene et al., 2009; Saitz, 2010; Whitlock, Polen, Green, Orleans, & Klein, 2004). A review conducted by Ballesteros and colleagues (2004) found that the number of hazardous/harmful drinkers within this setting needing to be treated before one person showed a benefit was between 8 and 12 (Ballesteros et al., 2004). Indeed a study estimated that if brief interventions were delivered to 25% of the at-risk population within primary care throughout Europe, 408,000 years of disability and premature death would be avoided, representing an estimated saving of €740 ($967) million each year (Chisholm, Rehm, Van Ommeren, & Monteiro, 2004). The evidence for the effectiveness of brief alcohol interventions in a primary care setting is so strong that the U.S. Preventive Services Task Force gave brief alcohol treatment a "B" recommendation meaning "there is strong evidence supporting the need for primary care providers to do it" (U.S. Preventive Services Task Force, 2010). Delivering brief interventions within a primary care setting enables capitalization upon the "teachable moment" wherein patients are able to consider their alcohol use within a context of an alcohol-related illness consultation and with a credible health care professional (Babor, Ritson, & Hodgeson, 1986).

While there is strong evidence for efficacy in males, many trials do not include sufficient female participants to provide conclusive results for the effect of brief interventions within female populations (Ballesteros et al., 2004; Kaner et al., 2007; Kaner, & Dickinson, 2009). The evidence for the efficacy of brief interventions for dependent drinkers is inconsistent with one review finding that the benefits cannot be extended to very heavy and dependent drinkers (Saitz, 2010), while another found evidence that brief interventions had a greater effect when applied to heavy drinkers than moderate drinkers (Ballesteros et al., 2004) as well as greater efficacy when applied to non-treatment seekers (Ballesteros et al., 2004). Extended brief interventions have generally not been found to be superior to brief interventions (Ballesteros et al., 2004; Kaner et al., 2007; Kaner, Dickinson, et al., 2009). There is some evidence that extended interventions may provide an additional benefit to male hazardous and harmful drinkers reporting low levels of readiness to change (Babor & Grant, 1992). However this finding was not supported by the SIPS trial, which found there was no additional benefit of delivering 5-minute brief advice or 20-minute brief lifestyle counseling when compared to providing a patient information leaflet (Kaner et al., 2013).

There is less evidence for brief interventions when delivered to other populations or in different settings. Nilsen and colleagues (2008) conducted a systematic review considering the effectiveness of alcohol brief interventions within emergency medicine (Nilsen et al., 2008). The review found that brief interventions had a significant effect upon alcohol intake, risky drinking practices, alcohol-related negative consequences, and injury frequency, when compared to a control group. A further systematic review however failed to find any evidence for superior efficacy of brief interventions (Havard, Shakeshaft, & Sanson-Fisher, 2008). A systematic review considering the effectiveness of brief interventions in general hospital settings (McQueen, Howe, Allan, Mains, & Hardy, 2011) found that compared to control interventions, brief intervention reduced alcohol consumption by 69 grams per week (95% CIs [10, 128]) at 6-month follow-up. A significant effect also was found at 12-month follow-up ($p = .02$). However, the small number of studies ($n = 3$) with comparable outcomes resulted in only weak evidence. While individual trials also have shown benefit for pregnant women (Handmaker et al., 2006) and within the workplace (Richmond, Kehoe, Heather, & Wodak, 2000), it should be noted this evidence is again based upon only a small number of studies; therefore no firm conclusions can be drawn.

Young People

Although there has been a great deal of evidence on primary prevention, which typically aims to delay the age that drinking begins and which uses general health education to prevent underage drinking, this body of work has been reported to be methodologically weak (Foxcroft, Lister-Sharp, & Lowe, 1997) and only a relatively small number of programs have reported clearly positive outcomes (Foxcroft & Tsertsvadze, 2011; Foxcroft, Ireland, Lister-Sharp, Lowe, & Breen, 2003). Thus targeting interventions at young people who are already drinking excessively may be a more effective strategy, since the intervention will have more salience for the individuals receiving them. Indeed, a recent review of interventions to reduce the harm associated with adolescent substance use outlined the positive potential of brief alcohol intervention (Toumbourou et al., 2007). Caution must be applied when considering these findings however as research into brief interventions with young people has generally included older adolescents in college settings. There also is a lack of evidence for brief interventions with young people in health care settings. This was in contrast with a lack of evidence for the efficacy of a range of treatment options. An important consideration however when comparing preventive and treatment interventions for young people is that those young people needing treatment often have numerous other difficulties including social, emotional, family, and criminological needs, which generally compound their alcohol needs and inefficacy of treatment interventions.

Most of the evidence base for brief interventions delivered with older adolescents is based within education settings, where there have now been around 16 controlled trials (Barnett & Read, 2005; Carey, Scott-Sheldon, Carey, & DeMartini, 2007; Hunter Fager & Mazurek Melnyk, 2004; Larimer & Cronce, 2007; Larimer, Cronce, Lee, & Kilmer, 2005; Walters & Neighbors, 2005). The key elements of the brief interventions were MI approaches and/or personalized feedback on alcohol consumption typically with a normative component (Larimer & Cronce, 2007; Moreira, Smith, & Foxcroft, 2009). The trials considered brief interventions predominately delivered in a single session, although a minority were extended to include two or more sessions. The duration of the intervention ranged from 30 minutes to 2 hours (modal duration one hour), delivered to varying sample sizes from 60 (Borsari & Carey, 2005) to over 500 young people (Carey, Carey, Maisto, & Henson, 2006). Trial participants were typically college students of White American ethnicity, aged 18 to 21 years (Natarajan & Kaner, 2007) and were highly motivated to receive alcohol intervention, although mandated participation resulting from alcohol-related disorder is increasingly prevalent in more recent studies (Borsari & Carey, 2005). Methodological quality of the trials varied; however, more recent trials are of improved quality and include larger samples with clear random assignment of study conditions (Larimer & Cronce, 2007).

Meta-analyses of brief intervention trials within education settings compared to control conditions of assessment only, have consistently shown that students who received brief interventions reduced their alcohol consumption (Carey et al., 2007; Larimer & Cronce, 2007). Furthermore, such brief interventions typically achieved small to medium effect sizes (Cohen, 1969) across multiple measures of alcohol consumption including quantity, frequency, and intensity of drinking. The effects of brief intervention seem to diminish over time. Indeed it has been noted that relatively few of the reduced drinking effects seemed to persist beyond 6 months following the intervention (Carey et al., 2007). This has resulted in booster or repeated brief intervention sessions being suggested as beneficial in college populations to help sustain positive changes in drinking behavior (Kaner & Bewick, 2010). Reductions in alcohol-related problems, which often took longer to emerge, were however reported in longer-term follow-up of 1 year to 18 months.

In contrast to the large amount of work in education settings, just one systematic review has focused on young people in health care settings alone. This review identified eight controlled trials (Jackson et al., 2009), seemingly of high methodological quality although two trials reported inadequate or unclear randomization and allocation concealment (Bailey, Baker, Webster, & Lewin, 2004; D'Amico, Miles, Stern, & Meredith, 2008). Sample sizes ranged from 34 to 655 young people aged between 12 and 24 years. Seven out of the eight trials were based in the United States, the remaining trial being Australian (Bailey et al., 2004). The study intervention was typically based upon MI, lasted 20 to 45 minutes, and was delivered over one or two sessions, although one trial included four motivational interventions delivered over a period of 1 month (Bailey et al., 2004).

Four trials reported significant positive effects of brief intervention on a number of varying alcohol consumption measures (Bailey et al., 2004; Monti et al., 1999, 2007; Spirito et al., 2004). A reduction in alcohol-related risk-taking behavior also was reported (Monti et al., 1999; Schaus, Sole, McCoy, Mullett, & O'Brien, 2009). However, a reduction in drinking levels was reported in both intervention and control conditions in three trials (Monti et al., 1999, 2007; Spirito et al., 2004). A further three trials did not find effect after brief intervention (D'Amico et al., 2008; Maio et al., 2005; Peterson, Baer, Wells, Ginzler, & Garrett, 2006). Lastly, one trial which included 12- to 17-year-old adolescents reported an adverse reaction wherein an increase in alcohol use and binge drinking among brief intervention subjects was observed (Boekeloo et al., 2004). No other trials reported adverse outcomes associated with brief intervention delivered in health care settings.

There are a number of challenges inherent in delivering brief interventions to young people who drink relating to both the setting in which the intervention can occur and its traditional face-to-face format. Brief interventions with adults have primarily been delivered in health settings; thus this approach often misses individuals who tend not to engage with health services such as young people (Roche & Freeman, 2004).

Moreover, some young people are reluctant to seek traditional services for alcohol problems; in part due to skepticism of the benefit of discussing their alcohol concerns directly with health practitioners. Thus it has been suggested that young people may prefer self-directed or minimal-contact methods or technically focused alcohol intervention (Kypri, Saunders, & Gallagher, 2003; Paperny, Aona, Lehman, Hammar, & Risser, 1990; Saunders, Kypri, Walters, Laforge, & Larimer, 2004).

New Technology

The technological advances of the 1980s offered the potential to develop electronic forms of brief intervention (Djikstra & DeVries, 1999; Skinner, Allen, McIntosh, & Palmer, 1985). Initially the limitations of the Internet (penetration, reliability, and speed) and security concerns led to the development of interventions using CD-ROM or DVD technologies. Improvements in and increasing use of the Internet and other technologies (Nilsen,2010) have resulted in a shift in the focus toward interventions delivered via the Internet and other mobile technologies (Cassell, Jackson, & Cheuvront, 1998). Indeed, electronically delivered brief interventions have been reported in North America (Doumas & Hannah, 2008; Lewis, Neighbors, Oster-Aaland, Kirkeby, & Larimer, 2007; Saitz et al., 2007; Chiauzzi, Green, Lord, Thum, & Goldstein, 2005), Australasia (Kypri et al., 2004; Kypri & McAnnally, 2005), and Europe (Bewick, Trusler, Mulhern, Barkham, & Hill, 2008; Bendtsen, Johansson, & Akerline, 2006). Most of the reviews considered university or college students either exclusively or within their study populations (Khadjesari, Murray, Hewitt, Hartley, & Godfrey, 2010; Kypri & McAnnally, 2005; Riper et al., 2009); one review included studies of e-health interventions which targeted adult population drinkers and excluded those which included student populations (Riper et al., 2011).

Seven reviews have examined computer- or web-based brief alcohol interventions (Bewick, Trusler, Barkham, & Hill, 2008; Elliott, Carey, & Bolles, 2008; Khadjesari et al., 2010; Kypri, Sitharthan, Cunningham, Kavanagh, & Dean, 2005; Riper et al., 2011; Riper et al., 2009; Walters & Neighbors, 2005). A number of reviews provide evidence that supports the use of electronic personalized interventions (Kypri et al., 2005; Walters & Neighbors, 2005), reporting small to modest effect sizes (Riper et al., 2011; Riper et al., 2009). However evidence for efficacy is only evident when compared to minimally active comparator groups, notably screening or assessment alone (Carey et al., 2007; Elliott et al., 2008; Khadjesari et al., 2010; Kypri et al., 2005), with no significant difference being observed when compared against other active intervention. The duration of effect is also unclear. A recent meta-analysis concluded that single sessions of personalized feedback, including those delivered electronically (without therapist input) can be effective in reducing problem drinking in the short term (with follow-up up to 9 months post-intervention), although further evidence is needed on long-term impact (Elliott et al., 2008; Riper et al., 2009). A further review found evidence for electronic interventions to be inconsistent (Bewick, Trusler, Barkham, & Hill, 2008) resulting in uncertainty as to whether electronic forms of brief interventions are as effective as those delivered by therapists.

Methodological weaknesses within studies (Khadjesari et al., 2010), heterogeneous study populations (Elliott et al., 2008), and control and study interventions (Bewick, Trusler, Barkham, & Hill, 2008) have been highlighted as potential sources of conflicting evidence within the research. Interventions often contain multiple components (Carey et al., 2007). Hence it is difficult to ascertain which components are effective. Within the published literature it is common for electronic forms of brief intervention to include alcohol education, feedback on drinking behavior and/or negative consequences, and normative comparisons (Bewick, Trusler, Barkham, & Hill, 2008; Bendtsen et al., 2006; Butler & Correia, 2009; Chiauzzi et al., 2005; Doumas & Hannah, 2008; Dimeff & McNeely, 2000; Kypri et al., 2004; Neighbors, Lewis, Bergstrom, & Larimer, 2006; Walters, Vader, & Harris, 2007). A recent review of social norms interventions concluded that personalized feedback, delivered either face-to-face or electronically, appeared to reduce excessive drinking and alcohol-related problems (Moreira et al., 2009). However, the evidence for interventions that did not personalize feedback was less convincing (Moreira et al., 2009). This evidence has recently been supported by additional research reporting significantly greater reductions in alcohol consumption in mandated students, required to attend an intervention, receiving personalized web-based brief intervention compared to those receiving web-based education without personalization (Doumas, McKinley, & Book, 2009).

The lack of effect found in some studies of electronic forms of brief interventions has been attributed to heterogeneity in study populations, with some trials including a high proportion of non-drinkers, light drinkers, or infrequent drinkers (Maio et al., 2005; Kypri & McAnnally, 2005; Bersamin, Paschall, Fearnow-Kenney, & Wyrick, 2007). Indeed some studies report reduced alcohol consumption in at-risk students but not among abstainers and light drinkers (Walters et al., 2007; Doumas & Hannah, 2008; Chiauzzi et al., 2005). Thus electronic forms of brief alcohol interventions may be most helpful for more heavily drinking young people or those who have experienced alcohol-related problems. Hence it is not clear whether it is the brief intervention that produces reductions in drinking or if this is due to an increased motivation for change following an adverse experience that causes the young person to go looking for help. Moreover, there are other groups of young people, with whom electronic forms of brief interventions may be less effective: young women compared to young men (Chiauzzi et al., 2005); young people who have already considered changing their alcohol consumption compared to those who have not considered change (Bendtsen et al., 2006); individuals who report higher intention to become intoxicated through drinking (Neighbors, Lee, Lewis, Fossos, & Walter, 2009); and those who report drinking for social reasons (Neighbors, Larimer, & Lewis, 2004).

TREATMENT

PSYCHOLOGICAL THERAPIES

There are largely two types of psychological therapies used to treat individuals with alcohol use disorders: therapies which have been developed to treat individuals with depression and adapted to individuals with alcohol (and other drug) disorders and those that have been developed specifically for individuals with alcohol and drug disorders. Cognitive behavioral therapy (CBT) is an example of a psychological therapy that was developed to treat individuals with depression. It is one of the most extensively researched psychotherapies (Butler, Chapman, Forman, & Beck, 2006), partially due to its extension and application to a wide range of disorders (Salkovskis, 1996). Based upon principles of social learning theory, CBT sees problematic alcohol use as being linked to other problems within the user's life. CBT assumes therefore that it is more effective to consider a range of difficulties rather than focus upon drinking alone (Longabaugh & Morgenstern, 1999). By addressing skill deficit and behaviors that precipitate relapse, including personal difficulties, individuals are trained to replace maladaptive coping mechanisms with other strategies.

Twelve-step facilitation is a type of psychological therapy developed to treat individuals with alcohol and drug disorders. Commonly confused with Alcoholics Anonymous (AA), twelve-step facilitation is a professional, manualized intervention designed to facilitate an individual's engagement in AA (Kelly, Magill, & Stout, 2009). In comparison, AA is a non-professional fellowship based upon a mutual aid philosophy wherein members access help through a network of informal meetings (Kelly et al., 2009). Both twelve-step facilitation and AA are grounded in the disease model of addiction wherein abstinence is viewed as the treatment goal. Twelve-step facilitation encourages attendance at AA and focuses upon steps one through five, in preparation for engagement in AA, wherein individuals will be required to progress through the full twelve steps of recovery.

A further type of psychotherapy developed specifically to treat individuals with alcohol and drug disorders is that based upon motivational psychology. Motivational interviewing (MI) and motivational enhancement therapy (MET) are closely related versions of psychotherapies which were developed following observations that the abstinence required from interventions such as twelve-step facilitation was often met by resistance (Woody, 2003). MI and MET do not challenge resistance but rather "roll with it" while employing a motivational approach to mobilizing the individual's own resources to effect change. Both MI and MET incorporate the components described within the FRAMES acronym above while MET is manualized and adopts a more directive style, includes a "check-up" form of assessment feedback (Miller & Sovereign, 1989) and a three-phase approach. Phase one is concerned with building motivation for change, phase two seeks to consolidate commitment, and phase three reviews progress and follow-through strategies (Miller, 1995).

Psychological Therapy Evidence Base

To date, 53 controlled trials have considered the impact of CBT on substance use and 23 specifically on alcohol use (Magill & Ray, 2009). A small but clinically significant effect of CBT was reported although its impact reduced over time from 6 months after the initial input (Magill & Ray, 2009). A large effect size was found for CBT compared to no treatment, although a smaller effect was found for other comparison conditions (e.g., usual care or another active treatment). CBT combined with other psychosocial treatment showed a larger effect size than CBT combined with pharmacologic treatment.

Meta-analyses of 30 controlled clinical trials (15 of which were with problem drinkers) found a small to medium effect size (Cohen, 1969) of MI on drinking outcomes, when compared to no treatment or placebo control (0.25–0.53) (Burke, Arkowitz, & Menchola, 2003). A systematic review of 59 MI trials (29 on alcohol abuse) found that MI had a significant impact in reducing substance misuse when compared to no intervention. The effect was greatest soon after intervention (standardized mean difference 0.79; 95% CIs [0.48, 1.09]) and reduced over time. For longer-term follow-up (12 months or longer), the effect was not significant (standardized mean difference 0.06; 95% CIs [0.16, 0.28]). However when compared to other active treatments the results rarely reached significance (Smedslund et al., 2011).

Evidence for twelve-step facilitation and AA is somewhat inconclusive and there is a lack of high quality randomized trials considering its effectiveness. Benefit has been suggested from AA's ability to provide access to free, long-term support (Kelly et al., 2009). However there is insufficient evidence to support efficacy (Ferri, Amato, & Davoli, 2009).

Given the absence of unequivocal evidence for the superiority of one psychotherapeutic intervention, the interaction between patient and treatment has been evaluated.

Project MATCH (Project Match Research Group, 1997) was a large randomized controlled trial (RCT) seeking to test a number of a priori hypotheses regarding the efficacy of assigning treatment approaches based upon the specific needs and characteristics of individuals with alcohol problems. Participants were randomly assigned to receive twelve-step facilitation, relapse prevention (based upon cognitive-behavioral coping skills), or MET over a 12-week treatment period. Drinking outcomes, quality of life, and service utilization were measured at 3-month intervals for one year. Project MATCH found little difference between the psychotherapy interventions. Similarly, the UK alcohol treatment trial compared social behavior and network therapy against MET and found that the two interventions did not differ significantly in effectiveness (UKATT Research Team, 2005).

One systematic review identified 30 studies that compared at least two psychological interventions against one another and included 3,503 participants within the meta-analysis (Imel, Wampold, Miller, & Fleming, 2008). The studies examined the efficacy of a range of therapies including twelve-step facilitation, behavior self-control training, MET, aversion therapy, relapse prevention, and psychodynamic treatment. Synthesis found no evidence of inferiority of a psychological therapy for alcohol use disorder. The seeming equivalence of varying psychological therapies can be partially explained by the presence of active components in each (Luborsky et al., 2002).

PHARMACOLOGIC THERAPIES

There is evidence that repeated detoxifications, which involve the managed removal of alcohol from the body, result in poor treatment outcomes in the longer term (Malcolm, Roberts, Wang, Myrick, & Anton, 2000), resulting in an emphasis being placed upon supporting and maintaining the change in drinking. In recent years, there has been an increase in the use of pharmacologic interventions used as an adjunct to traditional interventions such as detoxification (Mann, Lehert, & Morgan, 2004). Similarly, such interventions have been used in conjunction with or instead of psychological therapies. Three key pharmacologic therapies are typically used to promote abstinence or reduced consumption in problem drinkers. These are disulfiram (an alcohol antagonist) which has sensitizing agents that produce an unpleasant reaction when mixed with alcohol, and naltrexone (an opioid antagonist) and acamprosate (a glutamate antagonist) both of which have anti-craving properties. Gamma-hydroxybutyrate (GHB) also has been found to have alcohol-mimicking properties, which has been provided as a rationale for using it in alcohol addiction treatment as well as in the management of cravings (Gallimberti et al., 1989; Gallimberti, Ferri, Ferrara, Fadda, & Gessa, 1992).

Pharmacologic Therapy Evidence Base

A review of 24 trials of oral disulfiram and 14 trials of implanted disulfiram concluded that there is evidence to support the use of oral but not implanted disulfiram (Hughes & Cook, 1997). Intervention trials also have demonstrated efficacy of disulfiram in voluntary patients (Chick, 1992; Hughes & Cook, 1997) as well as those mandated by the court (Martin et al., 2003).

In 2010, two systematic reviews identified 24 acamprosate trials (Rösner, Hackl-Herrwerth, Leucht, Lehert, Vecchi, & Soyka, 2010) and 50 naltrexone trials (Rösner et al., 2010). Compared to placebo, acamprosate significantly reduced the risk of drinking (relative risk 0.86; 95% CIs [0.81, 0.91]) and the cumulative duration of abstinence reported by trial participants (mean difference 10.94; 95% CIs [5.08, 16.81]) with minimal side effects (Rösner et al., 2010). Naltrexone reduced the risk of heavy drinking compared to a placebo group (relative risk 0.83; 95% CIs [0.76, 0.90]) and significantly decreased the number of drinking days by about 4% (mean difference –3.89; 95% CIs –5.75, –2.04). Positive effects also were demonstrated for a number of secondary outcomes including heavy drinking days, total alcohol consumption, and gamma-glutamyltransferase (Rösner et al., 2010). However, side effects of naltrexone were mainly gastrointestinal problems and sedative effects (Rösner et al., 2010). Meta-analyses of 33 trials compared acamprosate and naltrexone on abstinence (Carmen, Angeles, Ana, & Maria, 2004). Compared to placebo, acamprosate showed significant results, while naltrexone failed to do so.

Meta-analyses conducted by Berglund (2005) found evidence of the additive effects of naltrexone when combined with CBT, wherein CBT was found to enhance the individual's ability to manage a craving. Adding CBT to acamprosate was not found to bring about additional benefits. There was also a statistically significant difference between naltrexone combined with acamprosate when compared to acamprosate alone and placebo alone however not naltrexone alone.

A recent Cochrane review identified 13 RCTs examining the efficacy of GHB in the treatment of alcohol withdrawal and relapse prevention (six evaluating the effect upon withdrawal and seven upon relapse prevention and maintaining abstinence) (Leone, Vigna-Taglianti, Avanzi, Brambilla, & Faggiano, 2011). The review found that while there was a small amount of evidence suggesting that GHB was more effective than placebo at managing alcohol withdrawal syndrome, it was insufficient to draw any confident conclusions. There was no evidence of the superiority of GHB in the treatment of alcohol withdrawal syndrome when compared to other drugs including benzodiazepines or clomethiazole. There was some evidence that GHB was better than naltrexone and disulfiram in preventing craving and maintaining abstinence between 3- and 12-month follow-up. However, the potential for adverse reactions including abuse of GHB also should be considered.

CONCLUSIONS

There is a large and robust evidence base for alcohol brief interventions aimed at reducing risk or harm when delivered to non-treatment seeking individuals attending generalist health settings which are not focused on substance-related problems. In particular, research demonstrates benefit for non-treatment seeking White adult males within primary care settings. There is a growing evidence base to support the use of brief intervention approaches for young people, primarily older adolescents within an educational setting as well as electronic forms of brief interventions. While brief interventions show promise with other groups and when extended to other settings, such research findings are inconsistent and therefore no conclusive evidence can be drawn.

Regarding treatment seeking individuals, there is evidence for efficacy of psychological therapies although effect sizes are typically small to medium. Furthermore, significance is frequently only found when compared to a non-active comparator such as stand-alone assessment. Active psychological therapies rarely outcompete each other when compared directly and so it is likely that an active behavior change component is present in each approach. However, an alternative explanation for equivalent effects of different therapies may be due to the attributes of the therapists delivering them as well as the treatment fidelity of the psychotherapeutic treatment (Tober, Clyne, Finnegan, Farrin, & Russell, 2008). Last, since the beneficial effects of psychological therapies often diminish over time, there may be a need for booster input to maintain effects.

While there is some evidence of the effects of anti-craving medication at preventing relapse, it is inconsistent thus preventing any confident conclusion. This is complicated somewhat by the potential for an adverse reaction, notably relating to naltrexone and GHB. Disulfiram has been found to be effective in maintaining abstinence when administered orally and therefore has a clear role in alcohol treatment (Fuller & Gordis, 2004). Finally, whilst the additive benefits of combining psychological and pharmacological therapies offer some promise, further research is needed (Anton et al., 2006).

REFERENCES

Anton, R., O'Malley, S., Ciraulo, D., Cisler, R., Couper, D., Donovan, D., … Combine Study Research Group. (2006). Combined pharmacotherapies and behavioural interventions for alcohol dependence. The COMBINE study: A randomized controlled trial. *Journal of the American Medical Association, 295*(17), 2003–2017.

Babor, R. F., & Grant, M. (1992). *Project on identification and management of alcohol related problems. Report on phase II: A randomised clinical trial of brief interventions in primary health care.* Geneva: World Health Organization.

Babor, T. F. (1994). Avoiding the horrid and beastly sin of drunkenness: Does dissuasion make a difference? *Journal of Consulting and Clinical Psychology, 62*(6), 1127–1140.

Babor, T. F., Ritson, E. B., & Hodgeson, R. J. (1986). Alcohol-related problems in the primary health care setting: A review of early intervention strategies. *British Journal of Addictions, 81*, 23–46.

Bailey, K. A., Baker, A. L., Webster, R. A., & Lewin, T. J. (2004). Pilot randomized controlled trial of a brief alcohol intervention group for adolescents. *Drug & Alcohol Review, 23*(2), 157–166.

Balakrishnan, R., Allender, S., Scarborough, P., Webster, P., & Rayner, M. (2009). The burden of alcohol-related ill health in the United Kingdom. *Journal of Public Health, 31*, 366–373.

Ballesteros, J. A., Duffy, J. C., Querejeta, I., Arino, J., & Gonzalez-Pinto, A. (2004). Efficacy of brief interventions for hazardous drinkers in primary care: Systematic review and meta-analysis. *Alcoholism, Clinical & Experimental Research, 28*(4), 608–618.

Bandura, A. (1997). *Social learning theory.* Englewood Cliffs, NJ: Prentice-Hall.

Barnett, N. P., & Read, J. P. (2005). Mandatory alcohol intervention for alcohol-abusing college students: A systematic review. *Journal of Substance Abuse Treatment, 29*, 147–158.

Bendtsen, P., Johansson, K., & Akerline, I. (2006). Feasibility of an email based electronic screening and brief intervention (eSBI) to college students in Sweden. *Addictive Behaviours, 31*, 777.

Berglund, M. (2005). A better widget? Three lessons for improving addiction treatment from a meta-analytical study. *Addiction, 100*, 742–750.

Bersamin, M., Paschall, M. J., Fearnow-Kenney, M., & Wyrick, D. (2007). Effectiveness of a web-based alcohol misuse and harm prevention course among high and low risk students. *Journal of American College Health, 55*, 247–254.

Bertholet, N., Daeppen, J.-B., Wietlisbach, V., Fleming, M., & Burnand, B. (2005). Brief alcohol intervention in primary care: Systematic review and meta-analysis. *Archives of Internal Medicine, 165*, 986–995.

Bewick, B. M., Trusler, K., Barkham, M., & Hill, A. J. (2008). The effectiveness of web-based interventions designed to decrease alcohol consumption – A systematic review. *Preventive Medicine, 47*(1), 17–26.

Bewick, B. M., Trusler, K., Mulhern, B., Barkham, M., & Hill, A. J. (2008). The feasibility and effectiveness of a web-based personalised feedback and social norms alcohol intervention in UK university students: A randomised control trial. *Addictive Behaviours, 33*, 1192–1198.

Boekeloo, B. O., Jerry, J., Lee-Ougo, W. I., Worrell, K. D., Hamburger, E. K., Russek-Cohen, E., & Snyder, M. H. (2004). Randomized trial of brief office-based interventions to reduce adolescent alcohol use. *Archives of Pediatrics & Adolescent Medicine, 158*(7), 635–642.

Borsari, B., & Carey, K. (2005). Two brief alcohol interventions for mandated college students. *Psychology of Addictive Behaviors, 19*, 296–302.

Burke, B. L., Arkowitz, H., & Menchola, M. (2003). The efficacy of motivational interviewing: A meta-analysis of controlled clinical trials. *Journal of Consulting and Clinical Psychology, 71*(5), 843–861.

Butler, A. C., Chapman, J. E., Forman, E. M., & Beck, A. T. (2006). The empirical status of cognitive-behavioral therapy: A review of meta-analyses. *Clinical Psychology Review, 26*, 17–31.

Butler, L. H., Correia, C. J. (2009). Brief alcohol intervention with college student drinkers: Face to face versus computerised feedback. *Psychology of Addictive Behaviours, 23*, 163–167.

Carey, K., Scott-Sheldon, L., Carey, M., & DeMartini, K. (2007). Individual-level interventions to reduce college student drinking: A meta-analytic review. *Addictive Behaviors, 32*, 2469–2494.

Carey, K. B., Carey, M. P., Maisto, S. A., & Henson, J. M. (2006). Brief motivational interventions for heavy college drinkers: A randomized controlled trial. *Journal of Consulting and Clinical Psychology, 74*, 943–954.

Carmen, B., Angeles, M., Ana, M., & Maria, A. J. (2004). Efficacy and safety of naltrexone and acamprosate in the treatment of alcohol dependence: A systematic review. *Addiction, 99*, 811–828.

Cassell, M. M., Jackson, C., & Cheuvront, B. (1998). Health communication on the internet: An effective channel for health behaviour change? *Journal of Health Communication, 3*, 71–79.

Chiauzzi, E., Green, T., Lord, S., Thum, C., & Goldstein, M. (2005). My student body: A high risk drinking prevention web site for college students. *Journal of American College Health, 53*(6), 263–274.

Chick, J. (1992). Disulfiram treatment of alcoholism. *British Journal of Psychiatry, 161*, 84–89.

Chisholm, D., Rehm, J., Van Ommeren, M., & Monteiro, M. (2004). Reducing the global burden of hazardous alcohol use: A comparative cost-effectiveness analysis. *Journal of Studies on Alcohol, 65*, 782–793.

Cohen, J. (1969). *Statistical power of analysis for the behavioural sciences.* New York, NY: Academic Press.

Cox, W. M., Rosenberg, H., Hodgins, C. H. A., Macartney, J. I., & Maurer, K. A. (2004). United Kingdom and United States healthcare providers' recommendations of abstinence versus controlled drinking. *Alcohol and Alcoholism, 39*, 130–134.

D'Amico, E. J., Miles, J. N., Stern, S. A., & Meredith, L. S. (2008). Brief motivational interviewing for teens at risk of substance use consequences: A randomized pilot study in a primary care clinic. *Journal of Substance Abuse Treatment, 35*(1), 53–61.

Dimeff, M. A., & McNeely, M. (2000). Computer enhanced primary care practitioner advice for high risk college drinkers in a student primary health care setting. *Cognitive and Behavioural Practice, 7*, 82–100.

Djikstra, A., & DeVries, H. (1999). The development of computer generated tailored interventions. *Patient Education and Counselling, 36*, 193–203.

Donovan, D., & Healther, N. (1997). Acceptability of the controlled-drinking goal among alcohol treatment agencies in New South Wales, Australia. *Journal of Studies of Alcohol, 58*, 253–256.

Doumas, D. M., & Hannah, E. (2008). Preventing high risk drinking in youth in the workplace: A web based normative feedback program. *Journal of Substance Abuse Treatment, 34*, 263–271.

Doumas, D. M., McKinley, L. L., & Book, P. (2009). Evaluation of two web based alcohol interventions for mandated college students. *Journal of Substance Abuse Treatment, 36*, 65–74.

Drummond, C., Oyefeso, A., Phillips, T., Cheeta, S., Deluca, P., Perryman, K., ... Christoupoulos, A. (2004). *Alcohol Needs Assessment Research Project (ANARP). The 2004 National needs assessment for England.* London: Department of Health and the National Treatment Agency.

Elliott, J. C., Carey, K. B., & Bolles, J. R. (2008). Computer based interventions for college drinking: A qualitative review. *Addictive Behaviours, 33*(8), 994–1005.

Ferri, M., Amato, L., & Davoli, M. (2009). Alcoholics Anonymous and other 12-step programmes for alcohol dependence. *Cochrane Database of Systematic Reviews*, (3), CD005032.

Fleming, M. F., Mundt, M. P., French, M. T., Manwell, L. B., Stauffacher, E. A., & Barry, K. L. (2002). Brief physician advice for problem drinkers: Long-term efficacy and benefit-cost analysis. *Alcohol Clinical and Experimental Research, 26*(1), 36–43.

Foxcroft, D. R., Ireland, D., Lister-Sharp, D. J., Lowe, G., & Breen, R. (2003). Longer-term primary prevention for alcohol misuse in young people: A systematic review. *Addiction, 98*, 397–411.

Foxcroft, D. R., Lister-Sharp, D., & Lowe, G. (1997). Alcohol misuse prevention for young people: A systematic review reveals methodological concerns and lack of reliable evidence of effectiveness. *Addiction, 92*(5), 531–537.

Foxcroft, D. R., & Tsertsvadze, A. (2011). Universal school-based prevention programs for alcohol misuse in young people (review). *Cochrane Collaboration Review Database.*

Fuller, R. K., & Gordis, E. (2004). Does disulfiram have a role in alcohol treatment? *Addiction, 99*, 21–24.

Gallimberti, L., Canton, G., Gentile, N., Ferri, M., Cibin, M., & Ferrara, S. D. (1989). Gamma-hydroxybutyric acid for treatment of alcohol withdrawal syndrome. *Lancet, 2*, 787–789.

Gallimberti, L., Ferri, M., Ferrara, S. D., Fadda, F., & Gessa, G. L. (1992). Gamma-hydroxybutyric acid in the treatment of alcohol dependence: A double-blind study. *Alcoholism, Clinical and Experimental Research, 16*, 673–676.

Handmaker, N. S., Rayburn, W. F., Meng, C., Bell, J. B., Rayburn, B. B., & Rappaport, V. J. (2006). Impact of alcohol exposure after pregnancy recognition on ultrasonographic fetal growth measures. *Alcoholism: Clinical and Experimental Research, 30*(5), 892–898.

Havard, A., Shakeshaft, A., & Sanson-Fisher, R. (2008). Systematic review and meta-analyses of strategies targeting alcohol problems in emergency departments: Interventions reduce alcohol-related injuries. *Addiction, 103*, 368–376.

Health Improvement Analytical Team, & Department of Health. (2008). *The cost of alcohol harm to the NHS in England: An update to the Cabinet Office (2003) study.* London: Department of Health.

Heather, N. (2007). A long-standing World Health Organization collaborative project on early identification and brief alcohol intervention in primary health care comes to an end. *Addiction, 102*, 679–681.

Hughes, J. C., & Cook, C. C. H. (1997). The efficacy of disulfiram: A review of outcome studies. *Addiction, 92*, 381–395.

Hunter Fager, J., & Mazurek Melnyk, B. (2004). The effectiveness of intervention studies to decrease alcohol use in college undergraduate students: An integrative analysis. *Worldviews on Evidence-Based Nursing, 1*(2), 102–119.

Imel, Z. E., Wampold, B. E., Miller, S. D., & Fleming, R. R. (2008). Distinctions without a difference: Direct comparisons of psychotherapies for alcohol use disorders. *Psychology of Addictive Behaviors, 22*(4), 533–543.

Jackson, R., Johnson, M., Campbell, F., Messina, J., Guillaume, L., Purshouse, R., ... Meier, P. (2009). *Screening and brief interventions: Effectiveness review to the national institute for health & clinical excellence.* Sheffield, UK: The University of Sheffield, School of Health and Related Research (ScHARR).

Jernigan, D. (2001). *Global status report: Alcohol and young people.* Geneva: World Health Organization.

Kaner, E. (2012). Health sector responses. In P. M. Anderson, L. Møller, & G. Galea (Eds.), *Alcohol in the European Union. Consumption, harm and policy approaches* (pp. 40–48). Copenhagen: World Health Organization.

Kaner, E., Beyer, F., Dickinson, H., Pienaar, E., Campbell, F., Schlesinger, C., ... Burnand, B. (2007). Effectiveness of brief alcohol interventions in primary care populations. *Cochrane Database of Systematic Reviews, 18*(2), CD004148. doi: 004110.001002/14651858.CD14654148.pub14651853

Kaner, E., Dickinson, H., Beyer, F., Pienaar, E., Schlesinger, C., Campbell, F., ... Heather, N. (2009). The effectiveness of brief alcohol interventions in primary care settings: A comprehensive review. *Drug and Alcohol Review, 28*, 301–323.

Kaner, E., Newbury-Birch, D., & Heather, N. (2009). Brief interventions. In P. Miller (Ed.), *Evidence-based addiction treatment* (Vol. Part 3 Treatment methods, Chapter 10). San Diego, CA: Elsevier.

Kaner, E. B. M., Cassidy, P., Coulton, S., Dale, V., DeLuca, P., Gilvarry, E., ... Drummond, C. (2013). Effectiveness of screening and brief alcohol intervention in primary care (SIPS trial): Pragmatic cluster randomised controlled trial. *BMJ (Clinical Research Ed.), 346*, e8501

Kaner, E. F. S., & Bewick, B. M. (2010). Brief alcohol intervention in young people. In J. B. Saunders & J. M. Rey (Eds.), *Young people and alcohol: Impact, policy, prevention, treatment (Chap. 9).* Queensland, Australia: Wiley-Blackwell Publishing.

Kelly, J. F., Magill, M., & Stout, R. L. (2009). How do people recover from alcohol dependence? A systematic review of the research on mechanisms of behavior change in Alcoholics Anonymous. *Addiction Research and Theory, 17*(3), 236–259.

Khadjesari, Z., Murray, E., Hewitt, C., Hartley, S., & Godfrey, C. (2010). Can stand-alone computer-based interventions reduce alcohol consumption? A systematic review. *Addiction, 106*, 267–282.

Kreitman, N. (1986). Alcohol consumption and the preventive paradox. *British Journal of Addictions, 81*, 353–363.

Kypri, K., & McAnnally, H. M. (2005). Randomised controlled trial of a web based primary care intervention for multiple health risk behaviours. *Preventive Medicine, 41*, 761–766.

Kypri, K., Saunders, J. B., & Gallagher, S. J. (2003). Acceptability of various brief intervention approaches for hazardous drinking among university students. *Alcohol and Alcoholism, 38*, 626–628.

Kypri, K., Saunders, J. B., Williams, S. M., McGee, R. O., Langley, J. D., Cashell-Smith, M. L., ... Gallagher, S. J. (2004). Web-based screening and brief intervention for hazardous drinking: A double-blind randomized controlled trial. *Addiction, 99*, 1410-1417.

Kypri, K., Sitharthan, T., Cunningham, J., Kavanagh, D., & Dean, J. (2005). Innovative approaches to intervention for problem drinking. *Current Opinion in Psychiatry, 18*, 229–234.

Larimer, M., & Cronce, J. (2007). Identification, prevention, and treatment revisited: Individual-focused college drinking prevention strategies 1999-2006. *Addictive Behaviours, 32*, 2439–2468.

Larimer, M. E., Cronce, J. M., Lee, C. M., & Kilmer, J. R. (2005). Brief intervention in college settings. *Alcohol Research and Health, 28*(2), 94–104.

Leone, M. A., Vigna-Taglianti, F., Avanzi, G., Brambilla, R., & Faggiano, F. (2011). Gamma-hydroxybutyrate (GHB) for treatment of alcohol withdrawal and prevention of relapses. *Cochrane Collaboration Review Database*, doi: 10.1002/14651858.CD14006266.pub14651852

Lewis, M. A., Neighbors, C., Oster-Aaland, L. O., Kirkeby, B. S., & Larimer, M. E. (2007). Indicated prevention for incoming freshmen: Personalised normative feedback and high risk drinking. *Addictive Behaviours, 32*, 2495–2508.

Littlejohn, C. (2006). Does socio-economic status influence the acceptibility of, attendance for, and outcome of, screening and brief interventions for alcohol misuse: A review. *Alcohol & Alcoholism, 41*(5), 540–545.

Longabaugh, R., & Morgenstern, J. (1999). Cognitive-behavioral coping-skills therapy for alcohol dependence. *Alcohol Research and Health, 23*(2), 78–85.

Luborsky, L., Rosenthal, R., Diguer, L., Andrusyna, T. P., Berman, J. S., & Levitt, J. T. (2002). The Dodo bird verdict is alive and well – mostly. *Clinical Psychology: Science and Practice, 9*, 2–12.

Magill, M., & Ray, L. (2009). Cognitive behavioural treatment with adult alcohol and illicit drug users: A meta-analysis of randomized controlled trials. *Journal of Studies on Alcohol and Drugs, 70*, 516–527.

Maio, R. F., Shope, J. T., Blow, F. C., Gregor, M. A., Zakrajsek, J. S., Weber, J. E., Nypaver, M. M. (2005). A randomized controlled trial of an emergency department-based interactive computer program to prevent alcohol misuse among injured adolescents. *Annals of Emergency Medicine, 45*(4), 420–429.

Malcolm, R., Roberts, J. S., Wang, W., Myrick, H., & Anton, R. F. (2000). Multiple previous detoxifications are associated with less responsive treatment and heavier drinking during an index outpatient detoxification. *Alcohol, 22*, 159–164.

Mann, K., Lehert, P., & Morgan, M. (2004). The efficacy of acamprosate in the maintenance of abstinence in alcohol-dependent individuals: Results of a meta-analysis. *Alcoholism, Clinical and Experimental Research, 28*(1), 51–63.

Martin, B., Clapp, L., Biakowski, D., Brodgeford, D., Amponsah, A., Lyons, L., & Beresford, T. P. (2003). Compliance to supervised disulfiram therapy: A comparison of voluntary and court-ordered patients. *American Journal on Addictions, 12*, 137–143.

McQueen, J., Howe, T., Allan, L., Mains, D., & Hardy, V. (2011). Brief interventions for heavy alcohol users admitted to general hospital wards. *Cochrane Database of Systematic Reviews*, (8), CD005191. doi: 005110.001002/14651858.CD14005191.pub14651853

Miller, W. R. (1995). *Motivational enhancement therapy with drug abusers*. University of New Mexico Press.

Miller, W., & Rollnick, S. (1991). *Motivational interviewing; preparing people to change addictive behavior*. New York, NY: Guildford Press.

Miller, W., & Sovereign, R. (1989). The check-up: A model for early intervention in addictive behaviors. In T. Loberg, W. Miller, P. Nathan, & G. Marlatt (Eds.), *Addictive behaviors: Prevention and early intervention* (pp. 219–231). Amsterdam: Swets & Zeitlinger.

Monti, P. M., Barnett, N. P., Colby, S. M., Gwaltney, C. J., Spirito, A., Rohsenow, D. J., & Woolard, R. (2007). Motivational interviewing versus feedback only in emergency care for young adult problem drinking. *Addiction, 102*(8), 1234–1243.

Monti, P. M., Spirito, A., Myers, M., Colby, S. M., Barnett, N. P., Rohsenow, D. J., … Lewander, W. (1999). Brief intervention for harm reduction with alcohol-positive older adolescents in a hospital emergency department. *Journal of Consulting and Clinical Psychology, 67*(6), 989–994.

Moreira, M. T., Smith, L.A., & Foxcroft, D. (2009). Social norms interventions to reduce alcohol misuse in university or college students (review). *Cochrane Database of Systematic Reviews*, (3), CD006748. doi: 006710.001002/14651858.CD14006748.pub14651852

Moyer, A., Finney, J. W., Swearingen, C. E., & Vergun, P. (2002). Brief interventions for alcohol problems: A meta-analytic review of controlled investigations in treatment-seeking and non-treatment-seeking populations. *Addiction, 97*(3), 279–292.

Natarajan, M., & Kaner, E. (2007). Brief alcohol interventions in young people: Evidence and applicability. In E. Gilvarry & P. McArdle (Eds.), *Alcohol, drugs and young people: Clinical approaches. Clinics in developmental medicine no. 172 (Chapter 15)*. London: McKeith Press.

National Audit Office. (2008). *Reducing alcohol harm: Health services in England for alcohol misuse*. London: The Stationary Office (TSO).

National Institute for Health and Clinical Excellence. (2010). *Alcohol-use disorders – Preventing the development of hazardous and harmful drinking*. Retrieved from http://guidance.nice.org.uk/PH24

Neighbors, C., Larimer, M.E., Lewis, M.A. (2004). Targeting misperceptions of descriptive drinking norms: Efficacy of a computer delivered personalised normative feedback intervention. *Journal of Consulting and Clinical Psychology, 72*, 434–447.

Neighbors, C., Lee, C.M., Lewis, M.A., Fossos, N., & Walter, T. (2009). Internet based personalised feedback to reduce 21st birthday drinking: A randomised controlled trial of an event-specific prevention intervention. *Journal of Consulting and Clinical Psychology, 77*, 51–63.

Neighbors, C., Lewis, M. A., Bergstrom, R. L., & Larimer, M. E. (2006). Being controlled by normative influences: Self determination as a moderator of a normative feedback alcohol intervention. *Health Psychology, 25*, 571–579.

Nilsen, P. (2010). Brief alcohol intervention – Where to from here? Challenges remain for research and practice. *Addiction, 105*(6), 954–959.

Nilsen, P., Baird, J., Mello, M., Nirenberg, T., Woolard, R., Bendtsen, P., & Longabaugh, R. (2008). A systematic review of emergency care brief alcohol interventions for injury patients. *Journal of Substance Abuse Treatment, 35*, 184–201.

Ockene, J., Adams, A., Hurley, T., Wheeler, E. V., & Hebert, J. R. (1999). Brief physician- and nurse practitioner-delivered counseling for high risk drinkers: Does it work? *Archives of Internal Medicine, 159*, 2198–2205.

Ockene, J., Reed, G., & Reiff-Hekking, S. (2009). Brief patient-centered clinician-delivered counselling for high-risk drinking: 4-year results. *Annals of Behavioral Medicine, 37*(3), 335–342.

Paperny, D. M., Aona, J. Y., Lehman, R. M., Hammar, S. L., & Risser, J. (1990). Computer-assisted detection and intervention in adolescent high-risk health behaviours. *Journal of Pediatrics, 116*, 456–462.

Peterson, P. L., Baer, J. S., Wells, E. A., Ginzler, J. A., & Garrett, S. B. (2006). Short-term effects of a brief motivational intervention to reduce alcohol and drug risk among homeless adolescents. *Psychology of Addictive Behaviors, 20*(3), 254–264.

Project Match Research Group. (1997). Matching alcoholism treatment to client heterogeneity: Project MATCH post-treatment drinking outcomes. *Journal of Studies on Alcohol, 58*, 7–29.

Richmond, R., Kehoe, L., Heather, N., & Wodak, A. (2000). Evaluation of a workplace brief intervention for excessive alcohol consumption: The Workscreen project. *Preventive Medicine, 30*, 51–63.

Riper, H., Spek, V., Boon, B., Conijn, B., Kramer, J., Martin-Abello, K., & Smit, F. (2011). Effectiveness of E-self-help interventions for curbing adult problem drinking: A meta-analysis. *Journal of Medical Internet Research, 13*(2), e42.

Riper, H., van Straten, A., Keuken, M., Smit, F., Schippers, G., & Cuijpers, P. (2009). Curbing problem drinking with personalised feedback interventions: A meta-analysis. *American Journal of Preventive Medicine, 36*, 247–255.

Roche, A. M., & Freeman, T. (2004). Brief interventions: Good theory but weak in practice. *Drug and Alcohol Review, 23*(1), 11–18.

Rose, G. (1981). Strategy of prevention: Lessons from cardiovascular disease. *British Medical Journal, 282*, 1847–1851.

Rösner, S., Hackl-Herrwerth, A., Leucht, S., Lehert, P., Vecchi, S., & Soyka, M. (2010). Acamprosate for alcohol dependence. *Cochrane Database of Systematic Reviews*, (8), CD004332. doi: 004310.001002/14651858.CD14004332.pub14651852

Rösner, S., Hackl-Herrwerth, A., Leucht, S., Vecchi, S., Srisurapanont, M., & Soyka, M. (2010). Opioid antagonists for alcohol dependence. *Cochrane Database of Systematic Reviews*, (12), CD001867. doi: 001810.001002/14651858.CD14001867.pub14651853

Saitz, R. (2010). Alcohol screening and brief intervention in primary care: Absence of evidence for efficacy in people with dependance or very heavy drinking. *Drug and Alcohol Review, 29*, 631–640.

Saitz, R., Palfai, T., Freedner, N., Winter, M., Macdonald, A., Lu, J., … Dejong, W. (2007). Screening and brief intervention online for college students: The ihealth study. *Alcohol & Alcoholism, 42*(1), 28–36.

Salkovskis, P. M. (Ed.). (1996). *Frontiers of cognitive therapy*. New York, NY: Guilford Press.

Saunders, J. B., Kypri, K., Walters, S. T., Laforge, R. G., & Larimer, M. E. (2004). Approaches to brief interventions for hazardous drinking in young people. *Alcoholism, Clinical and Experimental Research, 28*, 322–329.

Saunders, J. B., & Lee, N. K. (2000). Hazardous alcohol use: Its delineation as a subthreshold disorder, and approaches to its diagnosis and management. *Comprehensive Psychiatry, 41*(2), 95–103.

Schaus, J. F., Sole, M. L., McCoy, T. P., Mullett, N., & O'Brien, M. C. (2009). Alcohol screening and brief intervention in a college student health center: A randomized controlled trial. *Journal of Studies on Alcohol and Drugs, 16*(Supp.), 131–141.

Skinner, H. A., Allen, B. A., McIntosh, M. C., & Palmer, W. H. (1985). Lifestyle assessment: Applying microcomputers in family practice. *British Medical Journal, 290*, 212–214.

Smedslund, G., Berg, R., Hammerstrøm, K., Steiro, A., Leiknes, K., Dahl, H., & Kjetil, K., (2011). Motivational interviewing for substance abuse. *Cochrane Database of Systematic Reviews*, (5), CD008063. doi: 008010.001002/14651858.CD14008063.pub14651852

Spirito, A., Monti, P., Barnett, N., Colby, S., Sindelar, H., Rohsenow, D., ... Myers, M. (2004). A randomized clinical trial of a brief motivational intervention for alcohol-positive adolescents treated in an emergency department. *Journal of Pediatrics, 145,* 396–402.

Tober, G., Clyne, W., Finnegan, O., Farrin, A., & Russell, I. (2008). Validation of a scale for rating the delivery of psycho-social treatments for alcohol dependence and misuse: The UKATT process rating scale. *Alcohol and Alcoholism, 43*(6), 675–682.

Toumbourou, J., Stockwell, T., Neighbors, C., Marlatt, G., Sturge, J., & Rehm, J. (2007). Interventions to reduce harm associated with adolescent substance use. *Lancet, 369,* 1391–1401.

U.S. Preventive Services Task Force. (2010). Internet Citation: *Screening for obesity in children and adolescents,* Topic Page. January 2010. http://www.uspreventiveservicestaskforce.org/uspstf/uspschobes.htm

UKATT Research Team. (2005). Effectiveness of treatment for alcohol problems: Findings of the randomised UK alcohol treatment trial (UKATT). *British Medical Journal, 331*(7516), 541.

Walters, S. T., & Neighbors, C. (2005). Feedback interventions for college alcohol misuse: What, why and for whom? *Addictive Behaviours,* (30), 1168–1182.

Walters, S. T., Vader, A. M., & Harris, T. R. (2007). A controlled trial of web-based feedback for heavy drinking college students. *Prevention Science, 8,* 83–88.

Whitlock, E. P., Polen, M. R., Green, C. A., Orleans, T., & Klein, J. (2004). Behavioral counseling interventions in primary care to reduce risky/harmful alcohol use by adults: A summary of the evidence for the US Preventive Services Task Force. *Annals of Internal Medicine, 140,* 557–568.

Woody, G. E. (2003). Research findings on psychotherapy of addictive disorders. *American Journal on Addictions, 12,* S19–S26.

World Health Organization. (1992). *International classification of diseases* (10th revision ed.). Geneva.

World Health Organization. (2009). *Global health risks: Mortality and burden of disease related to selected major risks.* (Vol. ISBN 978 92 4 156387 1). Geneva: World Health Organization.

Wutzke, S., Conigrave, K., Saunders, J., & Hall, W. (2002). The long-term effectiveness of brief interventions for unsafe alcohol consumption: A 10-year follow-up. *Addiction, 97,* 665–675.

11

Reducing Stress to Improve Health

ELLEN A. DORNELAS
JONATHAN GALLAGHER
MATTHEW M. BURG

LEARNING OBJECTIVES

- Describe the relationship between stress and health behaviors.
- Review studies of the impact of stress management interventions on health behaviors.
- Summarize the component elements that can be incorporated into comprehensive stress management interventions.

Stress places people at higher risk for heart disease, cancer progression, and medical illness, and is associated with a host of unhealthy behaviors such as cigarette smoking, alcohol abuse, poor nutrition, and sedentary behavior. Health behaviors are difficult to regulate in a stressful context and negative health habits are familiar, accessible, predictable, and immediate ways for people to cope with difficult circumstances. Given the impact of stress on health and disease and on health-related behaviors and lifestyle, it is useful to have a strong understanding of its mechanism and how to intervene with patients to help them reduce stress and improve health. This chapter describes the prognostic importance of stress in terms of development and progression of illness. It also provides interventions that have been tested and shown to be effective in helping people to reduce stress as part of a healthier lifestyle.

WHAT IS STRESS?

The current colloquial use of the term "stress" has a negative connotation. However Hans Selye (1956) widely credited with having coined the term "stress" defined it in more biological terms, as the body's response to any demand made upon it. Conceptualized in this way, stress may be thought of as a human's level of physiological and mental arousal. Robert Yerkes and John Dodson (1908) conducted a series of studies demonstrating that people benefit from an optimal level of stress. Excessive arousal can lead to impairment in the ability to perform normal daily activities or role function. Excessive and uncontrollable stress also promotes negative mood and is associated with poor physical functioning. Unremitting stress can lead to feelings of helplessness and hopelessness (a core feature of depression). However, some level of arousal is energizing and necessary for optimal functioning according to the Yerkes–Dodson principle. If stress is conceptualized in terms of the degree of physiological and mental arousal, then all humans exist with some level of stress.

Selye's model of stress posited that humans respond to stress with an initial state of alarm, followed by resistance and finally, exhaustion. Later work devoted to the conceptualization of stress further considered cognitive appraisal as a determinant of whether something is perceived to be stressful (Lazarus & Folkman, 1984). The determination as to whether a situation is perceived as stressful or not is based on individual interpretation. For example, though public speaking tends to be perceived as a universally stressful experience, the degree to which this is perceived as stressful varies greatly depending on the audience, context, and traits of the speaker. Situations are generally perceived to be more stressful when they are unpredictable, uncontrollable, or ambiguous. In addition, this theory posits that reaction to stress also involves a secondary appraisal process, which incorporates a person's perception of the possible methods of coping or resources available to deal with the potentially stressful situation. This model provided a theoretical foundation for interventions that incorporate cognitive strategies as a key aspect of stress management.

EPIDEMIOLOGY AND SIGNIFICANCE OF STRESS

There is a burgeoning literature indicating that stress has a negative impact on progression of many physical illnesses and is associated with the onset of some health conditions. However, it is simplistic to state that stress "causes" medical illness. Instead, the evidence suggests that underlying biological vulnerability to certain health conditions interacting with excessive stress can lead to the development and progression of health problems.

STRESS AND HEART DISEASE

The relationship between stress and heart disease has been well documented. The INTERHEART trial was an international study with more than 11,000 patients with a first myocardial infarction (MI) and more than 13,000 sex matched control cases. Patients with MI had a higher prevalence of reported stress in the year prior to MI across all regions, ethnicities, and for both men and women. The 4-item assessment of stress was, by necessity, a simple epidemiological measure. The effect size of stress was roughly comparable to the prognostic import of hypertension and abdominal adiposity (Rosengren et al., 2004).

Sudden cardiac death also has long been linked with emotional stress. Early case series (Engel, 1971; Reich, DeSilva, Lown, & Murawski, 1981) describe individuals suffering cardiac arrest or sudden death in settings of acute grief, fear, or anger. Epidemiological studies have shown that sudden death increases in populations suffering emotionally devastating disasters such as earthquake or war (Leor, Poole, & Kloner, 1996; Meisel et al., 1991). Toivonen, Helenius, and Viitasalo (1997) observed arrhythmia associated changes in the electrocardiogram of healthy physicians exposed to the sudden stress of an on-call alarm. Ventricular arrhythmias, the most common cause of sudden death, are also influenced by emotional stress. For example, an increase in ventricular arrhythmias among patients with implantable cardioverter defibrillators (ICDs)—a device implanted for patients at risk of sudden cardiac death—was seen in the weeks following the terrorist attacks of 9/11, in both New York City

(Steinberg et al., 2004) and distant locales (Shedd et al., 2004). Sudden death is also more likely to occur in the morning hours during which individuals experience a circadian increase in cardiac sympathetic activity (Muller et al., 1987) while in working patients with ICDs, ventricular tachycardia occurs more frequently on the first day of the work week (Peters, McQuillan, Resnick, & Gold, 1996).

Anger appears to be a particularly "cardiotoxic" aspect of emotional stress. People who have a tendency to respond to stressful situations with anger are at greater than 3-fold increased risk of incident heart disease (Chida & Steptoe, 2009) while the experience of moderate-to-extreme anger in response to environmental stress increases the risk of an acute cardiac event more than 2-fold for the subsequent 2 hours (Mittleman et al., 1995; Strike, Perkins-Porras, Whitehead, McEwan, & Steptoe, 2006). Of note, patients with these "anger-triggered" cardiac events show a delayed recovery of the physiological stress response when exposed to psychological stress in the laboratory (Strike, Magid et al., 2006), while in other laboratory studies, the recall of a previous anger provoking experience causes "mental stress ischemia" in approximately half of patients with stable coronary disease (Burg & Soufer, 2007). Similarly among ICD patients, the experience of even moderate anger increases the likelihood of a ventricular arrhythmia that requires an ICD shock for termination (Burg, Lampert, Joska, Batsford, & Jain, 2004).

In summary, the literature linking stress to cardiovascular disease is voluminous, and whether stress is due to life events, low social support, finances, relationship problems, work, or time urgency, there are consistent findings that tie stress to the development and progression of heart disease (Lukens, Turkoglu, & Burg, 2012). There is also evidence indicating that stress reduction can prolong life in people with established heart disease (Orth-Gomér et al., 2009).

STRESS AND CANCER

Cancer is a blanket term that covers many hundreds of diseases with a multitude of causes. The evidence that stress leads to the development of cancer has been inconsistent, with some studies supporting that stress is linked to the development of cancer in initially healthy populations (Chida, Hamer, Wardle, & Steptoe, 2008) and other studies that fail to support this link (Duijts, Zeegers, & Borne, 2003). There is growing evidence to support that stress is a risk factor for tumor growth and proliferation in patients already diagnosed with cancer. Higher stress levels have been linked with poorer survival in patients with diagnosed cancer according to a meta-analysis based on 330 studies (Chida et al., 2008). The effectiveness of stress management interventions on cancer survival has been mixed. In 1989, Spiegel and colleagues published a study indicating that partaking in a stress management intervention was associated with better survival in breast cancer patients; however when the authors repeated the study many years later, they failed to replicate the findings (Spiegel, Bloom, Kraemer, & Gottheil, 1989; Spiegel et al., 2007). Stress management interventions have been disproportionately confined to certain types of diagnoses such as breast cancer, making it difficult to make generalizations. Interpreting the literature is challenging given the wide variability in operational definitions of "stress," tremendous heterogeneity in terms of diagnostic groups, and the fact that there is no consensus on the component parts of an optimal stress management intervention. Notwithstanding this, one recent study has shown how stress management may improve cancer prognosis (Antoni et al., 2012). A study of 199 women with stage 0 to stage III breast cancer enrolled in a randomized, controlled trial of cognitive-behavioral stress management (CBSM) demonstrated that this intervention reduced anxiety-related symptoms, increased positive emotions, decreased negative affect, and reduced intrusive thoughts about cancer. The intervention was a

10-week stress management group and, over one year, participants in this condition also reduced circulating cortisol levels, and increased stimulated production of interleukin 2 and interferon gamma compared to the control group. The investigators also demonstrated that the stress management intervention resulted in "switching off" expression of the genes responsible for anxiety-related increases in inflammation, thus clarifying a possible pathway by which reduced stress may lead to longer survival in patients with cancer (Antoni et al., 2012).

THE RELATIONSHIP BETWEEN STRESS AND DISEASE

Stress increases risk for the development and progression of a wide range of health problems from acne to cardiac arrest (Cohen, Janicki-Deverts, & Miller, 2007). It is difficult to think of diseases where stress has not been shown to play a role. There are multiple possible parallel pathophysiological and behavioral pathways by which stress could lead to development and progression of illness. The mechanisms by which stress more generally, and anger more specifically, contribute to the development of heart disease and the provocation of catastrophic cardiac events are based in the normal physiological response to environmental demand—to stress. These mechanisms are apparent throughout the animal kingdom, speaking to their utility for survival within a physically demanding context. For example, the sympathetic arm (sympathetic nervous system [SNS]) of the autonomic nervous system when activated has immediate effects, increasing heart rate and contractility, the force of cardiac contraction. The SNS also directly regulates the vascular system, causing localized changes in vasomotor tone so as to direct increases in blood flow to the muscles that require increased oxygenation. The catecholamines—epinephrine and norepinephrine—are the "messengers" of this activity, playing a role both within nerve pathways and the circulation. Concurrently, these stress hormones can cause subtle disruptions in cardiac electrical activity, while also increasing platelet activity—blood coagulability—in part so as to staunch blood flow at the site of an open wound. Under these conditions, the hypothalamic–pituitary–adrenal (HPA) "axis" working through its primary "messenger" cortisol, contributes to this overall systemic response to stress, while also influencing inflammatory pathways that are integral to the development and progression of coronary disease. Thus, while the autonomic and HPA axis response to stress allows the organism to respond effectively to environmental demands so as to survive another day, the more subtle and less physically demanding nature of environmental stress within modern society results in a systemic response that in some ways is more cardiotoxic than survival promoting.

Activation of the HPA axis is also associated with immune dysregulation. The immune system can become dysregulated by overreacting, underreacting, or both (Segerstrom & Miller, 2004). As an example, acute stress increases inflammation, marked by exaggerated platelet reactivity and higher levels of interleukin 6, a blood protein. Stress has also been shown to increase the expression of pro-inflammatory and metastasis-related genes and to decrease the expression of interferon-related genes which offer a protective effect in terms of cancer. "Given the unlikely role of a singular system in explaining the biological effects of stress pathways on cancer progression, during the last 10 years, the focus of mechanistic biobehavioral oncology research has broadened to include examination of the effects of stress on (a) tumor angiogenesis, (b) invasion and anoikis, (c) stromal cells in the tumor microenvironment and (d) inflammation" (Lutgendorf & Sood, 2011, p. 725). The review by Lutgendorf and Sood provides strong support that stress can play a role in cancer progression and spread.

The behavioral pathway linking stress to disease suggests that stress is associated with greater reliance on unhealthy behaviors such as alcohol abuse, smoking, and poor nutrition as ways to cope with stress and negative mood. In addition, people who report high stress levels are less likely to engage in health-promoting behaviors and have more difficulty complying with medical regimens such as taking medication or follow up with recommended screenings. Stress also has a negative effect on sleep and thus, sleep disturbance mediates the relationship between stress and some diseases (Reitav, 2012). Thus stress has both direct and indirect effects on the body.

PSYCHOSOCIAL ASPECTS OF STRESS

From a sociological perspective, people who face the highest levels of stress are marginalized with the lowest levels of education and income. In addition, those who are impoverished face greater environmental stressors such as living in dangerous communities, having fewer opportunities for economic advancement, more barriers to accessing the health care system, and greater likelihood of experiencing fragmented, inconsistent health care when utilizing publicly funded health insurance (Weaver, Rowland, Bellizzi, & Aziz, 2010). Across the lifespan, younger adults generally rate themselves to be more stressed than older adults and this is particularly true among people with medical illness. Women report higher levels of stress and negative mood compared to men, who are more likely to exhibit stress-related behaviors such as alcohol abuse, domestic violence, and suicide (Dornelas, 2008). It is clear that although everyone is vulnerable to stress, some population subgroups face environmental and situational difficulties that increase chronic stress, which is associated with the development and progression of disease.

CHALLENGES TO ADDRESSING STRESS

Stress management is often defined very broadly, with many interventions focused on the mind–body connection (e.g., diaphragmatic breathing, meditation, and yoga). Some stress management interventions broaden the reach by incorporating diet and exercise (Ornish et al., 1990). In Western culture, it is becoming more common for people to adopt stress management practices, for example, by attending a regular yoga class. Sonya Suchday and colleagues (Suchday, Dziok, Katzenstein, Kaplan, & Kahan, 2012) have made the point that the practice of a yoga and meditation lifestyle is *a way of living* that is common in Eastern cultures and often also includes a vegetarian diet, as well as living by the philosophy of karma. Many Eastern cultures make reference to the concept of "right living" which promotes a focus on achieving equanimity of the mind. In contrast, people in Western cultures often conceptualize stress management as an adjunctive health practice rather than a way of life. Given the widely differing conceptualizations of what is meant by "stress management," it is a challenge for health behavior interventionists to define clearly what type of stress is targeted, which behavioral changes are desired, and what constitutes an optimal outcome.

INTERVENTIONS TO REDUCE STRESS

COGNITIVE-BEHAVIORAL MODEL

The cognitive-behavioral model of stress posits that people respond to environmental stimuli through a cognitive appraisal of the demands of the stimulus, relative to the perception about the adequacy of resources that the person has available to respond to the demand. Individuals react to situational stressors with thoughts, emotions, and behaviors that each, in turn, can influence each other. Cognitive-behavioral therapy (CBT) interventions focus on improving mood by changing *thoughts* about how the situational stressor is appraised, and changing the *behaviors* associated with maintaining its stressful impact. The cognitive aspect of CBT interventions focuses on increasing recognition of maladaptive patterns of thinking though awareness of common cognitive distortions, maladaptive core beliefs, and automatic thoughts. Faulty thinking patterns lead to negative affect expressed through symptoms of anxiety, depression, or poor coping abilities. CBT interventions can be carried out as group or individual modalities. Cognitive interventions usually include an educational component about the hypothesized relationship between thoughts, mood, and bodily response; homework exercises to help the individual become more aware of dysfunctional thought patterns and resulting responses; and practice of cognitive strategies to learn to shift maladaptive cognitions. There is tremendous breadth to the types of cognitive interventions that might be introduced in a stress management program and these could include specific focus on skills training in areas such as problem solving skills, time management, or communication.

The *behavioral* aspect of CBSM interventions may focus on learning relaxation skills, promoting physical activity or behavior change that is tied to the source of stress (i.e., reducing work hours, increasing self-care activities, and increasing time spent on pleasurable activities). Relaxation therapies are described in detail later in the chapter, and exercise is covered thoroughly in Chapter 8 of this book; therefore this section of the discussion is limited to other types of behavior change. When people experience stress and have increased symptoms of anxiety and depression, they often reduce their time spent on pleasurable activities such that the decreased time spent in pleasurable activities leads to worsened mood, and this negative mood in turn decreases a person's motivation to engage in activities that were previously found pleasurable. Thus, a simple but key aspect of behavioral intervention is to work with an individual on planning and engaging in activities that they find pleasurable. Ideally such activities would have both a physical and/or social component. For example, reading may be a pleasurable activity but may not have the same stress reduction and mood improvement potential as brisk walking with a good friend.

EXERCISE

Exercise is a form of stress management in its own right. Exercise, which exposes the body to repeated bouts of physiological stress, consequently blunts the stress response by "lengthening the fuse" or helping a person become less reactive to stress (Khatri & Blumenthal, 2000). The metabolic demands associated with regular exercise help the body to resume a normal balanced energy conservation mode whereas the stress response is designed to be followed by a vigorous episode of muscular activity (Sapolsky, 2004). Moreover, regular exercise better facilitates regulation of stress hormones from the body by reducing resting adrenaline levels. Exercise discharges muscular tension which acts as a trigger for stress. Physical activity releases endorphins and has an analgesic effect. From a cognitive perspective, exercise also serves as a distraction and can interrupt the tendency to ruminate, thus decreasing negative mood. Fitness also increases strength, balance, flexibility, and energy levels, fostering better resilience against physical, immunological, social, and mental stress.

RELAXATION THERAPIES

There are many forms of relaxation therapies, and a truly comprehensive list is beyond the scope of this chapter. Various "families" of relaxation have been described by Smith (2007), and the following sections focus on mainstream relaxation techniques from each family: breathing, mindfulness meditation (MM), progressive muscle relaxation (PMR), hypnosis, and yoga. There is tremendous variability within each group and overlap between different relaxation types. The crucial components for relaxation techniques to be successful include the following:

- Duration of 15 to 20 minutes
- Quiet environment
- Passive attitude regarding distraction and frustration
- Consistent practice in order to have sustained and generalized effects

Diaphragmatic breathing is typically introduced first because all relaxation therapies tend to incorporate healthy breathing as either the anchor or the enhancing component of the technique.

Diaphragmatic Breathing

The foundation of all relaxation approaches in both Western and Eastern culture focuses on healthy breathing techniques. Eastern culture refers to *pranayama* or breath. Effective breathing is viewed as both integral for optimal living and the cornerstone of reducing stress. Improving breathing is one of the easiest lead-ins for people to embrace stress management as a way of life. With the amount of dead time in 21st century lifestyle (waiting in lines, time-consuming meetings, commercial breaks, and traffic) there is ample opportunity to practice diaphragmatic breathing on a regular basis.

Diaphragmatic breathing refers to breathing from the abdomen at a comfortable depth. Regular rhythmic breathing is characterized by the abdomen rising and falling. Diaphragmatic breathing is observed naturally in babies during sleep and is associated with decreased sympathetic arousal. As people relearn to breathe from the abdomen rather than the chest, to regulate their breathing into comfortable, regular intervals and to maintain this optimal state of breathing throughout the day, physiological aspects of tension and stress are reduced. Diaphragmatic breathing is antithetical to stress. Breathing patterns at the apex of stress (e.g., a panic attack) are in sharp contrast to the type of slow, regular breathing that is associated with deep relaxation. Regular over-learning of diaphragmatic breathing will stimulate the breathing pattern to remain in this mode, or closer to it, even in trying circumstances.

Mindfulness-Based Meditation

There are many types of meditation. Mindfulness meditation (MM) refers to the non-judgmental observation and attention to one's immediate experiences. Practitioners are encouraged to maintain an attitude of acceptance and focused attention on moment-to-moment reality without the accompanying automatic physical, cognitive, or emotional reaction. Many other types of meditation exist, for example, transcendental meditation (TM) which aims to transcend awareness of the present moment. The concept of mindfulness has deep and longstanding roots in Buddhist philosophy (Suchday et al., 2012). Bishop (2002) has noted that mindfulness reflects a "kind of meta-cognitive ability in which the participant has the capacity to observe his or her own mental processes. This process of "stepping back" and observing the flow of consciousness is thought to result in the recognition that each thought and feeling reflects a mental event with no more inherent value or importance other than what the practitioner affords them" (Bishop, 2002, pp. 74–75). More than 30 years ago, Jon Kabat-Zinn developed an 8-week mindfulness-based stress reduction program (MBSR) that teaches the concepts of mindfulness and emphasizes the practice of regular meditation (Kabat-Zinn, 1990). Many studies of MBSR have been conducted and in a review of 20 studies of rigorous quality, Grossman, Niemann, Schmidt, and Walach (2004) concluded that MBSR is effective at reducing stress in a variety of populations (e.g., cancer, cardiac disease, fibromyalgia, and chronic pain) with an effect size of 0.5. Eight years later, in a review of 39 studies that employed an MM treatment, Eberth and Sedlmeir found larger effect sizes for MBSR compared to treatments that utilized only meditation but did not include other stress management techniques. The authors raised the question of whether the robust effect sizes shown for MBSR may be partially attributable to component parts of the program that are not necessarily specific to MM. There is also evidence that neurobiological changes may be achieved through MM. Electroencephalographic studies have demonstrated a significant increase in alpha and theta activity that occurs during meditation (Chiesa & Serretti, 2010). Neuroimaging studies have also shown that long-term practitioners of MM show differences in areas of the brain involved in attention compared to matched controls (Aftanas & Golocheikine, 2003). Though more research is needed to better understand the potential mechanisms by which meditation may work, MBSR programs remain an extremely popular choice for people seeking relief from stress.

Progressive Muscle Relaxation

Progressive muscle relaxation (PMR) is a form of relaxation that involves tensing and relaxing muscles throughout the body. The premise that stress is associated with muscular tension is intuitive and consequently, PMR is relatively easy to teach. Practitioners of PMR focus on noticing the difference between the feeling of tension and relaxation in the muscle and the associated psychological experience of reduced anxiety. PMR should last approximately 30 minutes but abbreviated PMR sessions are most often employed in practice. The process refers to systematically tensing and then relaxing a series of up to 16 muscle groups so that localized sensations of relaxation are achieved progressively, and eventually coalesce into an overall relaxation response, with all its attendant physiological and psychological benefits. As well as being easier to teach, it is easier to learn for patients because it is simple and bodily oriented and is not cognitively taxing as meditation is often perceived to be by novice practitioners. Though strictly speaking, the cardinal benefits of PMR are to be gained during wakefulness, patients who use PMR often report that they find it easy to fall asleep and it is employed as a core component of effective non-pharmacological treatment of insomnia (Riemann & Perlis, 2009). As well as being physically relaxing, PMR can interrupt the racing mind that can inhibit sleep onset and upon early waking, it provides an enhanced sense of control, as achieving deep relaxation is the next best thing to uninterrupted refreshing sleep. Enhancing sleep is its own form of stress management and PMR can provide a technique to achieve this goal.

PMR is often incorporated as part of a multi-component behavioral intervention rather than utilized as a single therapeutic modality. Consequently, it is somewhat difficult to determine the efficacy of PMR as a stand-alone stress reduction intervention though it has been used for the treatment of a wide variety of health conditions including tension headache, chronic pain, hypertension, insomnia, multiple sclerosis, cancer, anxiety, and depression. In a review of 29 studies using an abbreviated PMR treatment, the average effect size was moderate and best results were associated with individual (rather than group) training, longer treatment duration, and greater number of sessions (Carlson & Hoyle, 1993).

Hypnosis

Hypnosis has been well studied and refers to a state of consciousness characterized by highly focused attention, similar to daydreaming and reduced awareness of external stimuli or sensations. There is a strong literature suggesting that hypnosis is effective for pain control in both chronic and acute pain, as well as medical procedures (Jensen & Patterson, 2006; Ketterhagen, VandeVusse, & Berner, 2002; Lutgendorf et al., 2007). People can induce their own hypnotic or trance state and practitioners of self-hypnosis are taught to relax with diaphragmatic breathing. The practitioner may use visual imagery techniques (i.e., count the steps down a staircase or through a path) thereby evoking a deeper state of relaxation and reduced awareness of external stimuli. Once the practitioner has reached a place that connotes feelings of relaxation in his or her imagination, attention may be focused on using all of the five senses to make the image as vivid as possible and thus making it more salient and easily retrievable in times of need. Sometimes affirmations or other statements designed to elicit feelings of comfort, peace, and security may be constructed. To end the hypnotic state, the practitioner usually counts backward or imagines the transition back (i.e., climbing the staircase or returning on the same path) to a state of refreshed alertness. There are fewer specific reviews about self-hypnosis, as distinct from hypnosis, but those that exist (Ketterhagen et al., 2002), suggest that self-hypnosis can be an effective method to cope with pain and stress (Landolt & Milling, 2011).

Yoga

Yoga, a form of stretching, has been practiced for thousands of years in Eastern cultures and Hatha yoga (a branch of Hindu yoga) is one of the most widely practiced in Western culture (Smith & Pukall, 2009). There are many different styles of Hatha yoga and each emphasizes different aspects of the practice. From a behavioral perspective, yoga refers to breathing techniques, bodily postures, stretching, alignment of the pose, and the development of strength and flexibility. From a philosophical perspective, hatha yoga aims to achieve integration of the mind, body, and spirit and was originally thought of as a practice through which to achieve enlightenment (Suchday et al., 2012). Yoga often incorporates mindful meditation. From a physiological perspective, yoga has been shown to enhance parasympathetic output and there is evidence that the practice of yoga is associated with improved sleep regulation, better cardiovascular functioning, and gains in strength and flexibility (Raub, 2002). When yoga is part of a stress management program, it often employs only very basic and non-challenging stretches; thus the effects for "pure" versions of technique are likely to be very distinct from yoga as part of a multi-modal intervention. In a review of 35 studies that examined the effects of yoga on anxiety and stress, Li and Goldsmith (2012) found that the literature suggests that yoga has benefit in terms of lowering stress but that the quality of the studies conducted to date is mixed and there is a need for further research in this area.

PATIENT-CENTERED AND SUPPORTIVE APPROACHES

There are a number of different approaches that have been used to engage patients in health behavior change. Patient-centered counseling is a counseling approach based on a collaborative partnership between the counselor and client that has been demonstrated to be effective in engaging patients in their own care and in helping individuals change health-related behaviors. Motivational interviewing is a specific patient-centered approach that was originally developed by William Miller and Steven Rollnick (1991) for the treatment of problem drinking. Over the past two decades, there has been a burgeoning literature suggesting that this counseling approach can be very effective in helping patients to change health risk behaviors such as diet, exercise, and alcohol (Dornelas, 2008). Motivational interviewing is more of a philosophical stance about how to engage people in behavioral change programs and not a direct intervention for stress. However, to the extent that people become very stressed and defensive about difficult-to-change health behaviors (e.g., sedentary lifestyle and poor nutrition) a motivational approach can be effective at reducing the stress experienced by participants in behavior change efforts. Similarly, other patient-centered approaches such as those developed by Ockene and colleagues (Ockene et al., 1994, 1999a, 1999b) designed to result in health behavior change have included a specific focus on increasing self-efficacy and a plan using the strengths and resources of the individual. They have been demonstrated to be very effective in helping people to stop smoking, change diet, or decrease drinking. Patient-centered approaches can be easily integrated into other therapies and educational programs and are frequently employed as a "warm-up" intervention prior to more intensive behavioral change programs. Most comprehensive stress management programs are informed by patient-centered principles related to increasing motivation, self-efficacy, and empowerment.

Pure "support groups" for stress management are difficult to find. Most stress reduction groups incorporate one or more of the relaxation techniques described above and it is rare to find a stress management group that relies only on interpersonal emotional support from the other members. Therefore, it is difficult to disentangle the relative contribution of support apart from other component aspects of stress management interventions. Social isolation and lack of emotional support are strong predictors of morbidity and mortality (Berkman, 1995). People who have strained interpersonal relationships or are socially isolated may experience stress due to practical matters (e.g., a ride to work when the car won't start), motivational issues (e.g., encouragement to stick to an exercise regimen), or direct effect on the body (e.g., increased heart rate following an argument). Social support found in a stress management group has tremendous potential to be of help to people lacking strong, healthy interpersonal relationships and people generally rate the emotional support gained from other group members as being key to the success of the intervention.

TECHNOLOGY/E-HEALTH STRATEGIES

Biofeedback

Biofeedback involves providing people with information about their own physiological state (e.g., skin temperature, heart rate, blood pressure) to increase the ability to self-regulate physiological signs of stress. Taking a pulse after a minute of diaphragmatic breathing is a simple form of biofeedback. Currently there are quite a few biofeedback approaches based on electromyographic (EMG) feedback, heart rate variability, blood pressure, thermal sensor, skin conductance, and respiration rate. There is strong evidence suggesting that biofeedback can be very effective at reducing blood pressure in hypertensives (Nakao, Yano, Nomura, & Kuboki, 2003) and is found to be superior to control conditions such as sham or non-specific behavioral intervention when it is combined with other relaxation techniques. A review of 14 studies examining biofeedback for heart rate variability has shown acute effects during biofeedback sessions but limited evidence of long-term effectiveness that carries beyond the session (Wheat & Larkin, 2010). EMG feedback has been shown to be more effective than relaxation therapies for tension type headache, to reduce anxiety in people with headache, and the treatment effects remain stable over more than one year, according to a meta-analysis conducted by Nestoriuc, Martin, Rief, and Andrasik (2008). Thermal biofeedback has been shown to be efficacious for Raynaud's phenomenon, which can be exacerbated by stress (Karavidas, Tsai, Yucha, McGrady, & Lehrer, 2006). One of the advantages of biofeedback is that many types of equipment can now be directly purchased by the user. In addition, some biofeedback technologies are deployed through a personal computer or mobile telephone as discussed in the sections that follow.

Web-Based Stress Management Therapies

The Internet offers a great deal of promise for stress management due to the accessibility, low cost, convenience, potential to be individually tailored, and anonymity offered through web-based interventions. Internet-based stress management programs that are interactive can engage people through self-tests, games, stress monitoring, personalized feedback and discussion groups, as well as a wide array of educational content. To the extent that effective stress management depends on changing perceptions, improving knowledge, and developing skills to cope effectively with stress, the Internet offers tremendous possibility for testing and refining interventions aimed at education and skill building. In addition web-based interventions extend stress management services to people who otherwise might not be treated in more traditional settings or might not engage with mental health or other professionals. An increasing number of insurance companies in the United States offer Internet-based health promotion programs or discounted fees for commercially available e-health programs to their participants.

High subject dropout rates and difficulties with compliance make it difficult to evaluate the effectiveness of stress management delivered via the Internet (Zetterqvist, Maanmies, Ström, & Andersson, 2003), and there is a need to better understand who is most likely to benefit from these types of interventions. Despite the fact that the majority of Americans are Internet users, there is a "digital divide" that separates older, low income, and less educated people from frequent users of the Internet. People who are impoverished and less educated face disproportionate stress and have great potential to benefit from web-based interventions; however it is just as difficult to engage and retain these populations in Internet-based programs as in traditional in-person stress management programs (Steinmark, Dornelas, & Fischer, 2006). Even among frequent Internet users, a primary difficulty with e-health strategies has been effective engagement and utilization. "People simply stop using technologies that do not correspond in any way with their daily lives, habits, or rituals" (van Gemert-Pijnen et al., 2011). Use of Internet technology as a persuasive medium to help engage, motivate, and bond with users is often overlooked (van Gemert-Pijnen et al., 2011). Since mobile telephone technologies may accomplish this goal to a greater degree than a personal computer, this type of technology may represent the next evolution in the delivery of computer-delivered stress management technologies.

Phone Apps

Mobile phone applications have become an increasingly popular and portable method of delivering interventions designed to improve mood, sleep, physical activity, and a host of other stress management efforts. Cellular telephones are everyday devices that offer opportunity for user discretion to engage in unobtrusive behaviors to lower stress. A person may subtly keep track of an activity log, thought or stress diary or may track tension in a manner as normative as texting or web browsing. Moreover, people enjoy their phones, as evidenced by the great amount of time spent engaged with this technology. Phone-delivered stress management programs could in the future explicitly incorporate Premack's principle (Premack, 1959), by requiring engagement in the behavioral change intervention prior to reinforcement with user-chosen, rewarding telephone activities. Mobile phones come equipped with personal digital assistants, Internet browser, MP3, and video player as well as a host of other technological options. These technologies offer a wide variety of resources, including the facility to remotely detect stress-related increases in heart rate, complete stress self-assessments and stress diaries, generate suggestions for disputing negative thoughts, and listen to relaxation audio tracks, educational/instructional material, and self-talk prompts. It is possible that phone applications may have greater potential to help people gain the visceral experience of stress relief compared to the Internet interventions delivered via personal computers because of the greater degree of engagement that people have with mobile phones. Smartphones can incorporate all of the same options that Internet-based, computer-delivered stress management programs can offer but can also offer mobility, which may increase the likelihood that the individual will both learn and practice relaxation in real-life settings. Though tablet computers offer the same mobility and ease, people often feel an attachment with their smart phones which might in turn lead to greater motivation, engagement, and compliance with stress management delivered via mobile technology.

An 8-session self-help stress management training delivered via mobile phone was tested with oncology nurses in Italy. This innovative study compared the stress management intervention with a control group, who watched neutral videos through their mobile phones. Stress management users had lower anxiety at the end of each session and the experimental group reduced trait anxiety and acquired stress management coping skills at the end of the protocol (Villani et al., 2012). The literature on stress management delivered via smart phones and phone applications is still sparse but these types of technology may be even more effective at engaging users than web-based interventions delivered on a personal computer due to the greater familiarity and attachment to mobile telephones.

MULTI-FOCAL INTERVENTIONS

Stress is often addressed in the context of interventions for other health-compromising behaviors (tobacco use, sedentary lifestyle, alcohol consumption, and unhealthy diet). Approaches may be sequential, first addressing stress before targeting behavioral change, or concurrent, addressing stress at the same time as intervening with other health behaviors. Both approaches have merit. A review of multiple meta-analyses (meta-synthesis) concluded that because stress management interventions have greater efficacy than other health behavior changes, it is easier to reduce stress than to achieve health behavior change (Johnson, Scott-Sheldon, & Carey, 2010). Because stress may present an obstacle to making health behavior change, there is a case to be made for addressing stress prior to intervening with other health behaviors. On the other hand, stress mediates relapse to health risk behaviors; thus most health behavior interventions incorporate some stress management strategies, such as teaching basic relaxation skills. Stress is often cited as a primary predisposing factor that precipitates relapse to smoking, alcohol abuse, unhealthy eating, and sedentary behavior. Exercise, good nutrition, adequate sleep, work–life balance, and cognitive flexibility are all key aspects of effective stress management but the relationship is complex and multi-directional. Stress is often a cause of obesity, fatigue, work overload, and rigidity in thought processes but is also a consequence of diet, sedentary behavior, lack of sleep, and work–life imbalance.

SUMMARY

Whereas cognitive strategies work best for psychological manifestations of stress, relaxation strategies are best utilized for physiological stress reduction and the combination of both techniques has been associated with the best outcomes (Jones & Johnston, 2000). People can develop greater stress resilience through changing underlying beliefs, attitudes, and thought patterns, as well as the practice of relaxation techniques. However, the concept that stress management is a way of living—similar to regular exercise—rather than something to be practiced as an ancillary part of disease recovery (Suchday et al., 2012) is slow to be adopted in Western medicine. People who survive a medical crisis such as cancer, heart attack, or other life-threatening illness sometimes find unforeseen benefit in these practices. These types of experiences act as a springboard for prioritizing wellness and integrating it into everyday life for many people. There are many other smaller, "teachable moments" in Western culture that could serve to introduce the philosophy of practicing a lifestyle designed to manage stress effectively.

CONCLUSIONS

In the years to come, stress management is likely to evolve in several areas. Scientists will continue to develop a better understanding of the pathophysiology of stress and the mechanisms by which stress leads to disease in both human and animal models. It seems likely that there will be a convergence of research that will demonstrate different parallel pathways linking stress to the development and progression of disease. With improved understanding of the underlying mechanisms by which stress is linked to health, there will come improved interventions for reducing stress. Improved stress management skills may become more widespread as the technology to teach and demonstrate these skills is widely available through mobile phones. In all facets of work, from the military to the corporate world, there is an increasing emphasis on cultivating stress resilience and stress management capacity in employees and leaders. Psychologists and behavioral health specialists who can develop effective stress management interventions that can be easily disseminated will hold great value. Building greater psychological reliance among people through improving their repertoire of stress management skills could greatly reduce the number of individuals suffering from distress and stress-related health problems.

REFERENCES

Aftanas, L. I., & Golocheikine, S. A. (2003). Changes in cortical activity in states of consciousness: The study of meditation by high resolution EEG. *Human Physiology, 29*, 143–151.

Antoni, M. H., Lutgendorf, S. K., Blomberg, B., Carver, C. S., Lechner, S., Diaz, A., & Cole, S. W. (2012). Cognitive-behavioral stress management reverses anxiety-related leukocyte transcriptional dynamics. *Biological Psychiatry, 71*, 366–372.

Berkman, L. (1995). The role of social relations in health promotion. *Psychosomatic Medicine, 57*, 245–254.

Bishop, S. R. (2002). What do we really know about mindfulness-based stress reduction? *Psychosomatic Medicine, 64*, 71–84.

Burg, M. M., Lampert, R., Joska, T., Batsford, W., & Jain, D. (2004). Psychological traits and emotion-triggering of ICD shock-terminated arrhythmias. *Psychosomatic Medicine, 66*, 898–902.

Burg, M. M., & Soufer, R. (2007). Mental stress-induced myocardial ischemia: Moving forward. *Journal of Nuclear Cardiology, 14*, 308–313.

Carlson, C. R., & Hoyle, R. H. (1993). Efficacy of abbreviated progressive muscle relaxation training: A quantitative review of behavioral medicine research. *Journal of Consulting and Clinical Psychology, 61*(6), 1059–1067.

Chida, Y., Hamer, M., Wardle, J., & Steptoe, A. (2008). Do stress-related psychosocial factors contribute to cancer incidence and survival? *Nature Clinical Practice Oncology, 5*(8), 466–475.

Chida, Y., & Steptoe, A. (2009). The association of anger and hostility with future coronary heart disease: A meta-analytic review of prospective evidence. *Journal of the American College of Cardiology, 53*, 936–946.

Chiesa, A., & Serretti, A. (2010). A systematic review of neurobiological and clinical features of mindfulness meditations. *Psychological Medicine, 40*, 1239–1252.

Cohen, S., Janicki-Deverts, D., & Miller, G. E. (2007). Psychological stress and disease. *Journal of the American Medical Association, 298*(14), 1685–1687.

Dornelas, E. A. (2008). *Psychotherapy for cardiac patients: Behavioral cardiology in practice*, Washington, DC: American Psychological Association.

Duijts, S. F., Zeegers, M. P., & Borne, B. V. (2003). The association between stressful life events and breast cancer risk: A meta-analysis. *International Journal of Cancer, 107*(6), 1023–1029.

Engel, G. L. (1971). Sudden and rapid death during psychological stress. *Annals of Internal Medicine, 74*, 771–782.

Grossman, P., Niemann, L., Schmidt, S., & Walach, H. (2004). Mindfulness-based stress reduction and health benefits. A meta-analysis. *Journal of Psychosomatic Research, 57*(1), 35–43.

Jensen, M., & Patterson, D. R. (2006). Hypnotic treatment of chronic pain. *Journal of Behavioral Medicine, 29*, 95–124.

Johnson, B. T., Scott-Sheldon, L. A. J., & Carey, M. P. (2010). Meta-synthesis of health behavior change meta-analyses. *American Journal of Public Health, 100*, 2193–2198.

Jones, M. C., & Johnston, D. W. (2000). Reducing distress in first level and student nurses: A review of the applied stress management literature. *Journal of Advanced Nursing, 32*, 66–74.

Kabat-Zinn, J. (1990). *Full catastrophe living: Using the wisdom of your body and mind to face stress, pain, and illness*. New York, NY: Bantam Dell.

Karavidas, M. K., Tsai, P-S., Yucha, C., McGrady, A., & Lehrer, P. M. (2006). Thermal biofeedback for primary Raynaud's phenomenon: A review of the literature. *Applied Psychophysiology and Biofeedback, 31*, 203–216.

Ketterhagen, D., VandeVusse, L., & Berner, M. A. (2002). Self-hypnosis: Alternative anesthesia for childbirth. *American Journal of Maternal Child Nursing, 27*, 335–341.

Khatri, P., & Blumenthal, J. (2000). Exercise. In G. Fink (Ed.), *Encyclopedia of stress* (vol. 2, p. 98). San Diego, CA: Academic Press.

Landolt, A. S., & Milling, L. S. (2011). The efficacy of hypnosis as an intervention for labor and delivery pain: A comprehensive methodological review. *Clinical Psychology Review, 31*(6), 1022–1031.

Lazarus, R. S., & Folkman, S. (1984). *Stress, appraisal, and coping*. New York, NY: Springer Publishing Company.

Leor, J., Poole, W. K., & Kloner, R. A. (1996). Sudden cardiac death triggered by an earthquake. *New England Journal of Medicine, 334*, 413–419.

Li, A. W., & Goldsmith, C. A. (2012). The effects of yoga on anxiety and stress. *Alternative Medicine Review, 17*(1), 21–35.

Lukens, C., Turkoglu, D., & Burg, M. M. (2012). Stress management with cardiac patients. In E. A. Dornelas (Ed.), *Stress proof the heart: Behavioral interventions for cardiac patients* (pp. 199–222). New York, NY: Springer.

Lutgendorf, S. K., Lang, E. V., Berbaum, K. S., Russell, D., Berbaum, M. L., Logan, H., …. Spiegel, D. (2007). Effects of age on responsiveness to adjunct hypnotic analgesia during invasive medical procedures. *Psychosomatic Medicine, 69*, 191–199.

Lutgendorf, S. K., & Sood, A. K. (2011). Biobehavioral factors and cancer progression: Physiological pathways and mechanisms. *Psychosomatic Medicine, 73*(9), 724–730.

Meisel, S. R., Kutz, I., Dayan, K. I., Pauzner, H., Chetboun, I., Arbel, Y., & David, D. (1991). Effect of Iraqi missile war on incidence of acute myocardial infarction and sudden death in Israeli civilians. *Lancet, 338*, 660–661.

Miller, W. R., & Rollnick, S. (1991). *Motivational interviewing: Preparing people to change addictive behavior.* New York, NY: Guilford Press.

Mittleman, M. A., Maclure, M., Sherwood, J. B., Mulry, R. P., Tofler, G. H., Jacobs, S. C., … Muller, J. E. (1995). Triggering of acute myocardial infarction onset by episodes of anger. Determinants of Myocardial Infarction Onset Study Investigators. *Circulation, 92*, 1720–1725.

Muller, J. E., Ludmer, P. L., Willich, S. N., Tofler, G. H., Aylmer, G., Klangos, I., & Stone, P. H. (1987). Circadian variation in the frequency of sudden cardiac death. *Circulation, 75*, 131–138.

Nakao, M., Yano, E., Nomura, S., & Kuboki, T. (2003). Blood pressure-lowering effects of biofeedback treatment in hypertension: A meta-analysis of randomized controlled trials. *Hypertension Research, 26*(1), 37–46.

Nestoriuc, Y., Martin, A., Rief, W., & Andrasik, F. (2008). Biofeedback treatment for headache disorders: A comprehensive efficacy review. *Applied Psychophysiology and Biofeedback, 33*(3), 125–140.

Ockene, I. S., Hebert, J. R., Ockene, J. K., Saperia, G. M., Stanek, E., Nicolosi, R., … Hurley, T. G. (1999a). Effect of physician-delivered nutrition counseling training and an office-support program on saturated fat intake, weight, and serum lipid measurements in a hyperlipidemic population: Worcester Area Trial for Counseling in Hyperlipidemia (WATCH). *Archives of Internal Medicine, 159*, 725–731.

Ockene, J. K., Adams, A., Hurley, T. G., Wheeler, E. V., & Hebert, J. R. (1999b). Brief physician- and nurse practitioner-delivered counseling for high-risk drinkers: Does it work? *Archives of Internal Medicine, 159*, 2198–2205.

Ockene, J. K., Kristeller, J., Pbert, L., Hebert, J. R., Luippold, R., Goldberg, R. J., … Kalan, K. (1994). The physician-delivered smoking intervention project: Can short-term interventions produce long-term effects for a general outpatient population? *Health Psychology, 13*, 278–281.

Ornish, D., Brown, S. E., Billings, J. H., Scherwitz, L. W., Armstrong, W. T., Ports, T. A., … Gould, K. L. (1990). Can lifestyle changes reverse coronary heart disease? The Lifestyle Heart Trial. *Lancet, 336*, 129–133.

Orth-Gomér, K., Schneiderman, N., Wang, H. X., Walldin, C., Blom, M., & Jernberg, T. (2009). Stress reduction prolongs life in women with coronary disease: The Stockholm Women's Intervention Trial for Coronary Heart Disease (SWITCHD). *Circulation: Cardiovascular Quality and Outcomes, 2*, 25–32.

Peters, R. W., McQuillan, S., Resnick, S. K., & Gold, M. R. (1996). Increased Monday incidence of life-threatening ventricular arrhythmias. *Circulation, 94*, 1346–1349.

Premack, D. (1959). Toward empirical behavior laws: I. Positive reinforcement. *Psychological Review, 66*, 219–233.

Raub, J. A. (2002). Psychophysiologic effects of Hatha Yoga on musculoskeletal and cardiopulmonary function: A literature review. *Journal of Alternative & Complementary Medicine, 8*(6), 797–812.

Reich, P., DeSilva, R. A., Lown, B., & Murawski, B. J. (1981). Acute psychological disturbances preceding life-threatening ventricular arrhythmias. *Journal of the American Medical Association, 246*, 233–235.

Reitav, J. (2012). Managing sleep problems among cardiac patients. In E. A. Dornelas (Ed.), *Stress proof the heart: Behavioral interventions for cardiac patients* (pp. 281–317). New York, NY: Springer.

Riemann, D., & Perlis, M. L. (2009). The treatments of chronic insomnia: A review of benzodiazepine receptor agonists and psychological and behavioral therapies. *Sleep Medicine Review, 13*(3), 205–214.

Rosengren, A., Hawken, S., Õunpuu, S., Sliwa, K., Zubaid, M., Almahmeed, W. A., … Yusuf, S. (2004). Association of psychosocial risk factors with risk of acute myocardial infarction in 11,119 cases and 13,648 controls from 52 countries (the INTERHEART study): Case-control study. *Lancet, 364*, 953–962.

Sapolsky, R. (2004). *Why zebras don't get ulcers.* New York, NY: Henry Holt & Company.

Sedlmeier, P., Eberth, J., Schwarz, M., Zimmermann, D., Haarig, F., Jaeger, S., & Kunze, S. (2012). The psychological effects of meditation: A meta-analysis. *Psychological Bulletin, 138*(6), 1139–1171.

Selye, H. (1956). *The stress of life.* New York, NY: McGraw Hill.

Segerstrom, S. C., & Miller, G. E. (2004). Psychological stress and the human immune system: A meta-analytic study of 30 years of inquiry. *Psychological Bulletin, 130*(4), 601–630.

Shedd, O. L., Sears, S. F., Harvill, J. L., Arshad, A., Conti, J. B., Steinberg, J. S., & Curtis, A. B. (2004). The World Trade Center attack: Increased frequency of defibrillator shocks for ventricular arrhythmias in patients living remotely from New York City. *Journal of the American College of Cardiology, 44*, 1265–1267.

Smith, J. C. (2007). The psychology of relaxation. In P. M. Lehrer, R. L. Woolfolk, & E. Sime (Eds.), *Principles and practice of stress management* (3rd ed., pp. 38–52). New York, NY: Guilford Press.

Smith, K. B., & Pukall, C. F. (2009). An evidence-based review of yoga as a complementary intervention for patients with cancer. *Psycho-Oncology, 18*(5), 465–475.

Spiegel, D., Bloom, J. R., Kraemer, H. C., & Gottheil, E. (1989). Effect of psychosocial treatment on survival of patients with metastatic breast cancer. *Lancet, 2,* 888–891.

Spiegel, D., Butler, L. D., Giese-Davis, J., Koopman, C., Miller, E., DiMiceli, S., … Kraemer, H. C. (2007). Effects of supportive-expressive group therapy on survival of patients with metastatic breast cancer: A randomized prospective trial. *Cancer, 110,* 1130–1138.

Steinberg, J. S., Arshad, A., Kowalski, M., Kukar, A., Suma, V., Vloka, M., … Rozanski, A. (2004). Increased incidence of life-threatening ventricular arrhythmias in implantable defibrillator patients after the World Trade Center attack. *Journal of the American College of Cardiology, 44,* 1261–1264.

Steinmark, A., Dornelas, E. A., & Fischer, E. H. (2006). Determinants and barriers to participation in an internet-based recovery program for cardiac patients. *Journal of Clinical Psychology in Medical Settings, 14*(4), 353–357.

Strike, P. C., Magid, K., Whitehead, D. L., Brydon, L., Bhattacharyya, M. R., & Steptoe, A. (2006). Pathophysiological processes underlying emotional triggering of acute cardiac events. *Proceedings from the National Academy of Science USA, 103,* 4322–4327.

Strike, P. C., Perkins-Porras, L., Whitehead, D. L., McEwan, J., & Steptoe, A. (2006). Triggering of acute coronary syndromes by physical exertion and anger: Clinical and sociodemographic characteristics. *Heart, 92,* 1035–1040.

Suchday, S., Dziok, M., Katzenstein, M., Kaplan, E., & Kahan, M. (2012). The effects of meditation and yoga on cardiovascular disease. In E. A. Dornelas (Ed.), *Stress proof the heart: Behavioral interventions for cardiac patients* (pp. 223–248). New York, NY: Springer.

Toivonen, L., Helenius, K., & Viitasalo, M. (1997). Electrocardiographic repolarization during stress from awakening on alarm call. *Journal of the American College of Cardiology, 30,* 774–779.

van Gemert-Pijnen, J., Nijland, N., van Limburg, M., Ossebaard, H. C., Kelders, S. M., Eysenbach, G., & Seydel, E. R. (2011). A holistic framework to improve the uptake and impact of eHealth technologies. *Journal of Medical Internet Research, 13*(4), e111.

Villani, D., Grassi, A., Cognetta, C., Toniolo, D., Cipresso, P., & Riva, G. (2012). Self-help stress management training through mobile phones: An experience with oncology nurses. *Psychological Services, 173,* 524–528.

Weaver, K. E., Rowland, J. H., Bellizzi, K. M., & Aziz, N. M. (2010). Forgoing medical care because of cost. *Cancer, 116,* 3493–3504.

Wheat, A. L., & Larkin, K. T. (2010). Biofeedback of heart rate variability and related physiology: A critical review. *Applied Psychophysiology and Biofeedback, 35*(3), 229–242.

Yerkes, R. M., & Dodson, J. D. (1908). The relation of strength of stimulus to rapidity of habit-formation. *Journal of Comparative Neurology and Psychology, 18,* 459–482.

Zetterqvist, K., Maanmies, J., Ström, L., & Andersson, G. (2003). Randomized controlled trial of internet-based stress management. *Cognitive Behaviour Therapy, 32,* 151–160.

12

Building a Science for Multiple-Risk Behavior Change

JUDITH J. PROCHASKA
JANICE M. PROCHASKA
JAMES O. PROCHASKA

LEARNING OBJECTIVES

- Recognize the high co-occurrence of risk behaviors and negative implications for health.
- Review the literature on multiple-risk behavior change (MRBC) interventions, both successes and limitations as well as identification of research gaps.
- Apply multiple approaches to analyzing change in multiple-risk behaviors.
- Appreciate factors relevant to the dissemination of interventions designed to treat multiple-risk behaviors.

Lions, tigers, and bears—oh my!

Admittedly, one's work would be simpler if focused on a single-risk behavior such as tobacco, alcohol, exercise, or diet and if, in turn, research participants and clients were simply viewed as smokers, alcoholics, or the obese. Yet, the reality is, people are multidimensional and most engage in multibehavioral risks (Fine, Philogene, Gramling, Coups, & Sinha, 2004; Pronk et al., 2004). Among smokers, over 90% engage in additional risks, such as poor diet, inactivity, and problematic alcohol or illicit drug use (Berrigan, Dodd, Troiano, Krebs-Smith, & Barbash, 2003; Fine et al., 2004).

Addressing multiple health behaviors brings real complexities as few individuals are prepared to take action on any single risk. For those who refuse targeted health interventions or relapse over time because they are not in that moment ready or able to change, might they be engaged and supported in the change process and their self-efficacy supported by addressing complementary risk behaviors of their own choosing? Even among those who successfully adopt a new health behavior, what about the risks that go unassessed and unaddressed? We would argue that failure to detect and treat a broader constellation of health-compromising behaviors represents missed opportunity for significant reductions in morbidity, mortality, and health care costs (Edington, Yen, & Witting, 1997).

Cancer, heart disease, stroke, and diabetes, the leading preventable causes of death, are influenced by smoking, alcohol, inactivity, poor diet, and stress. Using the analogy of an individual caged with a lion, tiger, and bear, certainly risk will be reduced if the lion is removed as a singular threat, yet the participant still faces real jeopardy from the threats that remain. Teaching people effective behavior change principles—providing the keys to freedom from a predatory cage—should lead to greater gains, reduced risks, and improved overall well-being.

With consideration of the prevalence and co-occurrence of multiple-risk behaviors and attending to key concerns and methodological questions, our chapter centers on building a science of multiple-risk behavior change (MRBC). We discuss the need for an evidence base of interventions that target multiple-risk behaviors. Recent innovative studies are presented, and methodological, analytic, and theoretical issues unique to MRBC interventions are discussed. We close with consideration of dissemination issues and our vision for this growing field.

BACKGROUND AND RATIONALE FOR MULTIPLE-RISK BEHAVIOR CHANGE

The 52-nation INTERHEART study identified tobacco use, obesity, high lipids, and psychosocial factors as accounting for about 90% of the population-attributable risks for myocardial infarction; fruit and vegetable consumption and exercise were identified as protective (Lanas et al., 2007; Yusuf et al., 2004). Mental illness, or stress and distress more broadly, also place a significant burden on health and productivity in the United States and globally (U.S. Department of Health & Human Services, 1999).

Individuals often struggle with multiple unhealthful behaviors, and there is evidence of co-occurrence among the risk factors. Analysis of data from the 2001 National Health Interview Study indicated that the majority of adults in the United States met criteria for two or more risk behaviors (Fine et al., 2004; Pronk et al., 2004). Tobacco users, in particular, tended to have poor behavioral profiles, with over 90% of smokers having at least one additional risk behavior (Fine et al., 2004; Klesges, Eck, Isbell, Fulliton, & Hanson, 1990; Pronk et al., 2004). In the United States, only 3% of adults met all four health behavior goals of being a nonsmoker, having a healthy weight, being physically active, and eating five or more fruits and vegetables a day (Reeves & Rafferty, 2005).

Among youth, there is evidence of a clustering of dietary patterns and physical activity (Sallis, Prochaska, & Taylor, 2000); tobacco use increases the likelihood of experimentation with illicit drug use (Lai, Lai, Page, & McCoy, 2000), and tobacco and other substance use is a highly predictive marker for youth engagement in multiple-risk behaviors, including bicycling without a helmet, perpetrating violence and carrying a weapon, not using a seatbelt, and having suicidal ideation (DuRant, Smith, Kreiter, & Krowchuk, 1999).

The health care burden is believed to multiply with an increasing number of risk factors in terms of both medical consequences and costs (Conry et al., 2011; Edington et al., 1997). Put simply, excess risks lead to excess costs. Figures 12.1 and 12.2 show the incremental gain in pharmaceutical and disability costs due to excess risks. Longitudinal data indicate that effectively treating two behaviors reduces medical costs by about $2,000 per year (Edington, 2001). Targeting multiple-risk behaviors for change offers the potential of greater health benefits, maximized health promotion opportunities, and reduced health care costs.

Lifestyle behaviors also may serve as a gateway to intervention on behaviors for which individuals have low motivation to change. Confidence or self-efficacy gained

FIGURE 12.1 Excess pharmaceutical costs due to excess risks, age and gender adjusted.

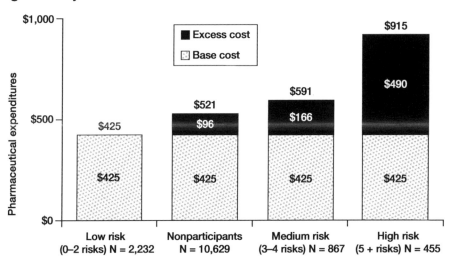

from making changes in one behavior may serve to support changes in additional risks. In a 3-year prospective study, individuals who quit smoking significantly increased their physical activity, whereas continued smokers did not (Perkins et al., 1993). Similar changes were not observed for diet or alcohol use. The change process appears to be similar for different health behaviors, and it may be efficient to work on multiple behaviors at the same time in a single intervention.

Given limited opportunity for health promotion contacts, interventions would ideally address all behaviors relevant to an individual's health profile. Researchers have emphasized that opportunities for intervening on multiple behaviors abound in the applied setting and have reasoned that specifically targeted interventions, even if effective, will be limited in their impact (Hayes, Barlow, & Nelson-Gray, 1999). A science of multibehavioral change is needed.

FIGURE 12.2 Excess disability costs due to excess risks.

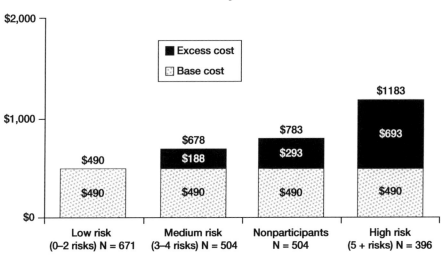

To identify motivators and challenges to growth of research on MRBC interventions, an anonymous online survey was conducted with 69 behavioral scientists and practitioners affiliated with the Society of Behavioral Medicine (Prochaska, Nigg, Spring, Velicer, & Prochaska, 2010). The survey assessed attitudes regarding potential strengths and limitations of MRBC research. Most respondents (83%) were engaged in MRBC research or practice. Overall, a sample majority rated nearly all 24 benefits as very to extremely important, whereas, only 1 of 31 barriers was rated as very to extremely important—the challenge of developing integrated delivery systems for health behavior change. Highest rated benefits centered on the potential for greater real-world applicability for patients, health care, and affiliated systems; greater health improvements; and providing information on effective treatments for behaviors that co-occur. Professionals engaged in MRBC gave significantly higher ratings to the benefits of MRBC research relative to individuals focused on single-behavior change. Respondents focused on single-behavior change rated the benefits and challenges of MRBC equally, whereas respondents engaged in MRBC rated the benefits significantly higher than the challenges. The findings indicated that individuals focused solely on single behaviors do not fully appreciate the benefits that impress MRBC researchers; it is not that substantial barriers are holding them back. Findings suggest that the benefits of MRBC interventions need emphasizing more broadly to advance this research area. The Society of Behavioral Medicine's Special Interest Group on Multiple Health Behavior Change is a professional network aimed specifically at fostering the science and scientific community around MRBC research and practice. The European Society for Prevention Research also has active interests in MRBC, and the International Society for Physical Activity and Nutrition is focused specifically on advancing and fostering excellence in research on nutrition behavior and physical activity.

DEFINITIONS

MRBC interventions can be defined as efforts to treat two or more risk behaviors effectively within a limited time period simultaneously or sequentially. By risk behaviors, we mean actions in which individuals engage that impact health. The impact can be negative, as with tobacco and other drug use and risky sexual behaviors, or positive, as with physical activity, fruit and vegetable consumption, and the wearing of helmets or seatbelts. Medical screening behaviors, such as mammography, colonoscopy, cholesterol testing, blood pressure screening, HIV tests, and glucose screening, also are clearly relevant to health and disease prevention and may be included as behavioral targets in MRBC interventions.

The field of MRBC research is still at an early stage, and its boundaries are being further expanded and refined. Historically, much of the research focused on changing multiple-risk behaviors within populations; fewer studies have targeted multiple risks within individuals; and the distinction is meaningful. When MRBC interventions are focused on populations, a program of interventions is offered to a community and community members receive intervention only on the behaviors for which they are identified as at risk. For example, only smokers in a community would receive the quit-smoking program, while individuals with high-fat diets would receive the nutrition intervention and individuals at risk for both smoking and high-fat diet would receive both intervention components. Changes are reported at the population level as a change in means or prevalence rates (e.g., smoking rates). With greater behavioral targets, the relevance of the intervention to the community and systems being served is increased as all members are likely to be at risk for at least one of the targeted behaviors.

When MRBC interventions target multiple risks in individuals, all individuals receive intervention on all targeted behaviors. The potential impact on an individual's health is increased, as are the behavior change demands. MRBC interventions within individuals may be relevant to only a select high-risk group, since participants need to be at risk for all targeted behaviors, though this may be less of an issue with behaviors that co-occur at high rates, such as alcohol and tobacco use or physical inactivity and poor diet. If the intervention promotes concurrent immediate action in multiple behaviors, it may be overwhelming and result in poor adherence. Sequencing change goals or matching intervention strategies to individuals' readiness to change may facilitate greater adherence and overall change.

To summarize, the main difference between MRBC interventions at the population level and similar interventions at the individual level is that the former matches the intervention strategies to the risk needs of the participants within the community, whereas the latter delivers all interventions to all participants. The former provides interventions more broadly to everyone in the community, while the latter focuses on a more select high-risk group.

REVIEWS OF MRBC INTERVENTION STUDIES

Though most health promotion research has addressed risk factors as categorically separate entities, given a window of intervention opportunity, a higher impact paradigm is to target multiple behaviors, and growing evidence suggests the potential for MRBC interventions to have much greater impact on public health than single-behavior interventions (Prochaska & Prochaska, 2011).

STUDIES OF MRBC INTERVENTIONS IN POPULATIONS

The concept of intervening on multiple-risk behaviors concurrently became a focus of attention in the early 1970s and was targeted at preventing cardiovascular disease (CVD) (Labarthe, 1998). One early proposal was a factorial design to evaluate the independent contributions and the joint effects of targeting diet, physical activity, and smoking habits in a single trial, named "Jumbo." The proposal was deemed too costly, however, and the trial was never conducted. Large-scale multifactorial CVD risk factor interventions that were conducted include the Multiple-Risk Factor Intervention Trial (MRFIT), the North Karelia Project, the Stanford Three-City and Five-City Projects, and the Pawtucket and Minnesota Heart Health Programs. Youth multifactor interventions also were developed, with a movement toward comprehensive school health programs.

The multibehavioral studies conducted over the past 30 years have had a range of outcomes, from favorable to unfavorable. The interventions have focused almost entirely on practitioner-based modalities such as health advice and counseling from a physician, dietician, or nurse; home visits; and group health education. Community-level promotional materials also have been incorporated. Significant changes were often seen in some but not all targeted behaviors (Emmons, Marcus, Linnan, Rossi, & Abrams, 1994; Sorensen et al., 1996). A Cochrane review of these large multifactor interventions estimated the net reduction in smoking prevalence at 20% (Ebrahim et al., 2011). Changes in dietary and physical activity behaviors, unfortunately, were not reported in the review. The pooled effects suggested that the MRBC interventions had no effect on mortality.

Another Cochrane review summarized findings from 21 youth obesity prevention studies that targeted physical activity and dietary change (Waters et al., 2011). The studies were conducted in schools and communities, with children and adolescents, in the United States and Europe, representing a diversity of ethnic groups and socioeconomic levels. Most of the studies followed a social learning or environmental theoretical framework. Only 3 of the 21 studies achieved significant changes in both dietary and physical activity behaviors, with the finding in one of the studies significant only for girls and not for boys (Gortmaker et al., 1999). The effects in the adolescent trial by Haerens and colleagues (2006) were reduced dietary fat consumption and reduced declines in light intensity physical activity; additionally, among boys, the intervention was associated with increased school-related physical activity. A trial conducted by Hamelink-Basteen and colleagues (2008) in primary schools reported increased fruit and vegetable consumption, decreased sweets, improvements in physical activity, and declines in sedentary behavior. Ten of the studies reported significant intervention reduction effects on BMI, one reported a significant increase, and 10 were nonsignificant. The overall effect on BMI was a standardized mean change of -0.18 (95% CI [-0.27, -0.09]).

In our review of the literature on randomized controlled trials of combined physical activity and nutrition interventions conducted with youth and published between 2004 and 2009 (Prochaska & Prochaska, 2011), we identified 31 unique trials in which the outcome was body mass index (9 studies with significant effects and 5 with effects in both gender groups) and 23 unique studies in which youth physical activity and dietary behaviors were the outcomes (3 studies with significant effects in both behaviors, 1 physical activity only, and 1 diet only). In the adult literature, we found that while single interventions were more effective at increasing the behaviors, the MRBC interventions were more effective for weight loss and weight gain prevention. Unfortunately, few of the adult trials reported on both behavioral and weight loss outcomes preventing direct investigation of this rather conflicting finding.

RECENT SUCCESSES IN POPULATION-BASED MRBC INTERVENTIONS

While many of the early attempts at achieving change in multiple-risk behaviors within populations met with limited success, the story does not end there. Here we describe several examples of innovative interventions that have succeeded in stimulating change in multiple-risk behaviors and discuss some of the potential reasons for their successes.

Historically, researchers and practitioners have used an action paradigm, prescribing immediate action in a risk behavior. Pushing individuals to make behavioral changes in more than one area, however, can have negative effects. For example, less than 10% of smokers are prepared to take action on more than one risk behavior (Prochaska, Velicer, Prochaska, Delucchi, & Hall, 2006). When instructed to change multiple behavioral risks, individuals can become overwhelmed, disillusioned, and ineffective at making any behavior changes.

Transtheoretical Model and Application to MRBC Interventions

In contrast to action-oriented paradigms, which promote immediate action among all participants, the Transtheoretical Model (TTM) of behavior change recommends tailoring of strategies to an individual's intention and readiness to change (Prochaska, DiClemente, & Norcross, 1992). Briefly, the TTM has identified five stages of change defined as precontemplation, not intending to change; contemplation, intending to change within the next 6 months; preparation, actively planning change within the next 30 days; action, overtly making changes; and maintenance, taking steps to sustain change and resist temptation to relapse. To begin action, individuals are required to meet some behavioral criterion for some minimal amount of time (e.g., quit smoking for 24 hours). With most behaviors, the action stage has been defined as lasting up to 6 months, at which time the individual enters maintenance. Other key TTM constructs are decisional balance, or the pros and cons of change, and self-efficacy, operationalized as situational confidence in changing a behavior and situational temptations to engage in a problem behavior. Using the TTM or stage-of-change paradigm, there is consistent evidence supporting MRBC (e.g., Jones et al., 2003; Johnson et al., 2006; Prochaska et al., 2004, 2005; Mauriello et al., 2010).

Three parallel TTM population-based MRBC studies targeted smoking, high-fat diet, and high-risk sun exposure (Prochaska et al., 2004, 2005; Velicer et al., 2004). The studies were conducted with employees in worksites, parents of high school students, and patients in primary care. The interventions used computerized expert system interventions delivering tailored individualized feedback based on participants' responses to measures of the key TTM constructs. The expert system was repeated at three time points over a 6-month period, and feedback was provided on the basis of both normative data and participants' earlier responses. Combined, the studies included nearly 10,000 participants. Participants assigned to the TTM intervention group received treatment for the behavior(s) for which they were identified as being at risk on the basis of their baseline stage of change. In all three studies, across all three behaviors, treatment effects were significant at 12- and 24-month follow-up, with the exception of smoking in the worksite study, which had a relatively small number of smokers. Importantly, the smoking cessation effects obtained in these TTM-based MRBC studies were comparable to previously reported intervention effects for TTM studies focused on smoking alone (Prochaska et al., 2006). Further, among smokers in the three trials, treatment of one or two coexisting risk factors (diet and/or sun exposure) did not decrease the effectiveness of smoking cessation treatment, and treatment for the coexisting factors was effective, as well. With a focus on youth, Mauriello and colleagues (2010) targeted MRBC for healthy weight management in 1,800 high school students, including exercise, fruits and vegetables, and limit TV viewing instead of emotional eating. There were treatment effects for each behavior with the most pronounced effects for fruits and vegetables and total risks across all time points.

Targeting adults with high cholesterol, another population-based TTM intervention reported significant effects on lipid medication adherence, physical activity, and dietary fat reduction. The treatment group was 50% more likely than the control group to make changes to reach the criterion for action on all three behaviors (Johnson et al., 2006). Approaching healthy weight management as an MRBC challenge, Johnson et al. (2008) proactively recruited 1,277 overweight or obese adults to a TTM computer tailored intervention (CTI) intervention for healthy eating, exercise, and emotional eating. An unusual result of recruiting was that so many men from a transportation company signed up that they had to get an administrative supplement from National Heart, Lung and Blood Institute (NHLBI) to reach their goal of 50% women. At 24-month follow-up, there were significant effects on each of the three treated behaviors and on fruit and vegetable consumption that received minimal treatment.

The unique advantage of TTM interventions for MRBC is that the likelihood of overwhelming participants is greatly reduced and the proportion of the at-risk population participating is likely to be greatly increased, since immediate action is not demanded. With proactive recruitment strategies such as random digit dialing, TTM studies have consistently reported participation rates of 80% or greater (Prochaska et al., 2004; Velicer et al., 2004). Importantly, strategies are matched to participants' readiness to change, and all participants at risk are supported through the change process. Moving the field beyond the old gold standard of efficacy trials with highly selected samples of motivated individuals with a single problem, the TTM has yielded evidence from effectiveness trials of large population samples with multiple problems (Prochaska, 2006).

Social Cognitive Theory and Application to MRBC Interventions

Social cognitive theory (SCT) focuses on the interaction of personal factors, behavior, and the environment (Bandura, 1986). For example, factors related to the individual such as knowledge, attitudes, values, and beliefs elicit certain behaviors and in turn, the outcome of those behaviors influences one's knowledge, attitudes, values, and beliefs. Similarly, the social environment has an influence on attitudes, values, and behavior, and when behavior leads to success or "failure," then perceptions about the environment are likely to be reinforced or altered (see Chapter 1 for a more in-depth discussion of SCT).

With some success, SCT has been applied to multiple-risk behaviors. PREVENT, a telephone-delivered intervention plus tailored materials, based on motivation to change and SCT, targeted six behavioral factors in determining colon cancer risk: red meat consumption, fruit and vegetable intake, multivitamin intake, alcohol, smoking, and physical inactivity (Emmons et al., 2005). Participants were 1,247 adults with recent diagnoses of adenomatous colorectal polyps. Intervention participants were more likely to change two or more risk behaviors than were those in the standard care condition. For the individual behaviors, intervention effects were significant for improved multivitamin intake and reduced red meat consumption, and there was less regression in physical activity levels among those receiving intervention over the course of the study. There were no between-condition differences in smoking, alcohol, or fruit and vegetable consumption.

The Mediterranean Lifestyle Program is another successful example of a population-level MRBC intervention (Toobert et al., 2007). This randomized clinical trial for postmenopausal women with type 2 diabetes employed social learning theory to guide intervention strategies to address healthful eating, physical activity, stress management, smoking cessation, and social support. At 12 and 24 months, intervention participants demonstrated improvements in all targeted lifestyle behaviors except smoking (there were too few smokers to analyze effects of the intervention on tobacco use). Additionally, significant treatment effects were seen in psychosocial measures of use of supportive resources, problem solving, self-efficacy, and quality of life.

RECENT STUDIES OF MRBC INTERVENTIONS IN INDIVIDUALS

Few studies have directly compared the effectiveness of multifactor interventions within individuals to that of single-factor interventions, and findings have been inconsistent. A 2004 review of MRBC interventions in primary care identified large gaps in the field's knowledge base (Goldstein, Whitlock, & DePue, 2004). The review emphasized the successes of interventions targeted on single risks, such as tobacco use, alcohol use, poor diet, and, to a lesser extent, physical inactivity, but acknowledged the dearth of studies in primary care aimed at treating multiple risks.

The strongest evidence for MRBC intervention in individuals has aimed at secondary rather than primary prevention, specifically interventions focused on individuals at high risk for or already diagnosed with CVD (Ketola, Sipila, & Makela, 2002) or diabetes (Norris, Engelgau, & Narayan, 2001). These interventions have targeted tobacco use, physical inactivity, and poor diet, as well as more specific disease management care, for example, adherence to lipid-lowering drugs and hypertensives for those with CVD and blood glucose monitoring and foot exams for those with diabetes. Even in these studies, while the evidence generally has been strong for short-term effects, sustained effects have been difficult to achieve.

A notable exception is the Lifestyle Heart Trial for patients with moderate to severe CVD. The intensive intervention promotes a 10% fat whole food vegetarian diet, aerobic exercise, stress management, and smoking cessation and provides group psychosocial support. In a small efficacy trial ($N = 48$), program adherence was reported as excellent and significant intervention effects were seen at 1 and 5 years for reductions in weight and LDL cholesterol, as well as reduction in arterial diameter stenosis and cardiac events (Ornish et al., 1998).

Individuals with drug and alcohol problems are another high-risk patient group of interest for multibehavioral change. In particular, rates of tobacco use are high, and tobacco is a primary cause of death among individuals treated for substance abuse (Hser, McCarthy, & Anglin, 1994; Hurt et al., 1996). The health effects of tobacco and other substance use appear synergistic, 50% greater than the sum of each individually (Bien & Burge, 1990). Historically, clinical lore has discouraged smoking cessation efforts during addiction treatment out of concern that sobriety would be compromised. Tobacco has been viewed as the last remaining vice among those in recovery and a necessary behavioral crutch. A meta-analysis examined this issue in 12 randomized controlled smoking cessation interventions delivered to individuals in substance abuse treatment (Prochaska, Delucchi, & Hall, 2004). The interventions were built on a variety of theoretical frameworks, including stage-based or motivational enhancement, cognitive-behavioral therapy, relapse prevention, and pharmacological treatments. Smoking cessation effects were significant at post-treatment but were not sustained at long-term follow-up. Importantly, exposure to the smoking cessation interventions was associated with a 25% increased likelihood of long-term abstinence from alcohol and illicit drugs. The study concluded that, contrary to previous concerns, smoking cessation interventions delivered during addictions treatment appeared to enhance rather than compromise long-term sobriety.

Tobacco treatment studies also have examined the impact of incorporating strategies to prevent weight gain, a common side effect and a potential deterrent to quitting smoking. Early studies suggested that a focus on caloric restriction may lead to greater relapse to smoking (Hall, Tunstall, Vila, & Duffy, 1992), and the 2008 tobacco treatment clinical practice guidelines discourage active weight control measures during a quit attempt (Fiore et al., 2008). As with tobacco cessation among substance users, the concern is with multiple intervention interference—that change in one behavior may negatively impact change in another. A 2009 meta-analysis of 10 trials of behavioral interventions aimed at treating tobacco and preventing weight gain, however, demonstrated increased abstinence (odds ratio [OR] = 1.29; 95% CI [1.01, 1.64]) and reduced weight gain (g = −0.30; 95% CI [−0.57, −0.02]) in the short term (less than 3 months) compared with patients who received smoking treatment alone (Spring et al., 2009). At long-term follow-up (greater than 6 months), differences in abstinence and weight control were no longer significant. A randomized controlled trial testing nutrition advice within a smoking cessation treatment, published since the meta-analysis, was nonsignificant for both weight gain prevention and abstinence (Leslie et al., 2012). Given the salient issue of weight gain among smokers, greater investigation is needed and particularly with attention to relapse prevention and long-term weight management.

Physical activity also has been studied as an adjunct to tobacco cessation interventions as a treatment strategy. In laboratory studies with smokers, physical activity has reduced withdrawal symptoms and cigarette cravings and enhanced mood (Haasova et al., 2012; Patterson, 2013; Roberts, Maddison, Simpson, Bullen, & Prapavessis, 2012).

Yet, in randomized controlled trials, the effect of exercise for supporting smoking cessation has not been encouraging. A Cochrane review concluded that while exercise promotion did not appear to harm smoking cessation efforts, there was limited evidence that it helped (Ussher, Taylor, & Faulkner, 2012). Only 1 of the 15 identified trials found evidence for exercise aiding smoking cessation at long-term follow-up (Marcus et al., 1999). Unfortunately, few of the studies reported changes in physical activity, limiting our understanding of the feasibility of efforts to help smokers make changes in their tobacco use and exercise patterns concurrently. Of note, the one study that had significant effects for both quitting smoking and increasing fitness was based on the TTM and matched exercise and smoking cessation strategies to participants' readiness to quit, rather than prescribing immediate action (Marcus et al., 1999).

SIMULTANEOUS VS. SEQUENTIAL INTERVENTIONS

When there is concern about multiple intervention interference, a sequential treatment approach may be undertaken. A study compared the effect of a dietary intervention implemented early in the quit attempt to those of an after-cessation effort and a no-diet control program (Spring et al., 2004). The study reported no difference in smoking cessation rates among the three groups, with some advantage in weight gain prevention among participants in the delayed diet group. Similarly, a study evaluating immediate and delayed smoking cessation among veterans in substance abuse treatment reported comparable quit smoking rates, with some apparent benefit to sobriety among participants treated for tobacco use in the delayed-treatment group (Joseph, Willenbring, Nugent, & Nelson, 2004).

One study examined the impact of simultaneous and sequential targeting of multiple risks and concluded that sequential targeting was not superior to, and may be inferior to, a simultaneous approach (Hyman, Pavlik, Taylor, Goodrick, & Moye, 2007). The trial used stage-based counseling and promoted changes in physical activity, dietary sodium intake, and tobacco use. Another study found equivocal effects between sequential and simultaneous approaches to targeting physical activity and dietary fat reduction using computerized stage-tailored interventions (Vandelanotte, Reeves, Brug, & de Bourdeaudhuij, 2008). The theoretical model employed and the types of behaviors targeted certainly may influence the efficacy of a simultaneous and a sequential approach. More research is needed to address this key intervention design issue.

In their qualitative article titled "Eating the Elephant Whole or in Slices...," Koshy, Mackenzie, Leslie, Lean, and Hankey (2012) summarized smokers' ($N = 40$) perspectives about efforts to change nutrition and activity patterns within a smoking cessation treatment. They found that while sequential behavior change was preferred by 1 in 4, nearly 1 in 2 simultaneously changed their smoking, diet, and physical activity patterns. Further, those who attempted concurrent behavior change were more successful at quitting smoking and at changing multiple behaviors compared to those who attempted changes sequentially. Identified mechanisms of change in these multiple-risk behaviors included improved confidence, improved taste sensation, ease of breathing, and more generally feeling healthier.

COACTION AND OPTIMAL TAILORING

One of the most exciting developments in our knowledge of simultaneously changing multiple behaviors is the phenomena of coaction. Coaction is the increased probability that if individuals take effective action on one behavior (like smoking) they are more likely to take action on a secondary behavior (like diet). Coaction was observed across three TTM-tailored cancer prevention studies and two healthy weight management projects (Johnson et al., 2008; Mauriello et al., 2010; Prochaska et al., 2004, 2005; Velicer et al., 2004). In more systematic analyses of coaction in these studies, we found that significant coaction typically occurs only in TTM treatment groups (Johnson et al., in press; Paiva et al., 2012) and not in control groups, suggesting it is likely to be treatment induced. A longitudinal survey study of youth physical activity and fruit and vegetable intake observed correlation in the two behaviors but not covariation over time and concluded that intervention is likely necessary to achieve coaction in health behaviors (Woolcott, Disman, Motl, Matthai, & Nigg, 2013).

Building on the emergent coaction phenomena, two TTM studies have applied optimal tailoring strategies to MRBC. With a sample of 3,391 adults recruited from 39 states, Prochaska and colleagues (2012) compared three groups: (1) full TTM tailoring online for stress management and stage tailoring only for exercise; (2) telephonic coaching with optimal tailoring on stage, pros and cons and self-efficacy for exercise and stage tailoring only for stress; and (3) controls. At 6 months, the outcome patterns for each of the target behaviors and untreated diet and depression were: exercise coaching > online stress > controls. Similar patterns were found for enhancement of behaviors of well-being (emotional health, physical health, overall well-being, and progress from struggling or suffering to thriving).

The second study compared two TTM-tailored computerized interventions designed to impact multiple substance use or energy balance behaviors in 20 middle schools ($N = 4{,}158$) (Velicer et al., 2013). The energy balance program targeted exercise as the behavior that received full TTM tailoring and fruits and vegetables and TV watching were secondary and alternated receiving tailoring on stage, pros and cons, and self-efficacy or just on stage. The other group received tailoring on profiles using pros, cons, and self-efficacy for smoking and alcohol use. Full energy balance TTM-tailored computerized interventions provided strong effects for physical activity, healthy diet, and reducing TV time. Despite no direct treatment, the energy balance group also showed significantly lower smoking and alcohol use over time than the substance use prevention group.

One important development that may help explain coaction is a meta-analysis of the pros and cons of changing related to stages of change for 48 health behaviors (Hall & Rossi, 2008). The same principles of progress seem to hold across very different behaviors, such as the pros increasing from precontemplation to contemplation, the cons decreasing from contemplation to action, and the pros increasing twice as much as the cons decrease. TTM treatments applying these principles may be teaching participants how to maximize change across two or more behaviors (coaction) by relying on common principles of change. Other common principles that have been identified are called the four effects, which predict long-term success across very different types of behaviors (Blissmer et al., 2010). Treatment, stage, severity, and effort are the four long-term predictors. Those in treatment are significantly more successful than controls; those in preparation were more successful than those in contemplation who are more successful than those in precontemplation; those with less severe problems are more likely to progress to action or maintenance for their problems; and those making better efforts (e.g., on the pros and cons of changing) at baseline are more likely to change. These effects can produce smarter goals early on to help clients complete treatment, progress from precontemplation to contemplation to preparation, to reduce severity, to make better efforts on TTM change variables, and to make more progress across multiple behaviors.

METHODOLOGICAL ISSUES

Methodological challenges with multibehavioral interventions include the increased time and participant demands for intervention and evaluation components and the lack of direction in the field on how best to conceptualize and analyze MRBC.

MEASURING CHANGES IN MULTIPLE-RISK BEHAVIORS

Approaches taken to minimize assessment and participant burden include efforts to simplify assessment tools, while maintaining rigorous psychometrics, and movement toward more technologically sophisticated and, one hopes, more objective assessment tools that ideally reduce the burden on participants for data collection. Health risk appraisals are an option for quickly assessing engagement in a wide range of risk behaviors (Smith, McKinlay, & McKinlay, 1989).

More objective, behavioral measures include biochemical measures of dietary changes (e.g., plasma carotenoid concentrations), tobacco (e.g., cotinine and anabasine), and other drug use; biometric measures of physical activity (pedometers and accelerometers) and fitness (VO_2 max); and computerized innovations to assess medication adherence (e.g., MEMS caps). All measures, of course, have their limitations. With biometrics, a metabolite's half-life may be too short to detect sustained behavioral changes, research costs can be high, and participants may not adhere to assessment protocols. In the tobacco arena, consensus guidelines have been developed recommending when bioinformation is and is not necessary (Society for Research on Nicotine and Tobacco, 2002).

Alternatively, rather than measuring changes separately for each targeted behavior, measures may be incorporated to conceptualize and assess overall health outcomes due to changes in multiple risks. Examples include changes in weight, blood pressure, cholesterol, or blood glucose due to changes in diet, exercise, and/or tobacco use. Self-report measures of overarching change may include health-related quality of life (Rasanen et al., 2006). The Mediterranean Life Program, for example, reported changes in behavioral, psychological, and quality of life measures (Toobert et al., 2007). Economic measures may include medical, pharmaceutical, and disability costs. If MRBC interventions ultimately aim to maximize health outcomes, then measures should assess these gains. Longer follow-up periods, however, will likely be necessary to detect changes in these more distal outcomes.

ANALYZING CHANGES IN MULTIPLE-RISK BEHAVIORS

Use of overarching, integrative measures also would serve to simplify analysis of outcomes in MRBC interventions. Historically, MRBC interventions have included separate measures for each risk behavior targeted, sometimes incorporating multiple measures for each behavior. The consequence is multiple significance testing with the potential for inflating the type I error rate, as well as creating confusion by describing inconsistent findings across the different outcomes.

Method 1: Summative Indices

Indices of MRBC have been proposed as a way of combining changes in separate risk behaviors, although no standard exists and selection (or modification) tends to be study specific. Examples include the Framingham Heart Study Risk Score, the Cooper Clinic

Mortality Risk Index, cancer risk indices, dietary quality indices, and an index of early problem behaviors (Janssen, Katzmarzyk, Church, & Blair, 2005; McGue, Iacono, & Krueger, 2006; Patterson, Haines, & Popkin, 1994; Wilson et al., 1998). Key considerations for MRBC indices include the number and types of behaviors and risks represented, the provision of credit for incremental change versus to-criterion behavioral adoption or cessation, equal versus weighted scoring (e.g., with respect to mortality risk), and full reliance on self-report versus combined self-report and biometric measures. Given variability in these study-specific parameters, comparison of risk score values between studies is difficult.

As an example, a relatively new index, the Prudence Score, assesses compliance with nonsmoking, physical activity, alcohol in moderation, six dietary behaviors, and body mass index. The total score ranges from 0 to 10 with each behavior scored "1" if meeting national health recommendations or "0" if not (Parekh, King, Owen, & Jamrozik, 2009). Designed for simplicity, the Prudence Score is categorical in scoring and equal weighted. In a study of elderly men, an 8-item version of the Prudence Score predicted an absolute reduction in cumulative mortality of 0.62% per single additional healthy behavior (Spencer, Jamrozik, Lawrence-Brown, & Norman, 2005). Use of the Prudence Score as the outcome measure in a recent MRBC trial intervening on diet, physical activity, smoking, and alcohol suggested significant overall effects; however, further examination of individual risks revealed significant changes were limited to three dietary behaviors (Parekh, Vandelanotte, King, & Boyle, 2012). Hence, the overrepresentation in the Prudence Score on dietary sub-behaviors may overshadow changes, or lack of changes, in the other measured risks.

Method 2: Standardized Change Score

Another alternative is creating a linear index of behavior change scores. If the behavioral measures to be combined are on different scales—for example, minutes of physical activity and servings of fruits and vegetables—a statistical transformation will be necessary. Standardized change scores can be created by subtracting baseline scores from the follow-up scores and then dividing by the standard deviation of the difference (i.e., z-score). The scores can then be summed into a combined behavioral index, which indicates the amount of increase or decrease in the combined behaviors from baseline to follow-up. Alternatively, standardized residuals from linear regressions of follow-up scores on baseline measures provide a simple change score adjusted for baseline variance. Residualized change scores are referred to as "base-free" measures of change (Tucker, Damarin, & Messick, 1966) and are viewed as superior to simple pretest–post-test differences in scores (Veldman & Brophy, 1974).

Method 3: Optimal Linear Combination

A third method, proposed by Goodman, Li, Bennett, Stoddard, and Emmons (2006), is to calculate an optimal linear combination of multiple behavioral risk factors (MRF score function), irrespective of individual demographic factors. The approach entails (1) setting the variables to an equivalent time scale (e.g., unit per week); (2) equating the meaning of a one-unit change across variables by standardizing the variables (i.e., subtracting the 5th percentile value from the original value and dividing by the difference between the 5th and 95th values); (3) and then running PROC PHREG in SAS/STATTM software to fit the conditional logistic regression model, conditioning out demographic characteristics, and forming a stratum for set matching of baseline and follow-up assessments for each individual. At each time point (pre- and post-intervention) each participant has a vector (containing the standardized multiple-risk behaviors) of covariates. Goodman et al. (2006) advised restricting step 3 to participants who received the intervention and with complete data for all targeted risk behaviors at all assessment points with the rationale of identifying an optimal linear combination that will show an intervention effect. The end product is a score function that combines each of the measured risk behaviors optimally weighted. The MRF score function can include main effects and interactions among the risk behaviors. Although the score is created utilizing only data from intervention participants, it can be applied to the full study sample with magnitude of change then compared between intervention and usual care groups. Goodman et al. (2006) noted that a limitation of this method is that the score weights are a direct function of the amount of change seen in the risk behavior either due to intervention effect and/or ease/burden of changing the risk behavior. The MRF score function is dependent on the risk behaviors measured and the chosen time scale making comparisons and attempts to synthesize findings across studies (e.g., in a meta-analysis) difficult. Further, because it is a composite, change in the score does not indicate which behavior(s) have contributed to the change.

Method 4: Latent Class/Transition Analysis

Another applicable method for examining multiple-risk behaviors in a sample is the application of latent class analysis (LCA), a subset of structural equation modeling used to find groups or subtypes of cases in multivariate categorical data. Unlike variable-centered approaches (e.g., correlations and regression), person-centered approaches, such as LCA, are ideal for clustering individuals based on similar responses to measured items (Nylund, Asparouhov, & Muthen, 2007). LCA can be used to identify meaningful classes (i.e., subgroups) of participants with distinct patterns of risk behaviors. A related method, latent transition analysis (LTA) allows one to estimate movement or transitions between subgroups over time.

Method 5: Impact Factor

The significance of intervention effects is moderated by the generalizability of the individuals willing to participate. An important outcome measure that incorporates intervention efficacy and participation rates is impact. Impact is increased by greater intervention efficacy and greater participation among individuals in the target population. For interventions targeting single-risk behaviors, impact has been measured as intervention efficacy (E) times participation (P) or $I = E \times P$. In MRBC interventions, measures for assessing impact need to account for the number of behaviors treated effectively. In MRBC interventions, impact may be considered as intervention efficacy times participation summed over the multiple behavioral targets, $I = \Sigma_{\text{# of behaviors(n)}} (E_n \times P_n)$. Here, P is the proportion of at-risk individuals participating in the intervention for each behavior. E is the estimate of efficacy for each behavior. Use of a common metric, such as the percentage no longer at risk (i.e., the percentage reaching Action or Maintenance), allows for summation across behaviors. This revised-impact equation provides a measure for assessing the impact of interventions for treating individuals and populations with multiple behavior risks (Table 12.1).

Use and Comparison Across Analytic Methods

A nonsystematic "scoping review" was conducted to describe the types of analyses used in research on multiple health behaviors (McAloney, Graham, Law, & Platt, 2013).

TABLE 12.1 Application of the Impact Formula for Quantifying Multiple-Risk Behavior Change Intervention Impact on Study Participants and the Overall Target Population

$$\text{Impact} = \Sigma_{\text{\# of behaviors (n)}}(E_{\text{fficacy}} \times P_{\text{articipation}})$$

STUDY	TARGET BEHAVIOR	PERCENTAGE AT RISK	EFFICACY AT 24 MO.	INDIVIDUAL IMPACT	IMPACT ON PARTICIPANTS	IMPACT ON POP.
Primary care patients (Prochaska et al., 2005) N=5407	Smoking	22%	25%	0.06	0.43	0.30
	Diet	68%	29%	0.20		RR=0.69
	Sun Exposure	71%	23%	0.17		
Parents of HS students (Prochaska et al., 2004) N=2460	Smoking	29%	22%	0.06	0.53	0.45
	Diet	74%	34%	0.25		RR=0.84
	Sun exposure	73%	30%	0.22		

The scoping review approach has its limitations: namely, it is not comprehensive in its search strategy. For example, MRBC intervention trials were not well represented. Nevertheless, the review identified two interesting trends: (1) a time trend with more publications on multiple risks published more recently, and (2) an analytic complexity effect with more recent publications applying more sophisticated methods. Though there was some inconsistency in the use of terminology, the earlier studies tended to be limited to examination of co-occurrence, which is calculated by dividing the observed prevalence by expected prevalence. This approach examines patterns of behavior rather than patterns of behavior change, with co-occurrence values greater than 1.00 indicating a greater prevalence than expected and values less than 1.00 indicating a lower than expected prevalence. Notably, more recent literature has applied more sophisticated analytic methods (e.g., LCA and factor analysis) with modeling of latent, or unobservable, patterns in associations among behaviors, including changes over time. No mention was made of use of the impact factor formula or other MRBC indices, though, again, few interventions were represented.

Carlson, Sallis, Ramirez, Patrick, and Norman, (2012) recently evaluated a physical activity and nutrition intervention and compared two analytic methods for summarizing MRBC outcomes: standardized residualized change scores and a behavioral index. The investigators concluded that while the residualized change score, as a continuous measure, had greater power to detect an effect, the behavioral index was more easily interpreted. Analyzing data from two cluster-randomized MRBC trials, Drake et al. (2013) compared summative, z-score, optimal linear combination, and impact scores and found comparable results with regard to overall behavior change outcomes regardless of method. The statistical significance of the individual risk behaviors, however, differed some by population and approach with effects less likely to be significant with the summative index, which dichotomized outcomes. Given the nascent stage of MRBC intervention research, particularly with regard to conceptualizing overall or global behavioral change, we encourage investigators to report outcomes utilizing multiple approaches to allow for comparison within and across trials.

THEORY TESTING ACROSS BEHAVIORS

Theories of behavior and behavior change have been applied across a wide variety of risk factors, demonstrating that the same skills can be applied to multiple behaviors. A model of lifestyle behavior change has suggested that with behaviors that co-occur (e.g., alcohol abuse and smoking), change in one may support change in the other (Wankel & Sefton, 1994). At this time, however, no theory of behavior change directly addresses the issue of how to intervene on more than one behavior simultaneously.

TTM, discussed earlier, was developed in the area of smoking cessation and has demonstrated relevance to over 48 problem or target behaviors (Hall & Rossi, 2008; Prochaska et al., 1994). Across multiple health behaviors, significant cross-sectional associations have been found with the TTM mediators of change. Among adults, the pros and cons for smoking were inversely associated with the pros and cons of exercising (King, Marcus, Pinto, Emmons, & Abrams, 1996). That is, individuals rating the benefits of smoking highly were less likely to endorse the benefits of physical activity as self-important. Self-efficacy for smoking cessation also was significantly related to self-efficacy for exercise. While the data were cross-sectional in nature, the authors concluded that the associations provide preliminary evidence for how change in one behavior may be related to change in another. Individuals working on increasing their physical activity seem motivated and confident about decreasing their smoking and vice versa. Similarly, Unger (1996) observed that adults in the later stages of change for smoking cessation had more healthful levels of alcohol use and exercised more than subjects in the earlier stages of change, suggesting people changing on their own may make improvements in several health behaviors concurrently. Lippke, Nigg, and Maddock (2012) analyzed co-occurrence in nutrition, physical activity, and smoking behaviors in three samples (total of 4,794 participants) from the United States and Germany and found that while correlations among risks were relatively weak ($r < 0.30$), individuals at a higher stage of change for one behavior were more likely to be at a higher stage for another behavior. The authors concluded success in one behavior may facilitate change in other behaviors and recommended that interventions target behavioral patterns rather than single behaviors.

The PREVENT trial, which utilized SCT, broadened intervention goals to include raising participants' self-efficacy for changing multiple risks by helping them recognize the natural intersections among their risky health habits. General cognitive and behavioral skills also were taught for application in changing any of their risk behaviors (Emmons et al., 2005).

CONSIDERATIONS FOR DISSEMINATION

Most of the early successes in MRBC interventions were achieved in research clinics or specialty settings, and serious considerations need to be taken into account when planning for dissemination. From the practitioner's perspective, there are legitimate concerns about addressing more than one behavioral risk at a time. It can be very challenging for health care professionals to try to impact behavioral changes through counseling or other forms of intervention within short medical appointments. A clever health message for promoting changes in multiple-risk behaviors is 0–5–10–25, indicating 0 cigarettes, 5 servings of fruits and vegetables, 10,000 steps, and a body mass index of less than 25 (Reeves & Rafferty, 2005).

In designing programs for dissemination, key considerations include: (1) involving the target population and organizations in intervention design and development; (2) reducing individual and organizational barriers to participation; and (3) being mindful of feasibility issues and the breadth of appeal of the intervention to the target system (Nigg, Allegrante, & Ory, 2002).

Experts in the field have concluded that using interactive behavior change technologies and tailored feedback are the current best practices for addressing multiple risks in primary care (Glasgow, Bull, Piette, & Steiner, 2004; Goldstein et al., 2004; Noar, Benac, & Harris, 2007). Interactive behavior change technologies have been praised for offering a viable solution to the otherwise overwhelming problem of addressing prevention effectively in primary care. Computer-tailored interventions are self-directed, generate tailored feedback to participants, maintain treatment fidelity, and are an important dissemination option.

Moving beyond the clinic, schools and worksites are becoming important channels for distribution of MRBCs. Computer-tailored interventions can reside on a school's web server. Teachers do not require additional training, as their main responsibility is to assist students in starting and completing the program. The programs provide a private interaction for youth to address sensitive issues such as experiences with bullying and experimentation with substance use. Because the programs are tailored to individuals' readiness to adopt or cease a risk behavior, they are broadly relevant to the populations served. Within a worksite, employees can take a comprehensive health risk appraisal online and then be guided to work on their identified risk behaviors. In addition to computer-tailored feedback, participants can be referred to personalized activity centers with activities to increase engagement in effective change processes.

As one example of success with disseminating MRBC interventions to clinics, schools, and worksites, Pro-Change Behavior Systems, with funding from the National Institutes of Health, has focused on developing and disseminating evidence-based behavior change programs. The programs utilize stage-based computer-tailored interventions to target multiple-risk behaviors, including weight gain (physical inactivity and poor diet), bullying, and high cholesterol. The programs have been disseminated nationally to more than 500 schools, 100 worksites, and 200,000 adults and youths. The programs have been well received and well used and have delivered significant impacts on multiple behavioral risks (Evers, Prochaska, Van Marter, Johnson, & Prochaska, 2007; Johnson et al., 2008; Mauriello et al., 2010; Velicer et al., 2013).

The Internet provides a convenient option for dissemination, but it still can be difficult to engage individuals. In the research literature, Internet-delivered intervention trials have reported participation rates as low as 2% to 10% and retention rates as low as 20% (Glasgow et al., 2007; Rothert et al., 2006). Through our research and dissemination practices, we have found that participation rates range greatly depending on the types of incentives employed (see Table 12.2).

CONCLUSIONS

Nearly 10 years ago, the need for multiple-risk, transbehavioral research models and paradigms was emphasized (Orleans, 2004). Specific research questions that remain include "whether, or in which situations, multiple-risk factor interventions are more effective or efficient at reducing risk than targeted single interventions" (Atkins & Clancy, 2004). For example, some attribute the success of tobacco cessation initiatives to a narrowly focused research and policy agenda. Research is needed to determine under what conditions multiple risks can be targeted without diminishing the effectiveness on any single behavior (Atkins & Clancy, 2004). Other areas in need of greater research are interventions that integrate efforts to change multiple-risk behaviors, as well as interventions that teach change strategies that can be generalized to multiple behavior change goals. With increased interest in MRBC interventions, the field will need ways to conceptualize

TABLE 12.2 Recruitment Incentives and Participation Rates

RECRUITMENT INCENTIVE	MECHANISM	PARTICIPATION RATE
Persuasive messages in letter or e-mails with or without a token incentive (e.g., T-shirt or $15 coupon)	Social influence	20%–30%
Positive reinforcement in the form of $150 to $300	Social influence	40%–50%
Personal outreach through face-to-face or phone call contact	Social influence	60%–70%
Negative reinforcement by requiring all nonparticipants to face some increase in financial payment for their health care plan for not participating	Social control	80%–90% (but do get negative reaction)

and analyze the issue of overall behavior change (Prochaska, Velicer, Nigg, & Prochaska, 2008).

If the challenge of MRBC intervention is met, health promotion and disease management programs will significantly affect entire populations. Such impacts require scientific and professional shifts from:

1. An action paradigm to a stage paradigm;
2. Reactive recruitment to a public health approach of proactive recruitment (that is, reaching out proactively to individuals and populations to engage them in MRBC interventions, rather than waiting passively in the clinic to react to the small proportion of patients who will seek services);
3. The expectation that participants must match the needs of programs to the understanding that programs must match their needs;
4. Clinic-based to population-based programs that are able to apply the field's most powerful individualized and interactive intervention strategies;
5. Single-behavior-change programs to MRBC programs for entire populations.

If the health behavior change field makes these paradigm shifts, a behavior health delivery system could be developed to reach many more people with behaviors that are the major killers and cost drivers in the United States. How can population approaches to health promotion be funded? Longitudinal data indicate that effectively treating two behaviors reduces health care costs by about $2,000 per year (Edington, 2001). For worksites, the return on investment (ROI) for employee participation in MRBC programs is estimated at 1.98 over three years' time, on the basis of reductions in absenteeism and workers' compensation hours, nearly a twofold ROI (Schultz et al., 2002). Population-based behavioral medicine is one of the few opportunities for health care systems to increase services that improve health and reduce health care costs. Over time, population-based prevention programs could pay for themselves.

We can envision a health care system in the near future where interactive MRBC interventions will be to behavioral medicine what pharmaceuticals are to biological medicine—one of the most cost-effective methods to bring optimal amounts of science to bear on multiple behavior problems, in entire populations, in a relatively user-friendly manner, without many of the side effects seen with pharmaceuticals.

REFERENCES

Atkins, D., & Clancy, C. (2004). Multiple-risk factors interventions. Are we up to the challenge? *American Journal of Preventive Medicine, 27*(2 Suppl.), 102–103.

Babyak, M., Blumenthal, J. A., Herman, S., Khatri, P., Doraiswamy, M., Moore, K., … Krishnan, K. R. (2000). Exercise treatment for major depression: Maintenance of therapeutic benefit at 10 months. *Psychosomatic Medicine, 62*(5), 633–638.

Bandura, A. (1986). *Social foundations of thought and action: A social cognitive theory.* Englewood Cliffs, NJ: Prentice-Hall.

Berrigan, D., Dodd, K., Troiano, R. P., Krebs-Smith, S. M., & Barbash, R. B. (2003). Patterns of health behavior in US adults. *Preventive Medicine, 36*(5), 615–623.

Bien, T. H., & Burge, R. (1990). Smoking and drinking: A review of the literature. *International Journal of Mental Health & Addiction, 25*(12), 1429–1454.

Blissmer, B., Prochaska, J. O., Velicer, W. F., Redding, C. A., Rossi, J. S., Greene, G. W., & Robbins, M. L. (2010). Common factors predicting long-term changes in multiple health behaviors. *Journal of Health Psychology, 15*, 201–214.

Burton, W. N., Chen, C. Y., Conti, D. J., Schultz, A. B., & Edington, D. W. (2003). Measuring the relationship between employees' health risk factors and corporate pharmaceutical expenditures. *Journal of Occupational and Environmental Medicine, 45*(8), 793–802.

Burton, W. N., Chen, C. Y., Conti, D. J., Schultz, A. B., Pransky, G., & Edington, D. W. (2005). The association of health risks with on-the-job productivity. *Journal of Occupational and Environmental Medicine, 47*(8), 769–777.

Carlson, J. A., Sallis, J. F., Ramirez, E. R., Patrick, K., & Norman, G. J. (2012). Physical activity and dietary behavior change in Internet-based weight loss interventions: Comparing two multiple-behavior change indices. *Preventive Medicine, 54*(1), 50–54.

Conry, M. C., Morgan, K., Curry, P., McGee, H., Harrington, J., Ward, M., & Shelley, E. (2011). The clustering of health behaviors in Ireland and their relationship with mental health, self-related health and quality of life. *BMC Public Health, 11*, 692–702.

Drake, B. F., Quintilliani, L. M., Sapp, A. L., Li, Y., Harley, A. E., Emmons, K. M., & Sorensen, G. (2013). Comparing strategies to assess multiple behavior change in behavioral intervention studies. *Translational Behavioral Medicine, 3*(1), 114–121.

DuRant, R. H., Smith, J. A., Kreiter, S. R., & Krowchuk, D. P. (1999). The relationship between early age of onset of initial substance use and engaging in multiple health risk behaviors among young adolescents. *Archives of Pediatric & Adolescent Medicine, 153*(3), 286–291.

Ebrahim, S., Taylor, F., Ward, K., Beswick, A., Burke, M., & Davey Smith, G. (2011). Multiple-risk factor interventions for primary prevention of coronary heart disease. *Cochrane Database of Systematic Reviews*, (1), CD001561. doi: 10.1002/14651858.CD001561.pub3

Edington, D. W. (2001). Emerging research: A view from one research center. *American Journal of Health Promotion, 15*(5), 341–349.

Edington, D. W., Yen, L. T., & Witting, P. (1997). The financial impact of changes in personal health practices. *Journal of Occupational & Environmental Medicine, 39*(11), 1037–1046.

Emmons, K. M., Marcus, B. H., Linnan, L., Rossi, J. S., & Abrams, D. B. (1994). Mechanisms in multiple-risk factor interventions: Smoking, physical activity, and dietary fat intake among manufacturing workers. Working Well Research Group. *Preventive Medicine, 23*(4), 481–489.

Emmons, K. M., McBride, C. M., Puleo, E., Pollak, K. I., Clipp, E., Kuntz, K., … Fletcher, R. (2005). Project PREVENT: A randomized trial to reduce multiple behavioral risk factors for colon cancer. *Cancer Epidemiology Biomarkers & Prevention, 14*(6), 1453–1459.

Evers, K. E., Prochaska, J. O., Van Marter, D., Johnson, J. L., & Prochaska, J. M. (2007). Transtheoretical-based bullying prevention effectiveness trial in middle schools and high schools. *Educational Research, 49*, 397–414.

Fine, L. J., Philogene, G. S., Gramling, R., Coups, E. J., & Sinha, S. (2004). Prevalence of multiple chronic disease risk factors. 2001 National Health Interview Survey. *American Journal of Preventive Medicine, 27*(2 Suppl.), 18–24.

Fiore, M. C., Jaen, C. R., Baker, T. B., et al. (2008). *Treating tobacco use and dependence: 2008 update. Clinical practice guideline.* Rockville, MD. From http://www.ahrq.gov/professionals/clinicians-providers/guidelines-recommendations/tobacco/clinicians/treating_tobacco_use08.pdf

Glasgow, R. E., Bull, S. S., Piette, J. D., & Steiner, J. F. (2004). Interactive behavior change technology. A partial solution to the competing demands of primary care. *American Journal of Preventive Medicine, 27*(2 Suppl.), 80–87.

Glasgow, R. E., Nelson, C. C., Kearney, K. A., Reid, R., Ritzwoller, D. P., Strecher, V. J., … Wildenhaus, K. (2007). Reach, engagement, and retention in an Internet-based weight loss program in a multi-site randomized controlled trial. *Journal of Medical Internet Research, 9*(2), e11.

Goldstein, M. G., Whitlock, E. P., & DePue, J. (2004). Multiple behavioral risk factor interventions in primary care. Summary of research evidence. *American Journal of Preventive Medicine, 27*(2 Suppl.), 61–79.

Gortmaker, S. L., Peterson, K., Wiecha, J., Sobol, A. M., Dixit, S., Fox, M. K., & Laird, N. (1999). Reducing obesity via a school-based interdisciplinary intervention among youth: Planet health. *Archives of Pediatric & Adolescent Medicine, 153*(4), 409–418.

Goodman, M. S., Li, Y., Bennett, G. G., Stoddard, A. M., & Emmons, K. M. (2006). An evaluation of multiple behavioral risk factors for cancer in a working class, multi-ethnic population. *Journal of Data Science, 4*, 291–306.

Haasova, M., Warren, F. C., Ussher, M., Janse Van Rensburg, K., Faulkner, G., Cropley, M., … Taylor, A. (2012). The acute effects of physical activity on cigarette cravings: Systematic review and meta-analysis with individual participant data. *Addiction, 108*, 26–37.

Haerens, L., Deforche, B., Maes, L., Stevens, V., Cardon, G., & De Bourdeaudhuij, I. (2006). Body mass effects of a physical activity and healthy food intervention in middle schools. *Obesity, 14*(5), 847–854.

Hall, K. L., & Rossi, J. S. (2008). Meta-analytic examination of the strong and weak principles across 48 health behaviors. *Preventive Medicine, 46*, 266–274.

Hall, S. M., Tunstall, C. D., Vila, K. L., & Duffy, J. (1992). Weight gain prevention and smoking cessation: Cautionary findings. *American Journal of Public Health, 82*(6), 799–803.

Hamelink-Basteen, K., Houben, F., Bun, C., & De Wit, N. (2008). Prevention and reduction of over-weight in primary school children. *Huisarts en Wetenschap, 51*(13), 651–656.

Hayes, S. C., Barlow, D. H., & Nelson-Gray, R. O. (1999). *The scientist practitioner: Research and accountability in the age of managed care* (2nd ed.). Boston, MA: Allyn & Bacon.

Hser, Y. I., McCarthy, W. J., & Anglin, M. D. (1994). Tobacco use as a distal predictor of mortality among long-term narcotics addicts. *Preventive Medicine, 23*(1), 61–69.

Hurt, R. D., Offord, K. P., Croghan, I. T., Gomez-Dahl, L., Kottke, T. E., Morse, R. M., & Melton, L. J., 3rd. (1996). Mortality following inpatient addictions treatment. Role of tobacco use in a community-based cohort. *Journal of the American Medical Association, 275*(14), 1097–1103.

Hyman, D. J., Pavlik, V. N., Taylor, W. C., Goodrick, G. K., & Moye, L. (2007). Simultaneous vs sequential counseling for multiple behavior change. *Archives of Internal Medicine, 167*(11), 1152–1158.

Janssen, I., Katzmarzyk, P. T., Church, T. S., & Blair, S. N. (2005). The Cooper Clinic Mortality Risk Index: Clinical score sheet for men. *American Journal of Preventive Medicine, 29*(3), 194–203.

Johnson, S. S., Driskell, M. M., Johnson, J. L., Dyment, S. J., Prochaska, J. O., Prochaska, J. M., & Bourne, L. (2006). Transtheoretical model intervention for adherence to lipid-lowering drugs. *Disease Management, 9*(2), 102–114.

Johnson, S. S., Paiva, A. L., Cummins, C. O., Johnson, J. L., Dyment, S. J., Wright, J. A., Prochaska, J. M., … Sherman, K. (2008). Transtheoretical model-based multiple behavior intervention for weight management: Effectiveness on a population basis. *Preventive Medicine, 46*, 238–246.

Jones, H., Edwards, L., Vallis, T. M., Ruggiero, L., Rossi, S. R., Rossi, J. S., … Diabetes Stages of Change (DiSC) Study. (2003). Changes in diabetes self-care behaviors make a difference in glycemic control: The Diabetes Stages of Change (DiSC) study. *Diabetes Care, 26*(3), 732–737.

Joseph, A. M., Willenbring, M. L., Nugent, S. M., & Nelson, D. B. (2004). A randomized trial of concurrent versus delayed smoking intervention for patients in alcohol dependence treatment. *Journal of Studies on Alcohol, 65*(6), 681–691.

Ketola, E., Sipila, R., & Makela, M. (2002). Effectiveness of individual lifestyle interventions in reducing cardiovascular disease and risk factors. *Annals of Medicine, 32*(4), 239–251.

King, T. K., Marcus, B. H., Pinto, B. M., Emmons, K. M., & Abrams, D. B. (1996). Cognitive behavioral mediators of changing multiple behaviors: Smoking and a sedentary lifestyle. *Preventive Medicine, 25*(6), 684–691.

Klesges, R. C., Eck, L. H., Isbell, T. R., Fulliton, W., & Hanson, C. L. (1990). Smoking status: Effects on the dietary intake, physical activity, and body fat of adult men. *American Journal of Clinical Nutrition, 51*(5), 784–789.

Koshy, P., Mackenzie, M., Leslie, W., Lean, M., & Hankey, C. (2012). Eating the elephant whole or in slices: Views of participants in a smoking cessation intervention trial on multiple behaviour changes as sequential or concurrent tasks. *BMC Public Health, 12*, 500.

Labarthe, D. R. (1998). *Epidemiology and prevention of cardiovascular disease: A global challenge.* Gaithersburg, MD: Aspen.

Lai, S., Lai, H., Page, J. B., & McCoy, C. B. (2000). The association between cigarette smoking and drug abuse in the United States. *Journal of Addictive Diseases, 19*(4), 11–24.

Lanas, F., Avezum, A., Bautista, L. E., Diaz, R., Luna, M., Islam, S., … INTERHEART Investigators in Latin America. (2007). Risk factors for acute myocardial infarction in Latin America: The INTER-HEART Latin American study. *Circulation, 115*(9), 1067–1074.

Leslie, W. S., Koshy, P. R., Mackenzie, M., Murray, H. M., Boyle, S., Lean, M. E., Walker, A., & Hankey, C. R. (2012). Changes in body weight and food choice in those attempting smoking cessation: A cluster randomised controlled trial. *BMC Public Health, 12*, 389.

Lippke, S., Nigg, C. R., & Maddock, J. E. (2012). Health-promoting and health-risk behaviors: Theory-driven analyses of multiple health behavior change in three international samples. *International Journal of Behavioral Medicine, 19*, 1–13.

Marcus, B. H., Albrecht, A. E., King, T. K., Parisi, A. F., Pinto, B. M., Roberts, M., … Abrams, D. B. (1999). The efficacy of exercise as an aid for smoking cessation in women: A randomized controlled trial. *Archives of Internal Medicine, 159*(11), 1229–1234.

Mauriello, L. M., Ciavatta, M. M., Paiva, A. L., Sherman, K. J., Castle, P. H., Johnson, J. L., & Prochaska, J. M. (2010). Results of a multi-media multiple behavior obesity prevention program for adolescents. *Preventive Medicine, 51*, 451–456.

McAloney, K., Graham, H., Law, C., & Platt, L. (2013). A scoping review of statistical approaches to the analysis of multiple health-related behaviors. *Preventive Medicine, 56*(6), 365–371.

McGue, M., Iacono, W. G., & Krueger, R. (2006). The association of early adolescent problem behavior and adult psychopathology: A multivariate behavioral genetic perspective. *Behavioral Genetics, 36*(4), 591–602.

Nigg, C. R., Allegrante, J. P., & Ory, M. (2002). Theory-comparison and multiple-behavior research: Common themes advancing health behavior research. *Health Education Research, 17*(5), 670–679.

Noar, S. M., Benac, C. N., & Harris, M. S. (2007). Does tailoring matter? Meta-analytic review of tailored print health behavior change interventions. *American Psychological Association Psychological Bulletin, 133*(4), 673–693.

Norris, S. L., Engelgau, M. M., & Narayan, K. M. (2001). Effectiveness of self-management training in type 2 diabetes: A systematic review of randomized controlled trials. *Diabetes Care, 24*(3), 561–587.

Nylund, K. L., Asparouhov, T., & Muthen, B. O. (2007). Deciding on the number of classes in latent class analysis and growth mixture modeling: A Monte Carlo simulation study. *Structural Equation Modeling: A Multidisciplinary Journal, 14*(4), 535–569.

Orleans, C. T. (2004). Addressing multiple behavioral health risks in primary care. Broadening the focus of health behavior change research and practice. *American Journal of Preventive Medicine, 27*(2 Suppl.), 1–3.

Ornish, D., Scherwitz, L. W., Billings, J. H., Brown, S. E., Gould, K. L., Merritt, T. A., … Brand, R. J.(1998). Intensive lifestyle changes for reversal of coronary heart disease. *Journal of the American Medical Association, 280*(23), 2001–2007.

Paiva, A. L., Prochaska, J. O., Yin, H. Q., Rossi, J. S., Redding, C. A., Blissmer, B., … Horiuchi, S. (2012). Treated individuals who progress to action or maintenance for one behavior are more likely to make similar progress on another behavior: Coaction results of a pooled data analysis of three trials. *Preventive Medicine, 54*(5), 331–334.

Parekh, S., King, D., Owen, N., & Jamrozik, K. (2009). Spousal concordance and reliability of the 'Prudence Score' as a summary of diet and lifestyle. *Australia & New Zealand Journal of Public Health, 33*(4), 320–324.

Parekh, S., Vandelanotte, C., King, D., & Boyle, F. M. (2012). Improving diet, physical activity and other lifestyle behaviours using computer-tailored advice in general practice: A randomised controlled trial. *International Journal of Physical Activity and Nutrition, 9*, 108.

Parker, G., & Crawford, J. (2007). Judged effectiveness of differing antidepressant strategies by those with clinical depression. *Australian & New Zealand Journal of Psychiatry, 41*(1), 32–37.

Patterson, F. (2013). Multiple health behaviour change in sequence: The case for physical activity and smoking cessation. *Journal of Health Behavior and Public Health, 3*(1), 1–4.

Patterson, R. E., Haines, P. S., & Popkin, B. M. (1994). Diet quality index: Capturing a multidimensional behavior. *Journal of the American Dietetic Association, 94*(1), 57–64.

Perkins, K. A., Rohay, J., Meilahn, E. N., Wing, R. R., Matthews, K. A., & Kuller, L. H. (1993). Diet, alcohol, and physical activity as a function of smoking status in middle-aged women. *Health Psychology, 12*(5), 410–415.

Prochaska, J. J., Delucchi, K., & Hall, S. M. (2004). A meta-analysis of smoking cessation interventions with individuals in substance abuse treatment or recovery. *Journal of Consulting & Clinical Psychology, 72*(6), 1144–1156.

Prochaska, J. J., Nigg, C. R., Spring, B., Velicer, W. F., & Prochaska, J. O. (2010). The benefits and challenges of multiple health behavior change in research and in practice. *Preventive Medicine, 50*, 26–29.

Prochaska, J. J., & Prochaska, J. O. (2011). A review of multiple health behavior change interventions for primary prevention. *American Journal of Lifestyle Medicine, 5*, 208–221.

Prochaska, J. J., Velicer, W. F., Nigg, C. R., & Prochaska, J. O. (2008). Methods of quantifying change in multiple-risk factor interventions. *Preventive Medicine, 46*, 260–265.

Prochaska, J. J., Velicer, W. F., Prochaska, J. O., Delucchi, K., & Hall, S. M. (2006). Comparing intervention outcomes in smokers treated for single versus multiple behavioral risks. *Health Psychology, 25*(3), 380–388.

Prochaska, J. O. (2006). Moving beyond the transtheoretical model. *Addiction, 101*, 768–778.

Prochaska, J. O., DiClemente, C. C., & Norcross, J. C. (1992). In search of how people change. Applications to addictive behaviors. *American Psychologist, 47*(9), 1102–1114.

Prochaska, J. O., Evers, K. E., Castle, P. H., Johnson, J. L., Prochaska, J. M., Rula, E. Y., ... Pope, J. E. (2012). Enhancing multiple domains of well-being by decreasing multiple health risk behaviors: A randomized clinical trial. *Population Health Management, 15*(5), 276–286.

Prochaska, J. O., Velicer, W. F., Redding, C., Rossi, J. S., Goldstein, M., DePue, J., ... Plummer, B. A. (2005). Stage-based expert systems to guide a population of primary care patients to quit smoking, eat healthier, prevent skin cancer, and receive regular mammograms. *Preventive Medicine, 41*(2), 406–416.

Prochaska, J. O., Velicer, W. F., Rossi, J. S., Goldstein, M. G., Marcus, B. H., Rakowski, W., ... Rossi, S. R. (1994). Stages of change and decisional balance for 12 problem behaviors. *Health Psychology, 13*(1), 39–46.

Prochaska, J. O., Velicer, W. F., Rossi, J. S., Redding, C. A., Greene, G. W., Rossi, S. R., ... Plummer, B. A. (2004). Multiple-risk expert systems interventions: Impact of simultaneous stage-matched expert system interventions for smoking, high-fat diet, and sun exposure in a population of parents. *Health Psychology, 23*(5), 503–516.

Pronk, N. P., Anderson, L. H., Crain, A. L., Martinson, B. C., O'Connor, P. J., Sherwood, N. E., & Whitebird, R. R. (2004). Meeting recommendations for multiple healthy lifestyle factors. Prevalence, clustering, and predictors among adolescent, adult, and senior health plan members. *American Journal of Preventive Medicine, 27*(2 Suppl.), 25–33.

Rasanen, P., Roine, E., Sintonen, H., Semberg-Konttinen, V., Ryynanen, O. P., & Roine, R. (2006). Use of quality-adjusted life years for the estimation of effectiveness of health care: A systematic literature review. *International Journal of Technology Assessment in Health Care, 22*(2), 235–241.

Reeves, M. J., & Rafferty, A. P. (2005). Healthy lifestyle characteristics among adults in the United States, 2000. *Archives of Internal Medicine, 165*(8), 854–857.

Roberts, V., Maddison, R., Simpson, C., Bullen, C., & Prapavessis, H. (2012). The acute effects of exercise on cigarette cravings, withdrawal symptoms, affect, and smoking behaviour: Systematic review update and meta-analysis. *Psychopharmacology, 222*, 1–15.

Rothert, K., Strecher, V. J., Doyle, L. A., Caplan, W. M., Joyce, J. S., Jimison, H. B., ... Roth, M. A. (2006). Web-based weight management programs in an integrated health care setting: A randomized, controlled trial. *Obesity (Silver Spring), 14*(2), 266–272.

Sallis, J. F., Prochaska, J. J., & Taylor, W. C. (2000). A review of correlates of physical activity of children and adolescents. *Medicine & Science in Sports & Exercise, 32*(5), 963–975.

Schultz, A. B., Lu, C., Barnett, T. E., Yen, L. T., McDonald, T., Hirschland, D., & Edington, D. W. (2002). Influence of participation in a worksite health-promotion program on disability days. *Journal of Occupational & Environmental Medicine, 44*(8), 776–780.

Singh, A. S., Paw, M. J., Brug, J., & van Mechelen, W. (2007). Short-term effects of school-based weight gain prevention among adolescents. *Archives of Pediatric & Adolescent Medicine, 161*(6), 565–571.

Smith, K. W., McKinlay, S. M., & McKinlay, J. B. (1989). The reliability of health risk appraisals: A field trial of four instruments. *American Journal of Public Health, 79*(12), 1603–1607.

Society for Research on Nicotine and Tobacco. (2002). Biochemical verification of tobacco use and cessation. *Nicotine & Tobacco Research, 4*(2), 149–159.

Sorensen, G., Thompson, B., Glanz, K., Feng, Z., Kinne, S., DiClemente, C., ... Lichtenstein, E. (1996). Worksite-based cancer prevention: Primary results from the Working Well Trial. *American Journal of Public Health, 86*(7), 939–947.

Spencer, C. A., Jamrozik, K., Lawrence-Brown, M., & Norman, P. E. (2005). Lifestyle still predicts mortality in older men with established vascular disease. *Preventive Medicine, 41*(2), 583–588.

Spring, B., Howe, D., Berendsen, M., McFadden, H. G., Hitchcock, K., Rademaker, A. W., & Hitsman, B. (2009). Behavioral intervention to promote smoking cessation and prevent weight gain: A systematic review and meta-analysis. *Addiction, 104*, 1472–1486.

Spring, B., Pagoto, S., Pingitore, R., Doran, N., Schneider, K., & Hedeker, D. (2004). Randomized controlled trial for behavioral smoking and weight control treatment: Effect of concurrent versus sequential intervention. *Journal of Consulting & Clinical Psychology, 72*(5), 785–796.

Toobert, D. J., Glasgow, R. E., Strycker, L. A., Barrera, M., Jr., Ritzwoller, D. P., & Weidner, G. (2007). Long-term effects of the Mediterranean lifestyle program: A randomized clinical trial for postmenopausal women with type 2 diabetes. *International Journal of Behavioral Nutrition & Physical Activity, 4*, 1–12.

Tucker, L. R., Damarin, F., & Messick, S. (1966). A base-free measure of change. *Psychometrika, 31*(4), 457–473.

Unger, J. B. (1996). Stages of change of smoking cessation: Relationships with other health behaviors. *American Journal of Preventive Medicine, 12*(2), 134–138.

U.S. Department of Health & Human Services. (1999). *Mental health: A report of the Surgeon General.* Washington, DC: Author.

Ussher, M., Taylor, A., & Faulkner, G. (2012). Exercise interventions for smoking cessation. *Cochrane Database of Systematic Reviews,* (1), CD002295. doi: 10.1002/14651858.CD002295.pub4

Vandelanotte, C., Reeves, M. M., Brug, J., & de Bourdeaudhuij, I. (2008). A randomized trial of sequential and simultaneous multiple behavior change interventions for physical activity and fat intake. *Preventive Medicine, 46*(3), 232–237.

Veldman, D. J., & Brophy, J. (1974). Measuring teacher effects on pupil achievement. *Journal of Educational Psychology, 66*(3), 319–324.

Velicer, W. F., Prochaska, J. O., Redding, C. A., Rossi, J. S., Sun, X., & Greene, G. W. (2004). Efficacy of expert system interventions for employees to decrease smoking, dietary fat, and sun exposure (Abstract). *International Journal of Behavioral Medicine, 11*(Suppl.), 277.

Velicer, W. F., Redding, C. A., Paiva, A. L., Mauriello, L. M., Blissmer, B., Oatley, K., ... Fernandes, A. C. (2013). Multiple behavior interventions to prevent substance abuse and increase energy balance behaviors in middle school students. *Translational Behavior Medicine, 3*, 82–93.

Waters, E., de Silva-Sanigorski, A., Hall, B. J., Brown, T., Campbell, K. J., Gao, Y., ... Summerbell, C. D. (2011). Interventions for preventing obesity in children. *Cochrane Database of Systematic Reviews,* (12), CD001871. doi: 10.1002/14651858.CD001871.pub3

Wankel, L. M., & Sefton, J. M. (Eds.). (1994). *Physical activity, fitness, and health: International proceedings and consensus statement.* Champaign, IL: Human Kinetics.

Wilson, P. W., D'Agostino, R. B., Levy, D., Belanger, A. M., Silbershatz, H., & Kannel, W. B. (1998). Prediction of coronary heart disease using risk factor categories. *Circulation, 97*(18), 1837–1847.

Woolcott, C. T., Disman, R. K., Motl, R. W., Matthai, C. H., & Nigg, C. R. (2013). Physical activity and fruit and vegetable intake: Correlations between and within adults in a longitudinal multiethnic cohort. *American Journal of Health Promotion.* Retrieved from http://www.ncbi.nlm.nih.gov/pubmed/?term=woolcott+disman+motl+nigg

Wright, D. W., Beard, M. J., & Edington, D. W. (2002). Association of health risks with the cost of time away from work. *Journal of Occupational and Environmental Medicine, 44*(12), 1126–1134.

Yusuf, S., Hawken, S., Ounpuu, S., Dans, T., Avezum, A., Lanas, F., ... INTERHEART Study Investigators. (2004). Effect of potentially modifiable risk factors associated with myocardial infarction in 52 countries (the INTERHEART study): Case-control study. *Lancet, 364*(9438), 937–952.

IV

Chronic Disease Management Interventions

The Centers for Disease Control and Prevention (CDC) states that chronic diseases "are among the most common, costly and preventable of all health problems in the U.S." As the population in the United States and elsewhere ages and health care innovations advance, self-care regimens for chronic illnesses often increase in complexity. Section IV highlights the challenges of maintaining positive health behavior and adherence while living with a chronic health condition. Despite experiencing negative health outcomes, adherence to a lifelong treatment regimen is often low. Recurring themes among the chapters are the need for multicomponent interventions and the importance of addressing health disparities. Research across all chronic illnesses consistently shows that disease- and treatment-focused education is insufficient to change behavior.

In Chapter 13, "Chronic Disease Management Interventions: Cardiovascular Disease," Hayman and Mruk discuss the challenges facing those with cardiovascular disease (CVD), one of the leading causes of death worldwide. They identify three multicomponent strategies for changing individual health behaviors related to CVD and place focus on secondary prevention of future CVD events and/or mortality through interventions targeting lifestyle changes and adherence to pharmacotherapy. They stress the importance of ongoing involvement of multidisciplinary teams of health care professionals to increase the potential for success in modifying adverse health behaviors.

Hood and colleagues address the complex and demanding management of diabetes in Chapter 14, "Diabetes Management Behaviors: The Key to Optimal Health and Quality of Life Outcomes." As the rates of diabetes incidence and mortality continue to grow, new technologies are being developed that could revolutionize future treatment. In the meantime, the authors note, the engagement in modification of multiple health-related behaviors is still the single best method for optimizing health and quality of life outcomes for those individuals suffering from the disease. For those with type 1 diabetes, challenges can include adherence to medication regimens and regulating carbohydrate intake. Those with type 2 diabetes often suffer from obesity, poor nutrition, and decreased physical activity, making it daunting to change related health behaviors to manage and control the disease. The authors discuss how breaking down barriers and fostering new skills through multicomponent interventions can lead to better health outcomes, and can include connecting the individual to family- and community-based interventions and use of motivational interviewing by the provider.

Key health behaviors relating to management of asthma and chronic obstructive pulmonary disease (COPD)—the two most common chronic respiratory diseases—are discussed by Welkom and colleagues in Chapter 15, "Behavioral Management of Chronic Respiratory Diseases: Examples from Asthma and Chronic Obstructive Pulmonary Disease." Technology-based interventions such as text messaging as a reminder to take daily asthma or COPD medication or to refill prescriptions are increasingly the focus of new interventions, while interventions targeting control of indoor and outdoor pollutants, including smoke exposure, are also key behavior change targets. Current research on behavioral interventions for both diseases, including educational, family-based, health care utilization, and shared decision making, is discussed, along with smoking cessation and pulmonary rehabilitation as key components for controlling COPD. The authors conclude by emphasizing the need for more interventions at the community level, such as those that partner health plans and utilize innovative technology, to broaden their impact. They call for greater attention to behavioral outcomes in research studies, such as medication adherence and smoking cessation, in addition to the traditional outcomes of symptom burden and health care use to better understand the mechanisms of efficacious interventions.

Management of health behaviors that affect those individuals suffering from HIV is discussed by Rhodes and colleagues in Chapter 16, "Chronic Infectious Disease Management Interventions," but new to this edition are other infectious diseases, including other sexually transmitted diseases and tuberculosis (TB). Infectious diseases are uniquely different from other chronic illnesses in that often there is no drug treatment to prescribe but rather the focus of community workers and health care providers is on encouraging actions that will prevent the transmission of the illness from one person to another, including safer sex practices and steps to prevent transmission from mother to child. When there are pharmacological therapies available, such as for HIV and TB, unusually high levels of adherence are necessary. The authors discuss a seven-step framework to maintain the health and well-being of individuals living with an infectious disease and also to prevent its transmission to others, as well as three other innovative approaches: natural helper interventions, provider-delivered interventions, and directly observed therapies. They conclude by addressing the importance and accessibility of vaccines, the need to reduce regimen complexity, and the importance of managing the diseases to reduce exposure to others.

In Chapter 17, "Adherence to Treatment and Lifestyle Changes Among People With Cancer," Peterman, Victorson, and Cella present the most current research in this field which has expanded exponentially since the previous edition of the Handbook. However, research on variables associated with treatment adherence and health behavior change among people with cancer continues to lag behind that for patients with other serious illnesses, and few intervention studies have been evaluated. As new regimens of oral chemotherapy become widespread, a person's individual responsibility for disease self-management has grown while the numbers of those receiving only intravenous treatment in a clinical setting are shrinking. Furthermore, as more cancers are "cured" the individual is expected to attend surveillance visits to monitor for recurrent or new cancers or negative late effects of treatment. The authors discuss cancer-related health behaviors and evolving therapies. Issues of adherence to lifestyle modifications are discussed, as is the need for interventions—including those involving health care providers, technological advances, motivational and educational components, as well as the use of patient navigators—to lead to better health outcomes. The authors highlight the dearth of information about adherence in children, adolescents, and the elderly with cancer.

In 2013, the American Medical Association announced that obesity would be henceforth classified as a disease. Although the declaration was controversial, it underscores obesity's significance to poor health and mortality in the United States and abroad. In Chapter 18, "Obesity," Burke and Turk discuss the challenges of lifestyle modification—"the cornerstone" of weight management—in managing obesity and overweight, and current research on a variety of interventions aimed at reducing weight and improving health. The combination of reduced energy intake, increased energy output, and standard behavioral treatment is described, as are interventions that include motivational interviewing, mobile technology, pharmacological treatment, and surgery, among other components. The emerging topics for research are the use of technology as a therapeutic approach, and the need for policy-level interventions and the need to translate efficacious interventions into real world clinical practice and communities.

13
Chronic Disease Management Interventions: Cardiovascular Disease

LAURA L. HAYMAN
MONIKA M. MRUK

LEARNING OBJECTIVES

- Describe the patterns and trends in the global prevalence of cardiovascular disease (CVD).
- Identify and discuss three strategies for changing CVD-related health behaviors in individuals with or at risk for CVD.
- Describe two implications for future research designed to enhance behavior change in individuals with CVD.

EPIDEMIOLOGY AND SIGNIFICANCE OF CARDIOVASCULAR DISEASE

Cardiovascular disease (CVD) remains a major cause of morbidity and premature mortality in women and men in the United States and globally (Roger et al., 2011). On a global level, the aging population, rapid urbanization, and population growth have contributed to major fundamental changes in disease patterns. Non-communicable diseases (NCDs), such as CVD and diabetes, currently exceed communicable/infectious diseases as the world's major disease burden (World Health Organization [WHO], 2011). Of note, CVD remains the number one global cause of death, accounting for 17.3 million deaths per year; this is expected to increase to 23.6 million deaths per year by 2030. Important to highlight in this context is that low- and middle-income countries bear an excess burden of CVD-related mortality where 80% of deaths occur and usually at younger ages than in higher-income countries (WHO, 2011).

Recognizing the global burden of CVD and with awareness of insufficient investment in sustainable global and national health policies necessary to prevent and control adverse health behaviors and established risk factors for CVD, the World Heart Federation (WHF) joined the NCD community in calling for a United Nations (UN) High-level Meeting held in September 2011. A Political Declaration, signed by heads of state resulted in governments committed to the development of specific measures to address the NCD burden in a well-defined timeline (WHO, 2011). Most recently, suggested global targets to address NCDs were embraced and recommended for adoption by UN Member States (WHO, 2012). Central to prevention and management of CVD, potentially modifiable targets for both high-risk and population-based efforts include physical inactivity, elevated blood pressure, salt/sodium intake, and tobacco use. Additional suggested targets that were originally proposed (in September 2011) and remain to be endorsed for adoption by all Member States include saturated fat intake, obesity, alcohol consumption, elevated cholesterol, drug therapy to prevent CVD, and essential/generic NCD medicines and basic technologies to treat major NCDs in both public and private facilities. Endorsed by the Global Cardiovascular Task Force that includes thought leaders from WHF, the American Heart Association (AHA), the American College of Cardiology Foundation (ACCF), the European Heart Network (EHN), and the European Society of Cardiology (ESC), a major goal of efforts initiated at the 2011 UN High-level Meeting on NCDs is to reduce premature mortality from NCDs by 25% by 2025. Strategies suggested for achieving these goals include both population-based and high-risk approaches to reducing adverse health behaviors and risk factors for CVD and other NCDs, implementing tactics that guide health policy, chronic disease plans, and ultimately, resources for national public health interventions (Smith et al., 2012).

The importance of reducing the global burden of CVD, a major contributor to premature mortality from NCDs, has been recognized by the World Health Organization (WHO) and the international community of cardiovascular professionals. Consistent with this effort, within the United States, the AHA has recently defined national goals for cardiovascular health promotion and disease reduction with emphasis on potentially modifiable health behaviors and health factors (Lloyd-Jones et al., 2010). Based on accumulated evidence, health behaviors and factors targeted for both prevention and management of CVD include smoking, physical activity, patterns of dietary intake, body mass index, total cholesterol, blood pressure, and fasting plasma glucose. These health behaviors and health factors are also recommended as targets for intervention in evidence-based guidelines issued by AHA/ACCF for secondary prevention of CVD (Smith et al., 2011).

BEHAVIORS INCLUDED IN MANAGING CARDIOVASCULAR DISEASE

Behaviors central to managing CVD include smoking cessation, adherence to heart-healthy patterns of dietary intake and physical activity, maintenance of appropriate body weight, adherence to gender-specific recommendations for alcohol consumption, and adherence to prescribed medications for blood pressure control, lipid management, glucose control, and anticoagulant therapy (Smith et al., 2011). Important to emphasize in this context is that health behaviors (smoke-free lifestyles, physical activity, and heart-healthy patterns of dietary intake) are the cornerstone of CVD management and likely will remain so even as evidence-based guidelines are revised. While adherence to therapeutic pharmacological agents will also continue to be emphasized, the specific medications recommended for CVD management may change as new evidence becomes available.

The central and essential role of patient adherence to lifestyle and pharmacological recommendations for management of CVD is well established. Adherence is defined as the extent to which an individual's behavior coincides with physician or health care provider recommendations. It is well established that adherence is a complex process influenced by many factors including but not limited to individual patient, health care provider, and health care system factors (Ockene, Schneider, Lemon, & Ockene, 2011). Although non-adherence may consist of stopping therapy (i.e., medications) altogether, there is also a significant problem with individual patients who remain in treatment but do not follow the regimen in sufficient quantity or appropriate intervals to derive the optimal benefit. Estimates of non-adherence vary considerably across studies and as a function of the length and complexity of the treatment regimen, setting and population, and method of assessment/measurement (Christensen, 2004). Accumulated data suggest that rates of non-adherence to therapeutic regimens for CVD management range from 20% to 80% (Dunbar-Jacob & Mortimer-Stephens, 2001; Kronish & Ye, 2013). A 2008 report indicated that 43% of adults with CVD or equivalent CVD risk adhere to medication recommendations for elevated low-density lipoprotein cholesterol (LDL-C), a major risk factor for CVD (Mann, Reynolds, Smith, & Muntner, 2008). Results of other studies underscore the challenge of non-adherence to medication prescriptions and indicate higher rates of non-adherence after 6 months of treatment: approximately 49% for lipid-lowering medications, 36% for anti-hypertensives, and 42% for oral anti-diabetic agents (Cramer, Benedict, Muszbek, Keskinaslan, & Khan, 2007).

Over the past several decades, numerous approaches have been suggested to increase patient adherence to preventive and therapeutic regimens. For CVD management, the responsibility is on the individual level; however, health care providers and systems of care are important targets for adherence-enhancement efforts. A recent report offers a summary of evidence-based strategies designed to assist providers in promotion of patient adherence to therapeutic regimens for CVD patients (Kronish & Ye, 2013). These include keeping adherence on the agenda, asking about it in a non-judgmental manner at every patient visit, and recalling that there are few definite predictors of who will be non-adherent; thus, it is best to directly ask patients. When health care providers identify non-adherence, being mindful of patient-centered communication and exploring patients' concerns about the treatment protocol may be key factors in improving adherence, particularly with medications. Additional suggestions include engaging the patient's social network and social support (i.e., spouse or partner), simplifying and tailoring the treatment regimen with consideration of the patient's literacy level, socio-cultural background, area of residence, preferences, and resources (Kronish & Ye, 2013).

INTERVENTIONS TO CHANGE BEHAVIORS FOCUSED ON MANAGEMENT OF CVD/SECONDARY PREVENTION OF CVD

Secondary prevention of CVD, the focus of this chapter, emphasizes interventions designed to reduce the likelihood of CVD events and/or mortality in individuals who have established disease. The major potentially modifiable targets in management of CVD in the setting of secondary prevention include health behaviors and established risk factors that are also part of primary prevention protocols. Important to note is that primary prevention focuses on reducing adverse health behaviors and CVD risk factors with the ultimate goal of preventing incident CVD. As discussed below, interventions to change behaviors in managing CVD include patient education, behavioral skills training, motivational techniques and strategies such as motivational interviewing (MI), and e-health technologies. Of note, multicomponent interventions that include and combine patient education and counseling, behavioral skills training, and e-health technologies focused on behaviors central to managing CVD such as smoking cessation, increasing physical activity and decreasing sedentary behaviors, enhancing heart-healthy dietary behaviors, and promoting adherence to therapeutic regimens including cardiac rehabilitation programs have shown to be highly effective in preventing recurring CVD events as well as maintenance of behavioral change. As discussed below, these multi-component interventions are most often provided by multidisciplinary teams of health care professionals.

EDUCATION: NECESSARY BUT NOT SUFFICIENT TO CHANGE CVD-RELATED HEALTH BEHAVIORS

Patient education and counseling focused on both prevention and management of CVD have been a central component of evidence-based guidelines. A meta-analytic review of controlled trials of cardiac patient education programs conducted in the early 1990s documented that the success of these programs in reducing established risk factors for CVD and improving health behaviors was more highly related to behavioral skill building rather than education alone (Mullen, Mains, & Velez, 1992). Of note, the majority of the trials included in this review were directed by nurses who used a variety of behavioral skills including patient goal setting, self-monitoring, and feedback/ reinforcement for positive behavior change. Subsequent comprehensive reviews of the literature focused on physician-directed, nurse case management and CVD risk reduction reaffirmed the importance of theory-based behavioral change strategies designed to include skills necessary for behavior change as well as impart knowledge about the major risk factors for CVD (Berra, 2011; Clark, Hartling, Vandermeer, & McAlister, 2005).

BEHAVIORAL STRATEGIES FOR MANAGING CARDIOVASCULAR DISEASE

Behavioral change strategies for managing CVD have emphasized key elements of Social Cognitive Theory (SCT) including goal setting, self-monitoring, self-efficacy enhancement, social support, and feedback provided by health care providers including reinforcement for positive behavior change (Bandura, 1986; Bandura, 1997). Discussed in detail elsewhere in this book, SCT-based behavioral change strategies have been effective in reducing single- and multiple-risk behaviors in the setting of secondary prevention of CVD. While research to date with regard to maintenance of behavioral change over time is more limited, results of selected studies indicate that key elements of SCT combined with other treatment modalities can be effective in long-term smoking cessation, and weight loss maintenance (Orth-Gomer, 2012; Weiner & Rabbani, 2009; Wing et al., 2005).

Motivational interviewing (MI) is a behavior change counseling strategy that emphasizes patient-centered approaches including eliciting patient priorities, needs and values; building rapport (i.e., reflective listening and empathy) and support for self-management (Miller & Rollnick, 2002). Motivational interviewing has been used in conjunction with the Transtheoretical Model of Stages of Change (Prochaska, DiClemente, & Norcross, 1992) to modify CVD-related health behaviors in patients who have experienced a cardiovascular event (Wood et al., 2008) and for individuals at increased CVD risk (Mochari-Greenberger, Terry, & Mosca, 2010; Steptoe et al., 1999). In both the setting of primary and secondary prevention of CVD, MI has also been widely used as an adjunctive strategy to modify physical activity and dietary behaviors for overweight and obese individuals (Armstrong et al., 2011).

Several recent clinical trials have demonstrated the efficacy of incorporating MI with other behavioral change strategies in individuals with or at risk for CVD. In the Family Intervention Trial for Heart Health, a 12-month, single site randomized controlled trial (RCT), MI was used (in person and by telephone) with Stages of Change to modify the intake of saturated fat, cholesterol, and other key nutrients among family members of hospitalized CVD patients. In this RCT, special intervention participants, family members of hospitalized CVD patients, in the contemplation stage at baseline experienced greater saturated fat and cholesterol reductions (-2.1% vs. $+0.3\%$ kcal; $p = .04$ and -34.0 vs. $+32.6$ mg/1,000 kcal; $p = .01$ respectively) as compared to participants in other stages and to controls. In addition, control intervention participants were more likely than special intervention participants to revert to lower levels on the stage-of-change continuum from baseline to 1 year (17% vs. 7%; $p = .002$). As illustrated in other studies, results indicate MI combined with Stages of Change and other behavioral change strategies can be effective in modifying CVD health behaviors (Martins & McNeil, 2009). Additional observations from these studies suggest that effectiveness of a stage-of-change matched educational intervention varies by baseline stage of change, is dynamic over time, and is positively influenced by dose and duration of MI interventions.

MULTICOMPONENT INTERVENTIONS: INTEGRATING BEHAVIORAL CHANGE STRATEGIES WITH EVIDENCE-BASED MULTIDISCIPLINARY CASE MANAGEMENT

Effective management of CVD, similar to other chronic conditions, is a complex process facilitated by multidisciplinary team approaches, multicomponent interventions, and integrated systems of care. In the setting of secondary prevention, individuals with documented CVD normally present with more than one adverse health behavior and multiple risk factors (Poulter, 1999; Smith et al., 2011; Yusuf, Giles, Croft, Anda, & Jasper, 1998). Substantial evidence indicates that a multidisciplinary collaborative care model that focuses on individually tailored, guideline-based, patient-centered interventions, family and social support, health care providers, community level factors (i.e., access to cardiac rehabilitation programs), and systems of care that enable coordination of care providers is highly effective in reducing multiple adverse health behaviors and risk factors and preventing recurring events (Fletcher, Berra, Fletcher, Gilstrap, & Wood, 2012; Smith et al., 2011). Based on results accumulated over the past several decades, recent evidence-based guidelines issued by the AHA and ACCF (Smith et al., 2011) as well as sections of the Affordable Care Act (PPACA, Public Law No. 111–148) focused on health care system redesign emphasize this integrated model of care delivery for persons with CVD as well as those with other chronic conditions.

The MULTIFIT program (DeBusk et al., 1994) was among the first to demonstrate the effectiveness of an integrated multidisciplinary team approach in changing adverse health behaviors and improving major modifiable risk factors in patients with CVD. Concomitantly, the Stanford Coronary Risk Intervention Program (SCRIP) demonstrated the effectiveness of a multidisciplinary team approach (consisting of physicians, nurses, psychologists, and nutritionists) in reducing total cardiovascular events, angiographically measured atherosclerosis, adverse health behaviors, and cardiovascular risk factors in men and women with documented coronary artery disease (Haskell, Alderman, & Fair, 1994). More recently, building on lessons learned in MULTIFIT and SCRIP and incorporating MI and selected e-health technologies, EUROACTION demonstrated the effectiveness of nurse-coordinated multidisciplinary, family-based interventions for patients with CVD and asymptomatic individuals at high risk of CVD (Wood et al., 2008). Conducted in eight European countries, EUROACTION was developed by the European Society of Cardiology (ESC) with the goal of helping patients with established coronary heart disease (CHD) and those with high multifactorial risk (outside specialist cardiac rehabilitation centers) to achieve lifestyle, risk factor, and therapeutic targets defined in the ESC prevention guidelines. A major aim of EUROACTION was to determine whether a nurse-coordinated, multidisciplinary, family-based, ambulatory preventive cardiology program (EUROACTION) in hospital and general practice could increase the proportions of patients and their families achieving the goals for CVD prevention compared with usual care.

EUROACTION, a matched, cluster-randomized controlled trial included six pairs of hospitals and six pairs of general practices assigned to an intervention (INT) program or usual care (UC). Primary endpoints measured at 1 year included family-based lifestyle change, management of blood pressure, lipids and blood glucose, as well as prescription of cardioprotective drugs. 1589 and 1499 patients with CHD in hospitals and 1189 and 1128 at high risk were assigned to INT and UC, respectively. In the hospitals, cardiologists and nurses recruited eligible patients and their families; a multidisciplinary team composed of a nurse, dietitian, and physiotherapist conducted a comprehensive guideline-based assessment of lifestyle behaviors and risk factors. Patients were given a personal record for lifestyle and risk factor targets. Couples attended a minimum of eight of sixteen sessions (held weekly) in which the multidisciplinary team reassessed their lifestyle behaviors and risk factors. Couples also attended group workshops focused on lifestyle behaviors and weight management and a supervised exercise class. At 16 weeks, patients and their partners were reassessed by the team and a report was sent to family physicians. A similar protocol was used in the general practice centers. All CVD patients and their partners as well as those identified as high risk and their partners were invited for reassessment at 1 year. Of note, both hospital-based and general practice INT groups incorporated stages of change and MI in individual and group-workshop assessments and interventions. Results indicated that of the CHD patients who smoked in the month prior to the event, 136 (58%) in the INT and 154 (47%) in the UC groups did not smoke 1 year afterwards (difference in change 10.4%, 95% CI [−0.3, 21.2], $p = .06$). Reduced consumption of saturated fat and increased consumption of fruits and vegetables and oily fish at the 1-year data point were significantly greater in the INT group. High-risk individuals and partners showed changes only for fruits and vegetables ($p = .005$). Of note, a blood pressure target of less than 140/90 mm was attained by both coronary (615 [65%] vs. 547 [55%]; 10.4%, 0.6 to 20.2, $p = .04$) and high-risk (586 [58%] vs. 407 [41%]; 16.9%, 2.0 to 31.8, $p = .03$) patients in the INT groups. Achievement of the guideline recommended target goal for total cholesterol (less than 5 mmol/L) did not differ between groups; however, in high-risk patients the difference in change from baseline to 1 year was 12.7% (2.4 to 23.0, $p = .02$) in favor of INT. Prescriptions for lipid-lowering medications in the hospital group were also higher in the INT group (810 [86%] vs. 794 [80%]; 6.0%, −0.5 to 11.5, $p = .04$) while in general practices in the INT groups, blood pressure medications and lipid-lowering medications were more frequently prescribed than in the UC groups. Taken together, the results of EUROACTION demonstrate that a nurse-coordinated, multidisciplinary prevention program that incorporates theory-based, guideline-directed lifestyle and pharmacological interventions can be effective in improving lifestyle behaviors and risk factors for patients with established CVD and those at high risk for CVD.

Other recent multidisciplinary, physician-directed, nurse-based case management studies have shown that individualized, systematic, guideline-based care results in reduction of cardiovascular-related morbidity and mortality (Berra, 2011; Fonarow, Gawlinski, Moughrabi, & Tillisch, 2001). Of note, these multidisciplinary team-based approaches were shown to be effective across settings including hospitalized patients, primary care patients, low-income clinics, and in community centers (Allen & Dennison, 2010; Berra 2011). Across studies (primarily RCTs), reduced mortality, recurrent events, and hospitalizations were observed in treatment compared to control groups/usual care. A systematic review of RCTs of secondary prevention programs reaffirmed these results indicating that in the majority of the 12 trials reviewed, patients randomized to multidisciplinary disease management programs were more likely to be prescribed efficacious medications, have improved health behaviors and risk factor profiles, and have better quality of life and functional status outcomes compared with individuals randomized to control groups/usual care (McAlister, Lawson, Teo, & Armstrong, 2001).

Noteworthy in this context is the importance of multicomponent behavioral interventions in modifying adverse health behaviors with attention to the dose and duration of respective interventions. In this context, dose refers to the intensity of the intervention while duration refers to the time allotted for the intervention (i.e., 2 vs. 4 hours of supervised exercise training per week for 8 weeks vs. 16 weeks). In addition, as summarized by Allen and Dennison (2010) and reaffirmed by others (Hayman et al., 2007; Orth-Gomer, 2012; Stuart-Shor, Berra, Kamau, & Kumanyika, 2012), the optimal combination of intervention components including specific strategy, mode of delivery, and frequency and duration for modifying individual and/or multiple adverse behaviors in patients with documented CVD remains unknown. The need for additional research in this important area of inquiry is clear and convincing. Particularly lacking are data relevant to modifying CVD-related health behaviors in the setting of secondary prevention of CVD for individuals from racially and ethnically diverse populations.

EVIDENCE-BASED GUIDELINES FOR SECONDARY PREVENTION AND RISK REDUCTION FOR PATIENTS WITH CORONARY AND OTHER ATHEROSCLEROTIC VASCULAR DISEASES

Reflecting evidence accumulated since the 2006 update of the AHA/ACCF guidelines on secondary prevention of CVD, the 2011 guidelines focus on major CVD risk factors and health-related behaviors. As illustrated in Tables 13.1 and 13.2, areas for intervention designate comprehensive risk-factor management including emphasis on CVD-related health behaviors. While not stated explicitly, evidence-based strategies for modifying individual and multiple risk behaviors and improving adherence to prescriptions for behavioral change and medication regimens are a central component of the recently revised AHA/ACCF guidelines. Based on accumulated evidence on the efficacy and effectiveness of cardiac rehabilitation/secondary prevention programs (CR/SPPs) that include multidisciplinary, multicomponent interventions for behavioral change and risk factor modification, these programs are also emphasized with the goal of reducing recurrent events in patients with CVD (Balady et al., 2012; Smith et al., 2011).

Despite the demonstrated benefits of CR/SPPs the use of these programs remains low. Of eligible patients, only 14% to 35% of heart attack survivors and approximately 31% of patients after coronary bypass grafting surgery participate in a CR/SPP (CDC, 2008; Suaya et al., 2007). Patients must be referred to participate in CR/SPP. Normally, this occurs prior to or soon after hospital discharge following a cardiac event. A review of patient, medical, and health care system factors suggests that variability in referral exists with women, the elderly, and individuals from racial/ethnic minority groups and low-income communities less likely to be referred to CR/SPP than their counterparts (Balady et al., 2012). The variability is explained in part by physician endorsement of CR/SPPs and failure of the hospital-based health care team to refer eligible patients (Grace et al., 2008). Brown and colleagues (2009) in a study of 72,819 hospitalized cardiac patients found that hospitals using the AHA's Get with the Guidelines program had a referral rate of 56%, higher than the national average. Of note, many patients who were referred do not enroll in a program. In one report, only 34% of those referred actually enrolled in CR/SPP (Mazzini, Stevens, Whalen, Ozonoff, & Balady, 2008). In addition, many who enroll do not complete the full course of CR/SPP which is generally 36 sessions over a 12-week period (Balady et al., 2012). A systematic review of literature demonstrates that the strength of evidence for any specific referral strategy is lacking; however, a combined approach using discharge order sets plus personal bedside provision of information and invitation to enroll offers the most promise (Grace et al., 2011).

TABLE 13.1 AHA/ACCF Secondary Prevention and Risk-Reduction Therapy for Patients With Coronary and Other Atherosclerotic Vascular Diseases: 2011 Update: Intervention Recommendations With Class of Recommendation and Level of Evidence

AREA FOR INTERVENTION	RECOMMENDATIONS
Smoking Goal: Complete cessation. No exposure to environmental tobacco smoke	**Class I** 1. Patients should be asked about tobacco use status at every office visit. (Level of Evidence: B) 2. Every tobacco user should be advised at every visit to quit. (Level of Evidence: A) 3. The tobacco user's willingness to quit should be assessed at every visit. (Level of Evidence: C) 4. Patients should be assisted by counseling and by development of a plan for quitting that may include pharmacotherapy and/or referral to a smoking cessation program. (Level of Evidence: A) 5. Arrangement for follow up is recommended. (Level of Evidence: C) 6. All patients should be advised at every office visit to avoid exposure to environmental tobacco smoke at work, home, and public places. (Level of Evidence: B) **Note: The writing committee did not think that the 2006 recommendations for blood pressure control (below) should be modified at this time. The writing committee anticipates that the recommendations will be reviewed when the updated JNC guidelines are released.**
Blood pressure control Goal: < 140/90 mmHg	**Class I** 1. All patients should be counseled regarding the need for lifestyle modification: weight control; increased physical activity; alcohol moderation; sodium reduction; and emphasis on increased consumption of fresh fruits, vegetables, and low-fat dairy products. (Level of Evidence: B) 2. Patients with blood pressure ≥ 140/90 mmHg should be treated, as tolerated, with blood pressure medication, treating initially with beta-blockers and/or ACE inhibitors, with addition of other drugs as needed to achieve targeted blood pressure. (Level of Evidence: A)

Lipid management

Goal: Treatment with statin therapy; use statin therapy to achieve an LDL-C of < 100 mg/dL; for very high-risk patients an LDL-C < 70 mg/dL is reasonable; if triglycerides are ≥ 200 mg/dL, non-HDL-C should be < 130 mg/dL, whereas non-HDL-C < 100 mg/dL for very high-risk patients is reasonable

Note: The writing committee anticipates that the recommendations will be reviewed when the updated ATP guidelines are released.

Class I

1. A lipid profile in all patients should be established, and for hospitalized patients, lipid-lowering therapy as recommended below should be initiated before discharge. (Level of Evidence: B)
2. Lifestyle modifications including daily physical activity and weight management are strongly recommended for all patients. (Level of Evidence: B)
3. Dietary therapy for all patients should include reduced intake of saturated fats (to < 7% of total calories), trans-fatty acids (to < 1% of total calories), and cholesterol (to < 200 mg/day). (Level of Evidence: B)
4. In addition to therapeutic lifestyle changes, statin therapy should be prescribed in the absence of contraindications or documented adverse effects. (Level of Evidence: A)
5. An adequate dose of statin should be used that reduces LDL-C to < 100 mg/dL and achieves at least a 30% lowering of LDL-C. (Level of Evidence: C)
6. Patients who have triglycerides ≥ 200 mg/dL should be treated with statins to lower non-HDL-C to < 130 mg/dL. (Level of Evidence: B)
7. Patients who have triglycerides > 500 mg/dL should be started on fibrate therapy in addition to statin therapy to prevent acute pancreatitis. (Level of Evidence: C)

Class IIa

1. If treatment with a statin (including trials of higher-dose statins and higher-potency statins) does not achieve the goal selected for a patient, intensification of LDL-C-lowering drug therapy with a bile acid sequestrant or niacin is reasonable. (Level of Evidence: B)
2. For patients who do not tolerate statins, LDL-C-lowering therapy with bile acid sequestrants and/or niacin is reasonable. (Level of Evidence: B)
3. It is reasonable to treat very high-risk patients with statin therapy to lower LDL-C to < 70 mg/dL. (Level of Evidence: C)
4. In patients who are at very high risk and who have triglycerides ≥200 mg/dL, a non-HDL-C goal of < 100 mg/dL is reasonable. (Level of Evidence: B)

Class IIb

1. The use of ezetimibe may be considered for patients who do not tolerate or achieve target LDL-C with statins, bile acid sequestrants, and/or niacin. (Level of Evidence: C)
2. For patients who continue to have an elevated non-HDL-C while on adequate statin therapy, niacin or fibrate therapy (Level of Evidence: B) or fish oil (Level of Evidence: C) may be reasonable.
3. For all patients, it may be reasonable to recommend omega-3 fatty acids from fish or fish oil capsules (1 g/d) for cardiovascular disease risk reduction. (Level of Evidence: B)

(continued)

TABLE 13.1 AHA/ACCF Secondary Prevention and Risk-Reduction Therapy for Patients With Coronary and Other Atherosclerotic Vascular Diseases: 2011 Update: Intervention Recommendations With Class of Recommendation and Level of Evidence (*continued*)

AREA FOR INTERVENTION	RECOMMENDATIONS
Physical activity Goal: At least 30 minutes, 7 days per week (minimum 5 days per week)	**Class I** 1. For all patients, the clinician should encourage 30 to 60 minutes of moderate–intensity aerobic activity, such as brisk walking, at least 5 days and preferably 7 days per week, supplemented by an increase in daily lifestyle activities (e.g., walking breaks at work, gardening, household work) to improve cardiorespiratory fitness and move patients out of the least fit, least active high-risk cohort (bottom 20%). (Level of Evidence: B) 2. For all patients, risk assessment with a physical activity history and/or an exercise test is recommended to guide prognosis and prescription. (Level of Evidence: B) 3. The clinician should counsel patients to report and be evaluated for symptoms related to exercise. (Level of Evidence: C) **Class IIa** 1. It is reasonable for the clinician to recommend complementary resistance training at least 2 days per week. (Level of Evidence: C)
Weight management Goals: Body mass index: 18.5–24.9 kg/m² Waist circumference: women < 35 inches (< 89 cm), men < 40 inches (< 102 cm)	**Class I** 1. Body mass index and/or waist circumference should be assessed at every visit, and the clinician should consistently encourage weight maintenance/reduction through an appropriate balance of lifestyle physical activity, structured exercise, caloric intake, and formal behavioral programs when indicated to maintain/achieve a body mass index between 18.5 and 24.9 kg/m². (Level of Evidence: B) 2. If waist circumference (measured horizontally at the iliac crest) is ≥ 35 inches (≥89 cm) in women and ≥ 40 inches (≥102 cm) in men, therapeutic lifestyle interventions should be intensified and focused on weight management. (Level of Evidence: B) 3. The initial goal of weight loss therapy should be to reduce body weight by approximately 5% to 10% from baseline. With success, further weight loss can be attempted if indicated. (Level of Evidence: C)

Type 2 diabetes mellitus management	**Note: Recommendations below are for prevention of cardiovascular complications.** **Class I** 1. Care for diabetes should be coordinated with the patient's primary care physician and/or endocrinologist. (Level of Evidence: C) 2. Lifestyle modifications including daily physical activity, weight management, blood pressure control, and lipid management are recommended for all patients with diabetes. (Level of Evidence: B) **Class IIa** 1. Metformin is an effective first-line pharmacotherapy and can be useful if not contraindicated. (Level of Evidence: A) 2. It is reasonable to individualize the intensity of blood-sugar-lowering interventions based on the individual patient's risk of hypoglycemia during treatment. (Level of Evidence: C) **Class IIb** 1. Initiation of pharmacotherapy interventions to achieve target HbA1c may be reasonable. (Level of Evidence: A) 2. A target HbA1c of ≤ 7% may be considered. (Level of Evidence: C) 3. Less stringent HbA1c goals may be considered for patients with a history of severe hypoglycemia, limited life expectancy, advanced microvascular or macrovascular complications, or extensive comorbidities, or those in whom the goal is difficult to attain despite intensive therapeutic interventions. (Level of Evidence: C)
Depression	**Class IIa** 1. For patients with recent coronary artery bypass graft surgery or myocardial infarction, it is reasonable to screen for depression if patients have access to case management, in collaboration with their primary care physician and a mental health specialist. (Level of Evidence: B) **Class IIb** 1. Treatment of depression has not been shown to improve cardiovascular disease outcomes but may be reasonable for its other clinical benefits. (Level of Evidence: C)

(continued)

283

TABLE 13.1 AHA/ACCF Secondary Prevention and Risk-Reduction Therapy for Patients With Coronary and Other Atherosclerotic Vascular Diseases: 2011 Update: Intervention Recommendations With Class of Recommendation and Level of Evidence (continued)

AREA FOR INTERVENTION	RECOMMENDATIONS
Cardiac rehabilitation	**Class I** 1. All eligible patients with ACS or whose status is immediately post coronary artery bypass surgery or post-percutaneous coronary intervention (PCI) should be referred to a comprehensive outpatient cardiovascular rehabilitation program either prior to hospital discharge or during the first follow-up office visit. (Level of Evidence: A) 2. All eligible outpatients with the diagnosis of ACS, coronary artery bypass surgery or PCI (Level of Evidence: A) chronic angina (Level of Evidence: B), and/or peripheral artery disease (Level of Evidence: A) within the past year should be referred to a comprehensive outpatient cardiovascular rehabilitation program. 3. A home-based cardiac rehabilitation program can be substituted for a supervised, center-based program for low-risk patients. (Level of Evidence: A) **Class IIa** 1. A comprehensive exercise-based outpatient cardiac rehabilitation program can be safe and beneficial for clinically stable outpatients with a history of heart failure. (Level of Evidence: B)

From Smith et al. (2011).

TABLE 13.2 Applying Classification of Recommendation and Level of Evidence

	Class I	Class IIa	Class IIb	Class III No Benefit or Class III Harm
	Benefit >>> Risk	Benefit >> Risk	Benefit >/= Risk	Procedure/Test — Treatment
	Procedure/Treatment **Should** be performed/administered	*Additional studies with focused objectives needed* **It is reasonable** to perform procedure/administer treatment	Additional studies with broad objectives needed; additional registry data would be helpful Procedure/Treatment **May be Considered**	CORIII No Benefit: Not Helpful — No Proven Benefit; CORIII Harm: Excess Cost w/o Benefit or Harmful — Harmful to Patients
Level A Multiple populations evaluated Data derived from multiple clinical trials or meta-analyses	• Recommendation that procedure or treatment is useful/effective • Sufficient evidence from multiple randomized trials or meta-analyses	• Recommendation in favor of treatment or procedure being useful/effective • Some conflicting evidence from multiple randomized trials or meta-analyses	• Recommendation's usefulness/efficacy less well established • Greater conflicting evidence from multiple randomized trials or meta-analyses	• Recommendation that procedure or treatment is not useful/effective and may be harmful • Sufficient evidence from multiple randomized wtrials or meta-analyses
Level B Limited populations evaluated Data derived from a single randomized trial or nonrandomized studies	• Recommendation that procedure or treatment is useful/effective • Sufficient evidence from single randomized trial or nonrandomized studies	• Recommendation in favor of treatment or procedure being useful/effective • Some conflicting evidence from single randomized trial or nonrandomized studies	• Recommendation's usefulness/efficacy less well established • Greater conflicting evidence from single randomized trial or nonrandomized studies	• Recommendation that procedure or treatment is not useful/effective and may be harmful • Sufficient evidence from single randomized trial or nonrandomized studies
Level C Very limited populations evaluated Only consensus opinion of experts, case studies, or standard care	• Recommendation that procedure or treatment is useful/effective • Only expert opinion, case studies, or standard care	• Recommendation in favor of treatment or procedure being useful/effective • Only diverging expert opinion, case studies, or standard care	• Recommendation's usefulness/efficacy less well established • Only diverging expert opinion, case studies, or standard care	• Recommendation that procedure or treatment is not useful/effective and may be harmful • Only expert opinion, case studies, or standard of care

Most recently, in a prospective cohort study designed to examine CR attendance and outcomes in coronary artery disease patients, Martin and colleagues (2012) assessed mortality rates, hospitalizations, cardiac hospitalizations, and emergency department visits among 5,886 individuals who had undergone cardiac catheterization and had detailed data collected at the time of index cardiac event. These patients were referred to a single community-based CR program within a year of the index event. Of note, more than 40% of eligible referred patients chose not to attend and an additional 9% enrolled but did not complete the program. Compared to CR completers, those who did not enroll or did not complete were older and had more comorbidities, were more likely to be women, and of lower socioeconomic status. The lowest mortality rate and hospitalization rate as well as emergency room visits were observed among the CR completers. Of the 3,454 individuals who started CR, information on the number of exercise sessions attended was available for 2,905 (84%) of individuals. Completers attended an average of 21.9 (*SD*, 10.2) sessions, and those who did not complete CR attended 6.7 (*SD*, 9.1; *p* < .0001) sessions. Cox proportional hazards models demonstrated that there was a 1% decrease in mortality with each additional session attended. Illustrating the critical importance of adherence to treatment as well as the dose–response relationship, this study merited a special call to action for health care providers on the importance of CR for reducing recurrent events and improving outcomes in patients with established CVD (Bittner, 2012).

CONCLUSIONS

While substantial progress has been made in reducing CVD mortality over the past several decades, CVD remains a major cause of death and disability in women and men in the United States and globally. Many population subgroups, defined by race, ethnicity, socioeconomic status, educational level, and area of residence, demonstrate an excess burden of CVD and its comorbidities (Stuart-Shor et al., 2012). Additional research is needed to guide and inform both clinical and public health efforts as well as multilevel policies designed to reduce disparities in both prevention and treatment of CVD.

Recent evidence-based guidelines for secondary prevention of CVD (Smith et al., 2012) place emphasis on behavioral-lifestyle change and assessment and management of risk factors as part of comprehensive risk-reduction strategies for individuals with established CVD. Accumulated evidence confirms that aggressive, comprehensive risk-factor management improves survival, reduces recurrent events, and improves quality of life for individuals with established heart disease. Adherence to provider recommendations for behavioral change and medication regimens is an essential component of achieving treatment goals and preventing recurrent events. Consistent with social-ecological models of health and behavior, evidence supports the need and potential for multilevel approaches for increasing adherence to therapeutic regimens. Additional research, however, is needed to guide and inform optimal adherence-enhancing strategies as well as treatment approaches for vulnerable individuals with documented CVD. With the goal of reducing CVD-related disparities and promoting health equity, such research should focus on individuals from racial and ethnic minority populations as well as those who reside in low-income communities and geographic areas.

As highlighted in this chapter, substantial evidence supports the effectiveness of multidisciplinary, multicomponent secondary prevention programs in reducing adverse health behaviors and CVD risk factors, recurrent events, and in improvement of quality of life in individuals with CVD. Key elements of successful programs identified are consistent with core components of the Chronic Care Model (Bodenheimer, Wagner, & Grumbach, 2002), supported in sections of the Affordable Care Act, and underscore the promise and potential of innovative models and integrated systems of care for reducing morbidity and mortality and improving the quality of life in diverse populations of patients with CVD.

REFERENCES

Allen, J. K., Blumenthal, R. S., Margolis, S., Young, D. R., Miller, E. R., III, & Kelly, K. (2002). Nurse case management of hypercholesterolemia in patients with coronary heart disease: Results of a randomized clinical trial. *American Heart Journal, 144,* 678–686. doi:10.1067/mhj.2002.124837

Allen, J. K., & Dennison, C. R. (2010). Randomized trials of nursing interventions for secondary prevention in patients with coronary artery disease and heart failure: Systematic review. *Journal of Cardiovascular Nursing, 25*(3), 207–220.

Armstrong, M. J., Mottershead, T. A., Ronksley, P. E., Sigal, R. J., Campbell, T. S., & Hemmelgarn, B. R. (2011). Motivational interviewing to improve weight loss in overweight and/or obese patients: A systematic review and meta-analysis of randomized controlled trials. *Obesity Reviews, 12*(9), 709–723. doi:10.1111/j.1467-789X.2011.00892.x

Balady, G. J., Ades, P. A., Bittner, V. A., Franklin, B. A., Gordon, N. F., Thomas, R. J., Tomaselli, G. F., & Yancy, C. W. (2012). Referral, enrollment and delivery of cardiac rehabilitation/secondary prevention programs at clinical centers and beyond: A presidential advisory from the American Heart Association. *Circulation, 124,* 2951–2960. doi:10.1161/CIR.0b013e31823b21e2

Bandura, A. (1986). *Social foundations of thought and action. A social cognitive theory.* Englewood Cliffs, NJ: Prentice Hall.

Bandura, A. (1997). *Self-efficacy: The exercise of self-control.* New York, NY: W.H. Freeman.

Berra, K. (2011). Does nurse case management improve implementation of guidelines for cardiovascular disease risk reduction? *Journal of Cardiovascular Nursing, 26*(2), 147–167. doi: 10.1097/JCN.0b013e31813ec 1337

Berra, K., Houston-Miller, N., & Jennings, C. (2011). Nurse-based models for cardiovascular disease prevention: From research to clinical practice. *Journal of Cardiovascular Nursing, 26*(4S), S46–S55. doi: 10.1097/JCN.0b013e318213ef5c

Bittner, V. (2012). Cardiac rehabilitation: A call to action for healthcare providers. *Circulation, 126,* 671–673.

Bodenheimer, T., Wagner, E. H., & Grumbach, K. (2002). Improving primary care for patients with chronic illness. *Journal of the American Medical Association, 288,* 1775–1779.

Brown, T. M., Hernandez, A. F., Bittner, V., Cannon, C. P., Ellrodt, G., Liang, L., … Fonarow, G. C., on behalf of American Heart Association Get with the Guidelines Investigators. (2009). Predictors of cardiac rehabilitation referral in coronary artery disease patients: Findings from the American Heart Association's Get with the Guidelines Program. *Journal of the American College of Cardiology, 34,* 515–521.

Campbell, N. C., Ritchie, L. D., Thain, J., Rawles, J. M., & Squair, J. L. (1998). Secondary prevention in coronary heart disease: A randomised trial of nurse led clinics in primary care. *Heart, 80,* 447–452.

Centers for Disease Control and Prevention (CDC). (2008). Recipient of outpatient cardiac rehabilitation among heart attack survivors – United States, 2003. *MMWR, Morbidity and Mortality Weekly Report, 57,* 89–94.

Christensen, A. J. (2004). *Patient adherence to medical treatment regimens: Bridging the gap between behavioral science and biomedicine.* New Haven, CT: Yale University Press.

Clark, A. M., Hartling, L., Vandermeer, B., & McAlister, F. A. (2005). Meta-analysis: Secondary prevention programs for patients with coronary artery disease. *Annals of Internal Medicine, 143*(9), 659–672.

Cramer, J. A., Benedict, A., Muszbek, N., Keskinaslan, A., & Khan, Z. M. (2007). The significance of compliance and persistence in the treatment of diabetes, hypertension, and dyslipidemia: A review. *Clinical Practice, 62,* 76–87.

Davies, P., Taylor, F., Beswick, A., Wise, F., Moxham, T., Rees, K., & Ebrahim, S. (2010). Promoting patient uptake and adherence in cardiac rehabilitation. *Cochrane Database Systematic Review.* CD 0007131.

DeBusk, R. F., Houston-Miller, N., Superko, H. R., Dennis, C. A., Thomas, R. J., Lew, H. T., … Taylor, C. B. (1994). A case-management system for coronary risk factor modification after acute myocardial infarction. *Annals of Internal Medicine, 120,* 721–729.

DiMatteo, M. R. (2004). Variations in patients' adherence to medical recommendations: A quantitative review of 50 years of research. *Medical Care, 42,* 200–209.

Dunbar-Jacob, J., & Mortimer-Stephens, M. K. (2001). Treatment adherence in chronic diseases. *Journal of Clinical Epidemiology, 54,* S57–S60.

Fletcher, G. F., Berra, K., Fletcher, B. J., Gilstrap, L., & Wood, M. J. (2012). The integrated team approach to the care of the patient with cardiovascular disease. *Current Problems in Cardiology, 37,* 369–397.

Fonarow, G. C., Gawlinski, A., Moughrabi, S., & Tillisch, J. H. (2001). Improved treatment of coronary heart disease by implementation of a Cardiac Hospitalization Atherosclerosis Management Program (CHAMP). *American Journal of Cardiology, 87*(7), 819–822.

Grace, S. L., Chessex, C., Arthur, H., Chan, S., Cyr, C., Dafoe, W., … Suskin, N. (2011). Systematizing inpatient referral to cardiac rehabilitation 2010: Canadian Association of Cardiac Rehabilitation and Canadian Society joint position paper. *Journal of Cardiopulmonary Rehabilitation Prevention, 31,* E1–E8.

Grace, S. L., Gravely-Witte, S., Brual, J., Monette, G., Suskin, N., Higginson, L., … Stewart, D. E. (2008). Contribution of patient and physician factors to cardiac rehabilitation enrollment: A prospective multilevel study. *European Journal of Cardiovascular Prevention and Rehabilitation, 15,* 548–546.

Haskell, W. L., Alderman, E. L., & Fair, J. M. (1994). Effects of intensive multiple risk factor reduction on coronary atherosclerosis and clinical cardiac events in men and women with coronary artery disease. The Stanford Coronary Risk Intervention Project (SCRIP). *Circulation, 89*(3), 975–990.

Hayman, L. L., Meininger, J. C., Daniels, S. R., McCrindle, B. W., Helden, L., Ross, J., … Williams, C. L. (2007). Primary prevention of cardiovascular disease in nursing practice: Focus on children and youth. *Circulation, 116*(3), 344–357.

Johnston, W., Bucsemi, B. A., & Coons, M. J. (2013). Multiple health behavior change: A synopsis and comment on "A review of multiple health behavior change interventions for primary prevention." *Translational Behavioral Medicine, 3*(1), 6–7. doi: 10.1007/s13142-013-0200-9

Kwan, G., & Balady, G. J. (2012). Cardiac rehabilitation 2012: Advancing the field through emerging science. *Circulation, 125,* e369–e373.

Lloyd-Jones, D. M., Hong, Y., Labarthe, D., Mozaffarian, D., Appel, L. J., Horn, L. V., … American Heart Association Strategic Planning Task Force and Statistics Committee. (2010). Defining and setting national goals for cardiovascular health promotion and disease reduction: The American Heart Association's strategic impact goal through 2020 and beyond. *Circulation, 121,* 586–613. doi: 10.1161.CIRCULATIONAHA.109.192703

Kronish, I. M., & Ye, S. (2013). Adherence to cardiovascular medications: Lessons learned and future directions. *Progress in Cardiovascular Diseases, 55,* 590–600.

Mann, D., Reynolds, K., Smith, D., & Muntner, P. (2008). Trends in statin use and low-density lipoprotein cholesterol levels among U.S. adults: Impact of the 2001 national Cholesterol Education Program Guidelines. *Annals of Pharmacotherapy, 42,* 1208–1215.

Martin, B. J., Hauer, T., Arena, R., Austford, L. D., Galbraith, P. D., Lewin, A. M., … Aggarwal, S. G. (2012). Cardiac rehabilitation attendance and outcomes in coronary artery disease patients. *Circulation, 126,* 677–687.

Martins, R. K., & Mc Neil, D. W. (2009). Review of motivational interviewing in promoting health behaviors. *Clinical Psychology Reviews, 29,* 283–293.

Mazzini, M. J., Stevens, G. R., Whalen, D., Ozonoff, A., & Balady, G. J. (2008). Effect of an American Heart Association Get with the Guidelines program-based clinical pathway on referral and enrollment into cardiac rehabilitation after acute myocardial infarction. *American Journal of Cardiology, 101,* 1084–1087.

McAlister, F. A., Lawson, F. M., Teo, K. K., & Armstrong, P. W. (2001). Randomised trials of secondary prevention programmes in coronary heart disease: Systematic review. *British Medical Journal, 323*(7319), 957–962.

Miller, W. R., & Rollnick, S. (2002). *Motivational interviewing: Preparing people for change* (2nd ed.). New York, NY: Guilford Press.

Mochari-Greenberger, H., Terry, M. B., & Mosca, L. (2010). Does stage of change modify the effectiveness of an educational intervention to improve diet among family members of hospitalized cardiovascular disease patients? *Journal of the American Dietetic Association, 110,* 1027–1035. doi: 10: 1016/jjada.2010.04.012

Mullen, P. D., Mains, D. A., & Velez, R. (1992). A meta-analysis of controlled trials of cardiac patient education. *Patient Education and Counseling, 19,* 143–162.

Ockene, J. K., Schneider, K. L., Lemon, S. C., & Ockene, I. S. (2011). Can we improve adherence to preventive therapies for cardiovascular health? *Circulation, 124,* 1276–1282.

Orth-Gomer, K. (2012). Behavioral interventions for coronary heart disease patients. *Biopsychosocial Medicine, 6,* 5.

Patient Protection and Affordable Care Act (PPACA), Public Law No. 111–146 124 Stat. 119 (March 23, 2010).

Poulter, N. (1999). Coronary heart disease is a multifactorial disease. *American Journal of Hypertension, 19,* 92S–95S.

Prochaska, J. O., DiClemente, C. C., & Norcross, J. C. (1992). In search of how people change: Applications to addictive behaviors. *American Psychologist, 47,* 1102–1114.

Roger, V. L., Go, A. S., Lloyd-Jones, D. M., Adam, D. M., Berry, J. D., Brown, T. M., ... Wylie-Rosett, J. (2011). Heart disease and stroke statistics-2011 update: A report from the American Heart Association. *Circulation, 123,* e18–e209.

Savage, P. D., Sanderson, B. K., Brown, T. M., Berra, K., & Ades, P. (2011). Clinical research in cardiac rehabilitation and secondary prevention: Looking back and moving forward. *Journal of Cardiopulmonary Rehabilitation and Prevention, 31*(6), 333–341. doi: 10.1097/HCR.0b013e31822d0d79

Smith, S. C., Jr., Benjamin, E. J., Bonow, R. O., Braun, L. T., Creager, M. A., Franklin, B. A., ... Taubert, K. A. (2011). AHA/ACCF secondary prevention and risk reduction therapy for patients with coronary and other atherosclerotic vascular disease: 2011 update: A guideline from the American Heart Association and American College of Cardiology Foundation endorsed by the World Heart Federation and the Preventive Cardiovascular Nurses Association. *Circulation, 124*(22), 2458–2473. doi: 10:.116/CIR.Ob13e31825eb4d

Smith, S. C., Jr., Collins, A., Ferrari, R., Holmes, D. R., Jr., Logstrup, S., Vaca McGhie, D., ... Zoghbi, W. A. (2012). Our time: A call to save preventable death from cardiovascular disease (Heart Disease and Stroke). *Circulation, 126.* doi: 10.1161/CIR.0b013e318267e99f

Spring, B., Moller, A., & Coons, M. (2012). Multiple health behaviors: Overview and implications. *Journal of Public Health, 34,* i3–i10.

Steptoe, A., Doherty, S., Rink, E., Kerry, S., Kendrick, T., & Hilton, S. (1999). Behavioral counseling in general practice for the promotion of healthy behavior among adults at increased risk of coronary heart disease: Randomized trial. *British Medical Journal, 319,* 943–948.

Stuart-Shor, E. M., Berra, K. A., Kamau, M. W., & Kumanyika, S. K. (2012). Behavioral interventions for cardiovascular risk reduction in diverse and underserved racial/ethnic groups. *Circulation, 125,* 171–184. doi: 10:111/CIRCULATIONAHA.110.968495

Suaya, J. A., Shepard, D. S., Normand, S. L., Ades, P. A., Prottas, J., & Stason, W. B. (2007). Use of cardiac rehabilitation by Medicare beneficiaries after myocardial infarction or coronary bypass surgery. *Circulation, 106,* 1653–1662.

United Nations General Assembly. (2011). Sixty-sixth session. Follow-up to the outcome of the Millennium Summit: Draft resolution submitted by the President of the General Assembly. A/66/L.1. Retrieved from http://www.un.org/ga/search/view_doc.asp?symbol=A/66/L.1

Weiner, S. D., & Rabbani, L. E. (2009). Secondary prevention strategies for coronary heart disease. *Journal of Thrombosis and Thrombolysis, 29,* 8–24.

Wing, R. R., & Phelan, S. (2005). Long term weight loss maintenance. *American Journal of Clinical Nutrition, 82*(Suppl. 1), 222S–225S.

Wood, D. A., Kotseva, K., Connolly, S., Jennings, C., Mead, A., Jones, J., ... Faergmann, O. (2008). Nurse-coordinated multidisciplinary, family-based cardiovascular disease prevention program (EURO-ACTION) for patients with coronary heart disease and asymptomatic individuals at high risk of cardiovascular disease: A paired, cluster-randomised controlled trial. *Lancet, 371,* 1999–2012.

World Health Organization. (2007). *Prevention of cardiovascular disease: Pocket guidelines for assessment and management of cardiovascular risk* [Brochure]. Geneva, Switzerland: Author.

World Health Organization. (2011). *WHO Discussion Paper: A comprehensive global monitoring framework and voluntary global targets for the prevention and control of NCDs.* Retrieved from http://www.who.int/nmh/events/2011/consultation_dec_2011/WHO_Discussion_Paper_FINAL.pdf

World Health Organization. (2012). *Sixty-Fifth World Health Assembly: Second report of Committee A.* Retrieved from http://apps.who.int/gb/ebwha/pdf_files/WHA65/A65_54Draft-en.pdf

Yusuf, H., Giles, W., Croft, J., Anda, R., & Jasper, M. (1998). Impact of multiple risk factor profiles on determining cardiovascular disease risk. *Preventive Medicine, 27,* 1–9.

14

Diabetes Management Behaviors: The Key to Optimal Health and Quality of Life Outcomes

KOREY K. HOOD
JENNIFER K. RAYMOND
MICHAEL A. HARRIS

LEARNING OBJECTIVES

- Increase understanding of the critical nature of diabetes care behaviors for optimal diabetes health outcomes.
- Provide case examples that illustrate how to use the evidence base to facilitate health behavior change in people with diabetes.
- Demonstrate how to take advantage of new and existing technologies to improve and facilitate health behaviors in people with diabetes.

The landscape of diabetes and its management has changed dramatically since the first results of the landmark Diabetes Control and Complications Trial (DCCT) were published in 1993. The DCCT transformed the notion of intensive diabetes management and fostered a new approach that focuses on performing multiple daily behaviors to optimize short- and long-term health. A host of other seminal studies have been published since documenting new therapeutics and technologies aimed at reducing patient burden and maximizing health outcomes. There is work under way to perfect our models of prevention for all types of diabetes, and to produce an artificial pancreas that would relieve the patient of chronic decision making and problem solving around diabetes. Until these projects and programs are fully realized, the engagement in multiple behaviors to treat diabetes is still the single best method for optimizing health and quality of life outcomes in patients with diabetes. This chapter provides a review of the important background and context of diabetes, and highlights the critical nature of health behaviors to diabetes management and outcomes. In addition, barriers to conducting these behaviors and interventions aimed at breaking down these barriers while simultaneously promoting effective problem-solving and coping skills will be highlighted.

DIABETES 101

TYPES OF DIABETES

Diabetes is a chronic disease caused by a relative deficiency in insulin. This manifests in one of two ways; either the body is unable to produce sufficient insulin (type 1 diabetes) or the body does not respond appropriately to insulin (type 2 diabetes). In the acute setting, elevated blood sugars can be deadly. Over the long term, chronic elevated blood sugars can result in damage to multiple body systems.

Type 1 diabetes is an autoimmune disease in which the immune system attacks the pancreatic beta cells, which make insulin. A combination of genetic, environmental, and biological factors is hypothesized to lead to the development of type 1 diabetes (Atkinson & Eisenbarth, 2001; Bluestone, Herold, & Eisenbarth, 2010). Type 2 diabetes has previously been characterized as adult-onset or non-insulin dependent diabetes; however, these are no longer appropriate. Children are diagnosed with type 2 diabetes (Liese et al., 2006), and patients with type 2 diabetes may require insulin treatment. Overweight, obesity, decreased physical activity, and older age are associated with type 2 diabetes. Type 2 diabetes accounts for approximately 90% of all cases of diabetes (Centers for Disease Control and Prevention [CDC], 2011).

PUBLIC HEALTH IMPACT OF DIABETES

Diabetes is a serious public health issue. Almost 26 million people in the United States have diabetes (CDC, 2011). As per the World Health Organization (WHO), 347 million people worldwide have diabetes. The rates of diabetes in U.S. adults vary with location. In 2010, the lowest percentage of the population having diabetes was in Vermont (5.8%) and the highest percentage was in Mississippi (11.3%). In the United States, diabetes disproportionately affects the "diabetes belt" in the southeastern United States. The higher diabetes rates are potentially due to increased prevalence of obesity, poor nutrition, decreased physical activity, and genetics (CDC, 2011).

Diabetes that is poorly controlled, for whatever reasons, can result in significant morbidity and mortality. In 2004, an estimated 3.4 million people in the world died from diabetes complications. More than 80% of diabetes deaths occur in low- and middle-income countries around the world, and the WHO projects that diabetes deaths will increase by 66% between 2008 and 2030 (WHO, 2012). Overall, the risk for death among people with diabetes is about twice the risk of people of similar age without diabetes.

Diabetes can also result in significant morbidity via acute and chronic complications. Uncontrolled diabetes causes increased susceptibility to illness and difficulty overcoming routine infections. Over time, elevated blood glucose levels can damage multiple organ systems, leading to cardiac, kidney, and eye complications. Adults with diabetes have 2 to 4 times higher risk of stroke and death from heart disease compared to adults without diabetes. Additionally, diabetes is the leading cause of kidney failure and new cases of blindness among adults (CDC, 2011).

EPIDEMIC OF DIABETES: INCREASING PREVALENCE AND INCIDENCE

The prevalence (the total number of existing diagnoses) and incidence (the number of new cases diagnosed each year) of diabetes are increasing in the United States and worldwide. In those less than 20 years of age in the United States, the incidence of type 2 diabetes is increasing, but type 1 diabetes is still the most common diagnosis. There is also a significant rise in the cases of type 1 diabetes, leading some to call it an "epidemic" (Forlenza & Rewers, 2011). In 2010, approximately 1.9 million new cases of diabetes were diagnosed in people aged 20 years or older. If current trends continue, 1 in 3 adults in the United States will have diabetes by 2050 (CDC, 2011; Imperatore et al., 2012).

There are several factors contributing to the increasing incidence of diabetes diagnoses. The American population is aging, which is impacting the rates of diabetes diagnoses. Additionally, the minority population in the United States is growing, and these groups have a higher risk of diabetes. Finally, the U.S. population is becoming increasingly overweight and sedentary, which are risk factors for the development of diabetes. However, the increasing rates of diabetes are not just related to increasing type 2 diabetes diagnoses. The incidence of type 1 diabetes is increasing by 3% to 5% per year in the United States, and the prevalence of type 1 diabetes is projected to double within the next 14 to 23 years (D'Angeli et al., 2010; Imperatore et al., 2012). There are multiple hypotheses regarding the reason for the increased rates of type 1 diabetes, including environmental triggers, in utero and early life exposures, and various infections. However, none of these hypotheses have been able to explain the etiology of the increasing prevalence and incidence of type 1 diabetes.

MANAGEMENT OF DIABETES

DIFFERENCES AND SIMILARITIES BY TYPE

The daily management of diabetes will vary with patients across types of diabetes (e.g., type 1 vs. type 2 diabetes); however, within types, there are often many similarities. The required and hallmark component to the daily management of type 1 diabetes is insulin. Insulin is administered by multiple daily injections or continuous subcutaneous insulin infusion (CSII; i.e., insulin pump). Insulin is typically injected or administered through an insulin pump more than 4 times per day. People with type 1 diabetes are also required to check their blood glucose levels multiple times daily by pricking the end of a finger and applying the blood sample to a glucose meter. It is typically recommended for this to happen at least 4 times daily, but those in optimal diabetes control can check 10 or more times daily. These tasks are demanding enough, but the complexity rises when the individual has to coordinate insulin administration with blood glucose levels, dietary intake, and physical activity. It is a delicate balance and is aimed at preserving short-term health and quality of life, as well as for the long term.

The treatment of type 2 diabetes is more variable and patient dependent. The first-line treatment is lifestyle modification. These alterations include a healthier diet, increased physical activity, and weight loss. In addition to required lifestyle changes, oral medications may be used to improve the body's sensitivity to insulin or increase insulin secretion. Over time, poor control of type 2 diabetes can progress to an insulin deficient state necessitating use of insulin (by injection or insulin pump); management then becomes similar to patients with type 1 diabetes.

In both type 1 and type 2 diabetes, glucose, blood pressure, and lipid control are critical. It is recommended that patients with diabetes have thorough evaluations by their endocrinologist 3 to 4 times per year. They are also required to have routine screenings for diabetes complications, including close monitoring of their heart, kidneys, eyes, and other systems impacted by elevated blood glucose levels. Of note, prior to becoming pregnant and during their pregnancy, patients with type 1 diabetes must have even tighter control of their diabetes and more intensive management.

ADHERENCE TO PRESCRIBED MANAGEMENT REGIMENS

Behavioral adherence to the type 1 diabetes regimen varies with task (Johnson, 1992; Kutz, 1990; McNabb, 1997). For example, rates of adherence to blood glucose monitoring and the regulation of carbohydrate intake tend to be the lowest (39%), while rates of adherence to insulin administration tend to be the highest (Peyrot, Rubin, Lauritzen, & Skovlund et al., 2005). Patients on insulin pumps tend to experience both a clinical benefit in terms of adherence and control (Phillip et al., 2007), as well as quality of life (Barnard, Thomas, Royle, Noyes, & Waugh, 2010; Weissberg-Benchell et al., 2003). There are a variety of factors that have been linked to poor adherence in individuals with type 1 diabetes. For example, those with depression have lower rates of adherence (Gonzalez et al., 2008). In addition, a lack of social support is related to poorer levels of adherence (Delamater, 2006). Further, background contextual factors such as family structure, access to resources and health care, and support within their family are also related to adherence rates (Modi et al., 2012).

As the management regimen for type 2 diabetes focuses (at least initially) on lifestyle modifications in the form of increased physical activity and decrease in caloric intake, adherence to lifestyle modifications is highly variable (Peyrot, Rubin, Lauritzen, & Snoek et al., 2005). Research on individuals with type 2 diabetes has demonstrated that adherence to the prescribed meal plan is around 37% and adherence to the prescribed physical activity recommendations is 35%. When the disease progresses beyond lifestyle modifications as the only treatment option, adherence rates still vary considerably. Adherence to oral medication to treat type 2 diabetes is highest, at 78%; however, adherence to daily blood glucose monitoring is 39% in those treated with insulin and only 5% in those who are not taking insulin (Peyrot, Rubin, Lauritzen, & Snoek et al., 2005). Thus, both type 1 and type 2 represent complex medical regimens that are difficult to follow as prescribed.

LINK BETWEEN ADHERENCE AND HEALTH OUTCOMES

After the DCCT was first published in 1993 for patients with type 1 diabetes and similar data were published by the United Kingdom Prospective Diabetes Study (UKPDS) for patients with type 2 diabetes in 1995, the diabetes world has had a hard, biological measure of a patient's overall level of diabetes control. This measure is the hemoglobin A1C value, which reflects the prior 8 to 12 weeks of glucose "control." The reference range for people without diabetes is 4% to 6% and treatment targets for people with diabetes are below 7.0% for adults (19 and older), and 7.5% to 8.5% for children and adolescents (American Diabetes Association 2005, 2012). However, the majority of patients do not meet these targets (Danne et al., 2001; Svoren et al., 2007; Weinger et al., 2005).

There are a number of factors that contribute to A1C values, but the variable assumed to be the largest contributor is adherence to the management regimen. Data from pediatric and adult patients, across type 1 and type 2 diabetes, highlight that 30% to 50% of overall control can be attributed to adherence (Hood, Peterson, Rohan, & Drotar, 2009; Weinger, Butler, Welch, & La Greca, 2005; Winkley, Ismail, Landau, & Eisler, 2006).

The remaining contributors cut across contextual variables such as access to health care, family structure, social support, and other psychosocial variables. Further, in youth, growth and puberty play a major role in A1C outcomes (Moreland et al., 2004).

BARRIERS TO EFFECTIVE DIABETES MANAGEMENT

As noted previously, diabetes management includes a set of complex and demanding behaviors that must be carried out multiple times daily. While there are a number of barriers to ongoing chronic disease management covered in other chapters in this text, there are diabetes-specific considerations or variants of those barriers. One set of barriers to carrying out diabetes management tasks cuts across habits and routines, and competing needs and priorities. Consider this situation:

Frank, a 49-year-old man, was just diagnosed with type 2 diabetes. He knew for several years that he was at risk for type 2 diabetes given his family history, and he tried to eat a healthier diet and walk for 60 minutes 3 to 4 times per week. There were large gaps where he was not able to do these positive lifestyle behaviors because of arriving home late from work and not having them scheduled in to his daily plans. He also saw no incentive for walking or eating healthier because he did not physically feel very different and never noticed any weight loss. Frank's diabetes care team decided to put him on an oral medication (metformin) twice daily to help with glucose control. Mindful of the difficulties making lifestyle changes previously, his diabetes care team set up a system of reminders and support around management. For example, the team helped him set reminders in his phone to take his pills. Further, they paired eating breakfast, something he always does at the same time, with checking his blood sugar. They had him leave his blood glucose meter by the breakfast food cabinet in his kitchen. They were able to embed these behaviors into his daily life by combining them with existing, and routine events.

The story of this patient is similar to many attempting to engage in positive diabetes management behaviors and not having success, and the need for more structured behaviors. Few are successful at embedding these behaviors into daily life and breaking down this significant behavior without the structure and direction of the team and support.

EMOTIONAL BARRIERS AND IMPACT ON DIABETES MANAGEMENT

Depression

There are clear data that diabetes doubles an individual's likelihood of being depressed (Anderson et al., 2001) and that depression can significantly impact a person's ability to manage diabetes (Gonzalez et al., 2008; McGrady, Laffel, Drotar, Repaske, & Hood, 2009). It is also the case that depression places a person at increased risk for type 2 diabetes, possibly because it impairs an individual's ability to carry out generally healthy behaviors (Golden et al., 2008). Whether depression started before or after the diagnosis of diabetes, depression can make the challenging lifestyle modifications and daily management behaviors seem overwhelming.

Consider the situation noted above, but with an additional twist:

After making progress taking his medications and checking his blood sugar, Frank reported feeling unsupported in his diabetes management during one of his medical visits. His team, mindful of his history of depression, referred him to a psychosocial group for adults newly diagnosed with diabetes. The aim of the group was to promote coping with diabetes and its management and address emotional barriers like depression. In this group, there was a focus on diabetes problem solving and cognitive restructuring. Specifically, a four-step method of solving problems related to diabetes was taught along with attempts to challenge irrational beliefs about diabetes (e.g., "I cannot live with this disease" and "it is always getting the best of me"). Frank learned to effectively identify problems related to his diabetes (Step 1), come up with possible solutions (Step 2), develop a plan to address barriers and work toward resolution of the problem (Step 3), and how to evaluate and rework potential solutions if needed (Step 4). Frank made significant progress in diabetes-specific problem solving, felt less stressed about diabetes and in general, and was better at integrating diabetes management in to his daily life.

Later in the intervention section, more details about the components of an intervention like the one Frank participated in to break down behavioral and emotional barriers through problem solving will be reviewed.

Diabetes Burnout and Psychological Insulin Resistance

A related emotional barrier to effective diabetes management has been termed "diabetes burnout" (Polonsky et al., 1995). Diabetes burnout occurs when a person feels "overwhelmed by diabetes and by the frustrating burden of diabetes self-care" (Polonsky et al., 1995). These emotions may be different from feelings of depression, but because of their diabetes-specific nature, they are often just as destructive and have implications for diabetes care.

A phenomenon unique to type 2 diabetes is the patient's resistance to initiate insulin therapy, also known as "psychological insulin resistance" (Polonsky, Fisher, Guzman, Villa-Caballero, & Edelman, 2005; Polonsky, 2007). Patients with type 2 diabetes often interpret initiating insulin therapy as a failure of the previous regimen. In addition, patients are resistant to insulin therapy because of the belief that their diabetes is not "serious" enough to begin insulin therapy. Polonsky and his associates (2005) demonstrated that of 708 patients with type 2 diabetes, 28% were unwilling to take insulin to treat their diabetes. Of those patients who were unwilling to initiate insulin therapy to treat their diabetes, 55% believed that needing to be on insulin indicated they failed in properly controlling their diabetes with oral agents. Likewise, 56% believed that being on insulin would restrict their lives and 53% believed that once they started insulin therapy it would be a permanent change in their regimen. Research has shown that health care providers who treat individuals with type 2 diabetes also have beliefs and attitudes about the initiation of insulin therapy that present obstacles to patients being willing to use insulin to treat their diabetes. For example, the initiation of insulin therapy in patients with type 2 diabetes is often used as a threat to patients in motivating them to adhere more closely to the diabetes regimen (typically to no avail). In addition, health care providers believe that insulin therapy for patients with type 2 diabetes is only for those whose diabetes is poorly controlled (Peyrot, Rubin, Lauritzen, Skovlund, et al., 2005). Thus, barriers to the initiation of insulin therapy in patients with type 2 diabetes exist for both patients and health care providers and are largely attitudinal.

Fear of Hypoglycemia

Fear of hypoglycemia (low blood glucose) is considered one of the major barriers to optimal glucose control in type 1, and advanced type 2, diabetes. Hypoglycemia is common; studies show that patients with type 1 diabetes experience approximately two episodes of hypoglycemia per week and one severe hypoglycemic episode per year (MacLeod, Hepburn, & Frier, 1993). Cryer (2008) reported that 6% to 10% of all deaths in people with type 1 diabetes were the result of hypoglycemia.

A review by Barnard et al. (2010) examining the fear of hypoglycemia in parents with young children (less than 12 years of age) with type 1 diabetes concluded fear of hypoglycemia impacted parental health and quality of life. Direct effects on regimen adherence were less clear, but the review did support the hypothesis that hypoglycemia avoidance by parents adversely impacts glucose control. They are more likely to underdose insulin when fears of hypoglycemia are present, resulting in higher blood sugar levels. Barnard et al.'s findings are consistent with a study by Clarke, Gonder-Frederick, Snyder, and Cox (1998) in adults with type 1 diabetes that found an association between fear of hypoglycemia and higher glucose levels. Wild et al. (2007) reviewed the literature on fear of hypoglycemia and concluded there is evidence that fear of hypoglycemia has a negative impact on diabetes management. The authors hypothesized interventions, including blood glucose awareness and cognitive behavioral therapy, may reduce levels of fear and improve diabetes management. Wild et al. (2007) recommended addressing the fear of hypoglycemia during clinic visits and diabetes education.

FAMILY BARRIERS

There are several well-studied family barriers that interfere with behavior management of diabetes, in addition to the factors outlined in Chapter 5 of this text. These diabetes-specific family barriers include a lack of adequate support around management, conflict between patients and families, and poor communication between patients and their families around the treatment regimen. The interpersonal conflict that emerges around diabetes can, and often does result in significant declines in diabetes self-care behaviors and, in turn, results in poorer glucose control (Wysocki, 1993).

Of the family factors that impact health behaviors and health status of youths with diabetes, family conflict emerges as a primary issue that needs attention (DiMatteo, 2004). Many of the conflictual interactions between patients and family often revolve around how the patient is managing his or her diabetes. Anderson and Coyne (1991) outlined a process known as "miscarried helping" for understanding how interpersonal conflict emerges in families of individuals with a chronic illness. Anderson and Coyne (1991) highlight how good intentions on the part of caregivers result in interpersonal conflict between the patient with diabetes and other family members, further polarizing the two parties and putting the patient's diabetes at greater risk. There are several reasons why the family is the primary focus for examining miscarried helping. First, those closest to an individual with diabetes are family members who are most likely to assist with day-to-day demands of the treatment regimen. Second, family members are the most likely to advise or influence a patient with diabetes around issues of disease management and general health care (DiMatteo, 2004). Finally, the family represents a model for health behaviors including diet, exercise, and interactions with the health care team. Thus, involvement from family in diabetes management can result in poor health behaviors via a lack of adequate support, increased interpersonal conflict, and poor communication about how best to manage diabetes (Coyne, Wortman, & Lehman, 1988; Harris et al., 2008; Pierce, Sarason, Sarason, Joseph, & Henderson, 1996).

FACILITATING EFFECTIVE MANAGEMENT OF DIABETES

THE EVIDENCE BASE

Over two decades of research in the behavioral management of diabetes leads us to conclude that (1) providing education for diabetes management is important, but not sufficient for optimal outcomes, and (2) breaking down barriers and fostering new skills serve as the most powerful interventions. These two points lead to a larger conclusion; multi-component interventions that focus on behavior change and the facilitators of those changes will have the most robust effect on quality of life and health outcomes for people with diabetes. These can be carried out in the clinical setting, within families, and in the communities where the patients with diabetes reside. The following section draws on the evidence base to highlight the best ways to facilitate behavior change in the management of diabetes.

Multi-Component Interventions

In a recent meta-analysis of nearly 1,000 youth and young adults with type 1 diabetes, the interventions that included components that directly attempted to increase management behaviors (e.g., blood glucose monitoring) and addressed the facilitators of those behaviors (e.g., better communication in the family) were the only interventions that had a positive effect on hemoglobin A1c values (Hood, Rohan, Peterson, & Drotar, 2010). Those interventions provided direct education and support around management behaviors while promoting better coping and problem-solving skills. The interventions that just focused on one or the other were far less effective in changing A1c values. Similarly, other problem-solving interventions not included in that meta-analysis have been shown to change behaviors and A1c values (Mulvaney et al., 2010).

Problem-solving interventions are popular in adults as well and these interventions cut across type 1 and type 2 diabetes. A systematic review by Hill-Briggs and Gemmell (2007) synthesized findings from nearly 40 studies on problem solving with adults with diabetes. Only about 50% of the adult studies had a significant impact on A1c values, but most did change health behaviors positively. The most effective interventions were those that focused on diabetes-specific problem solving, not just a general framework for solving everyday problems. Further, those that focused on decision making utilizing diabetes examples were particularly effective. Potential reasons for not observing as widespread an effect on A1c from these studies included too short of a time to follow-up to see whether the behaviors had been embedded in daily lives (to have an effect on A1c values). The results, however, are promising given their relative low intensity and large effects (for about half those sampled).

An example of an evidence-based problem-solving intervention for adults with diabetes comes from the work of Fisher and colleagues (Glasgow, Fisher, Skaff, Mullan, & Toobert, 2007). The major goals of their intervention are to decrease the distress and negative impact associated with diabetes (i.e., diabetes burnout), increase coping skills, and minimize the likelihood of similar problems re-occurring in the future. This problem-solving intervention includes educating patients, via a live diabetes counselor, about the impact of distress and burnout on diabetes (and vice versa), making a list of problems associated with diabetes and distress, prioritizing them, and, over a series of sessions, devising problem-solving strategies to address each. Adults with diabetes participating in this intervention receive two in-person sessions and four live phone calls across 5 months. Then they receive a supplemental in-person booster session and four more live calls across the remaining 6 months. They are taught an eight-step process to identify and define diabetes distress/burnout, establish realistic goals, generate ways to meet these goals, weigh the pros and cons of each, choose and evaluate solutions, create a diabetes distress action plan, evaluate outcome, and engage in pleasant activities. Also, through summary reports, this intervention permits ongoing feedback to primary providers to foster doctor/patient communication and facilitate ongoing clinical care.

Motivational Interviewing

Motivational interviewing (MI) is a clinical care approach, which allows providers and patients to work together to decide on treatment interventions. MI offers a brief, practical method for helping patients increase their motivation or readiness to change (Berg-Smith et al., 1999). The MI process is composed of establishing a relationship; setting an agenda; assessing importance, confidence, and readiness; exploring importance; helping patients select a plan of action; and building their confidence in their ability to change (Rollnick, Mason, & Butler, 1999). The main goal of MI is for patients and providers to collaboratively decide on the patient's next steps in a supportive, empathetic way.

Multiple MI interventions have been successful in both patients with type 1 and type 2 diabetes. In 2007, Channon and colleagues completed a multicenter trial investigating MI in teenagers with type 1 diabetes. At the end of the intervention (12 months), the mean A1C in the MI group was significantly lower than the control group. At 24 months, the difference between A1C values was maintained. The MI group also reported more positive well-being and improved quality of life. MI has also been effective in populations with type 2 diabetes. A 2012 randomized controlled trial by Chen and colleagues found MI resulted in improved self-management, psychological outcomes, and glycemic control in patients with type 2 diabetes. These note promising results for MI and highlight the need to engage people with diabetes and evaluate what has worked in the past to facilitate management, and why it has broken down due to barriers.

Family-Based Interventions

There have been many family-based interventions designed to improve behavioral management of diabetes in youth with diabetes. Several studies have examined the efficacy of involving multiple family members in the psychosocial treatment of individuals with diabetes. For example, previous research has examined the efficacy of involving parents in a crisis intervention program upon diagnosis of their child with diabetes. Findings from this study support the involvement of multiple family members in promoting positive health behaviors in youths with diabetes (Galatzer, Amir, Gil, Karp, & Laron, 1982). Other studies have examined separate psychosocial intervention sessions for youths with diabetes and their parents. Thus, there is evidence that involvement from family in diabetes management can result in better metabolic control and increased treatment adherence in individuals with diabetes (Anderson, Wolf, Burkhart, Cornell, & Bacon, 1989).

Several researchers have tested a clinic-based family intervention that involved collaborative problem solving ("Teamwork") between adolescents with type 1 diabetes and their parents (Auslander, 1993; Anderson, Brackett, Ho, & Laffel, 1999; Laffel et al., 2003). The Teamwork intervention involves family problem solving around three key areas: (1) examining the multiple causes for high blood sugars during early adolescence; (2) establishing realistic expectations for blood sugar values during adolescence; and (3) ongoing involvement from parents in diabetes management without shaming or blaming the youth. Youth and care providers spent approximately 20 to 30 minutes before or after each routine medical visit discussing these topics. During those meetings, a researcher provided information about the specific topic of focus and encouraged family-based discussion regarding pertinent issues. Also, each family was assisted in the process of developing a responsibility-sharing plan. The intervention proved effective in reducing diabetes-related conflict coupled with significant improvements in glycemic control.

Wysocki and colleagues (2000, 2006, 2007, 2008) conducted a series of randomized clinical trials examining the efficacy of a family-based psychosocial intervention (Behavioral Family Systems Therapy for Diabetes [BFST-D]) for adolescents with type 1 diabetes. BFST-D is a skills-based intervention for families that addresses four primary areas of family functioning: (1) problem solving, (2) communication, (3) strong beliefs, and (4) family structure, with additional sessions involving parent simulation of diabetes and nurse-directed identification of blood glucose patterns. Results from this series of randomized controlled trials have demonstrated that participation in BFST-D can result in significant improvements in glycemic control, treatment adherence, diabetes-related problem solving, and diabetes-related family conflict. Harris and colleagues (2003, 2005) conducted two studies examining a home-based version of BFST-D with adolescents with poorly controlled diabetes. Results from these two studies demonstrated that implementation of BFST-D in the home can result in significant decreases in general family conflict, decreases in diabetes-related family conflict, decreases in behavior problems, increases in diabetes treatment adherence, and improvements in glycemic control. Figure 14.1 highlights the components and sets expectations for families as they start this manualized, evidence-based family-based intervention.

Community-Based Interventions

Many of the multi-component interventions highlighted in the preceding section were delivered in the context of the clinic setting. Some were conducted at the time of quarterly diabetes care visits and others anchored intervention sessions around those visits, but offered more sessions in between. Community-based interventions are fundamentally different in that they are purposefully carried out away from the clinical setting. The aim is to promote generalization of learned skills and new education in the setting where these behaviors are conducted.

As noted throughout this chapter, diabetes management is complex and demanding. Lack of social support has been identified as a risk factor for poor diabetes management and increased morbidity and mortality (Brownson & Heisler, 2009). Peer

FIGURE 14.1 What can you expect during BFST sessions?

Your family will participate in 12 sessions of BFST that will be conducted by a highly trained psychologist or social worker. It will be important that teenagers and parents participate fully in order to learn how restructure family rules and roles in a way that family members can grow as individuals without disrupting the stability of your family. In addition, the therapist will be trying to understand how the other parts of your life, such as school, your community, and your medical team, can play a role in your ability to take care of your diabetes. The therapists will plan and carry out four components of the BFST approach that will be tailored to your family's specific needs. The four components of BFST are:

1. Problem-solving training: The therapist will teach your family to use a structured approach to problem solving. This will help you to define problems clearly, brainstorm a variety of possible solutions, and reach an agreement as a family on solutions to problems. You will practice these skills at home as well as in the sessions. You will be asked to monitor your problem-solving plan, evaluate the success or failure of the plan, and redefine the plan as needed. A nurse will be participating in sessions 6 and 7 to teach advanced problem solving using blood glucose data. The nurse also will train parents to simulate living with diabetes for one week. Parents will give themselves injections of sterile saline, test their blood glucose, follow a meal plan, test for ketones, and manage one unexpected simulated episode of hypoglycemia.

2. Communication skills training: In each of the 12 sessions, the therapist will ask you to talk together as a family about problems like you might at home. The therapist will offer you alternative ways to communicate in order to facilitate good family problem solving. The therapist will also give you feedback about your communication skills during the sessions to help you express your thoughts and feelings in a more clear and less threatening way. You may be asked to practice new communication skills in your session. In addition, your family will be given "homework assignments" to help you practice at home what you have learned in the sessions.

3. Strong belief restructuring: Along with communication skills and problem solving, there is another basic aspect of family interactions that determines how families get along. Sometimes parents and teenagers have strong beliefs, attitudes, and opinions about each other's behaviors and intentions. These beliefs are sometimes so strong that they get in the way of dealing more effectively with conflict. The therapist will help you to identify and "soften" strong beliefs to help you to communicate and problem-solve better as a family.

4. Family structuring: The way a family structures itself can determine how well the other components of BFST are implemented. Every family has specific roles for its members and rules to follow. These are often unspoken, but all family members are aware of them. The therapist will help families vocalize these roles and rules and determine if some of them need to change. The therapist will also explain some of the basic developmental stages of pre-teens and teens. This will help families understand that some of their child's behavioral changes are normal and necessary for growth.

support can provide the additional understanding and reinforcement individuals need to manage their diabetes. Additionally, peer-support interventions are more cost-effective and efficient than traditional diabetes management approaches. Based on a review of peer-support interventions by Heisler (2007), five models of peer-support have been identified, including (1) face-to-face group self-management programs, (2) peer coaches or mentors, (3) community health workers, (4) telephone-based peer support, and (5) Internet or e-mail-based peer support. Heisler concluded that no specific peer-support intervention could be identified as positively impacting diabetes control more than others; however, peer-support interventions were at least as effective, if not more effective, than standard clinical care models. Participant satisfaction was generally positive in all interventions, which may facilitate longer-term "buy-in" to the programs.

A large, community-based, peer-support program that has successfully decreased the risk of developing diabetes in at-risk patient populations is the Diabetes Prevention Program (DPP, 2002). DPP sessions are conducted in communities, and results show that intensive lifestyle interventions can result in weight loss and reduce the risk of developing diabetes. The intervention was accomplished through multiple methods, including (1) individual case managers or "lifestyle coaches," (2) frequent behavioral self-management strategies for weight loss and physical activity, (3) structured, state-of-the-art, 16-session core-curriculum teaching behavioral self-management strategies for weight loss and physical activity, (4) supervised physical activity sessions, (5) a more flexible maintenance intervention combining group and individual approaches, motivational campaigns, and "restarts," (6) individualization through a "toolbox" of adherence strategies, (7) tailoring of materials and strategies to address ethnic diversity, and (8) an extensive network of training, feedback, and clinical support.

The large-scale DPP can be resource-heavy and may not generalize to all community settings; thus it has been successfully translated into smaller settings, which offer more feasible interventions. A faith-based study by Boltri et al. (2008) found decreases in fasting glucose, weight, and systolic and diastolic blood pressures over 4 months in patients 18 years of age or older. The DPP has also been successfully adapted through partnerships with YMCA (Ackermann and Marrero, 2007; Ackermann, Finch, Brizendine, Zhou, & Marrero, 2008). The YMCA was found to be an inexpensive, effective way to impact the health of the community.

A large review of diabetes education in community settings by Norris and colleagues (2002) concluded different types of interventions effectively improve glycemic control in adults and pediatric patients. In adults, interventions delivered in community gathering places were effective. Interventions conducted in the home were effective for children and adolescents with type 1 diabetes. More research is needed to identify which community interventions are most effective in various populations, result in sustained behavior changes, and are the most cost-effective.

System-Based Interventions

System-based interventions are another example of multi-component diabetes interventions. System-based interventions have a focus beyond patients. They intervene with policy makers, public health officials, medical providers, and health centers caring for patients with diabetes, government, and institutions conducting diabetes research. There are examples of system-based interventions at national, state, and institutional levels. Many of the higher level, system-based interventions filter down to community-level interventions, which were reviewed in a previous section. However, more research needs to be conducted to determine the direct impact on the everyday lives of people with diabetes who are reached through these interventions.

At the national level, the CDC works to reduce the burden of preventable diabetes diagnoses and complications (www.cdc.gov). The CDC addresses their goals through public health leadership, partnerships, research, policies, and programs to translate science into practice. The CDC's Division of Diabetes Translation (DDT) focuses on public health surveillance, research delivery in clinical and public health practices, development and maintenance of effective state-based diabetes prevention and control programs, and closure of health gaps among the population most severely affected by diabetes (www.cdc.gov/diabetes).

South Carolina's Department of Health and Environmental Control has organized a state-level, system-based intervention to address diabetes (www.scdhec.gov/health /chcdp/diabetes/health_systems.htm). The state's Diabetes Division's Health System directs their efforts toward prevention of diabetes and reduction of diabetes-related complications. Their focus is on high-risk populations, such as the African American, Hispanic/Latino, and elderly populations. The Diabetes Division partners with other diabetes-focused health care organizations to ensure evidence-based diabetes prevention, screening, diagnosis, treatment, and control interventions are distributed to the community. This information is disseminated to health care providers through professional education sessions, symposia, and support of recognized diabetes self-management education programs. They also have a Diabetes Advisory Council that assists with the determination of minimum standards of medical care for patients with diabetes in South Carolina.

The Michigan Diabetes Research and Training Center (MDRTC) is one example of an institutional, system-based intervention to address the diabetes burden (www.med .umich.edu/mdrtc). The MDRTC provides a Behavioral, Clinical, and Health Systems Intervention Research Core (BCHS). It is an avenue for collaboration, training, and tangible resources to support high-quality diabetes-focused research. The BCHS provides interdisciplinary review and suggestions for research studies. It provides a route for translation of research from bench to bedside, and it supports collaboration that will increase the likelihood of successful research efforts.

The Task Force of Community Preventive Services (the Task Force) is an independent, nonfederal group focusing on public health recommendations and guidelines. In 2002, the Task Force developed the *Guide to Community Preventive Services* with support from the U.S. Department of Health and Human Services, and a portion of their guide focused on diabetes interventions. From a health care system intervention viewpoint, the Task Force strongly recommended disease management and case management to improve the performance of health care systems and providers delivering care to people with diabetes.

All of these system-based interventions, and the resultant community-based or direct clinic-based interventions, are aimed at improving outcomes for people with diabetes. Given the complexity of diabetes and its management, and the multiple contributors to quality of life and health outcomes, improvements in mortality and morbidity require a multi-pronged approach. The core component of all of these multi-component interventions and approaches is an attempt to change health behaviors.

ROLE OF TECHNOLOGY

In addition to the substantial improvements of existing technologies such as the insulin pump and continuous glucose monitoring systems over the past decade, the advent of new technologies and applications serves as adjunct strategies for improving diabetes management and outcomes. For example, applications such as *Glucose Buddy* are available for free download for most smartphones. In this program and others like it, a patient's blood glucose meter is directly linked to an application that synthesizes data and highlights trends in blood glucose (e.g., common occurrence of hypoglycemia each morning). Other programs synthesize these important data and connect the user to a social media forum where they can communicate about their diabetes with others with diabetes. Emerging technologies such as *CareCoach*, developed by Verilouge, Inc., focus on patient–provider communication and help patients know how to phrase questions to their diabetes care providers and set goals based on provider recommendations. These programs are ultimately aimed at taking advantage of the tech-savvy and connected nature of most individuals in the United States to ease management and see trends that previously were left to providers to develop. The programs that link that to recommendations and goal setting appear most promising and poised to facilitate diabetes management behaviors.

While promising and exciting, the documentation of the effectiveness of these applications to facilitate behavior change lags behind the pace that these applications hit the marketplace. Thus, few data are available about their effectiveness and impact on management and outcomes. The available data suggest that mobile phone applications are effective at increasing self-management behaviors and lowering hemoglobin A1C

(Liang et al., 2011). The meta-analysis was focused on adults, most with type 2 diabetes; however, there are data on adolescents and young adults as well. Mulvaney et al. (2010) have shown the utility of a mobile and web-based program called YourWay to improve the management and glycemic outcomes of adolescents with type 1 diabetes. There are other programs as well and several recent papers have focused on this topic (Harris, Hood, & Mulvaney, 2012). While no data exist yet to support this conclusion, the current evidence base and what is understood about health behavior change suggest the following: technology and applications that provide a scaffolding for patients to internalize the salience and routine of specific health behaviors, with clear contingencies in place for positive reinforcement, are most likely to increase and sustain diabetes management behaviors.

CONCLUSIONS

The conduct and coordination of multiple management behaviors remain the best way to optimize health outcomes and quality of life in people with diabetes. Given the substantial individual and public health burden of diabetes, and the trajectory toward an even greater burden in the future, a focus on facilitating behavior change in people with diabetes is timely and important. The evidence base indicates that diabetes-specific barriers to effective diabetes management include feeling distressed and burned out about diabetes, fear of hypoglycemia, and family conflict. Each of these directly contributes to the conduct, frequency, and durability of multiple diabetes management behaviors, which have been linked with poorer outcomes. Identification of these barriers is the first step in determining how to best facilitate behavior change. Once identified, there are appropriate and applicable interventions.

The evidence-based interventions that facilitate behavior change in people with diabetes range from individual programs to larger, systems-based interventions. In general, multi-component interventions are more effective at changing behavior than those that just provide education and support for specific behaviors, or the facilitators of those behaviors. Both components are necessary. Problem-solving interventions that help people with diabetes develop a framework for identifying diabetes-specific problems, solutions to those problems, goal setting, and an ability to evaluate outcomes. Motivational interviewing can also be effective at engaging and facilitating behavior change for diabetes-specific barriers to management. A number of family-based interventions have been shown to be effective at positively changing behaviors, particularly in pediatric diabetes. The most notable family-based interventions combine problem solving, coping, and the use of a diabetes-specific context for implementation of those newly learned skills. Community- and system-based interventions are also effective, but the specific components that trickle down to individuals are not well understood. Finally, technologies and applications can serve as scaffolding to and facilitators of behavior change. Their initial uptake and feasibility seem strong, but the sustainability for maintenance of diabetes management has yet to be established.

In sum, current evidence and clinical expertise indicate that diabetes-specific behavior change is most likely to occur when interventions are offered that break down barriers, promote problem solving, and engage patients in a way that synthesizes data from management. Given the complex and demanding, and lifelong nature of diabetes management, efforts to facilitate diabetes management are likely to promote better health and quality of life outcomes for people with diabetes.

REFERENCES

Ackermann, R. T., Finch, E. A., Brizendine, E., Zhou, H., & Marrero, D. G. (2008). Translating the Diabetes Prevention Program into the community. The DEPLOY Pilot Study. *American Journal of Preventive Medicine, 35*(4), 357–363.

Ackermann, R. T., & Marrero, D. G. (2007). Adapting the Diabetes Prevention Program lifestyle intervention for delivery in the community: The YMCA model. *Diabetes Educator, 33*(1), 69–77.

American Diabetes Association, Silverstein, J. H, Klingensmith, G., Copeland, K., Plotnick, L., Kaufman, F., … Clark, N. (2005). Care of children and adolescents with type 1 diabetes: A statement of the American Diabetes Association. *Diabetes Care, 28*(1), 186–212.

American Diabetes Association. (2012). Clinical practice recommendations. *Diabetes Care, 35*(Suppl. 1).

Anderson, B. J., Auslander, W. F., Jung, K. C., Miller, J. P., & Santiago, J. V. (1990). Assessing family sharing of diabetes responsibilities. *Journal of Pediatric Psychology, 15*, 477–492.

Anderson, B. J., Brackett, J., Ho, J., & Laffel, L. (1999). An office-based intervention to maintain parent-adolescent teamwork in diabetes management: Impact on parent involvement, family conflict, and subsequent glycemic control. *Diabetes Care, 22*, 713–721.

Anderson, B. J., & Coyne, J. C. (1991). "Miscarried helping" in families of children and adolescents with chronic diseases. In J. H. Johnson & S. B. Johnson (Eds.), *Advances in child health psychology*. Gainesville, FL: University of Florida Press.

Anderson, R. J., Freedland, K. E., Clouse, R. E., & Lustman, P. J. (2001). The prevalence of comorbid depression in adults with diabetes: A meta-analysis. *Diabetes Care, 24*(6), 1069–1078.

Anderson, B. J., Ho, J., Brackett, J., Finkelstein, D., & Laffel, L. (1997). Parental involvement in diabetes management tasks: Relationships to blood glucose monitoring adherence and metabolic control in young adolescents with insulin-dependent diabetes mellitus. *Journal of Pediatrics, 130*, 257–265.

Anderson, B. J., Wolf, F. M., Burkhart, M. T., Cornell, R. G., & Bacon, G. E. (1989). Effects of peer-group intervention on metabolic control of adolescents with IDDM: Randomized outpatient study. *Diabetes Care, 12*, 179–183.

Atkinson, M., & Eisenbarth, G. (2001). Type 1 diabetes: New perspectives on disease pathogenesis and treatment. *Lancet, 358*(9277), 221–229.

Auslander, W. F. (1993). Brief family interventions to improve family communication and cooperation regarding diabetes management. *Diabetes Spectrum, 6*, 330–331.

Barnard, K., Thomas, S., Royle, P., Noyes, K., & Waugh, N. (2010). Fear of hypoglycaemia in parents of young children with type 1 diabetes: A systematic review. *BMC Pediatrics, 10*, 50.

Berg-Smith, S. M., Stevens, V. J., Brown, K. M., Van Horn, L., Gernhofer, N., & Peters, E. (1999). A brief MI to improve dietary adherence in adolescents. *Health Education Research, 14*, 399–410.

Bluestone, J. A., Herold, K., & Eisenbarth, G. (2010). Genetics, pathogenesis, and treatment in type 1 diabetes. *Nature, 464*(7293), 1293–1300.

Boltri, J. M., Davis-Smith, Y. M., Seale, J. P., Shellenberger, S., Okosun, I. S., & Cornelius, M. E. (2008). Diabetes prevention in a faith-based setting: Results of translational research. *Journal of Public Health Management and Practice 14*(1), 29–32.

Brownson, C. A., & Heisler, M. (2009). The role of peer support in diabetes care and self-management. *The Patient, 2*(1), 5–17.

Burroughs, T. E., Harris, M. A, Pontious, S. L, & Santiago, J. V. (1997). Research on social support in adolescents with IDDM: A critical review. *Diabetes Educator, 23*, 438–448.

Centers for Disease Control and Prevention (CDC). (2011). *National diabetes fact sheet: National estimates and general information on diabetes and prediabetes in the United States, 2011*. Atlanta, GA: U.S. Department of Health and Human Services, Centers for Disease Control and Prevention.

Centers for Disease Control and Prevention (CDC). (2013). *Diabetes public health resource*. Retrieved from http://www.cdc.gov/diabetes

Channon, S. J., Huws-Thomas, M. V., Rollnick, S., Hood, K., Canning-John, R. L., Rogers, C., & Gregory, J. W. (2007). A multicenter randomized controlled trail of motivational interviewing in teenagers with diabetes. *Diabetes Care, 30*(6), 1390–1395.

Chen, S. M., Creddy, D., Lin, H. S., & Wollin, J. (2012). Effects of motivational intervention on self-management, psychological, and glycemic outcomes in type 2 diabetes: A randomized controlled trial. *International Journal of Nursing Studies, 49*(6), 637–644.

Clarke, W. L., Gonder-Frederick, A., Snyder, A. L., & Cox, D. J. (1998). Maternal fear of hypoglycemia in their children with insulin dependent diabetes mellitus. *Journal of Pediatric Endocrinology & Metabolism, 11*(Suppl. 1), 189–194.

Coyne, J. C., Wortman, C. B, & Lehman D. R. (1988). The other side of support: Emotional overinvolvement and miscarried helping. In B. H. Gottlieb (Ed.), *Marshalling social support: Formats, processes, and effects*. Newbury Park, NY: Sage Publications.

Cryer, P. E. (2008). The barrier of hypoglycemia in diabetes. [Research Support, N.I.H., Extramural Research Support, Non-U.S. Gov't Review]. *Diabetes, 57*(12), 3169–3176. doi:10.2337/db08-1084

D'Angeli, M. A., Merzon, E., Valbuena, L. F., Tirschwell, D., Paris, C. A., & Mueller, B. A. (2010). Environmental factors associated with childhood-onset type 1 diabetes mellitus: An exploration of the hygiene and overload hypotheses. [Research Support, N.I.H., Extramural Research Support, Non-U.S. Gov't]. *Archives of Pediatrics & Adolescent Medicine, 164*(8), 732–738. doi: 10.1001/archpediatrics.2010.115

Danne, T., Mortensen, H. B., Hougaard, P., Lynggaard, H., Aanstoot, H. J., Chiarelli, F., ... Hvidøre Study Group on Childhood Diabetes. (2001). Persistent differences among centers over 3 years in glycemic control and hypoglycemia in a study of 3,805 children and adolescents with type 1 diabetes from the Hvidøre Study Group. *Diabetes Care, 24*(8), 1342–1347.

Delamater, A. M. (2006). Improving patient adherence. *Clinical Diabetes, 24*(2), 71–77.

Diabetes Prevention Program (DPP) Research Group. (2002). The Diabetes Prevention Program (DPP): Description of lifestyle intervention. [Research Support, Non-U.S. Gov't Research Support, U.S. Gov't, P.H.S.]. *Diabetes Care, 25*(12), 2165–2171.

DiMatteo, M. R. (2004). Social support and patient adherence to medical treatment: A meta-analysis. *Health Psychology, 23*, 207–218.

Ershow, A. G., Peterson, C. M., Riley, W. T., Rizzo, A. S., & Wansink, B. (2011). Virtual reality technologies for research and education in obesity and diabetes: Research needs and opportunities. *Journal of Diabetes Science and Technology, 5*(2), 212–224.

Forlenza, G. P., & Rewers, M. (2011). The epidemic of type 1 diabetes: What is it telling us? *Current Opinion in Endocrinology, Diabetes, and Obesity, 18*(4), 248–251.

Galatzer, A., Amir, S., Gil, R., Karp, M., & Laron, Z. (1982). Crisis intervention program in newly diagnosed diabetic children. *Diabetes Care, 5*, 414–419.

Glasgow, R. E., Fisher, L., Skaff, M., Mullan, J., & Toobert, D. J. (2007). Problem solving and diabetes self-management: Investigation in a large, multiracial sample. *Diabetes Care, 30*(1), 33–37.

Golden, S. H., Lazo, M., Carnethon, M., Bertoni, A. G., Schreiner, P. J., Diez Roux, A. V., ... Lyketsos, C. (2008). Examining a bidirectional association between depressive symptoms and diabetes. *Journal of the American Medical Association, 299*(23), 2751–2759. doi: 10.1001/jama.299.23.2751

Gonzalez, J. S., Pierrot, M., McCarl, L. A., Collins, E. M., Serpa, L., Mimiaga, M. J., & Safren, S. A. (2008). Depression and diabetes treatment nonadherence: A meta-analysis. *Diabetes Care, 31*(12), 2398–2403.

Hanson, C. L., DeGuire, M. J., Schinkel, A. M., & Kolterman, O. G. (1995). Empirical validation for a family-centered model of care. *Diabetes Care, 18*, 1347–1356.

Harris, M. A., Antal, H., Oelbaum, R., Buckloh, L. M., White, N. H., & Wysocki, T. (2008). Good intentions gone awry: Assessing parental "miscarried helping" in diabetes. *Families, Systems & Health, 26*(4), 393–403.

Harris, M. A., Greco, P., Wysocki, T., Elder-Danda, C., & White, N. H. (1999). Adolescents with diabetes from single-parent, blended, and intact families: Health-related and family functioning. *Families, Systems & Health, 17*, 181–196.

Harris, M. A., Harris, B. S., & Mertlich, D. (2005). Brief report: In-home family therapy for adolescents with poorly controlled diabetes: Failure to maintain benefits at 6-month follow-up. *Journal of Pediatric Psychology, 30*, 683–688.

Harris, M. A., Hood, K. K., & Mulvaney, S. A. (2012). Pumpers, skypers, surfers and texters: Technology to improve the management of diabetes in teenagers. *Diabetes Obesity & Metabolism, 14*(11), 967–972.

Harris, M. A., & Mertlich, D. (2003). Piloting home-based behavioral family systems therapy for adolescents with poorly controlled diabetes. *Child Health Care, 32*, 65–79.

Harris, M. I. (2001). Frequency of blood glucose monitoring in relation to glycemic control in patients with type 2 diabetes. *Diabetes Care, 24*, 979–982.

Heisler, M. (2007). Overview of peer support models to improve diabetes self-management and clinical outcomes. *Diabetes Spectrum, 20*(4), 214–221. doi: 10.2337/diaspect.20.4.214

Hill-Briggs, F., & Gemmell, L. (2007). Problem solving in diabetes self-management and control: A systematic review of the literature. *Diabetes Educator, 33*(6), 1032–1050; discussion 1051–1052.

Hood, K. K., Peterson, C. M., Rohan, J. M., & Drotar, D. (2009). Association between adherence and glycemic control in pediatric type 1 diabetes: A meta-analysis. *Pediatrics, 124*(6), e1171–e1179.

Hood, K. K., Rohan, J. M., Peterson, C. M., & Drotar, D. (2010). Interventions with adherence-promoting components in pediatric type 1 diabetes: Meta-analysis of their impact on glycemic control. *Diabetes Care, 33*(7), 1658–1664.

Imperatore, G., Boyle, J. P., Thompson, T. J., Case, D., Dabelea, D., Hamman, R. F., … SEARCH for Diabetes in Youth Study Group. (2012). Projections of type 1 and type 2 diabetes burden in the U.S. population aged <20 years through 2050: Dynamic modeling of incidence, mortality, and population growth. *Diabetes Care, 35*(12), 2515–2520.

Johnson, S. B. (1992). Methodological issues in diabetes research: Measuring adherence. *Diabetes Care, 15*, 1658–1667.

Kutz, S. M. (1990). Adherence to diabetes regimens: Empirical status and clinical applications. *Diabetes Educator, 16*, 50–56.

Laffel, L. M., Vangsness, L., Connell, A., Goebel-Fabbri, A., Butler, D., & Anderson, B. J. (2003). Impact of ambulatory, family-focused teamwork intervention on glycemic control in youth with type 1 diabetes. *Journal of Pediatrics, 142*(4), 409–416.

Liang, X., Wang, Q., Yang, X., Cao, J., Chen, J., Mo, X., … Gu, D. (2011). Effect of mobile phone intervention for diabetes on glycaemic control: A meta-analysis. *Diabetic Medicine: A Journal of the British Diabetic Association, 28*(4), 455–463. doi: 10.1111/j.1464-5491.2010.03180.x

Liese, A. D., D'Agostino, R. B., Jr., Hamman, R. F., Kilgo, P. D., Lawrence, J. M., Liu, L. L., … Williams, D. E. (2006). The burden of diabetes mellitus among US youth: Prevalence estimates from the SEARCH for Diabetes in Youth Study. *Pediatrics, 118*(4), 1510–1518.

MacLeod, K. M., Hepburn, D. A., & Frier, B. M. (1993). Frequency and morbidity of severe hypoglycaemia in insulin-treated diabetic patients. [Comparative Study Research Support, Non-U.S. Gov't]. *Diabetic Medicine: A Journal of the British Diabetic Association, 10*(3), 238–245.

McGrady, M. E., Laffel, L., Drotar, D., Repaske, D., & Hood, K. K. (2009). Depressive symptoms and glycemic control in adolescents with type 1 diabetes: Mediational role of blood glucose monitoring. *Diabetes Care, 32*(5), 804–806.

McNabb, W. L (1997). Adherence in diabetes: Can we define it and can we measure it? *Diabetes Care, 20*, 215–218.

University of Michigan Health System. (2013). *Michigan diabetes research and training center.* Retrieved from http://www.med.umich.edu/mdrtc/

Miller-Johnson, S., Emery, R. E., Marvin, R. S., Clarke, W., Lovinger, R., & Martin, M. (1994). Parent-child relationships and the management of insulin-dependent diabetes mellitus. *Journal of Consulting and Clinical Psychology, 62*, 603–610.

Modi, A. C., Pai, A. L., Hommel, K. A., Hood, K. K., Cortina, S., Hilliard, M. E., Guilfoyle, S. M., … Drotar, D. (2012). Pediatric self-management: A framework for research, practice, and policy. *Pediatrics, 129*(2), e473–e485. doi: 10.1542/peds.2011-1635.

Moreland, E. C., Tovar, A., Zuehlke, J. B., Butler, D. A., Milaszewski, K., & Laffel, L. M. (2004). The impact of physiological, therapeutic and psychosocial variables on glycemic control in youth with type 1 diabetes mellitus. *Journal of Pediatric Endocrinology & Metabolism, 17*(11), 1533–1544.

Mulvaney, S. A., Rothman, R. L., Wallston, K. A., Lybarger, C., & Dietrich, M. S. (2010). An internet-based program to improve self-management in adolescents with type 1 diabetes. *Diabetes Care, 33*(3), 602–604. doi: 10.2337/dc09-1881.

Nansel, T. R., Anderson, B. J., Laffel, L., Simons-Morton, B. G., Weissberg-Benchell, J., Wysocki, T., … Lochrie, A. S. (2009). A multisite trial of a clinic-integrated intervention for promoting family management of pediatric type 1 diabetes: Feasibility and design. *Pediatric Diabetes, 10*, 105–115.

Norris, S. L., Nichols, P. J., Caspersen, C. J., Glasgow, R. E., Engelgau, M. M., Jack, L., … McCulloch, D. (2002). Increasing diabetes self-management education in community settings. A systematic review. [Review]. *American Journal of Preventive Medicine, 22*(4 Suppl.), 39–66.

Pierce, G. R., Sarason, B. R., Sarason, I. G., Joseph, H. J., & Henderson, C. A. (1996). Conceptualizing and assessing social support in the context of the family. In G. R. Pierce, B. R. Sarason, & I. G. Sarason (Eds.), *Handbook of social support and the family* (pp. 3–23). New York, NY: Plenum Press.

Peyrot, M., Rubin, R. R., Lauritzen, T., Skovlund, S. E., Snoek, F. J., Matthews, D. R., … International DAWN Advisory Panel. (2005). Resistance to insulin therapy among patients and providers. *Diabetes Care, 28*(11), 2673–2679.

Peyrot, M., Rubin, R. R., Lauritzen, T., Snoek, F. J., Matthews, D. R., & Skovlund, S. E. (2005). Psychosocial problems and barriers to improved diabetes management: Results of the cross-national diabetes attitudes, wishes, and needs (DAWN) study. *Diabetic Medicine, 22*, 1379–1385.

Phillip, M., Battelino, T., Rodriguez, H., Danne, T., Kaufman, F., European Society for Paediatric Endocrinology, … European Association for the Study of Diabetes. (2007). Use of insulin pump therapy in the pediatric age-group: Consensus statement from the European Society for Paediatric Endocrinology, the Lawson Wilkins Pediatric Endocrine Society, and the International Society for Pediatric and Adolescent Diabetes, endorsed by the American Diabetes Association and the European Association for the Study of Diabetes. *Diabetes Care, 30*(6), 1653–1662.

Polonsky, W. H. (2007). Psychological insulin resistance: The patient perspective. *Diabetes Educator, 33*(7), 241S–244S.

Polonsky, W. H., Anderson, B. J., Lohrer, P. A., Welch, G., Jacobson, A. M., Aponte, J. E., & Schwartz, C. E. (1995). Assessment of diabetes-related distress. *Diabetes Care, 18*(6), 754–760.

Polonsky, W. H., Fisher, L., Guzman, S., Villa-Caballero, L., & Edelman, S. V. (2005). Psychological insulin resistance in patients with type 2 diabetes. *Diabetes Care, 28*(10), 2543–2548.

Rollnick, S., Mason, P., & Butler, C. (1999). *Health behavior change: A guide for practitioners.* London: Churchill Livingstone.

South Carolina Department of Health and Environmental Control. (2013). *Diabetes prevention and control.* Retrieved from http://www.scdhec.gov/health/chcdp/diabetes/health_systems.htm

Svoren, B. M., Volkening, L. K., Butler, D. A., Moreland, E. C., Anderson, B. J., & Laffel, L. M. (2007). Temporal trends in the treatment of pediatric type 1 diabetes and impact on acute outcomes. *Journal of Pediatrics, 150*(3), 279–285.

Weinger, K., Butler, H. A., Welch, G. W., & La Greca, A. M. (2005). Measuring diabetes self-care: A psychometric analysis of the self-care inventory-revised with adults. *Diabetes Care, 28*(6), 1346–1352.

Weissberg-Benchell, J., Antisdel-Lomaglio, J., & Seshadri, R. (2003). Insulin pump therapy: A meta-analysis. *Diabetes Care, 26*(4), 1079–1087.

World Health Organization. (2012). Retrieved October 30, 2012, from http://www.who.int/mediacentre/factsheets/fs312/en/index.html

Wild, D., von Maltzahn, R., Brohan, E., Christensen, T., Clauson, P., & Gonder-Frederick, L. (2007). A critical review of the literature on fear of hypoglycemia in diabetes: Implications for diabetes management and patient education. [Research Support, Non-U.S. Gov't Review]. *Patient Education and Counseling, 68*(1), 10–15. doi: 10.1016/j.pec.2007.05.003

Winkley, K., Ismail, K., Landau, S., & Eisler, I. (2006). Psychological interventions to improve glycaemic control in patients with type 1 diabetes: Systematic review and meta-analysis of randomised controlled trials. *British Medical Journal (Clinical Research Ed.), 8*, 333(7558), 65.

Wysocki, T. (1993). Associations among teen-parent relationships, metabolic control, and adjustment to diabetes in adolescents. *Journal of Pediatric Psychology, 18*, 441–452.

Wysocki, T., Harris, M. A., Buckloh, L. M., Mertlich, D., Lochrie, A. S., Mauras, N., & White, N. H. (2007). Randomized trial of behavioral family systems therapy for diabetes: Maintenance of effects on adolescents' diabetes outcomes. *Diabetes Care, 30*, 555–560.

Wysocki, T., Harris, M. A., Buckloh, L. M., Mertlich, D., Lochrie, A. S., Taylor, A., … White, N. H. (2006). Effects of behavioral family systems therapy for diabetes on adolescents' family relationships, treatment adherence, and metabolic control. *Journal of Pediatric Psychology, 31*, 928–938.

Wysocki, T., Harris, M. A., Buckloh, L. M., Mertlich, D., Lochrie, A. S., Taylor, A., … White, N. H. (2008). Randomized controlled trial of behavioral family systems therapy for diabetes: Maintenance and generalization of effects on parent-adolescent communication. *Behavior Therapy, 39*, 33–46.

Wysocki, T., Harris, M. A., Greco, P., Bubb, J., Danda, C. E., Harvey, L. M., … White, N. H. (2000). Randomized controlled trial of behavior therapy for families of adolescents with insulin-dependent diabetes mellitus. *Journal of Pediatric Psychology, 25*, 23–33.

Wysocki, T., Miller, K., Greco, P., Harris, M. A., Harvey, L., Taylor, A., … White, N. H. (1999). Behavior therapy of families of adolescents with diabetes: Effects on directly observed family interactions. *Behavior Therapy, 30*, 507–525.

15

Behavioral Management of Chronic Respiratory Diseases: Examples From Asthma and Chronic Obstructive Pulmonary Disease

JOSIE S. WELKOM
KRISTIN A. RIEKERT
MICHELLE N. EAKIN
CYNTHIA S. RAND
MARISA E. HILLIARD

LEARNING OBJECTIVES

- Identify behaviors associated with managing chronic respiratory diseases (CRDs).
- Understand the research support for behavioral interventions in improving adherence in asthma and chronic obstructive pulmonary disease (COPD).
- Recognize gaps in the literature and future directions needed to advance adherence outcomes in asthma and COPD.

EPIDEMIOLOGY AND SIGNIFICANCE

Chronic respiratory diseases (CRDs) are widespread, impacting millions of people across the lifespan (American Lung Association, 2012). The combined expenses related to the treatment, management, and complications of CRDs reach into the billions, primarily attributable to health care costs and lost wages from missed work or school. In 2009, the total financial cost of CRDs in the United States was approximated at $177.4 billion, of which $113.6 billion was attributable to direct medical costs (Weiss & Sullivan, 2001). The financial burden of CRDs is growing rapidly and will continue to balloon as diagnoses become increasingly prevalent (American Lung Association, 2012). The price tag for CRDs is expected to reach over $800 billion by 2021 (DeVol et al., 2007).

Key health behaviors in CRD management include adherence to a range of medications and therapies in addition to avoiding environmental exposures that trigger CRD symptoms and exacerbations. These health behaviors impact CRD morbidity and mortality and may be influenced by a range of factors including disease self-management skills, psychological functioning, disease knowledge, symptom perceptions, and health beliefs (Jain & Lolak, 2009; Ritz, Meuret, Trueba, Fritzsche, & von Leupoldt, 2012). Health behaviors related to the two most common CRDs, asthma and chronic obstructive pulmonary disease (COPD), will be the focus of this chapter.

ASTHMA

Asthma is a chronic inflammatory disorder of the airways that is characterized by airway hyper-responsiveness, airflow limitation, wheezing, coughing, and dyspnea or shortness of breath. The onset is typically in childhood and persists throughout one's life. Asthma is the most common chronic disease in children (Malveaux, 2009), affecting approximately 8% of the U.S. population (Centers for Disease Control and Prevention [CDC], 2011). Worldwide estimates of asthma prevalence in children and adults are around 300 million, and an additional 100 million people are anticipated to be diagnosed by 2025 (Masoli, Fabian, Holt, & Beasley, 2004). Serious disparities in asthma prevalence exist, with African Americans being at highest risk and displaying the fastest rates of growth (i.e., around 50% increase between 2001 and 2009; Centers for Disease Control and Prevention, 2011).

ASTHMA SELF-MANAGEMENT BEHAVIORS

Asthma self-management includes administration of asthma medications, environmental control practices (ECPs) to reduce exposure to asthma triggers, and routine medical monitoring.

Medication

The primary aims of pharmacological treatment are to prevent and control symptoms, reduce the frequency and severity of asthma exacerbations, and reverse airflow obstruction (National Heart, Lung, and Blood Institute [NHLBI], 2007). Asthma medications are categorized into two general classes: long-term controllers and quick-relief or rescue medications. Controller medications are taken daily to maintain control of persistent asthma by reducing and preventing inflammation, and rescue medications are taken as needed to provide immediate relief of acute airflow obstruction (i.e., during an asthma attack). Prescribed regimens may include rescue medications alone or in combination with a controller medication. Published rates suggest that adherence to controller medications is approximately 50% in children (Bender et al., 2000) and as low as 25% in adults (Janson, Earnest, Wong, & Blanc, 2008; Park et al., 2010). It is important to note that because rescue medications are often taken on an as needed basis, rates of adherence cannot be determined. Poor adherence to medication overall is associated with more frequent asthma exacerbations in both children and adults (Anis et al., 2001).

Most medications are delivered by inhalation, and proper technique (i.e., simultaneous actuation of the inhaler and inhalation by the patient) is an essential aspect of medication effectiveness. Technical inhalation administration errors are common and have been shown to be associated with poor asthma control and decreased treatment efficacy (Giraud & Roche, 2002; Molimard et al., 2003). Given the critical impact of proper and complete medication administration on asthma control, health care utilization, and health care costs (Bender & Rand, 2004), interventions targeting increased medication adherence and proper technique are essential.

Environmental Control

Allergens and environmental irritants are known to trigger asthma symptoms and exacerbations (American Lung Association, 2012). Exposure to inhaled irritants leads to an increase in inflammation, airway hyper-responsiveness, and levels of eosinophils. Common environmental irritants and allergens that can impact asthma symptoms include tobacco smoke, dust mites, cockroach antigen, animal dander, and mold. Environmental control practices (ECPs) are recommended to reduce exposure to irritants and allergens (American Lung Association, 2012). Specific guidelines include limiting exposure to outdoor irritants (e.g., trees, grass, and pollen) to which individuals may be sensitive in addition to reducing exposure to indoor irritants such as rodent and animal allergens, mites, and mold (American Lung Association, 2012). Results from the National Asthma Survey suggest that only 17% of households reported comprehensive use of ECPs. For example, only 20% of families are willing to remove a pet and up to 55% continue to be exposed to secondhand smoke (Eakin & Rand, 2012; Halterman et al., 2008; Marks et al., 2006). Moreover, decreased adherence to ECPs is associated with poorer collaboration between the family and health care provider (McQuaid, Walders, Kopel, Fritz, & Klinnert, 2005), resulting in even higher health risks among children with greater exposure to environmental triggers. More research is needed to understand and promote adherence to ECP guidelines to reduce exposure.

Medical Monitoring

Regular follow-up with a physician is necessary to monitor symptoms and response to treatment, and is essential to achieving optimal disease management. Follow-up visits are recommended every 1 to 6 months depending on the level of asthma control, and after an emergency department (ED) visit. During these visits, individualized asthma action plans are developed outlining daily self-management and how to recognize and respond to worsening symptoms. Research has shown that rates of adherence to following up with pediatric primary care following an ED visit were 16% and 26% in the ensuing 7 and 30 days, respectively (Liberman, Shelef, He, McCarter, & Teach, 2012). Therefore, it appears that even after a crisis event many patients and families with asthma do not follow guidelines for medical visits.

INTERVENTIONS TO CHANGE ASTHMA ADHERENCE

The NHLBI recommends that individualized interventions be provided to all patients with asthma to promote engagement in self-monitoring and daily management and to recognize worsening symptoms (NHLBI, 2007). Research in this area has emphasized educational and behavioral strategies to promote medication adherence in asthma, and these strategies are often combined into multicomponent interventions to target both asthma knowledge and self-management behaviors. Environmental control practices (ECPs) have also been the target of several asthma interventions. As described below, health behavior interventions for patients with asthma can be provided in a variety of settings including the hospital, clinic, school, and home. In addition, the target of these interventions can be either the individual patient, family, or group.

Educational Interventions

Asthma education programs have been most common and have demonstrated positive impact on medication adherence and asthma control. A systematic review of educational interventions reported improvements in children's lung function and self-efficacy, and reductions in symptoms, activity restrictions, and ED visits (Guevara, Wolf, Grum, & Clark, 2003). Research suggests that the content of asthma education influences the effectiveness of the intervention. For example, single-session educational interventions that focus on specific health behaviors such as allergen and trigger avoidance (Bobb, Ritz, Rowlands, & Griffiths, 2010) have shown a greater improvement in asthma outcomes than those that provide general asthma knowledge (Gibson et al., 2002).

Self-Management Education

Educational interventions that teach self-management skills including disease knowledge, objective monitoring of symptoms, and avoiding triggers have been shown to reduce morbidity, lower health care expenditures, and improve health care practices (Hurd & Lenfant, 1992; NHLBI, 2007). In particular, education on daily self-management skills has been shown to be an effective intervention for improving both asthma health outcomes (Powell & Gibson, 2003) and adherence (Janson et al., 2008). Multicomponent self-management education programs which include a combination of information provision, symptom monitoring, medical follow-up, and written asthma action plans have been shown to have the greatest benefit for health outcomes (Gibson, Coughlan, & Abramson, 1999; Powell & Gibson, 2003). Improvement in medication adherence has been postulated as the mechanism through which self-management education improves health outcomes (Janson et al., 2008). In particular, comparing a tailored self-management education intervention which included behavioral strategies and self-monitoring to self-monitoring alone found that those in the intervention group maintained greater rates of adherence to inhaled corticosteroids over the course of 24 weeks and were 3 times as likely to achieve greater than 60% adherence at the end of the study (Janson et al., 2008). In addition, Schaffer and Tian (2004) reported that even a brief educational intervention resulted in a 15% to 19% improvement in pharmacy-verified adherence rates among adults with asthma, an impressive finding in stark comparison to reported declines up to 22% in individuals who did not receive the intervention (Schaffer & Tian, 2004).

School-Based Asthma Education

Providing asthma education within the school setting emphasizes teaching children skills to manage asthma as opposed to relying on parents (Coffman, Cabana, & Yelin, 2009). School-based interventions have the added benefit of broadly and systematically intervening to improve asthma management. A recent meta-analysis indicated that school-based asthma education interventions resulted in overall improved health outcomes (Guevara et al., 2003). Clark et al. (2004) developed an intervention which consisted of disease management training, classmate education, introduction and management of asthma for principals and counselors, identifying and remediating environmental triggers with custodial staff, question and answer sessions for parents at school fairs, and communication with primary care providers (PCPs; Clark et al., 2004). Results of this comprehensive intervention included reductions in daytime symptoms and asthma-related school absences in addition to improvements in illness management by parents (Clark et al., 2004). Bruzzese et al. (2011) developed a school-based intervention for adolescents and their medical providers to improve asthma self-management and reduce asthma morbidity. Adolescents participated in three group sessions and five weekly individualized tailored coaching sessions in which they learned asthma management and coping skills. The provider portion of the intervention consisted of academic detailing, an educational presentation led by experts either in person or by phone (Bruzzese et al., 2011). Compared to the control condition, intervention participants had significantly less asthma morbidity at the 12-month follow-up (Bruzzese et al., 2011).

Behavioral Interventions

A number of asthma self-management interventions aim to promote adherence and improve asthma control by using behavioral strategies, such as teaching problem solving and coping skills. Targeting an individual's psychological functioning and motivation to make behavior changes has been another area of focus for behavioral interventions, using techniques such as cognitive behavioral therapy (CBT) and motivational interviewing (MI). In addition, several other strategies including directly observed therapies (DOTs), communication and decision making, adherence monitoring and feedback, family training, and technology will be reviewed.

BEHAVIORAL SKILLS TRAINING

Problem-solving skills training is commonly composed of the following components: defining the problem, generating alternative solutions, deciding on a solution, and implementing and evaluating the solution. Problem-solving techniques can provide individuals with the skills to navigate and overcome barriers to optimal disease self-management. Pulgaron, Salamon, Patterson, and Barakat (2010) developed a problem-solving intervention for children with persistent asthma attending a pediatric summer camp. While children who received the problem-solving intervention showed improvements in disease knowledge and problem-solving abilities, the impact on adherence and asthma health outcomes was not reported (Pulgaron et al., 2010). Walders et al. (2006) included brief problem-solving skill training in their interdisciplinary intervention which aimed to reduce asthma symptoms over the course of 12 months. Results were mixed; whereas there were no changes in symptomatology or quality of life (QOL), reductions in health care utilization were noted (Walders et al., 2006). Apter et al. (2011) compared an individualized problem-solving intervention to asthma education for improving adherence to inhaled corticosteroids (ICS) and asthma outcomes. Whereas results revealed no differences in adherence among those receiving the problem-solving versus the asthma education intervention, electronic monitoring of ICS use in both groups improved health outcomes (Apter et al., 2011).

Given the impact of stress on suboptimal asthma adherence and risk for asthma exacerbations, coping skills training has been another focus of self-management skills interventions (Long et al., 2011). For example, Velsor-Friedrich et al. (2012) reported that a school-based coping skills training and asthma education intervention were equally effective in improving asthma symptoms, asthma-related QOL, knowledge, and self-efficacy and decreasing asthma-related school absenteeism. However, medication adherence data was not reported (Velsor-Friedrich et al., 2012).

FAMILY-BASED INTERVENTIONS

Behavioral asthma interventions often involve family members for maximum impact on children's health behaviors. Family interaction characteristics such as limited displays of affection, poor communication, and reactive approaches to illness management have been shown to be associated with poor medication adherence (Bender, Milgrom,

Rand, & Ackerson, 1998; Fiese & Wamboldt, 2003). In contrast, families who incorporated medication management into their daily routines demonstrate better adherence (Fiese, Wamboldt, & Anbar, 2005). Duncan et al. (2012) compared a parent–youth teamwork intervention, designed to increase adolescent disease management responsibility while concurrently fading parental involvement to a developmentally appropriate level, to standard care plus asthma education. Patients in the intervention group achieved a medication adherence rate greater than 80% compared to the 50% adherence rate in the education group (Duncan et al., 2012).

MOTIVATIONAL STRATEGIES

MI is a patient-centered approach addressing motivation and ambivalence about change that has demonstrated positive impact on adherence and other health behaviors in a variety of health conditions (Erickson, Gerstle, & Feldstein, 2005; Martins & McNeil, 2009). There is a small but growing body of research examining its impact on asthma self-management (Knight, McGowan, Dickens, & Bundy, 2006). For example, Riekert, Borrelli, Bilderback, and Rand (2011) developed a five-session, home-based MI intervention to promote adherence in adolescents with asthma. Results of this pilot study were promising, indicating improved adolescent-reported motivation and readiness to adhere to the medication regimen. Though the intervention did not demonstrate a direct effect on self-reported medication adherence, lack of a control group and objective indicators of adherence may have limited the ability to detect change (Riekert et al., 2011). Schmaling, Blume, and Afari (2001) compared the efficacy of an education only intervention to education plus MI. Participants in both conditions demonstrated an improvement in asthma knowledge and skills. However, the participants in the MI intervention showed a stable or increased level of readiness to adhere to their medications whereas those receiving education alone showed a decrease over time (Schmaling et al., 2001). Halterman et al. (2012) evaluated a telephone- and home-based MI intervention to improve medication adherence confidence, importance, and motivation. Adolescents receiving the intervention demonstrated significant improvements in their self-reported confidence, perceived importance, and motivation to take daily preventative medications in comparison to baseline (Halterman et al., 2011). These three studies (Halterman et al., 2011; Riekert et al., 2011; Schmaling et al., 2001) were all promising in that they reported improvements in specific motivational factors (e.g., readiness and perceived importance), yet it is important to note that their impact on objective medication adherence has not been established. Finally, Gamble, Stevenson, and Heaney (2011) examined whether targeting motivation among patients with poor adherence could improve outcomes. Patients received either a concordance interview (i.e., collaboratively developing a treatment plan to address poor adherence) or an MI+CBT intervention. Patients receiving the MI+CBT intervention improved their adherence rates from 37.6% to 61.9% compared to those in the concordance interview group with rates declining from 31.7% to 28.8% over 12 months (Gamble, Stevenson, & Heaney, 2011). Together these studies suggest that MI is a promising intervention to promote self-management behaviors and health outcomes in patients with asthma.

SHARED DECISION MAKING

Interactions among patients and providers have consequences for patient satisfaction, utilization, outcomes, and adherence (Beach et al., 2005). In particular, the frequency (Yawn, 2011) and quality (Wilson et al., 2010) of communication have been associated with adherence to therapy. Wilson et al. (2010) examined the impact of a shared decision making (SDM) intervention consisting of providing information, communicating about preferences, identifying the pros and cons to each option, and agreeing to a treatment plan and its effect on adherence among patients with poorly controlled asthma. Compared to patients whose treatment was guided by clinician decision making, patients in the SDM group demonstrated significantly higher adherence to their medication regimen (Wilson et al., 2010). Clark, Ko, Gong, and Johnson (2012) examined the impact of a negotiated asthma treatment plan on medication adherence in adult patients. Patients who reported that they worked collaboratively with their doctor to develop a plan to adjust medications according to symptom changes were more than twice as likely than those without a negotiated plan to report that they "usually" took their prescribed medications as opposed to "sometimes or rarely" (Clark et al., 2012).

Interventions targeted at providers have also demonstrated benefits for patients' medication adherence. Brown, Bratton, Cabana, Kaciroti, and Clark (2004) examined the impact of an intervention aimed at improving guideline-based clinical practice, patient teaching, and communication. At the 2-year follow-up, patients of physicians who received the intervention were more likely to report having received and filled a prescription for inhaled anti-inflammatory therapy and having received a written asthma treatment plan than patients of providers who did not receive the intervention (Brown et al., 2004). Clark, Cabana, Kaciroti, Gong, and Sleeman (2008) developed the Physician Asthma Care Education (PACE) program, an educational intervention aimed at teaching communication techniques and improving the delivery of asthma educational messages for families. Patients of physicians in the PACE program had fewer ED visits and hospitalizations and made fewer calls to the doctor's office in comparison to their baseline health care utilization (Clark et al., 2008). Moreover, Williams et al. (2010) compared the impact of patient–provider communication education on adherence to specific instruction on the interpretation of ePrescribing adherence data on patient ICS adherence. Although there were no significant differences in overall adherence, greater improvement in adherence was found among patients whose providers accessed more detailed ePrescribing information about their patients (Williams et al., 2010). These results further support the importance of patient–provider communication and SDM on patient adherence to medical regimens.

ADHERENCE MONITORING AND FEEDBACK

Monitoring a patient's medication adherence and providing them with feedback and reinforcement have been shown to be an important behavioral strategy for improving self-management. Intervention studies utilizing adherence monitoring and feedback with both children (Otsuki et al., 2009) and adults (Onyirimba et al., 2003) have demonstrated benefits. For example, Burgess, Sly, and Devadason (2010) provided children with an electronic monitoring device and informed families that the usage would be recorded. One group had their electronic monitoring data reviewed with them by one of the providers and achieved an average adherence rate of 79%, and the control group did not receive any feedback and demonstrated an average adherence rate of 57.9% over the course of 4 months (Burgess et al., 2010). Similarly, Otsuki et al. (2009) developed a home-based monitoring and feedback intervention for high-risk inner city children with asthma. Results revealed improvements in adherence for the intervention group during the study period. However, these rates declined after the intervention was withdrawn (Otsuki et al., 2009). Another study found that in comparison to standard care, adults who received direct feedback on their medication usage demonstrated an improvement from 61% to 80% over the course of the trial. Adherence for the patients in the control group decreased over time (Onyirimba et al., 2003). In sum, adherence monitoring and feedback have demonstrated significant improvement in adherence outcomes. Further research is needed to examine the sustainability of this type of intervention over time.

DIRECTLY OBSERVED THERAPY

Visual monitoring of medication ingestion typically by a health care worker is referred to as directly observed therapy (DOT). Halterman et al. (2011) examined the impact of a school-based DOT intervention that included dose adjustments combined with a home-based environmental tobacco smoke (ETS) reduction program and found reductions in asthma morbidity. As such, Halterman et al. (2012) went on to develop technology for screening symptoms, generating reports, and obtaining authorization from PCPs in the schools (Halterman et al., 2012). Children within the intervention group demonstrated improvements in symptoms, rescue medication use, school absenteeism, and interference with family activities. In addition, the parents, PCPs, and school personnel reported both satisfaction and ease of the intervention program (Halterman et al., 2012). Gerald et al. (2009) examined the impact of a school-based, supervised therapy intervention versus usual care in children over a 15-month period. Children receiving the intervention were supervised by study staff in the school on the use of their ICS daily and were provided with education on the proper technique as needed. Though results revealed no group differences between the baseline and follow-up periods, for those participants receiving the intervention, the odds of experiencing an episode of poor asthma control were approximately 1.6 times greater during the baseline period than during the subsequent follow-up period (Gerald et al., 2009). In sum, these studies suggest that DOT is a promising intervention for improving asthma control.

TECHNOLOGY-BASED BEHAVIORAL INTERVENTIONS

Recent innovations in intervention delivery include the use of mobile health technologies such as eHealth education, interactive voice recognition (IVR), and texting to deliver health care. Incorporating technology into the delivery of adherence-promotion interventions has many benefits including its interactive nature and the ability to reach a wider population base, address literacy concerns, and improve efficiency. Gustafson et al. (2012) investigated the effects of an automated eHealth intervention (i.e., educational modules which provided general asthma-related information, strategies to improve adherence, decision-making tools, and support services) combined with nurse case management on medication adherence and asthma control delivered by phone. Although the intervention did not result in improved medication adherence, there were some indications of improvement in asthma control (Gustafson et al., 2012). Vollmer et al. (2011) evaluated the impact of IVR intervention that prompted medication refills on ICS adherence in comparison to usual care. More specifically, IVR consisted of refill reminder phone calls, such as when patients had less than 30 days medication supply remaining or were greater than 30 days tardy for a refill, which were tailored to the participants based on information gathered through electronic medical records (Vollmer et al., 2011). Results of the intervention indicated a significant though small improvement on medication adherence. Of note, participants who were directly reached through the reminder calls showed a threefold improvement in medication adherence (Vollmer et al., 2011).

Due to its widespread reach, instantaneous delivery, and cost-efficiency, text messaging interventions have become more frequently incorporated as either a stand-alone or part of a multicomponent intervention. In an effort to provide a personalized, easily accessible motivational intervention to adolescents and adults with asthma, Petrie, Perry, Broadbent, and Weinman (2012) recently conducted a study examining the effect of daily text messaging individualized to each participant's illness and medication beliefs. Results indicated that self-reported medication adherence significantly improved over time (Petrie et al., 2012) suggesting that this format for a motivational intervention holds promise. In an effort to improve medication adherence, Strandbygaard, Thomsen, and

Backer (2010) randomized patients to either receive daily text messages over the course of 12 weeks reminding them to take their medication or to a control group. Whereas patients in the control group demonstrated a 14.2% reduction in adherence, patients in the intervention group demonstrated a 3.6% nonsignificant trend toward improved medication adherence. Over the course of 12 weeks, the mean adherence difference between the two groups was significant, averaging 17.8% (Strandbygaard et al., 2010). Similarly, Britto et al. (2012) tested the feasibility, acceptability, and utility of a text message medication reminder intervention for adolescents over the course of 4 months. Participants were able to tailor the reminders with regard to frequency, format, and content. Results revealed high feasibility, ease, and satisfaction among participants. However, self-reported asthma symptoms did not change, which may be due in part to the sample's limited size and unique characteristics. A recent study conducted with low-income and minority adolescents diagnosed with asthma delivered a multicomponent technology-based adherence intervention which integrated problem-solving skills training, MI, and tailored text messaging (Seid et al., 2012). Although medication adherence was not reported as an outcome, clinically important differences were detected with respect to long-term improvements in patient activation, intention, motivation to change, health-related quality of life (HRQOL), and reported barriers and symptoms. The added convenience and ease of technological advances appear useful for both patients and providers. However, it is important to note that the impact of texting interventions on objective indicators of adherence and health outcomes has not been established.

Environmental Control Interventions

Interventions focused on reducing environmental exposure to allergens and irritants have been shown to be effective in improving asthma health outcomes. Environmental interventions are cost-effective and do not require expertise to implement (Kattan et al., 2005; Wu & Takaro, 2007). Environmental control practices (ECPs) can target indoor or outdoor allergens and irritants, yet research suggests that the most benefit is derived when multiple allergens are targeted (Morgan et al., 2004). However, numerous barriers can make it difficult to reduce environmental exposures. For example, caregivers of children living in an urban setting have cited financial constraints, lack of support from property managers in making the needed alterations to rental properties, and an inability to control triggers within the school setting (Laster, Holsey, Shendell, Mccarty, & Celano, 2009). To address these and other barriers, Krieger, Takaro, Song, and Weaver (2005) developed a community health worker intervention to reduce indoor allergens in the households of low-income children, including in-home environmental assessment, education, support for behavior change (i.e., encouragement and social support), and home resources to reduce exposure. Results of this study included improved caregiver quality of life and decreased acute care utilization (Krieger et al., 2005). However, very little is known about the degree to which patients and families adhere to ECP recommendations or what intervention strategies can promote ECP adoption.

Health Care Utilization Interventions

Guideline-based follow-up care with PCPs is critical to monitoring asthma disease progression and resulting outcomes. In particular, following up with one's PCP following an ED presentation is important for optimal disease management (Baren et al., 2006). Baren et al. (2006) examined the impact of an intervention which included (1) free medication, transportation vouchers, and telephone reminders,

(2) a scheduled PCP appointment, or (3) usual discharge procedures. Patients who received a scheduled appointment were 2.8 times more likely to obtain a PCP follow-up visit in the subsequent 30 days compared to the other groups (Baren et al., 2006). There was no impact on rates of future utilization or health outcomes. Eakin et al. (2012) compared the impact of four intervention conditions: (1) Breathmobile, a mobile medical clinic, (2) a home-based asthma education and communication skills training, (3) a combined intervention, and (4) treatment as usual. Many of the barriers to receiving preventative care were removed in conditions 1 through 3, yet there were no improvements in asthma management or morbidity (Eakin et al., 2012). Furthermore, Nelson et al. (2011) evaluated the impact of a parental coaching intervention on ED utilization and hospitalizations in urban minority children. The intervention, based on the transtheoretical model of behavior change, was delivered by female lay coaches with expertise in asthma and focused on improving asthma management by avoiding environmental triggers, adhering to medications, maintaining an updated asthma action plan, regular follow-up with their PCP, and developing a collaborative partnership with their PCP (Nelson et al., 2011). Results indicated that whereas the intervention was successful in increasing self-reported use of asthma action plans and PCP utilization, rates of ED utilization and hospitalizations were not decreased (Nelson et al., 2011). Smith et al. (2006) combined parental coaching with monetary incentives to parents of children presenting to the ED in an effort to improve PCP follow-up. Results revealed no differences in PCP follow-up in the subsequent 2 weeks post-ED presentation in those families receiving the coaching intervention in comparison to usual care (Smith et al., 2006). Though it is well recognized that adherence to primary care follow-up is important, rates remain low. Furthermore, many interventions that have been developed and evaluated have not been effective in changing health care utilization. Thus, a better understanding of the mechanisms which contribute to poor follow-up and the subsequent development of interventions to address those barriers are needed.

CHRONIC OBSTRUCTIVE PULMONARY DISEASE (COPD)

COPD is a disease of the airways and lungs characterized by persistent airflow limitation and enhanced chronic inflammatory response to noxious particles or gases (Global Initiative for Chronic Obstructive Lung Disease [GOLD], 2013). COPD tends to present in mid-life and results from an interaction between one's environment and genetic risk. COPD affects more than 210 million people worldwide (Pauwels, Buist, Ma, Jenkins, & Hurd, 2001), 24 million in the United States (Mannino, Ford, & Redd, 2003), and is projected to be the fourth leading cause of mortality by 2030 (Mathers & Loncar, 2006). Cigarette smoking is the most common risk factor for COPD, with other environmental contributors including secondhand smoke exposure, indoor and outdoor air pollution, organic and inorganic dust, chemical agents, and fumes.

COPD SELF-MANAGEMENT BEHAVIORS

The primary components of COPD self-management include a combination of preventative behaviors including environmental control (i.e., smoking cessation or avoidance of smoke exposure), medication therapy, and pulmonary rehabilitation (GOLD, 2013). In order to assess disease progression, it is recommended that patients with COPD receive lung function screening and routine medical follow-up at least annually. In comparison to the general population, individuals with COPD experience more psychological distress (Wagena, Arrindell, Wouters, & van Schayck, 2005) and higher rates of major depressive disorder (Schneider, Jick, Bothner, & Meier, 2010), independent of disease severity, which may interfere with self-management.

Medication

Patients with COPD are responsible for self-administration of inhaled medications and oxygen if prescribed. The pharmacological treatment regimen for COPD is complex and based on the severity of symptoms, airflow limitation, and severity of exacerbations. Inhaled bronchodilator medications can be prescribed daily, long term, or as needed and are used to treat acute symptoms. Combination therapy may also include antibiotics and anti-inflammatory drugs. Oxygen therapy may also be prescribed as a supplement to other pharmacotherapies for COPD. Research suggests that 40% to 60% of patients with COPD are adherent to their prescribed pharmacological treatment (Cecere et al., 2012; George, Kong, Thoman, & Stewart, 2005; Restrepo et al., 2008). Moreover, medication adherence rates may be associated with medication class as research has shown that patients prescribed a long-acting beta agonist were more adherent than those prescribed inhaled corticosteroids (Cecere et al., 2012).

Pulmonary Rehabilitation

The American Thoracic Society (ATS, 2005) defines pulmonary rehabilitation as, "a multidisciplinary program of care for patients with chronic respiratory impairment that is individually tailored and designed to optimize physical and social performance and autonomy." Exercise training is the primary intervention in pulmonary rehabilitation to improve muscle function in COPD (Bernard et al., 1999; Sala et al., 1999) and consists of both endurance and strength training. However, comprehensive programs also include education, psychological support, nutrition counseling, outcome assessment, and relapse prevention. Smoking cessation interventions may be incorporated as needed. A recent Cochrane review found support for pulmonary rehabilitation in the following areas: symptom relief, improvement in exercise tolerance, and improvement in health status which includes emotional functioning. In comparison to standard care, completion of a pulmonary rehabilitation program has been shown to reduce length of hospital stays and frequency of home visits (Griffiths et al., 2000). However, data on rates of adherence to COPD regimens is scarce (Bender, 2012). Research suggests that less than 75% of patients will attend an initial assessment and only 40% will complete the program (Hogg et al., 2012). Patient characteristics associated with drop-out include increased social isolation and a greater likelihood of being a smoker (Young, Dewse, Fergusson, & Kolbe, 1999).

Environmental Control and Vaccination

It is important for patients with COPD to reduce their exposure to environmental risk factors such as tobacco smoke, occupational dust, fumes, gases, and indoor and outdoor air pollutants. Following diagnosis of COPD, approximately 30% of patients continue to smoke (CDC, 2013). Guidelines recommend that patients with COPD receive the pneumococcal and influenza vaccine which has been associated with decreased morbidity and mortality, especially in the elderly (Poole, Chacko, Wood-Baker, & Cates, 2006). Although rates of adherence to vaccinations in COPD are not well established, research with the elderly suggests that less than 70% of elderly patients with COPD receive vaccinations (Poole et al., 2006).

INTERVENTIONS TO CHANGE COPD ADHERENCE

There is very limited research examining the effectiveness of behavioral interventions on patient adherence. The data regarding the modest body of research regarding behavioral adherence promoting interventions and important avenues for future research will be detailed below.

Educational Interventions

ATS recommends that the core components of an education intervention curriculum for COPD should emphasize self-management, and should also include development of an action plan for prevention and early treatment of exacerbations, end-of-life decision making, and breathing strategies (ATS, 2005; Nici et al., 2006). A recent systematic review found inconclusive results with regard to the impact of self-management education on outcomes (Monninkhof et al., 2003). However, several limitations were noted including the limited research base and range of outcome measures as contributing factors (Monninkhof et al., 2003). Harris, Smith, and Veale (2008) indicated that increased COPD knowledge, improvement in patient self-efficacy, and systematic program development based in principles of behavior change were critical characteristics of COPD educational interventions. Specifically, it was recommended that developing a program which explores mechanisms of change and incorporates patient identification of goals, barriers, and facilitators would be more likely to succeed in improving outcomes (Harris et al., 2008).

SELF-MANAGEMENT EDUCATION

Managing COPD can be a complex task comprising both preventative behaviors and treatment. Fan et al. (2012) developed a self-management intervention titled Comprehensive Care Management Program (CCMP), to reduce the risk of COPD-related hospitalizations. CCMP consisted of four individual education sessions which included instruction on COPD in general, self-monitoring of symptoms, self-initiation of an antibiotic or prednisone for exacerbations, breathing and coughing techniques, energy conservation, anxiety reduction, medication adherence, smoking cessation, nutrition, and exercise (Fan et al., 2012). Participants also participated in a group session, received phone calls from a case manager, and were provided an individually tailored action plan. This study was stopped after 24 months due to an increase in all-cause mortality in the intervention group, highlighting the importance of Data and Safety Monitoring Boards (DSMB) in clinical research. However, results from the enrolled participants indicated that there was a small improvement in prednisone (but not antibiotic) use during COPD exacerbations (Fan et al., 2012). These results differed from two similar self-management interventions which resulted in decreased health care utilization and improved health outcomes (Bourbeau et al., 2003; Rice et al., 2010). Khdour, Kidney, Smyth, and McElnay (2009) examined the impact of a clinical-pharmacist-led disease and medicine management program on medication adherence, hospitalizations, ED visits, and HRQOL. More specifically, the intervention included education on COPD, medications, and breathing techniques. After 12 months there was a significant improvement in adherence to medication in the intervention versus control groups (i.e., 77.8% and 60.0%, respectively). In addition, both ED visits and hospitalizations were reduced, knowledge was increased, and aspects of HRQOL improved (Khdour et al., 2009). Given the mixed results of self-management interventions in COPD, more research is needed to understand if self-management interventions for COPD are efficacious and safe.

Behavioral and Multicomponent Interventions for Smoking Cessation

Smoking is the leading risk factor for developing COPD (Anthonisen et al., 1994; Xu, Dockery, Ware, Speizer, & Ferris, 1992) and individuals with COPD exhibit higher rates of daily cigarette use and subsequently higher physical dependency than the general population (Shahab, Jarvis, Britton, & West, 2006). Among those with established COPD, smoking cessation is the most effective intervention for slowing disease progression. Whereas low intensity interventions such as counseling achieve smoking cessation rates at approximately 9%, high intensity interventions which include a combination of behavioral strategies with pharmacological interventions achieve quit rates of up to 35% (Christenhusz, Prenger, Pieterse, Seydel, & van der Palen, 2012). Results of a systematic review of the efficacy of smoking cessation programs for patients with COPD found that the most efficacious smoking cessation intervention in sustaining prolonged abstinence was a combination of pharmacotherapy and individual counseling (Coronini-Cronberg, Heffernan, & Robinson, 2011; van der Meer, Wagena, Ostelo, Jacobs, & van Schayck, 2003; Wagena, van der Meer, Ostelo, Jacobs, & van Schayck, 2004).

Smoking cessation has been shown to reduce the rate of FEV_1, decline diminish symptoms, improve health status, and reduce exacerbations (Burchfiel et al., 1995). The delivery and/or components of smoking cessation interventions can vary widely to include any combination of self-help, individual/group/telephone counseling, and adjunctive pharmacological therapies such as nicotine replacement therapy (NRT) or bupropion SR. Although smokers with COPD attempt to quit smoking at higher rates than the general population, there are no reported differences in success rates (Schiller & Ni, 2006).

TECHNOLOGY-BASED SMOKING CESSATION

Technology is increasingly being used to support smoking cessation among people with COPD. Free et al. (2011) developed a smoking cessation intervention delivered via mobile text messaging. Participants in the intervention condition received text messages providing motivational encouragement, positive feedback, information regarding the benefits and consequences, social approval, and instruction on behavioral strategies to limit environmental cues (Free et al., 2011). Results revealed a significant increase in abstinence at 6 months in the intervention group (10.7%) versus those in the control group (4.9%; Free et al., 2011). Researchers have hypothesized that this intervention would likely be a cost-effective means to providing smoking cessation support in patients with COPD, calling for additional research on technologies to promote smoking cessation in individuals with COPD (Guerriero et al., 2013).

PROVIDER-DIRECTED INTERVENTIONS

It is important to understand the role of health care providers in providing behavioral interventions. Whereas there is no research to date examining the impact of provider-directed interventions on medication adherence or pulmonary rehabilitation for people with COPD, there is research to support the effectiveness of provider-directed smoking cessation interventions. Smokers without COPD have been shown to benefit from even brief simple advice to quit smoking from physicians as opposed to no advice (Stead, Bergson, & Lancaster, 2008), and the Global Initiative for COPD recommends offering brief advice to patients with COPD who smoke. However, approximately 20% of patients with COPD do not receive smoking cessation counseling during medical visits (Schiller & Ni, 2006). Thus, more work is needed related to health care provider encouragement of smoking cessation, as part of a multi-level approach to health behavior promotion in patients with COPD.

MAINTENANCE AND RELAPSE PREVENTION

Interventions which aim to maintain cessation and reduce the likelihood of relapse are important for long-term behavioral change. The Lung Health Study (LHS) was a longitudinal, multi-center trial of 5,887 adults with evidence of early stage COPD participating in a 10-week smoking cessation and ipratropium bromide inhalation intervention on lung function decline (Wise et al., 2003). A subset of patients participated in an individual or group Restart program following relapse, and results revealed that of those enrolled, men's smoking status 5 years post-intervention was related to their participation in the program but these results did not hold for women (Murray et al., 1997). These findings indicate that developing interventions which specifically target relapse has the potential to result in sustained cessation. More research is needed regarding the specific aspects of relapse prevention programs that contribute to cessation adherence.

Pulmonary Rehabilitation Interventions

Although the short-term benefits of exercise training have been shown to be effective in COPD, the rates of adherence to these programs following pulmonary rehabilitation are unclear (Nici et al., 2006). The National Emphysema Treatment Trial (NETT) examined factors associated with pulmonary rehabilitation adherence in more than 1,200 patients over the course of 2 years (Fan, Giardino, Blough, Kaplan, & Ramsey, 2008). Results revealed that patients who underwent lung volume reduction surgery and patients with better lung function were more likely to attend at least one session, and more highly educated patients were more likely to complete rehabilitation (Fan et al., 2008). In contrast, depressive and anxiety symptoms and greater distance from the rehabilitation center were associated with lower likelihood of adhering to rehabilitation (Fan et al., 2008). Research has suggested that pulmonary rehabilitation services could be integrated into routine clinical practice and achieve similar results to that of clinical trials (Hogg et al., 2012).

There is mixed support for the effectiveness of maintenance interventions on sustaining the benefits of pulmonary rehabilitation long term. Telephone support and repeating a course of pulmonary rehabilitation have shown modest, short-term benefit (Foglio, Bianchi, & Ambrosino, 2001; Ries, Kaplan, Myers, & Prewitt, 2003). Whereas strong support for the maintenance of HRQOL up to 2 years following rehabilitation has been established, there is limited research supporting its impact on other long-term outcomes (Bestall et al., 2003; Cambach, Wagenaar, Koelman, van Keimpema, & Kemper, 1999; Foglio et al., 1999; Troosters, Gosselink, & Decramer, 2000). Moreover, in light of the low rates of medication adherence in patients with COPD (Cecere et al., 2012), it will be an important future direction for pulmonary rehabilitation programs to target adherence to the program as a clinical outcome.

CONCLUSIONS

As the prevalence of CRDs continues to increase, advances are needed to grow the impact of clinical research and care on respiratory health. As evidenced throughout this chapter, relatively little data has been published regarding the impact of interventions on adherence and self-management behaviors of people with CRDs. This is particularly evident in the COPD literature, in which studies on medication adherence for COPD were scarce. Although interventions often aim to improve health-promoting behaviors such as medication adherence, engagement in physically active lifestyles, and smoking cessation, reported outcomes tend to be quality of life, symptoms, health care use, or variables thought to be proxy measures for adherence (e.g., disease knowledge and self-efficacy). While these are critically important outcomes, the absence of measures of actual self-management practices hinders our ability to determine the direct impact of interventions on health behavior change. It is essential for future research to specifically measure adherence and evaluate whether behavior change resulting from particular intervention strategies mediates the link between intervention delivery and health outcomes including asthma and COPD control.

Health technologies hold great potential to build upon existing interventions to both measure and intervene on targeted health behaviors such as medication adherence in CRDs. For example, Asthmapolis (Madison, WI) has developed a GPS-enabled sensor that snaps onto many inhalers used in the treatment of asthma and COPD. The associated software tracks when and where the device is activated, and users can receive educational materials and monitor their data through applications accessed via the Internet or mobile devices. Similarly, Exco InTouch (Exco InTouch Ltd., Nottingham, UK) has developed a Bluetooth-enabled inhaler and mobile app for people with COPD with functions that include access to educational material and tools to track symptoms and monitor medication adherence. Ongoing development and testing of these and other health technologies hold the potential for clinicians and researchers to collect objective behavioral data and to impact health behavior through the provision of real-time feedback.

In light of growing disparities in asthma and COPD (Keppel, 2007), efforts to expand the reach of existing interventions to underserved populations are a top priority. The educational, behavioral, and psychological interventions described in this chapter have generally been designed and tested in relatively small-scale settings, thus limiting their broader impact. Adherence-promotion interventions may benefit from adopting community-based strategies such as Wee Wheezers (Wilson et al., 1996) in pediatric asthma and rehabilitation-based COPD programs such as NETT (Fan et al., 2008) to extend the reach and impact on public health. Health behavior interventions for people with CRDs must now take the example of these school- and rehabilitation-based programs to scale up for maximum impact on public health. To successfully implement interventions at the community level, health behavior interventions must become more accessible, for example, through delivery in settings where individuals receive care (e.g., primary or urgent care settings) or through policy changes that promote prevention and reduce the financial and system barriers to accessing behavioral health care. For example, health plans and technology companies may partner to disseminate their services to members with CRDs and thus systematically promote health behavior change.

REFERENCES

American Lung Association. (2012). *Estimated prevalence and incidence of lung disease.* Retrieved from http://www.lung.org/finding-cures/our-research/trend-reports/estimated-prevalence.pdf

American Thoracic Society / European Respiratory Society Task Force. (2005). *Standards for the diagnosis and management of patients with COPD, Version 1.2.* Retrieved from http://www.thoracic.org/go/copd.

Anis, A. H., Lynd, L. D., Wang, X. H., King, G., Spinelli, J. J., Fitzgerald, M., Bai, T., & Pare, P. (2001). Double trouble: Impact of inappropriate use of asthma medication on the use of health care resources. *Canadian Medical Association Journal, 164*, 625–631.

Anthonisen, N. R., Connett, J. E., Kiley, J. P., Altose, M. D., Bailey, W. C., Buist, A. S., … O'Hara, P. (1994). Effects of smoking intervention and the use of an inhaled anticholinergic bronchodilator on the rate of decline of FEV1. The Lung Health Study. *Journal of the American Medical Association, 272*, 1497–1505.

Apter, A. J., Wang, X., Bogen, D. K., Rand, C. S., McElligott, S., Polsky, D., …Ten Have, T. (2011). Problem solving to improve adherence and asthma outcomes in urban adults with moderate or severe asthma: A randomized controlled trial. *Journal of Allergy and Clinical Immunology, 128*, 516–523.

Baren, J. M., Boudreaux, E. D., Brenner, B. E., Cydulka, R. K., Rowe, B. H., Clark, S., & Camargo, C.A. (2006). Randomized controlled trial of emergency department interventions to improve primary care follow-up for patients with acute asthma. *Chest, 129*, 257–265.

Beach, M. C., Sugarman, J., Johnson, R. L., Arbelaez, J. J., Duggan, P. S., & Cooper, L. A. (2005). Do patients treated with dignity report higher satisfaction, adherence, and receipt of preventive care? *Annals of Family Medicine, 3*, 331–338.

Bender, B., Milgrom, H., Rand, C., & Ackerson, L. (1998). Psychological factors associated with medication nonadherence in asthmatic children. *Journal of Asthma, 35*, 347–353.

Bender, B., Wamboldt, F. S., O'Connor, S. L., Rand, C., Szefler, S., Milgrom, H., & Wamboldt, M. Z. (2000). Measurement of children's asthma medication adherence by self report, mother report, canister weight, and Doser CT. *Annals of Allergy Asthma & Immunology, 85*, 416–421.

Bender, B. G. (2012). Nonadherence to COPD treatment: What have we learned and what do we do next? *COPD, 9*, 209–210.

Bender, B. G., & Rand, C. (2004). Medication non-adherence and asthma treatment cost. *Current Opinion in Allergy and Clinical Immunology, 4*, 191–195.

Bernard, S., Whittom, F., Leblanc, P., Jobin, J., Belleau, R., Berube, C., … Maltais, F. (1999). Aerobic and strength training in patients with chronic obstructive pulmonary disease. *American Journal of Respiratory and Critical Care Medicine, 159*, 896–901.

Bestall, J. C., Paul, E. A., Garrod, R., Garnham, R., Jones, R. W., & Wedzicha, A. J. (2003). Longitudinal trends in exercise capacity and health status after pulmonary rehabilitation in patients with COPD. *Respiratory Medicine, 97*, 173–180.

Bobb, C., Ritz, T., Rowlands, G., & Griffiths, C. (2010). Effects of allergen and trigger factor avoidance advice in primary care on asthma control: A randomized-controlled trial. *Clinical and Experimental Allergy, 40*, 143–152.

Bourbeau, J., Julien, M., Maltais, F., Rouleau, M., Beaupre, A., Begin, R., … Collet, J. P. (2003). Reduction of hospital utilization in patients with chronic obstructive pulmonary disease: A disease-specific self-management intervention. *Archives of Internal Medicine, 163*, 585–591.

Britto, M. T., Munafo, J. K., Schoettker, P. J., Vockell, A. L., Wimberg, J. A., & Yi, M. S. (2012). Pilot and feasibility test of adolescent-controlled text messaging reminders. *Clinical Pediatrics, 51*, 114–121.

Brown, R., Bratton, S. L., Cabana, M. D., Kaciroti, N., & Clark, N. M. (2004). Physician asthma education program improves outcomes for children of low-income families. *Chest, 126*, 369–374.

Bruzzese, J. M., Sheares, B. J., Vincent, E. J., Du, Y., Sadeghi, H., Levison, M. J., … Evans, D. (2011). Effects of a school-based intervention for urban adolescents with asthma. A controlled trial. *American Journal of Respiratory and Critical Care Medicine, 183*, 998–1006.

Burchfiel, C. M., Marcus, E. B., Curb, J. D., Maclean, C. J., Vollmer, W. M., Johnson, L. R., … Buist, A. S. (1995). Effects of smoking and smoking cessation on longitudinal decline in pulmonary function. *American Journal of Respiratory and Critical Care Medicine, 151*, 1778–1785.

Burgess, S. W., Sly, P. D., & Devadason, S. G. (2010). Providing feedback on adherence increases use of preventive medication by asthmatic children. *Journal of Asthma, 47*, 198–201.

Cambach, W., Wagenaar, R. C., Koelman, T. W., van Keimpema, A. R., & Kemper, H. C. (1999). The long-term effects of pulmonary rehabilitation in patients with asthma and chronic obstructive pulmonary disease: A research synthesis. *Archives of Physical Medicine and Rehabilitation, 80*, 103–111.

Cecere, L. M., Slatore, C. G., Uman, J. E., Evans, L. E., Udris, E. M., Bryson, C. L., & Au, D. H. (2012). Adherence to long-acting inhaled therapies among patients with chronic obstructive pulmonary disease (COPD). *COPD, 9*, 251–258.

Centers for Disease Control and Prevention (CDC). (2011). *CDC Vital Signs; Asthma in the US*. Retrieved from http://www.cdc.gov/vitalsigns/asthma/

CDC. (2013). *Behavioral Risk Factor Surveillance System Data*. Retrieved from http://www.cdc.gov/brfss/

Christenhusz, L. C., Prenger, R., Pieterse, M. E., Seydel, E. R., & van der Palen, J. (2012). Cost-effectiveness of an intensive smoking cessation intervention for COPD outpatients. *Nicotine & Tobacco Research, 14*, 657–663.

Clark, N. M., Brown, R., Joseph, C. L., Anderson, E. W., Liu, M., & Valerio, M. A. (2004). Effects of a comprehensive school-based asthma program on symptoms, parent management, grades, and absenteeism. *Chest, 125*, 1674–1679.

Clark, N. M., Cabana, M., Kaciroti, N., Gong, M., & Sleeman, K. (2008). Long-term outcomes of physician peer teaching. *Clinical Pediatrics, 47,* 883–890.

Clark, N. M., Ko, Y. A., Gong, Z. M., & Johnson, T. R. (2012). Outcomes associated with a negotiated asthma treatment plan. *Chronic Respiratory Disease, 9,* 175–182.

Coffman, J. M., Cabana, M. D., & Yelin, E. H. (2009). Do school-based asthma education programs improve self-management and health outcomes? *Pediatrics, 124,* 729–742.

Coronini-Cronberg, S., Heffernan, C., & Robinson, M. (2011). Effective smoking cessation interventions for COPD patients: A review of the evidence. *JRSM Short Reports, 2,* 78.

DeVol, R., Bedroussian, A., Charuworn, A., Chatterjee, A., Kim, I., Kim, S., & Klowden, K. (2007). *An unhealthy America: The economic burden of chronic disease—Charting a new course to save lives and increase productivity and economic growth.* Retrieved from http://www.milkeninstitute.org/pdf /ES_ResearchFindings.pdf

Duncan, C. L., Hogan, M. B., Tien, K. J., Graves, M. M., Chorney, J. M., Zettler, M. D., ... Portnoy, J. (2012). Efficacy of a parent-youth teamwork intervention to promote adherence in pediatric asthma. *Journal of Pediatric Psychology,* doi: 10.1093/jpepsy/jss123

Eakin, M. N., & Rand, C. S. (2012). Improving patient adherence with asthma self-management practices: What works? *Annals of Allergy, Asthma & Immunology, 109,* 90–92.

Eakin, M. N., Rand, C. S., Bilderback, A., Bollinger, M. E., Butz, A., Kandasamy, V., & Riekert, K. A. (2012). Asthma in Head Start children: Effects of the Breathmobile program and family communication on asthma outcomes. *Journal of Allergy and Clinical Immunology, 129,* 664–670.

Erickson, S. J., Gerstle, M., & Feldstein, S. W. (2005). Brief interventions and motivational interviewing with children, adolescents, and their parents in pediatric health care settings: A review. *Archives of Pediatrics & Adolescent Medicine, 159,* 1173–1180.

Fan, V. S., Gaziano, J. M., Lew, R., Bourbeau, J., Adams, S. G., Leatherman, S., ... Fiore, L. (2012). A comprehensive care management program to prevent chronic obstructive pulmonary disease hospitalizations: A randomized, controlled trial. *Annals of Internal Medicine, 156,* 673–683.

Fan, V. S., Giardino, N. D., Blough, D. K., Kaplan, R. M., & Ramsey, S. D. (2008). Costs of pulmonary rehabilitation and predictors of adherence in the National Emphysema Treatment Trial. *COPD, 5,* 105–116.

Fiese, B. H., & Wamboldt, F. S. (2003). Tales of pediatric asthma management: Family-based strategies related to medical adherence and health care utilization. *Journal of Pediatrics, 143,* 457–462.

Fiese, B. H., Wamboldt, F. S., & Anbar, R. D. (2005). Family asthma management routines: Connections to medical adherence and quality of life. *Journal of Pediatrics, 146,* 171–176.

Foglio, K., Bianchi, L., & Ambrosino, N. (2001). Is it really useful to repeat outpatient pulmonary rehabilitation programs in patients with chronic airway obstruction? A 2-year controlled study. *Chest, 119,* 1696–1704.

Foglio, K., Bianchi, L., Bruletti, G., Battista, L., Pagani, M., & Ambrosino, N. (1999). Long-term effectiveness of pulmonary rehabilitation in patients with chronic airway obstruction. *European Respiratory Journal, 13,* 125–132.

Free, C., Knight, R., Robertson, S., Whittaker, R., Edwards, P., Zhou, W., ... Roberts, I. (2011). Smoking cessation support delivered via mobile phone text messaging (txt2stop): A single-blind, randomised trial. *Lancet, 378,* 49–55.

Gamble, J., Stevenson, M., & Heaney, L. G. (2011). A study of a multi-level intervention to improve nonadherence in difficult to control asthma. *Respiratory Medicine, 105,* 1308–1315.

George, J., Kong, D. C., Thoman, R., & Stewart, K. (2005). Factors associated with medication nonadherence in patients with COPD. *Chest, 128,* 3198–3204.

Gerald, L. B., McClure, L. A., Mangan, J. M., Harrington, K. F., Gibson, L., Erwin, S., Atchison, J., & Grad, R. (2009). Increasing adherence to inhaled steroid therapy among schoolchildren: Randomized, controlled trial of school-based supervised asthma therapy. *Pediatrics, 123,* 466–474.

Gibson, P. G., Coughlan, J., & Abramson, M. (1999). Self-management education for adults with asthma improves health outcomes. *Western Journal of Medicine, 170,* 266.

Gibson, P. G., Powell, H., Coughlan, J., Wilson, A. J., Hensley, M. J., Abramson, M., Bauman, A., & Walters, E. H. (2002). Limited (information only) patient education programs for adults with asthma. *Cochrane Database Systematic Reviews,* CD001005.

Giraud, V., & Roche, N. (2002). Misuse of corticosteroid metered-dose inhaler is associated with decreased asthma stability. *European Respiratory Journal, 19,* 246–251.

Global Initiative for Chronic Obstructive Lung Disease (GOLD). (2013). *Global strategy for the diagnosis, management, and prevention of COPD.* Retrieved from http://www.goldcopd.org

Griffiths, T. L., Burr, M. L., Campbell, I. A., Lewis-Jenkins, V., Mullins, J., Shiels, K., ... Turnbridge, J. (2000). Results at 1 year of outpatient multidisciplinary pulmonary rehabilitation: A randomised controlled trial. *Lancet, 355*, 362–368.

Guerriero, C., Cairns, J., Roberts, I., Rodgers, A., Whittaker, R., & Free, C. (2013). The cost-effectiveness of smoking cessation support delivered by mobile phone text messaging: Txt2stop. *European Journal of Health Economics, 14*, 789–797.

Guevara, J. P., Wolf, F. M., Grum, C. M., & Clark, N. M. (2003). Effects of educational interventions for self management of asthma in children and adolescents: Systematic review and meta-analysis. *BMJ (Clinical Research Ed.), 326*, 1308–1309.

Gustafson, D., Wise, M., Bhattacharya, A., Pulvermacher, A., Shanovich, K., Phillips, B., ...Kim, J. S. (2012). The effects of combining Web-based eHealth with telephone nurse case management for pediatric asthma control: A randomized controlled trial. *Journal of Medical Internet Research, 14*, e101.

Halterman, J. S., Borrelli, B., Tremblay, P., Conn, K. M., Fagnano, M., Montes, G., & Hernandez, T. (2008). Screening for environmental tobacco smoke exposure among inner-city children with asthma. *Pediatrics, 122*, 1277–1283.

Halterman, J. S., Fagnano, M., Montes, G., Fisher, S., Tremblay, P., Tajon, R., Sauer, J., & Butz, A. (2012). The school-based preventive asthma care trial: Results of a pilot study. *Journal of Pediatrics, 161*, 1109–1115.

Halterman, J. S., Riekert, K., Bayer, A., Fagnano, M., Tremblay, P., Blaakman, S., & Borrelli, B. (2011). A pilot study to enhance preventive asthma care among urban adolescents with asthma. *Journal of Asthma, 48*, 523–530.

Harris, M., Smith, B. J., & Veale, A. (2008). Patient education programs–Can they improve outcomes in COPD? *International Journal of Chronic Obstructive Pulmonary Disease, 3*, 109–112.

Hogg, L., Garrod, R., Thornton, H., McDonnell, L., Bellas, H., & White, P. (2012). Effectiveness, attendance, and completion of an integrated, system-wide pulmonary rehabilitation service for COPD: Prospective observational study. *COPD, 9*, 546–554.

Hurd, S. S., & Lenfant, C. (1992). The National Heart, Lung and Blood Institute asthma program. *Chest, 101*, 359S–361S.

Jain, A., & Lolak, S. (2009). Psychiatric aspects of chronic lung disease. *Current Psychiatry Reports, 11*, 219–225.

Janson, S. L., Earnest, G., Wong, K. P., & Blanc, P. D. (2008). Predictors of asthma medication nonadherence. *Heart Lung, 37*, 211–218.

Kattan, M., Stearns, S. C., Crain, E. F., Stout, J. W., Gergen, P. J., Evans, R., III, ... Mitchell, H. E. (2005). Cost-effectiveness of a home-based environmental intervention for inner-city children with asthma. *Journal of Allergy and Clinical Immunology, 116*, 1058–1063.

Keppel, K. G. (2007). Ten largest racial and ethnic health disparities in the United States based on Healthy People 2010 Objectives. *American Journal of Epidemiology, 166*, 97–103.

Khdour, M. R., Kidney, J. C., Smyth, B. M., & McElnay, J. C. (2009). Clinical pharmacy-led disease and medicine management programme for patients with COPD. *British Journal of Clinical Pharmacology, 68*, 588–598.

Knight, K. M., McGowan, L., Dickens, C., & Bundy, C. (2006). A systematic review of motivational interviewing in physical health care settings. *British Journal of Health Psychology, 11*, 319–332.

Krieger, J. W., Takaro, T. K., Song, L., & Weaver, M. (2005). The Seattle-King County Healthy Homes Project: A randomized, controlled trial of a community health worker intervention to decrease exposure to indoor asthma triggers. *American Journal of Public Health, 95*, 652–659.

Laster, N., Holsey, C. N., Shendell, D. G., Mccarty, F. A., & Celano, M. (2009). Barriers to asthma management among urban families: Caregiver and child perspectives. *Journal of Asthma, 46*, 731–739.

Liberman, D. B., Shelef, D. Q., He, J., McCarter, R., & Teach, S. J. (2012). Low rates of follow-up with primary care providers after pediatric emergency department visits for respiratory tract illnesses. *Pediatric Emergency Care, 28*, 956–961.

Long, K. A., Ewing, L. J., Cohen, S., Skoner, D., Gentile, D., Koehrsen, J., ... Marsland, A. L. (2011). Preliminary evidence for the feasibility of a stress management intervention for 7- to 12-year-olds with asthma. *Journal of Asthma, 48*, 162–170.

Malveaux, F. J. (2009). The state of childhood asthma: Introduction. *Pediatrics, 123*(Suppl. 3), S129–S130.

Mannino, D. M., Ford, E. S., & Redd, S. C. (2003). Obstructive and restrictive lung disease and functional limitation: Data from the Third National Health and Nutrition Examination. *Journal of Internal Medicine, 254*, 540–547.

Marks, G. B., Mihrshahi, S., Kemp, A. S., Tovey, E. R., Webb, K., Almqvist, C., …. Leeder, S. R. (2006). Prevention of asthma during the first 5 years of life: A randomized controlled trial. *Journal of Allergy and Clinical Immunology, 118*, 53–61.

Martins, R. K., & McNeil, D. W. (2009). Review of Motivational Interviewing in promoting health behaviors. *Clinical Psychology Review, 29*, 283–293.

Masoli, M., Fabian, D., Holt, S., & Beasley, R. (2004). The global burden of asthma: Executive summary of the GINA Dissemination Committee report. *Allergy, 59*, 469–478.

Mathers, C. D., & Loncar, D. (2006). Projections of global mortality and burden of disease from 2002 to 2030. *PLoS Medicine, 3*, e442.

McQuaid, E. L., Walders, N., Kopel, S. J., Fritz, G. K., & Klinnert, M. D. (2005). Pediatric asthma management in the family context: The family asthma management system scale. *Journal of Pediatric Psychology, 30*, 492–502.

Molimard, M., Raherison, C., Lignot, S., Depont, F., Abouelfath, A., & Moore, N. (2003). Assessment of handling of inhaler devices in real life: An observational study in 3811 patients in primary care. *Journal of Aerosol Medicine, 16*, 249–254.

Monninkhof, E., van der Valk, P., van der Palen, J., van Herwaarden, C., Partridge, M. R., & Zielhuis, G. (2003). Self-management education for patients with chronic obstructive pulmonary disease: A systematic review. *Thorax, 58*, 394–398.

Morgan, W. J., Crain, E. F., Gruchalla, R. S., O'Connor, G. T., Kattan, M., Evans, R., … Mitchell, H. (2004). Results of a home-based environmental intervention among urban children with asthma. *New England Journal of Medicine, 351*, 1068–1080.

Murray, R. P., Voelker, H. T., Rakos, R. F., Nides, M. A., McCutcheon, V. J., & Bjornson, W. (1997). Intervention for relapse to smoking: The Lung Health Study restart programs. *Addictive Behaviors, 22*, 281–286.

National Heart, Lung, and Blood Institute. (2007). National Asthma Education and Prevention Program: Expert Panel 3: Guidelines for the diagnosis and management of asthma. Bethesda, MD. NIH Publication No. 07-4051.

Nelson, K. A., Highstein, G. R., Garbutt, J., Trinkaus, K., Fisher, E. B., Smith, S. R., & Strunk, R. C. (2011). A randomized controlled trial of parental asthma coaching to improve outcomes among urban minority children. *Archives of Pediatrics & Adolescent Medicine, 165*, 520–526.

Nici, L., Donner, C., Wouters, E., ZuWallack, R., Ambrosino, N., Bourbeau, J., … Troosters, T. (2006). American Thoracic Society/European Respiratory Society statement on pulmonary rehabilitation. *American Journal of Respiratory and Critical Care Medicine, 173*, 1390–1413.

Onyirimba, F., Apter, A., Reisine, S., Litt, M., McCusker, C., Connors, M., & ZuWallack, R. (2003). Direct clinician-to-patient feedback discussion of inhaled steroid use: Its effect on adherence. *Annals of Allergy, Asthma & Immunology, 90*, 411–415.

Otsuki, M., Eakin, M. N., Rand, C. S., Butz, A. M., Hsu, V. D., Zuckerman, I. H., … Riekert, K. A. (2009). Adherence feedback to improve asthma outcomes among inner-city children: A randomized trial. *Pediatrics, 124*, 1513–1521.

Park, J., Jackson, J., Skinner, E., Ranghell, K., Saiers, J., & Cherney, B. (2010). Impact of an adherence intervention program on medication adherence barriers, asthma control, and productivity/daily activities in patients with asthma. *Journal of Asthma, 47*, 1072–1077.

Pauwels, R. A., Buist, A. S., Ma, P., Jenkins, C. R., & Hurd, S. S. (2001). Global strategy for the diagnosis, management, and prevention of chronic obstructive pulmonary disease: National Heart, Lung, and Blood Institute and World Health Organization Global Initiative for Chronic Obstructive Lung Disease (GOLD): Executive summary. *Respiratory Care, 46*, 798–825.

Petrie, K. J., Perry, K., Broadbent, E., & Weinman, J. (2012). A text message programme designed to modify patients' illness and treatment beliefs improves self-reported adherence to asthma preventer medication. *British Journal of Health Psychology, 17*, 74–84.

Poole, P. J., Chacko, E., Wood-Baker, R. W., & Cates, C. J. (2006). Influenza vaccine for patients with chronic obstructive pulmonary disease. *Cochrane Database Systematic Reviews*, CD002733.

Powell, H., & Gibson, P. G. (2003). Options for self-management education for adults with asthma. *Cochrane Database Systematic Reviews*, CD004107.

Pulgaron, E. R., Salamon, K. S., Patterson, C. A., & Barakat, L. P. (2010). A problem-solving intervention for children with persistent asthma: A pilot of a randomized trial at a pediatric summer camp. *Journal of Asthma, 47*, 1031–1039.

Restrepo, R. D., Alvarez, M. T., Wittnebel, L. D., Sorenson, H., Wettstein, R., Vines, D. L., … Wilkins, R. L. (2008). Medication adherence issues in patients treated for COPD. *International Journal of Chronic Obstructive Pulmonary Disease, 3*, 371–384.

Rice, K. L., Dewan, N., Bloomfield, H. E., Grill, J., Schult, T. M., Nelson, D. B., … Niewoehner, D. E. (2010). Disease management program for chronic obstructive pulmonary disease: A randomized controlled trial. *American Journal of Respiratory and Critical Care Medicine, 182*, 890–896.

Riekert, K. A., Borrelli, B., Bilderback, A., & Rand, C. S. (2011). The development of a motivational interviewing intervention to promote medication adherence among inner-city, African-American adolescents with asthma. *Patient Education Counselling, 82*, 117–122.

Ries, A. L., Kaplan, R. M., Myers, R., & Prewitt, L. M. (2003). Maintenance after pulmonary rehabilitation in chronic lung disease: A randomized trial. *American Journal of Respiratory and Critical Care Medicine, 167*, 880–888.

Ritz, T., Meuret, A. E., Trueba, A. F., Fritzsche, A., & von Leupoldt, A. (2012). Psychosocial factors and behavioral medicine interventions in asthma. *Journal of Consulting and Clinical Psychology, 8*, 231–250.

Sala, E., Roca, J., Marrades, R. M., Alonso, J., Gonzalez De Suso, J. M., Moreno, A., … Wagner, P. D. (1999). Effects of endurance training on skeletal muscle bioenergetics in chronic obstructive pulmonary disease. *American Journal of Respiratory and Critical Care Medicine, 159*, 1726–1734.

Schaffer, S. D., & Tian, L. (2004). Promoting adherence: Effects of theory-based asthma education. *Clinical Nursing Research, 13*, 69–89.

Schiller, J. S., & Ni, H. (2006). Cigarette smoking and smoking cessation among persons with chronic obstructive pulmonary disease. *American Journal of Health Promotion, 20*, 319–323.

Schmaling, K. B., Blume, A. W., & Afari, N. (2001). A randomized controlled pilot study of motivational interviewing to change attitudes about adherence to medications for asthma. *Journal of Clinical Psychology in Medical Settings, 8*, 167–172.

Schneider, C., Jick, S. S., Bothner, U., & Meier, C. R. (2010). COPD and the risk of depression. *Chest, 137*, 341–347.

Seid, M., D'Amico, E. J., Varni, J. W., Munafo, J. K., Britto, M. T., Kercsmar, C. M., Drotar, D., …Darbie, L. (2012). The in vivo adherence intervention for at risk adolescents with asthma: Report of a randomized pilot trial. *Journal of Pediatric Psychology, 37*, 390–403.

Shahab, L., Jarvis, M. J., Britton, J., & West, R. (2006). Prevalence, diagnosis and relation to tobacco dependence of chronic obstructive pulmonary disease in a nationally representative population sample. *Thorax, 61*, 1043–1047.

Smith, S. R., Jaffe, D. M., Highstein, G., Fisher, E. B., Trinkaus, K. M., & Strunk, R. C. (2006). Asthma coaching in the pediatric emergency department. *Academic Emergency Medicine, 13*, 835–839.

Stead, L. F., Bergson, G., & Lancaster, T. (2008). Physician advice for smoking cessation. *Cochrane Database Systematic Reviews*, CD000165.

Strandbygaard, U., Thomsen, S. F., & Backer, V. (2010). A daily SMS reminder increases adherence to asthma treatment: A three-month follow-up study. *Respiratory Medicine, 104*, 166–171.

Troosters, T., Gosselink, R., & Decramer, M. (2000). Short- and long-term effects of outpatient rehabilitation in patients with chronic obstructive pulmonary disease: A randomized trial. *American Journal of Medicine, 109*, 207–212.

van der Meer, R. M., Wagena, E. J., Ostelo, R. W., Jacobs, J. E., & van Schayck, C. P. (2003). Smoking cessation for chronic obstructive pulmonary disease. *Cochrane Database Systematic Reviews*, CD002999.

Velsor-Friedrich, B., Militello, L. K., Richards, M. H., Harrison, P. R., Gross, I. M., Romero, E., & Bryant, F. B. (2012). Effects of coping-skills training in low-income urban African-American adolescents with asthma. *Journal of Asthma, 49*, 372–379.

Vollmer, W. M., Feldstein, A., Smith, D. H., Dubanoski, J. P., Waterbury, A., Schneider, J. L., …Rand, C. (2011). Use of health information technology to improve medication adherence. *American Journal of Managed Care, 17*, SP79–SP87.

Wagena, E. J., Arrindell, W. A., Wouters, E. F., & van Schayck, C. P. (2005). Are patients with COPD psychologically distressed? *European Respiratory Journal, 26*, 242–248.

Wagena, E. J., van der Meer, R. M., Ostelo, R. J., Jacobs, J. E., & van Schayck, C. P. (2004). The efficacy of smoking cessation strategies in people with chronic obstructive pulmonary disease: Results from a systematic review. *Respiratory Medicine, 98*, 805–815.

Walders, N., Kercsmar, C., Schluchter, M., Redline, S., Kirchner, H. L., & Drotar, D. (2006). An interdisciplinary intervention for undertreated pediatric asthma. *Chest, 129*, 292–299.

Weiss, K. B., & Sullivan, S. D. (2001). The health economics of asthma and rhinitis. I. Assessing the economic impact. *Journal of Allergy and Clinical Immunology, 107*, 3–8.

Williams, L. K., Peterson, E. L., Wells, K., Campbell, J., Wang, M., Chowdhry, V. K., … Pladevall, M. (2010). A cluster-randomized trial to provide clinicians inhaled corticosteroid adherence information for their patients with asthma. *Journal of Allergy and Clinical Immunology, 126*, 225–31, 231.

Wilson, S. R., Latini, D., Starr, N. J., Fish, L., Loes, L. M., Page, A., & Kubic, P. (1996). Education of parents of infants and very young children with asthma: A developmental evaluation of the Wee Wheezers program. *Journal of Asthma, 33*, 239–254.

Wilson, S. R., Strub, P., Buist, A. S., Knowles, S. B., Lavori, P. W., Lapidus, J., & Vollmer, W. M. (2010). Shared treatment decision making improves adherence and outcomes in poorly controlled asthma. *American Journal of Respiratory and Critical Care Medicine, 181*, 566–577.

Wise, R. A., Kanner, R. E., Lindgren, P., Connett, J. E., Altose, M. D., Enright, P. L., & Tashkin, D. P. (2003). The effect of smoking intervention and an inhaled bronchodilator on airways reactivity in COPD: The Lung Health Study. *Chest, 124*, 449–458.

Wu, F., & Takaro, T. K. (2007). Childhood asthma and environmental interventions. *Environmental Health Perspectives, 115*, 971–975.

Xu, X., Dockery, D. W., Ware, J. H., Speizer, F. E., & Ferris, B. G., Jr. (1992). Effects of cigarette smoking on rate of loss of pulmonary function in adults: A longitudinal assessment. *American Review of Respiratory Disease, 146*, 1345–1348.

Yawn, B. P. (2011). The role of the primary care physician in helping adolescent and adult patients improve asthma control. *Mayo Clinic proceedings. Mayo Clinic, 86*, 894–902.

Young, P., Dewse, M., Fergusson, W., & Kolbe, J. (1999). Respiratory rehabilitation in chronic obstructive pulmonary disease: Predictors of nonadherence. *European Respiratory Journal, 13*, 855–859.

16

Chronic Infectious Disease Management Interventions

SCOTT D. RHODES
AIMEE M. WILKIN
CLAIRE ABRAHAM
LAURA H. BACHMANN

LEARNING OBJECTIVES

- List and outline the burden of main chronic infectious diseases.
- Describe three promising approaches to chronic infectious disease management.
- Delineate future directions for research for chronic infectious disease management.

Infectious diseases are caused by pathogenic microorganisms, such as bacteria, viruses, parasites, or fungi. These diseases can be spread, directly or indirectly, from one person to another. Accurate numbers of persons infected with infectious diseases are difficult to determine because many of these diseases are endemic in developing countries, where many people do not have access to modern medical care, and epidemiologic surveillance may be insufficient. Globally, however, approximately half of all deaths caused by infectious diseases each year are attributed to three diseases: HIV/AIDS, tuberculosis, and malaria. In this chapter, we present an overview of the epidemiology of selected chronic infectious diseases, including sexually transmitted infections (STIs; specifically, human papilloma virus [HPV], hepatitis B virus [HBV], and hepatitis C virus [HCV]), HIV, and tuberculosis (TB). We also explore factors related to their transmission and intervention strategies that have been used or may be promising to manage infection with these diseases or prevent transmission of these diseases to others. We recommend directions for future research that may be necessary to increase their effective management and reduce the morbidity and mortality associated with STIs, HIV, and TB.

EPIDEMIOLOGY

SEXUALLY TRANSMITTED INFECTIONS AND HIV

Sexual risk behavior is a leading cause of morbidity in the United States and throughout the world (Institute of Medicine & Committee on Prevention and Control of Sexually Transmitted Diseases, 1997; Naughton & Rhodes, 2009). Sexual risk can be defined in a number of ways. The most obvious way is according to the risk behavior itself: unprotected vaginal, oral, or anal intercourse. Sexual risk behavior may take several forms, including a high number of sexual partners, high-risk sexual practices (such as "fisting" [insertion of the hand into the rectum or vagina]), and sex under the influence of substances such as alcohol or other drugs. However, it may be difficult to discern what behaviors are occurring within a population, and thus contributing to disease burden, given the sensitivity and stigma related to many of these behaviors. A second way may refer to the nature of the sex partner such as those at increased risk including persons living with HIV/AIDS (PLWHA), persons who inject drugs, or nonexclusive partners.

Consequences of sexual risk behavior include exposure to, and transmission of, STIs, including HIV infection. Worldwide, more than 1 million people become infected with an STI each day. In the United States, 19 million new STIs occur each year, and about half of these infections occur in people aged 15 to 24 years (Satterwhite et al., 2013). Important STIs include HPV, HBV, and HIV. HCV may be sexually transmitted, especially among specific populations (e.g., men who have sex with men [MSM]; Fox et al., 2008; Rauch et al., 2005; Rhodes, DiClemente, Yee, & Hergenrather, 2001b; Rhodes & Yee, 2006; Urbanus et al., 2009; van de Laar et al., 2009).

HUMAN PAPILLOMA VIRUS

HPV is the most common STI in the United States. An estimated 20 million persons are currently infected, and an estimated 6.2 million new HPV infections occur annually. HPV infection is common among adolescents and young adults. Although women who begin having sex at an early age or who have had "many" sexual partners are considered to be at increased risk for HPV and cervical cancer, a woman can be infected with HPV even if she has had only one sexual partner. HPV infections are common in healthy women and typically cleared by the immune system; rarely does the infection persist and lead to cervical cancer. Persistence of HPV infection and progression to cancer is influenced by many factors including high parity, long-term use of oral contraceptives, tobacco use, and immunosuppression (American Cancer Society [ACS], 2013).

HPV causes the two most common types of cervical cancer worldwide: (1) squamous cell carcinoma and, less commonly, (2) adenocarcinoma. Over 11,000 new cases of cervical cancer are diagnosed in the United States each year (ACS, 2013), and approximately 3,870 women will die as a result of cervical cancer.

HPV infection is also common in men. Among heterosexual men in clinic-based studies, prevalence of genital HPV infection is often greater than 20%. However, prevalence is highly dependent on the anatomic sites sampled and method of specimen collection (Dunne, Nielson, Stone, Markowitz, & Giuliano, 2006). Gay and bisexual men, non-self-identifying MSM, and men with weakened immune systems, including those with HIV, are more likely to develop HPV-related health problems. For example, gay and bisexual men and other MSM are estimated to be up to 20 times more likely to develop anal cancer than men who have sex only with women (Machalek et al., 2012).

Recent research also suggests that incidence is increasing for cancers of the oropharynx among both women and men. These cancers are associated with the transmission of HPV during oral sexual contact (ACS, 2011).

The lack of available curative treatments for HPV infection emphasizes the importance of prevention. Two highly effective HPV vaccines are currently available for administration to males and females aged 9 to 26 years and should be implemented as part of routine care. Although it is optimal to administer the vaccine prior to sexual debut, sexually experienced individuals also may benefit from the vaccine (Centers for Disease Control and Prevention [CDC], 2010a, 2010b). Unfortunately HPV vaccination rates in the United States are low; for example, only about one-third of eligible females have received the vaccine (Darden et al., 2013).

HEPATITIS B VIRUS

HBV is highly transmissible, and thus, is one of the most common infectious diseases globally and an important cause of acute and chronic liver disease. It has been estimated that there are 350 million chronic HBV carriers worldwide (Hou, Liu, & Gu, 2005). The prevalence of chronic HBV infection varies geographically. In the United States, HBV infects 5% to 7% of the population, and about 800,000 to 1.4 million persons are living with chronic infection (Lee & Park, 2010).

In adults, approximately half of newly acquired HBV infections are symptomatic, with 1% of reported cases resulting in acute liver failure and death. Risk for chronic infection is inversely related to age at infection; approximately 90% of infected infants and 30% of infected children aged ≤ 5 years become chronically infected, compared with 2% to 6% of adults (CDC, 2010c). There is no specific treatment available for acute HBV. Instead, it is recommended that those infected avoid infecting others by taking precautions to prevent them from coming into contact with contaminated blood and bodily fluids (Heymann, 2008).

HBV is efficiently transmitted by percutaneous or mucous membrane exposure to infectious blood or bodily fluids that contain blood. Although HBV infection is uncommon among adults in the general population (the lifetime risk of infection is less than 20%) in the United States, it is more prevalent in certain groups, including heterosexuals who have contact with infected persons or multiple partners, injection-drug users, health care workers, patients who require regular blood transfusion or hemodialysis, and gay and bisexual men and MSM (Rhodes, DiClemente, Yee, & Hergenrather, 2001a). Persons with chronic infection are often asymptomatic and may not be aware that they are infected; however, they are capable of infecting others and have been referred to as "carriers." Chronic infection is responsible for most HBV-related morbidity and mortality, including chronic hepatitis, cirrhosis, liver failure, and hepatocellular carcinoma. An estimated 3,000 to 4,000 persons die of hepatitis B-related cirrhosis each year in the United States. Persons with chronic HBV infection are at 12 to 300 times higher risk of hepatocellular carcinoma than non-carriers. An estimated 1,000 to 1,500 persons die each year in the United States of HBV-related liver cancer (CDC, 2010c).

Vaccination against HBV has resulted in decreased numbers of HBV cases in the United States. However, full vaccination requires completion of three doses over several months, and in the United States less than 40% of adults have been vaccinated against HBV (CDC, 2006; Lu, Byrd, Murphy, & Weinbaum, 2011; Pollack et al., 2011). This percentage may increase, however, as schools increasingly require proof of HBV vaccination for students based on vaccination recommendations of the Advisory Committee on Immunization Practices (ACIP; Mast et al., 2005).

HEPATITIS C VIRUS

Although less efficiently transmitted sexually than HBV, HCV infection is the most common blood-borne infection in the United States. HCV is a major global disease with an estimated prevalence of 170 to 200 million persons infected, and an estimated 3.2 million persons in the United States have chronic HCV infection (Armstrong et al., 2006). The most effective treatment of chronic HCV has been a combination therapy of ribavirin and slow release interferon though newer protease inhibitors are now available with higher cure rates (Ghany, Nelson, Strader, Thomas, & Seeff, 2011; Heymann, 2008).

HCV is most commonly transmitted through blood-to-blood contact, that is, when blood from a person infected with the HCV enters the body of someone who is not infected. Before 1992, when widespread screening of the blood supply began in the United States, HCV was also commonly spread through blood transfusions and organ transplants. Individuals are primarily infected with HCV through: (1) sharing needles, syringes, or other equipment to inject drugs; (2) needle-stick injuries in health care settings; and (3) being born to a mother who has HCV. Less commonly, sharing personal care items that may have come in contact with another's blood, such as razors or toothbrushes, and having sexual contact with an individual infected with HCV can transmit HCV.

Furthermore, studies have reported an association between acquiring HCV infection and exposure to a sex contact with HCV infection or exposure to multiple sex partners (CDC, 2011; Rhodes et al., 2001b). Surveillance data indicate that 15% to 20% of persons reported with acute HCV infection had a history of sexual exposure in the absence of other risk factors. Mounting evidence suggests that among MSM with HIV, HCV may be transmitted during high-risk sexual practices (such as "fisting") (Garg, Taylor, Grasso, & Mayer, 2013).

Sixty percent to 70% of those newly infected with HCV are asymptomatic or have a mild clinical illness. Of every 100 persons infected with HCV, approximately 75 to 85 will develop chronic infection, 60 to 70 will develop chronic liver disease, 5 to 20 will develop cirrhosis over a period of 20 to 30 years, and 1 to 5 will die from the consequences of chronic infection (liver cancer or cirrhosis) (ACS, 2011). Hepatitis C mediated cirrhosis is one of the most common indications for liver transplantation in the United States (Mukherjee & Sorrell, 2008).

HCV can be treated effectively, but adherence to treatment is challenging because of the lengthy duration, complex regimen (including high pill burden and lengthy treatment), active substance use, lack of social support, frequent side effects, and the presence of cirrhosis in some cases (Sun et al., 2012). Adherence rates tend to range from 70% to 85%; however, studies vary based on population, for example, injection-drug users may have lower rates of adherence. Furthermore, adherence rates differ based on therapies prescribed, and studies have not been consistent in how adherence is measured and defined (Brett Hauber, Mohamed, Beam, Medjedovic, & Mauskopf, 2011; Sun et al., 2012).

HIV

HIV, which has multiple modes of transmission but most often is sexually transmitted (Heymann, 2008), continues its impact, with an estimated 34 million people living with HIV/AIDS worldwide, and 0.8% of adults aged 15 to 49 years old are living with HIV worldwide; 2.5 million people are newly infected and 1.7 million deaths occur each year (Joint United Nations Programme on HIV/AIDS, 2012). In the United States, an estimated 1 million people are living with HIV/AIDS currently and over 50,000 new infections occur each year (CDC, 2013).

Gay and bisexual men and MSM carry a disproportionate burden of HIV infection in the United States and incidence has been increasing within this group since the mid-1990s (Nanin et al., 2009; Naughton & Rhodes, 2009; Wolitski, Valdiserri, Denning, & Levine, 2001). Sixty-five percent of new HIV infections in 2011 were attributable to MSM contact (including injection-drug using MSM) and 27% to heterosexual contact. Rates of HIV are higher in African American/Blacks and in Hispanic/Latinos as well, and the majority of new AIDS cases among all MSM are diagnosed in racial/ethnic-minority men (CDC, 2013). For example, in a 2005 study of five large U.S. cities, 46% of African American/Black MSM were HIV positive, compared to 21% of White MSM. In 2001, the AIDS case rate for Hispanic/Latino men was triple that of White men, and Hispanic/Latino MSM aged 23 to 29 years have twice the rate of HIV infection of their White peers (CDC, 2005).

Although it can be transmitted through blood-to-blood contact through needle and/or syringe sharing, HIV is commonly sexually transmitted. Besides blood, HIV can be transmitted through semen, vaginal fluids, and breast milk of a person infected with HIV. Unfortunately, a vaccine or cure for HIV is several years, perhaps decades, away (WHO-UNAIDS Consultation, 2001). However, advances in medical treatments have improved the outcomes for most persons with HIV/AIDS who are able to access antiretroviral therapy and medical care. Dramatic improvements in HIV treatment came in 1996, when highly active antiretroviral therapy (HAART) became available. The advent of HAART has changed the lives of many of those with HIV/AIDS in the United States (Rhodes, Hergenrather, Wilkin, & Wooldredge, 2009), turning HIV/AIDS from a uniformly fatal disease into a chronic disease for which strict adherence to a drug regimen is necessary (Heymann, 2008). A recent study found that early treatment with antiretroviral therapy yielded benefits not only for the individual, in terms of reduction in morbidity and mortality, but also conferred benefit to the public's health in that it reduced sexual transmission of HIV by 96%, reiterating the importance of linkage to and retention in HIV care and the benefits of adherence to antiretroviral therapy (Cohen et al., 2011).

To maximize its benefit, antiretroviral therapy requires unusually high levels of adherence when compared to other medications. In fact, individuals on antiretroviral therapy regimens must adhere to their schedule 95% of the time to achieve an 80% likelihood of having an undetectable viral load. This translates into missing no more than three doses a month of a twice-a-day regimen. An undetectable viral load is usually defined as 50 or fewer copies of HIV per milliliter of blood, and is an accepted surrogate marker for effectiveness of an antiretroviral regimen in controlling disease progression. Lower viral loads are preferred because low viral loads mean that less HIV is replicating within the body. With less than 95% adherence, the probability of suppression to undetectable levels can drop to less than 50%. Unfortunately, non-adherence to antiretroviral therapy is common. The average rate of adherence varies with the method used to measure adherence and the population studied, but appears to be approximately 70%, and in the United States only 19% to 28% of those taking antiretrovirals achieve viral suppression (Zuniga & Young, 2013). In one prospective study, for example, 140 individuals in a public hospital HIV clinic were followed for 1 year after initiation of antiretroviral therapy. Adherence was assessed using three methods: (1) a computer chip embedded in a specially designed pill-bottle cap to record the time and duration of each bottle opening (microelectronic monitoring system [MEMS], or MEMS caps), (2) pill count, and (3) self-report. The investigators calculated a composite adherence rate including the three measures and identified a mean adherence rate of 71%. Only 6% of the patients took ≥ 95% or more of their medications, the optimal level for durable virological and clinical success (Golin et al., 2002). International studies conducted in Canada, Europe, and developed countries in Latin America have identified similar rates of adherence (Barroso et al., 2003).

Besides maintaining one's own health through adhering to medical regimens, people with HIV can prevent spread to others through various strategies. In the United States, perinatal transmission has been dramatically lowered by implementing U.S. Public Health Service guidelines to reduce transmission from pregnant women to their children. Without antiretroviral therapy, approximately 25% of pregnant women infected with HIV will transmit the virus to their children (Connor et al., 1994). Despite success in reducing perinatal transmission, 100 to 200 infants in the United States are infected with HIV annually. Most of these infections involve women who were not tested early enough in their pregnancy or did not receive prevention services (CDC, 2013).

"Safer sex" is another strategy to prevent transmission of HIV from an infected partner to another partner during sexual intercourse. Safer sex refers to sexual intercourse that prevents the exchange of infectious bodily fluids (i.e., semen, vaginal secretions, human breast milk, and blood). One of the most common ways of preventing transmission of HIV and some other STIs during sexual intercourse is the use of latex condoms. Despite the high level of knowledge in the United States about HIV and STI transmission, condom use remains low; in fact, although the prevalence of sexual risk behavior generally declines following HIV diagnosis, a substantial proportion of HIV-positive people continue to engage in unprotected intercourse. For example, in a sample of HIV-positive women in the United States, 36.5% reported having engaged in any unprotected sexual intercourse during the past 3 months (Carvalho et al., 2011). Similarly, a substantial proportion of HIV-positive MSM also report not adhering to condom use recommendations to prevent HIV transmission to others. In a study of HIV-infected (predominately) MSM attending an Alabama-based HIV clinic, investigators found condom use rates to be about 38% during anal intercourse (Bachmann et al., 2009).

TUBERCULOSIS

TB is second only to HIV/AIDS as the greatest killer worldwide due to a single infectious agent, and nearly a third of the world's population is infected with *Mycobacterium tuberculosis*, the bacterium that causes TB, although active TB disease develops in only a fraction of these people. In 2011, an estimated 8.7 million people were newly infected with TB and 1.4 million people died from TB globally (World Health Organization [WHO], 2012). Although 95% of TB cases and TB-related deaths are in developing countries, TB has re-emerged in the United States. This resurgence is attributable to a variety of factors including increased rates of HIV infection, the development of multi-drug resistant TB, increased immigration from countries where TB is endemic, and national and international neglect toward the elimination and treatment of the disease (CDC, 2008; Institute of Medicine, 2000).

Risk factors for TB infection include being in close personal contact with an individual with infectious TB disease, immigration from areas of the world with high rates of TB (e.g., China, India, and Russia), children less than 5 years of age who have a positive TB test, individuals with silicosis, those living with HIV, and poor nutrition and low body weight. Overcrowding is associated with TB because individuals are in close proximity, have poor nutrition, and lack health care services. Locations particularly vulnerable to overcrowding include homeless shelters, correctional facilities, and other types of residential homes (WHO, 2012).

M. tuberculosis most often attacks the lungs, but can affect any part of the body such as the kidney, spine, and brain. If not treated properly, active TB can be fatal. TB is spread through the air from one individual to another, transmitted on small airborne droplets that are produced when an individual with TB of the lungs, throat, or larynx coughs, sneezes, or talks.

TB can be treated with a combination of drugs that vary depending on the specific strain of the infected individual. Because of the long duration of the therapy, there is a risk of non-adherence or "default" that contributes to prolonged infectiousness, drug resistance, relapse, and death. Globally, adherence to treatment is about 80% on average but well below this mean in many of the countries with the highest burden of TB (WHO, 2011). When possible, it is recommended that the patient should use a facemask to cover their nose and mouth to prevent spread, or at least be taught to cover the nose and mouth while coughing and sneezing (Heymann, 2008).

INTERVENTION SCIENCE TO MANAGE CHRONIC INFECTIOUS DISEASES

The primary prevention of STIs, including HPV, HBV, HCV, and HIV, and other infections like TB, is clearly preferable as opposed to their management. Prevention includes immunization against vaccine preventable diseases (i.e., routine infant HBV immunization and HPV vaccination of individuals aged 9 to 26 years), adequate sterilization of all syringes and needles, the use of condoms in sexual intercourse, and education of the public in proper prevention measures (such as mode of spread of TB and the importance of prompt diagnosis and treatment; Heymann, 2008).

Furthermore, after infection, the management of these chronic infectious diseases can be challenging. Interventions should support the ongoing management of the chronic infectious disease to reduce morbidity and mortality and reduce transmission of the infection to others. This is a unique characteristic of the management of chronic infectious diseases: the need to try to maintain the health and well-being of those living with an infectious disease and also to prevent its transmission to others.

A seven-step framework to support adherence has been developed. This framework includes: (1) developing patient-centered relationships, (2) using motivational interviewing techniques, (3) addressing the known impediments to adherence, (4) screening regularly for poor adherence, (5) utilizing adherence aids, (6) expanding pharmacy services or directly observed therapy, and (7) creating an adherence program to formalize attention to this issue (Machtinger & Bangsberg, 2007). Because it is clear that a single approach will not suit everyone, strategies to match adherence interventions to the populations or individuals most likely to benefit from them are needed.

Although practical and potentially useful strategies to improve adherence to care and treatment regimens are being used with some success, including medication reminder devices such as beepers, pill boxes, and supportive reminder telephone calls, there are key types of innovative interventions around which evidence of efficacy and effectiveness is being shown to be successful in the ongoing management of chronic infectious diseases. These interventions creatively blend components of the seven-step framework to support adherence described above. In this subsequent section, we describe three types of innovative and promising interventions to support those living with a chronic infectious disease. These interventions are natural helper interventions, provider-delivered interventions, and directly observed therapies.

NATURAL HELPER INTERVENTIONS

An intervention strategy that has gained the interest of both researchers and practitioners includes the selection, training, and support of lay community members to promote health. Natural helper interventions have been used internationally quite often as an approach to disseminate information and resources and facilitate access to health care. In this case, natural helpers can ensure efficient use of resources particularly in countries in which resources are scarce. However, these types of interventions are becoming more important in developed countries as these developed countries are faced with both limited health care resources and awareness that community "insiders" may be able to reach other community members to facilitate the best care possible.

These trained community members are "natural helpers" and often are known as village health workers, community health workers, volunteer health workers, community outreach workers, community health service volunteers, patient navigators, public health aides, peer health promoters, peer leaders, community health representatives, community health advocates, or lay health advisors (LHAs). These types of interventions are intuitively appealing because for the most part they are based in the existing social networks of community members. Natural helpers are theoretically effective because they are experientially similar to those whom they are working with; are naturally relied on for advice, emotional support, and tangible aid by others; possess an intimate understanding of community assets, priorities, and needs; understand what is meaningful to their communities; communicate in a similar language; and can effectively incorporate culture (e.g., cultural identity, spiritual coping, and traditional health practices) to promote health. Natural helper interventions have been broadly used in primary prevention and the evidence supporting their use is growing. Only more recently have these interventions been applied to support ongoing disease management (Eng, 1993; Eng, Rhodes, & Parker, 2009; Israel, 1985; Paskett et al., 2012).

In practice, natural helpers serve as health advisors and referral sources, connect community members to needed services and help community members navigate these services, distribute materials, serve as role models, and advocate on behalf of community members. Often they themselves are living with disease and have become successful at managing their own disease (Eng, Parker, & Harlan, 1997; Eng et al., 2009; Lorhan et al., 2012; Nonzee et al., 2012; Paskett et al., 2012; Ramirez et al., 2013; Rhodes, Foley, Zometa, & Bloom, 2007; Viswanathan et al., 2010). Patient navigators may be effective because they understand barriers faced by those living with disease and may provide the most tailored and culturally congruent messages to increase meaningfulness of messages and approaches to motivate others (Institute of Medicine & Committee on Prevention and Control of Sexually Transmitted Diseases, 1997; Rhodes et al., 2007; Viswanathan et al., 2010).

Traditionally these types of interventions have tended to be more pragmatic than theoretic; however, this is changing as social support, community capacity development, organizational change, education, and empowerment theories and models are increasingly incorporated into public health. Much of this movement from the pragmatic to the theoretic results from the need to positively affect the health of marginalized populations. Thus, natural helper interventions may be ideal for improving the management of chronic infectious diseases among populations, especially those populations that are more difficult for providers and practitioners to reach and yet experience disproportionate disease burden.

Patient navigator interventions have been found to improve patient satisfaction and follow-up rates. Despite a broad literature base, evidence of patient navigators to effect longer-term health outcomes associated with disease management is limited (Bradford,

Coleman, & Cunningham, 2007; Lorhan et al., 2012; Nonzee et al., 2012; Paskett et al., 2012; Pruthi et al., 2013; Ramirez et al., 2013; Vargas & Cunningham, 2006). Often the evaluation of natural helper interventions focuses on changes within the natural helper (e.g., how did the knowledge, attitudes, and skills change). It is rare to find evaluations of outcomes based on changes in knowledge, attitudes, and behaviors of members of their social networks.

However, given the stigma associated with chronic infectious diseases and the disproportionate burden borne by some populations, natural helper interventions may have considerable promise in supporting those with chronic infectious diseases. For example, patient navigators who are successfully managing their own HIV status could be trained to work with those who are newly diagnosed. These patient navigators could reduce barriers to ongoing care and treatment. Their activities with those who are more recently diagnosed or those more recently linked to care may include ongoing education about HIV prevention, care, and treatment; medical and other service appointment coordination; transportation and contingency planning; medication reminders; and motivational interviewing (Bradford et al., 2007; Vargas & Cunningham, 2006). Natural helpers could also support behavioral changes that would reduce the risk of transmission of HIV to others through increasing knowledge about infectious disease transmission, changing attitudes about risk taking, and working with individuals to develop skills to troubleshoot risky situations (e.g., condom negotiation and use).

PROVIDER-DELIVERED INTERVENTIONS

Integrating behavioral interventions into settings in which patients receive their primary care provides recurring opportunities to assess and reinforce care and treatment and to address other behaviors that may negatively influence individual health (e.g., substance use). Several provider-delivered interventions have demonstrated feasibility and effectiveness to improve HIV disease management among persons with HIV in primary care. Based on these studies, consensus has been reached regarding the need to implement these risk assessment and tailored interventions into the care and treatment of persons with HIV (Bachmann et al., 2013; Fisher et al., 2006; Gardner et al., 2008; Milam et al., 2005; Myers et al., 2010).

A computer-assisted "expert system" programmed to perform a detailed sexual risk assessment, synthesize the data, and generate theory-based messages to assist providers with interacting with their patients to address sexual risk reduction has been shown to lessen the burden on providers and perhaps lend itself to sustainability of risk reduction interventions in the primary care setting (Bachmann et al., 2013). The intervention, entitled Providers Advocating for Sexual Health Initiative (PASHIN), was developed, implemented, and evaluated as part of a multi-site Health Resources and Services Administration (HRSA)-sponsored Special Projects of National Significance (SPNS) initiative (Myers et al., 2010). PASHIN was designed to increase condom use during sex, decrease numbers of sexual partners among those with multiple partners, and increase HIV serostatus disclosure to all sex partners.

Before seeing a provider during each quarterly primary care visit, each patient completed an audio computer-assisted self-interview (ACASI)-administered assessment that measured risk behaviors that could transmit HIV to others through sexual behaviors or injection-drug use. Based on the information provided during the assessment, providers received feedback from a computerized assessment in the form of an "advice sheet" that served as a prompt to assist the provider with intervention delivery. The advice sheet was based on a carefully constructed pre-programmed algorithm and guided the brief intervention. The tailored advice sheets were printed for use by the provider during the clinical encounter along with a three-point, targeted behavioral risk reduction "prescription" which recapped the provider's intervention messages and was given to each patient to take home. The provider advice sheet and the behavior prescription focused on one targeted behavior at a time, or a sequential approach to changing multiple health risk behaviors. In addition, a separate substance abuse and depression "flag" sheet was generated for the provider if such issues were detected based on data collected at each visit.

The computer-assisted, expert system provider-delivered intervention was tested among gay and bisexual men and MSM. PASHIN was found efficacious to reduce unprotected anal sex and reduce numbers of sex partners (Bachmann et al., 2013). Thus, this intervention represents an important step for efforts designed to reduce transmission of infectious diseases to others. The next challenge will be to further optimize such an intervention for full incorporation into the primary care setting in a way that enhances clinic patient flow.

DIRECTLY OBSERVED THERAPY

Directly observed therapy is the delivery of every scheduled dose of medication by a health care provider. The provider directly administers, observes, and documents the patient's ingestion or injection of the medication. Directly observed therapy is particularly appropriate for TB treatment, given the potential for incomplete treatment to lead to further spread and multi-drug resistance (Volmink & Garner, 2007). For example, health care providers often are hesitant to initiate TB treatment unless they feel sure that a patient will complete the treatment protocol (Institute of Medicine, 2000). The process of having to show up and present oneself to a health care provider for directly observed therapy may increase adherence because it reinforces the importance of the treatment regimen for some populations (Garner, Smith, Munro, & Volmink, 2007). This ongoing "checking in" may prove invaluable to ensure increased understanding of infectivity and disease progression, and trust of medicine among patients.

It has been reported that more than 30 million patients with TB have been treated with directly observed therapy, resulting in cure rates of over 80% worldwide (Frieden & Sbarbaro, 2007). However, results of directly observed therapy among individuals with HIV have been mixed. Although few studies have been conducted studying the efficacy of this kind of treatment among those with HIV, studies that focused on youth, a commonly non-adherent group, received positive feedback from participants. For example, in one study, participants with HIV (median age = 21 years) reported that meeting with the facilitator of their directly observed therapy was easy, directly observed therapy increased their motivation to take medications, they felt sad when directly observed therapy ended, and 100% would recommend directly observed therapy to a friend. This study also indicated that while directly observed therapy is safe, feasible, and acceptable, the benefits of directly observed therapy appear to be short term (Gaur et al., 2010).

FUTURE APPROACHES TO CHRONIC INFECTIOUS DISEASE MANAGEMENT

Although care and treatment for the management of chronic infectious diseases continue to evolve, vaccination development to prevent infection with STIs, HIV, and TB is clearly a potentially effective approach to reduce infection and the impact of these chronic infectious diseases and thus the need for disease management. Strides are being made in the development of vaccines but to date, for many infectious diseases, efficacious vaccines are a long way off. Vaccinations for some STIs have been developed, including HPV and HBV; however, there are no efficacious vaccines for HCV and HIV and studies are being conducted. Only a few HIV vaccines have been tested in clinical efficacy trials. It is difficult to make a vaccine for HIV for several reasons: HIV mutates, or changes, much more rapidly than most other viruses and targeting a vaccine to a rapidly changing virus is challenging, and HIV damages the cells of the immune system. To be effective, a vaccine must trigger the immune system to fight the disease agent. Thus, a challenge for HIV vaccine research is to develop a vaccine for HIV that must interact with the immune system in a way that is very different from the natural behavior of the virus. To date, researchers have developed several candidate HIV vaccines, but none has performed well enough in clinical trials to be approved.

Currently, there is a vaccine for TB, Bacille Calmette-Guérin (BCG). However, the vaccine is not widely used in the United States, but it is often given to infants and small children in other countries where TB is endemic. BCG does not always protect against TB and in fact the immunity it induces wanes within a decade (Rhodes, 2009). Current studies are testing approaches designed to replace BCG or enhance the immunity induced by BCG (Lawn & Zumla, 2011).

Furthermore, it is important to note that vaccines, like treatment for those with an infectious chronic disease, first require availability and access to the vaccine before adherence to vaccination guidelines can become a priority. Generally, adherence to BCG tends to be low. For example, a study of a targeted vaccination of at-risk children in France reported a 44% to 60% vaccination rate (Guthmann et al., 2009; Rossignol et al., 2011).

Finally, while medical therapy for HIV infection has evolved tremendously over the last decade, innovations in TB therapy lag behind. Treatment of TB requires a minimum of 6 to 9 months of daily therapy for maximum effectiveness, depending on the drug combination. This is a prolonged period of adherence for some populations, particularly some vulnerable populations that may be more likely to have TB. Increased multi-drug resistant TB argues for shorter, simpler, and less toxic regimens for treatment. However, limited drug development research is currently being undertaken to develop alternatives to TB treatment due in part to the perceived limited market of patients with active TB in the United States. Although investigators in academia and the biotechnology industry explore how to translate basic knowledge into pragmatic applications, industry decision makers, who influence drug development efforts, may base their priorities on the perceived economics of the potential market. The prevention, care, and treatment of TB are not viewed as profitable, thus, disincentivizing the development of new medications and new combinations of existing drugs and their regimens being explored.

CONCLUSIONS

Maintaining health while living with a chronic infectious disease includes adhering to pharmacological treatment regimens, clinical and treatment appointments, and in the case of STIs and HIV, safer sex and safer drug use recommendations. Furthermore, lifestyle changes are often necessary which may be challenging for those living with a chronic infectious disease. Common lifestyle changes include reducing or terminating alcohol use, staying healthy through a diet rich in fruits and vegetables, regular exercise, and sufficient sleep.

Further research is needed to understand disease management among those with STIs, HIV, and TB, including their adherence to medication, medical appointments, and other behavioral recommendations. Future research must also address a variety of important issues facing disease management, including: (1) how to help patients decide when to initiate therapy (e.g., identifying when the patient is psychologically ready to commit to strictly adhering to a potentially lifelong regimen); (2) the rapidly advancing treatment options facing those with infectious diseases and their providers; (3) the evolving intervention science; and (4) the potential of continual or ongoing adherence intervention in contrast to the traditional approach of a short-term or limited intervention for the promotion of long-term adherence.

Furthermore, research must continue to improve the medical regimens for those living with chronic infectious diseases in order to improve the management of chronic infectious diseases through reduced regimen complexity. Moreover, further development of vaccines is needed; however, the development of vaccines will require strategies to ensure vaccine uptake. Finally, chronic infectious diseases have an added challenge. Not only is it necessary to manage disease, but by definition these diseases are infectious and thus require those with these diseases to change their behaviors and adopt prevention behaviors to reduce exposure to others.

REFERENCES

American Cancer Society. (2011). *Cancer facts & figures for Hispanics/Latinos 2009–2011*. Atlanta, GA: Author.

American Cancer Society. (2013). *Cancer facts & figures*. Atlanta, GA: Author.

Armstrong, G. L., Wasley, A., Simard, E. P., McQuillan, G. M., Kuhnert, W. L., & Alter, M. J. (2006). The prevalence of hepatitis C virus infection in the United States, 1999 through 2002. *Annals of Internal Medicine, 144*(10), 705–714.

Bachmann, L. H., Grimley, D. M., Chen, H., Aban, I., Hu, J., Zhang, S., … Hook, E. W., 3rd. (2009). Risk behaviours in HIV-positive men who have sex with men participating in an intervention in a primary care setting. *International Journal of STD & AIDS, 20*(9), 607–612.

Bachmann, L. H., Grimley, D. M., Gao, H., Aban, I., Chen, H., Raper, J. L., … Hook, E. W. (2013). Impact of a computer-assisted, provider-delivered intervention on sexual risk behaviors in HIV-positive men who have sex with men (MSM) in a primary care setting. *AIDS Education and Prevention, 25*(2), 87–101.

Barroso, P. F., Schechter, M., Gupta, P., Bressan, C., Bomfim, A., & Harrison, L. H. (2003). Adherence to antiretroviral therapy and persistence of HIV RNA in semen. *Journal of Acquired Immune Deficiency, 32*(4), 435–440.

Bradford, J. B., Coleman, S., & Cunningham, W. (2007). HIV system navigation: An emerging model to improve HIV care access. *AIDS Patient Care STDS, 21*(Suppl. 1), S49–S58.

Brett Hauber, A., Mohamed, A. F., Beam, C., Medjedovic, J., & Mauskopf, J. (2011). Patient preferences and assessment of likely adherence to hepatitis C virus treatment. *Journal of Viral Hepatitis, 18*(9), 619–627.

Carvalho, F. T., Goncalves, T. R., Faria, E. R., Shoveller, J. A., Piccinini, C. A., Ramos, M. C., & Medeiros, L. R. (2011). Behavioral interventions to promote condom use among women living with HIV. *Cochrane Database Systematic Reviews (Online)*, (9), CD007844.

Centers for Disease Control and Prevention (CDC). (2005). HIV prevalence, unrecognized infection, and HIV testing among men who have sex with men – Five U.S. cities, June 2004–April 2005. *MMWR. Morbidity and Mortality Weekly Report, 52*(24), 597–601.

CDC. (2006). Hepatitis B vaccination coverage among adults – United States, 2004. *MMWR. Morbidity and Mortality Weekly Report, 55*(18), 509–511.

CDC. (2008). Trends in tuberculosis – United States, 2007. *MMWR. Morbidity and Mortality Weekly Report, 57*(11), 281–285.

CDC. (2010a). FDA licensure of bivalent human papillomavirus vaccine (HPV2, Cervarix) for use in females and updated HPV vaccination recommendations from the Advisory Committee on Immunization Practices (ACIP). *MMWR. Morbidity and Mortality Weekly Report, 59*(20), 626–629.

CDC. (2010b). FDA licensure of quadrivalent human papillomavirus vaccine (HPV4, Gardasil) for use in males and guidance from the Advisory Committee on Immunization Practices (ACIP). *MMWR. Morbidity and Mortality Weekly Report, 59*(20), 630–632.

CDC. (2010c). Hepatocellular carcinoma – United States, 2001–2006. *MMWR. Morbidity and Mortality Weekly Report, 59*(17), 517–520.

CDC. (2011). Sexual transmission of hepatitis C virus among HIV-infected men who have sex with men – New York City, 2005–2010. *MMWR. Morbidity and Mortality Weekly Report, 60*(28), 945–950.

CDC. (2013). HIV Surveillance Report, 2011. Atlanta, GA: US Department of Health and Human Services.

Cohen, M. S., Chen, Y. Q., McCauley, M., Gamble, T., Hosseinipour, M. C., Kumarasamy, N., ... HPTN 052 Study Team. (2011). Prevention of HIV-1 infection with early antiretroviral therapy. *New England Journal of Medicine, 365*(6), 493–505.

Connor, E. M., Sperling, R. S., Gelber, R., Kiselev, P., Scott, G., O'Sullivan, M. J., ... Jacobson R. L. (1994). Reduction of maternal-infant transmission of human immunodeficiency virus type 1 with zidovudine treatment. Pediatric AIDS Clinical Trials Group Protocol 076 Study Group. *New England Journal of Medicine, 331*(18), 1173–1180.

Darden, P. M., Thompson, D. M., Roberts, J. R., Hale, J. J., Pope, C., Naifeh, M., & Jacobson, R. M. (2013). Reasons for not vaccinating adolescents: National Immunization Survey of Teens, 2008-2010. *Pediatrics, 131*(4), 645–651.

Dunne, E. F., Nielson, C. M., Stone, K. M., Markowitz, L. E., & Giuliano, A. R. (2006). Prevalence of HPV infection among men: A systematic review of the literature. *Journal of Infectious Diseases, 194*(8), 1044–1057.

Eng, E. (1993). The Save our Sisters Project. A social network strategy for reaching rural black women. *Cancer, 72*(3 Suppl.), 1071–1077.

Eng, E., Parker, E., & Harlan, C. (1997). Lay health advisor intervention strategies: A continuum from natural helping to paraprofessional helping. *Health Education & Behavior, 24*(4), 413–417.

Eng, E., Rhodes, S. D., & Parker, E. A. (2009). Natural helper models to enhance a community's health and competence. In R. J. DiClemente, R. A. Crosby, & M. C. Kegler (Eds.), *Emerging theories in health promotion practice and research* (Vol. 2, pp. 303–330). San Francisco, CA: Jossey-Bass.

Fisher, J. D., Fisher, W. A., Cornman, D. H., Amico, R. K., Bryan, A., & Friedland, G. H. (2006). Clinician-delivered intervention during routine clinical care reduces unprotected sexual behavior among HIV-infected patients. *Journal of Acquired Immune Deficiency, 41*(1), 44–52.

Fox, J., Nastouli, E., Thomson, E., Muir, D., McClure, M., Weber, J., & Fidler, S. (2008). Increasing incidence of acute hepatitis C in individuals diagnosed with primary HIV in the United Kingdom. *AIDS (London, England), 22*(5), 666–668.

Frieden, T. R., & Sbarbaro, J. A. (2007). Promoting adherence to treatment for tuberculosis: The importance of direct observation. *World Hospitals and Health Services, 43*(2), 30–33.

Gardner, L. I., Marks, G., O'Daniels, C. M., Wilson, T. E., Golin, C., Wright, J., ... Thrun, M. (2008). Implementation and evaluation of a clinic-based behavioral intervention: Positive steps for patients with HIV. *AIDS Patient Care and STDS, 22*(8), 627–635.

Garg, S., Taylor, L. E., Grasso, C., & Mayer, K. H. (2013). Prevalent and incident hepatitis C virus infection among HIV-infected men who have sex with men engaged in primary care in a Boston community health center. *Clinical Infectious Diseases, 56*(10), 1480–1487.

Garner, P., Smith, H., Munro, S., & Volmink, J. (2007). Promoting adherence to tuberculosis treatment. *Bulletin of the World Health Organization, 85*(5), 404–406.

Gaur, A. H., Belzer, M., Britto, P., Garvie, P. A., Hu, C., Graham, B., ... Pediatric AIDS Clinical Trials Group P1036B Team. (2010). Directly observed therapy (DOT) for nonadherent HIV-infected youth: Lessons learned, challenges ahead. *AIDS Research and Human Retroviruses, 26*(9), 947–953.

Ghany, M. G., Nelson, D. R., Strader, D. B., Thomas, D. L., & Seeff, L. B. (2011). An update on treatment of genotype 1 chronic hepatitis C virus infection: 2011 practice guideline by the American Association for the Study of Liver Diseases. *Hepatology, 54*(4), 1433–1444.

Golin, C. E., Liu, H., Hays, R. D., Miller, L. G., Beck, C. K., Ickovics, J., ... Wenger, N. S. (2002). A prospective study of predictors of adherence to combination antiretroviral medication. *Journal of General Internal Medicine, 17*(10), 756–765.

Guthmann, J. P., de La Rocque, F., Boucherat, M., van Cauteren, D., Fonteneau, L., Lecuyer, A., ... Levy-Bruhl, D. (2009). BCG vaccine coverage in private medical practice: First data in children below two years old, seven months after the end of compulsory vaccination in France. *Archives de Pédiatrie, 16*(5), 489–495.

Heymann, D. L. (2008). *Control of communicable diseases manual* (19th ed.). Washington, DC: APHA.

Hou, J., Liu, Z., & Gu, F. (2005). Epidemiology and prevention of hepatitis B virus infection. *International Journal of Medical Sciences, 2*(1), 50–57.

Institute of Medicine. (2000). *Ending neglect: The elimination of tuberculosis in the United States.* Washington, DC: National Academy Press.

Institute of Medicine, & Committee on Prevention and Control of Sexually Transmitted Diseases. (1997). *The hidden epidemic: Confronting sexually transmitted diseases.* Washington, DC: National Academy Press.

Israel, B. A. (1985). Social networks and social support: Implications for natural helper and community level interventions. *Health Education Quarterly, 12*(1), 65–80.

Joint United Nations Programme on HIV/AIDS. (2012). *Global Report: UNAIDS Report on the Global AIDS Epidemic 2012.* Geneva, Switzerland: UNAIDS.

Lawn, S. D., & Zumla, A. I. (2011). Tuberculosis. *Lancet, 378*(9785), 57–72.

Lee, H., & Park, W. (2010). Public health policy for management of hepatitis B virus infection: Historical review of recommendations for immunization. *Public Health Nursing, 27*(2), 148–157.

Lorhan, S., Cleghorn, L., Fitch, M., Pang, K., McAndrew, A., Applin-Poole, J., …Wright, M. (2012). Moving the agenda forward for cancer patient navigation: Understanding volunteer and peer navigation approaches. *Journal of Cancer Education, 28*(1), 84–91.

Lu, P. J., Byrd, K. K., Murphy, T. V., & Weinbaum, C. (2011). Hepatitis B vaccination coverage among high-risk adults 18–49 years, U.S., 2009. *Vaccine, 29*(40), 7049–7057.

Machalek, D. A., Poynten, M., Jin, F., Fairley, C. K., Farnsworth, A., Garland, S. M., … Grulich, A. E. (2012). Anal human papillomavirus infection and associated neoplastic lesions in men who have sex with men: A systematic review and meta-analysis. *Lancet Oncology, 13*(5), 487–500.

Machtinger, E. L., & Bangsberg, D. R. (2007). Seven steps to better adherence: A practical approach to promoting adherence to antiretroviral therapy. *AIDS Reader, 17*(1), 43–51.

Mast, E. E., Margolis, H. S., Fiore, A. E., Brink, E. W., Goldstein, S. T., Wang, S. A., … Advisory Committee on Immunization Practices (ACIP). (2005). A comprehensive immunization strategy to eliminate transmission of hepatitis B virus infection in the United States: Recommendations of the Advisory Committee on Immunization Practices (ACIP) part 1: Immunization of infants, children, and adolescents. *MMWR. Recommendations and reports: Morbidity and Mortality Weekly Repor, 54* (RR-16), 1–31.

Milam, J., Richardson, J. L., McCutchan, A., Stoyanoff, S., Weiss, J., Kemper, C., … Bolan, R. (2005). Effect of a brief antiretroviral adherence intervention delivered by HIV care providers. *Journal of Acquired Immune Deficiency, 40*(3), 356–363.

Mukherjee, S., & Sorrell, M. F. (2008). Controversies in liver transplantation for hepatitis C. *Gastroenterology, 134*(6), 1777–1788.

Myers, J. J., Shade, S. B., Rose, C. D., Koester, K., Maiorana, A., Malitz, F. E., . . . Morin, S. F. (2010). Interventions delivered in clinical settings are effective in reducing risk of HIV transmission among people living with HIV: Results from the Health Resources and Services Administration (HRSA)'s Special Projects of National Significance initiative. *AIDS and Behavior, 14*(3), 483–492.

Nanin, J., Osubu, T., Walker, J., Powell, B., Powell, D., & Parsons, J. (2009). "HIV is still real": Perceptions of HIV testing and HIV prevention among black men who have sex with men in New York City. *American Journal of Men's Health, 3*(2), 150–164.

Naughton, M. J., & Rhodes, S. D. (2009). Adoption and maintenance of safer sex practices. In S. A. Shumaker, J. K. Ockene, & K. Riekert (Eds.), *The handbook of health behavior change* (3rd ed., pp. 253–269). New York, NY: Springer.

Nonzee, N. J., McKoy, J. M., Rademaker, A. W., Byer, P., Luu, T. H., Liu, D., … Simon, M. A. (2012). Design of a prostate cancer patient navigation intervention for a Veterans Affairs hospital. *BMC Health Services Research, 12*(1), 340.

Paskett, E. D., Katz, M. L., Post, D. M., Pennell, M. L., Young, G. S., Seiber, E. E., … Ohio Patient Navigation Research Program. (2012). The Ohio Patient Navigation Research Program: Does the American Cancer Society patient navigation model improve time to resolution in patients with abnormal screening tests? *Cancer Epidemiology, Biomarkers & Prevention, 21*(10), 1620–1628.

Pollack, H., Wang, S., Wyatt, L., Peng, C. H., Wan, K., Trinh-Shevrin, C., … Kwon, S. (2011). A comprehensive screening and treatment model for reducing disparities in hepatitis B. *Health Affairs (Project Hope), 30*(10), 1974–1983.

Pruthi, S., Stange, K. J., Malagrino, G. D., Jr., Chawla, K. S., Larusso, N. F., & Kaur, J. S. (2013). Successful implementation of a telemedicine-based counseling program for high-risk patients with breast cancer. *Mayo Clinic proceedings. Mayo Clinic, 88*(1), 68–73.

Ramirez, A. G., Perez-Stable, E. J., Penedo, F. J., Talavera, G. A., Carrillo, J. E., Fernandez, M. E., … Gallion, K. (2013). Navigating Latinas with breast screen abnormalities to diagnosis: The Six Cities Study. *Cancer, 119*(7), 1298–1305.

Rauch, A., Rickenbach, M., Weber, R., Hirschel, B., Tarr, P. E., Bucher, H. C., ... Swiss HIV Cohort Study. (2005). Unsafe sex and increased incidence of hepatitis C virus infection among HIV-infected men who have sex with men: The Swiss HIV Cohort Study. *Clinical Infectious Diseases, 41*(3), 395–402.

Rhodes, S. D. (2009). Tuberculosis, sexually transmitted diseases, HIV, and other infections among farmworkers in the eastern United States. In T. A. Arcury & S. A. Quandt (Eds.), *Latino farmworkers in the Eastern United States: Health, safety and justice* (pp. 131–152). New York, NY: Springer.

Rhodes, S. D., DiClemente, R. J., Yee, L. J., & Hergenrather, K. C. (2001a). Correlates of hepatitis B vaccination in a high-risk population: An Internet sample. *American Journal of Medicine, 110*(8), 628–632.

Rhodes, S. D., DiClemente, R. J., Yee, L. J., & Hergenrather, K. C. (2001b). Factors associated with testing for hepatitis C in an internet-recruited sample of men who have sex with men. *Sexually Transmitted Diseases, 28*(9), 515–520.

Rhodes, S. D., Foley, K. L., Zometa, C. S., & Bloom, F. R. (2007). Lay health advisor interventions among Hispanics/Latinos: A qualitative systematic review. *American Journal of Preventive Medicine, 33*(5), 418–427.

Rhodes, S. D., Hergenrather, K. C., Wilkin, A. M., & Wooldredge, R. (2009). Adherence and HIV: A lifetime commitment. In S. A. Shumaker, J. K. Ockene, & K. Riekert (Eds.), *The handbook of health behavior change* (3rd ed., pp. 659–675). New York, NY: Springer.

Rhodes, S. D., & Yee, L. J. (2006). Public health and gay and bisexual men: A primer for practitioners, clinicians, and researchers. In M. Shankle (Ed.), *The handbook of lesbian, gay, bisexual, and transgender public health: A practitioner's guide to service* (pp. 119–143). Binghamton, NY: Haworth.

Rossignol, L., Guthmann, J. P., Kerneis, S., Aubin-Auger, I., Lasserre, A., Chauvin, P., ... Blanchon, T. (2011). Barriers to implementation of the new targeted BCG vaccination in France: A cross sectional study. *Vaccine, 29*(32), 5232–5237.

Satterwhite, C. L., Torrone, E., Meites, E., Dunne, E. F., Mahajan, R., Ocfemia, M. C., ... Weinstock, H. (2013). Sexually transmitted infections among US women and men: Prevalence and incidence estimates, 2008. *Sexually Transmitted Diseases, 40*(3), 187–193.

Sun, X., Patnode, C. D., Williams, C., Senger, C. A., Kapka, T. J., & Whitlock, E. P. (2012). Interventions to improve patient adherence to hepatitis C treatment: Comparative effectiveness. *Comparative Effectiveness Review No. 91. AHQ Publication No. 13–EHC009-EF* (Vol. Agency for Healthcare Research and Quality). Rockville, MD.

Urbanus, A. T., van de Laar, T. J., Stolte, I. G., Schinkel, J., Heijman, T., Coutinho, R. A., & Prins, M. (2009). Hepatitis C virus infections among HIV-infected men who have sex with men: An expanding epidemic. *AIDS, 23*(12), F1–F7.

van de Laar, T., Pybus, O., Bruisten, S., Brown, D., Nelson, M., Bhagani, S., ... Danta, M. (2009). Evidence of a large, international network of HCV transmission in HIV-positive men who have sex with men. *Gastroenterology, 136*(5), 1609–1617.

Vargas, R. B., & Cunningham, W. E. (2006). Evolving trends in medical care-coordination for patients with HIV and AIDS. *Current HIV/AIDS Reports, 3*(4), 149–153.

Viswanathan, M., Kraschnewski, J. L., Nishikawa, B., Morgan, L. C., Honeycutt, A. A., Thieda, P., ... Jonas, D. E. (2010). Outcomes and costs of community health worker interventions: A systematic review. *Medical Care, 48*(9), 792–808.

Volmink, J., & Garner, P. (2007). Directly observed therapy for treating tuberculosis. *Cochrane Database Systematic Reviews,* (4), CD003343.

WHO-UNAIDS Consultation. (2001). Future access to HIV vaccines. Report from a WHO-UNAIDS Consultation, Geneva, 2–3 October 2000. *AIDS, 15*(7), W27–W44.

Wolitski, R. J., Valdiserri, R. O., Denning, P. H., & Levine, W. C. (2001). Are we headed for a resurgence of the HIV epidemic among men who have sex with men? *American Journal of Public Health, 91*(6), 883–888.

World Health Organization. (2011). *Guidelines for the programmatic management of drug-resistant tuberculosis – 2011 update.* Geneva, Switzerland: Author.

World Health Organization. (2012). *Global Tuberculosis Report 2012.* Geneva, Switzerland: WHO Press.

Zuniga, J. M., & Young, B. (2013). Achieving improvements across the HIV treatment cascade: A clinical management algorithm based on IAPAC's entry into and retention in care and antiretroviral therapy adherence guidelines. *Journal of the International Association of Providers of AIDS Care, 12*(1), 15–17.

17

Adherence to Treatment and Lifestyle Changes Among People With Cancer

AMY H. PETERMAN
DAVID VICTORSON
DAVID CELLA

LEARNING OBJECTIVES

- Identify four adherence-related behaviors that may facilitate successful cancer treatment.
- Explain the primary difference between adherence to traditional (i.e., intravenously administered) chemotherapy and newer oral chemotherapy agents.
- Describe the role of patient navigation (PN) interventions in promoting cancer treatment adherence.

EPIDEMIOLOGY AND SIGNIFICANCE OF CANCER AND CANCER MANAGEMENT BEHAVIORS

According to the American Cancer Society (ACS, 2013), more than 1.6 million people will be diagnosed with cancer and almost 600,000 people will die from it in 2013 alone. It is the second leading cause of death in the United States and is responsible for approximately 25% of all deaths. The ACS also estimates that 13.7 million people in the United States have a current or former cancer diagnosis: this is approximately 10% of the entire U.S. population.

Despite this, research on treatment adherence and health behavior change among people with cancer continues to lag behind that among patients with other serious illnesses or the general population. A large portion of the existing literature with cancer patients is focused simply on documenting rates of adherence to treatment. Significantly less attention has been paid to variables associated with adherence or, importantly, to interventions designed to improve it. One potential reason for the relative lack of attention to adherence in this population is the widely held assumption that patients facing a possibly terminal illness like cancer should adhere without question to whatever recommendations are made. That is, health professionals have assumed that patients will adhere if they believe that the likely alternative is death. However, comparisons of adherence rates among diseases varying in severity do not confirm this assumption (DiMatteo, 2004).

Another factor that may contribute to a limited focus on cancer-related adherence is that, until fairly recently, almost all cancer treatment was administered intravenously (IV) in a hospital or outpatient clinic setting. Specialized skills are required for IV administration and there was a pressing need for close patient observation to prevent life-threatening side effects or complications. There were simply fewer opportunities for the kind of self-management that characterizes treatment for other conditions. However, improved supportive care (e.g., anti-nausea medications and white and red blood cell growth factors), reduced insurance coverage for inpatient stays, and the development of numerous oral cancer therapies have changed the cancer treatment landscape considerably. In short, people with cancer now have a much greater personal responsibility for adherence to cancer treatment recommendations; the performance of health behaviors to support quality of life during and after treatment; and to follow up with appropriate surveillance to detect recurrences, metastases, and late treatment effects as early as possible.

Despite this, DiMatteo's (2004) authoritative review of 50 years of medical adherence research estimated that about one-fifth of cancer patients do not adhere to some part of their prescribed treatment. Such failure can carry high personal costs, such as higher mortality rates, shorter disease-free survival, greater likelihood of cancer recurrence, and the delayed identification of possible complications of treatment (e.g., osteoporosis) (Adsay et al., 2004; Ballantyne, 2003; de Csepel, Tartter, & Gajdos, 2002; Hershman & Narayanan, 2004; McCready et al., 2000; Van Gerpen & Mast, 2004). On the societal level, cancer-related non-adherence can result in the waste of vast amounts of health care resources and can also create misleading or incorrect results from clinical research (Dunbar-Jacob & Mortimer-Stephens, 2001; Halfdanarson & Jatoi, 2010).

This chapter presents an overview of the literature on cancer-related health behaviors and behavior change *among people who have already received a cancer diagnosis*. For the general population, professional organizations and cancer advocacy groups publish guidelines for screening and early detection tests (ACS, 2013). Although cancer screening and prevention behavior are not covered in this chapter that is focused on people already diagnosed with cancer, they are a crucial component of the fight against this disease. (Also see Section II of this book for chapters on health behaviors linked to cancer risk reduction.)

The chapter is organized as follows. First, the various cancer-related health behaviors are outlined, along with a discussion of the potential significance of each for treatment success and an overview of current estimates of adherence rates for these behaviors. Next, interventions to improve adherence to cancer treatment, lifestyle changes, and follow-up recommendations are examined. The chapter concludes with a discussion of future directions for research.

CANCER MANAGEMENT BEHAVIORS

Similar to other serious illnesses, the behaviors required for good management of a cancer diagnosis are many and varied. Once a cancer has been diagnosed, additional diagnostic tests may be required to determine if the cancer has spread and, if so, the location of the metastasis. Treatment recommendations will then be discussed with the patient who will be asked to participate in the decision-making process, then to adhere to a course that could include surgery, chemotherapy, other anti-cancer drugs or supportive medications, and radiation therapy. The care regimen may require the patient to attend multiple appointments for treatment and checkups, to take oral or IV medications, to make lifestyle changes, and, finally, to attend specified follow-up visits after treatment completion. In the upcoming sections, we will consider various aspects of adherence/self-management in these three categories of cancer-related behavior: cancer treatment, lifestyle changes, and follow-up surveillance to detect possible recurrence or late complications of cancer therapy.

Cancer Treatment

The bottom-line significance of adherence to cancer treatment regimens is assumed to be increased likelihood of treatment success, which should translate into improved physical health, better quality of life, and longer survival. Indeed, a great deal of cancer research is directed toward identifying treatment schedules (e.g., weekly doses rather than every-3-week dosing) and supportive medications (e.g., growth factors for white and red blood cells) that will allow more intense and dense treatment regimens to be administered without intolerable side effects (e.g., Desai et al., 2007; Gridelli et al., 2007; Lyman, Barron, Natoli, & Miller, 2012). In addition, the dosing schedule is a crucial component of the effectiveness of some medications. Thus, if non-adherence contributes to a patient receiving less than optimal treatment, such non-adherence may lead to a poorer outcome.

INTRAVENOUS CHEMOTHERAPY

The treatment context and demands differ greatly between chemotherapy administered intravenously in an oncology clinic and oral antineoplastic therapies that the patient is responsible for taking on a daily basis. The former is still more common and evokes a traditional image popular in the medical literature, of a passive patient compliantly receiving treatment. In fact, relatively high rates of adherence have been demonstrated for this form of cancer treatment. This is particularly true for people being treated for early stage cancer. For example, a report of a four-arm treatment trial for Stage II and III colon cancer reported that 88.4% of randomized subjects received the treatment as it was specified by the trial (Haller et al., 2005). Importantly, treatment adherence did not differ between the treatment arms. The issue of differential compliance between treatments is an important one, however, as it impacts the analysis and interpretation of clinical trial results. For example, von Minckwitz et al. (2006) reported on a trial for early stage breast cancer. In it, 97.7% of subjects completed the three cycles of a combination chemotherapy, but only 75.4% of subjects completed the other prescribed regimen.

Investigations of adherence to IV chemotherapy for more advanced cancers have reported significantly lower adherence rates. For example, a clinical trial was specifically designed to answer the question of whether the continuation of chemotherapy longer than 12 weeks for late stage lung cancer resulted in better outcomes (i.e., longer survival, better quality of life) than 12 weeks of chemo followed by monitoring only until relapse (Socinski et al., 2002). There was no difference in survival or health-related quality of life between the two treatment arms, demonstrating that more treatment is not necessarily better in this particularly setting. However, this trial also spoke to the difficulty of adherence to a treatment protocol among patients with advanced cancer: approximately equal numbers of patients on each arm of the trial stopped receiving chemotherapy before 12 weeks. Only 42% of patients actually received more than four cycles of chemotherapy, even though this was the main difference between the two treatment arms. The reasons were varied and included serious treatment toxicity such that the physician deemed the treatment not in the patient's best interests, death, transition to hospice care, and patient choice not to continue the trial often because of worsening illness or significant treatment side effects.

Research specifically investigating rates and consequences of non-adherence to IV chemotherapy is complicated by the relationship between poor baseline health, treatment toxicity, comorbidities, adherence, and treatment outcome. For example, a study of IV chemotherapy in patients with gynecologic cancer found that only 27.5% of older patients and 39% of younger patients received all six prescribed cycles of chemotherapy, but that the small overall survival difference between adherers and non-adherers was not statistically or clinically meaningful (Jorgensen et al., 2012). Rather, baseline physical health and age were the strongest independent predictors of survival, independent of treatment adherence.

ORAL ANTI-CANCER MEDICATION

Beginning with anti-hormonals such as tamoxifen for breast cancer, there has been exponential growth in the availability of oral medications for cancer. Oral antineoplastic therapies (i.e., pills) are changing expectations of the cancer patient, making them more responsible for their own treatment and health than ever before. Such treatments are taken on a regular schedule, similar to any other prescription and, therefore, are likely to be subject to the same difficulties with adherence and persistence. In considering potential difficulties with taking oral anti-cancer medications as prescribed, it is important to distinguish between persistence and adherence. Persistence is defined as whether or not a patient continues to take a medication for the entire length of time for which it is prescribed, whether that is several weeks or years. Therefore, 100% persistence for a 5-year course of tamoxifen would mean that a patient took tamoxifen for the entire 5 years. This is usually measured by examining prescription refills: if someone continues to refill their prescription, they are presumed to be persistent. Adherence is the behavior of taking the medication *as it was prescribed* on a regular basis. Thus, if someone took tamoxifen once daily every day for 5 years, she would be 100% adherent. Obviously, problems with either persistence and/or adherence will lead to the receipt of a lower-than-prescribed cumulative dosage. Several studies have documented the association between poor adherence, poor persistence, and poorer cancer outcomes for various cancer types, including breast cancer and chronic myelogenous leukemia (CML).

Indeed, Nilsson et al. (2006) reported on the use of clinical pharmacy records to obtain the rates at which people with cancer refilled their prescriptions. The majority of these prescriptions were for hormonal antagonist treatments (86%), with the remainder for oral chemotherapies (8.5%) and hormones (5.5%). Of their sample of 141 cancer-related prescriptions, about 14% were filled less than 80% of the recommended times; the authors calculated that those 14% had a median treatment gap of 39 days. Fifty-six percent of prescriptions were filled appropriately and 30% were actually filled more often than recommended. Contrary to the authors' expectations, these rates did not differ significantly from refill adherence rates for all other (noncancer) medications.

Oral medication for hormone receptor positive breast cancer (e.g., tamoxifen, aromatase inhibitors) has been in existence for several decades and major clinical trials have documented the survival advantage of taking these medications for at least 5 years (Dowsett et al., 2010), rather than 2 or 3 years (Early Breast Cancer Trialists' Collaborative Group, 2005). Although patient adherence was not specifically evaluated in these trials, their findings have been generalized to support a role for adherence in treatment outcome.

However, pharmacy records were examined for a large ($n = 8,769$) cohort of women treated for early stage breast cancer in a captive health system (Hershman et al., 2011).

These records indicated that 32% of women discontinued adjuvant hormonal treatment by 4.5 years into the 5 years for which the medication was prescribed. Twenty-eight percent of the remaining 68% of the total were not completely adherent. Importantly, both early discontinuation and non-adherence were significant predictors of poorer 10-year survival, even after adjusting for clinical and demographic variables.

Despite these known benefits, several studies have reported suboptimal adherence rates over a 5-year period. Partridge, Wang, Winer, and Avorn (2003) examined adherence to tamoxifen among 2,378 women beginning tamoxifen for primary breast cancer. Although filled prescriptions were relatively higher during the first year (87%), this decreased to less than 50% of the time by year 4. Another study investigated patterns of tamoxifen use among 516 women with estrogen receptor positive breast cancer (Fink, Gurwitz, Rakowski, Guadagnoli, and Silliman, 2004). They found that 17% stopped by the second year and that the majority of those who stopped took it less than 1 year. Similarly, Lash, Fox, Westrup, Fink, and Silliman (2006) reported that 31% of their sample of older women diagnosed with stage I–IIIA breast cancer (N = 462) stopped taking tamoxifen by 5 years. A study examined tamoxifen use among a cohort of 881 women with stage I or II disease (Kahn, Schneider, Malin, Adams, & Epstein, 2007). Findings indicated that roughly 21% stopped taking tamoxifen by year 4, while 54% of those who stopped did so between the first and third year. This available evidence suggests that adherence is decidedly suboptimal for this type of oral treatment for breast cancer.

The number of non-hormonal, oral chemotherapies for other cancers has skyrocketed in the past 10 years, with an estimated 25% of all chemotherapy now given as oral prescriptions. Some traditional chemotherapy agents are now available in oral form (e.g., capecitabine for breast and colon cancers) and many new, "targeted" therapies are only available that way (e.g., gefitinib for non-small-cell lung cancer). In some cases, these oral agents have better side-effect profiles than IV chemotherapy because of the drugs' targeted nature. However, this is not true across the board: Barton (2011) provides a nice overview of current oral anti-cancer treatments, along with their typical side effects and important interactions with food and with other commonly prescribed medications.

There is a wide range of estimates for adherence/persistence with targeted oral medications, with higher rates seen in clinical trials than in community samples. For example, patients enrolled in a clinical trial of imatinib for CML had a persistence rate of 91% at 19 months; far lower rates were recorded for the same drug prescribed in general practice (56% at 12 months and 41% at 24 months) (Hohneker, Shah-Mehta, & Brandt, 2011).

The consequences of low persistence and/or non-adherence appear to be similar to those with oral hormonal treatment, although they obviously vary by disease and drug. For example, a major molecular response at 6 years was seen in 94.5% of patients who had greater than 90% adherence to imatinib for CML, but in only 28.4% of patients who were less than 90% adherent (Noens et al., 2009). The significance of continued research into adherence to oral agents is highlighted by the expanding availability of oral anti-tumor agents, the likelihood of adherence and persistence problems, and the relationship between drug exposure and treatment outcome.

In summary, it can be quite difficult to judge the significance of non-adherence, as there are multiple factors affecting outcome, only one of which is adherence. Frequently, the current state of scientific knowledge does not allow an accurate assessment of the impact of treatment. Adjuvant chemotherapy, for example, is given in the absence of any visible evidence of disease. As such, there is no way to reliably monitor the success of treatment, unless the treatment fails and there is a recurrence. Additionally, it is very difficult to specify what a particular patient must do to ensure a response from a treatment: dosage recommendations are made on the basis of group data, and any particular individual may need more or less treatment for the cure or control of disease (Barofsky, 1984). Thus, while adherence and persistence are likely to play important roles, they are but two of many factors affecting treatment outcomes.

Follow-Up Surveillance After Cancer Treatment

After treatment ends, cancer survivors are asked to adhere to recommended follow-up surveillance, which can include appointments, exams, imaging, and other tests in order to detect cancer recurrences, metastases, cancers secondary to treatment, or late effects of treatment. As with other types of treatment-related behaviors, adherence to follow-up visits varies widely. In a recent study of 8,500 people with health insurance who had received treatment with curative intent for breast or colon cancer, 87% of breast cancer survivors but only 55% of colon cancer survivors received the recommended physical examinations in the 18 months after cancer treatment ended (Salloum et al., 2012). In addition, 65% of breast cancer survivors and 73% of colon cancer survivors received additional tests for metastatic disease that are NOT recommended by the guidelines. Another population-based study of colorectal cancer survivors found that level of adherence varied with type of recommended follow-up procedure (Sisler et al., 2012). In the 3 years after treatment ended, approximately 80% of survivors had a colonoscopy. However, only 47% and 22% had the recommended liver imaging and a blood test for carcinoembryonic antigen (CEA), respectively. All three of these tests are part of the recommended surveillance strategy for colorectal cancer survivors, but only 12.3% of this cohort received all of them. These investigations did not address the source of the non-adherence, leaving open the question of whether patients are adhering well to recommendations, but physicians are not following surveillance guidelines.

Does adherence to recommended follow-up surveillance result in better outcomes? Research findings are equivocal. It appears that more intensive follow-up is associated with earlier detection of recurrence and more successful treatment of new primary cancers, particularly in colon cancer (Jeffery, Hickey, & Hider, 2007). However, the impact on cancer-related mortality and survival is less clear, with several investigations into the utility of intensive follow-up after cancer treatment having failed to show a benefit to more frequent checkups (Secco et al., 2000) or the use of state-of-the-art imaging MRI technology in areas where recurrence is most likely (Titu, Nicholson, Hartley, Breen, & Monson, 2006). A Cochrane systematic review evaluated survival and disease-free survival based on the intensity of the follow-up schedule after primary treatment for Stage I–III breast cancer (Rojas et al., 2005). No difference was found for these outcomes in the more than 3,000 women enrolled in these trials.

A recent article reviewed outcomes of randomized controlled trials (RCTs) of follow-up surveillance in four cancer types that differ in the availability of effective treatments for recurrence. Furman, Lambert, Sullivan, and Whalen (2013) examined the possibility that intensive surveillance would be more effective in breast and colorectal cancer—for which adequate follow-up treatments do exist—than in non-small-cell lung carcinoma or pancreatic cancer for which adequate follow-up treatments do not exist. After reviewing existing trials, the authors concluded that the current state of the literature does not clearly support the need for intensive follow-up to detect recurrence in any of these cancers. However, earlier diagnosis of a new primary cancer through such surveillance does improve patient outcomes (Furman et al., 2013).

Adherence to Recommendation Not to Seek Definitive Cancer Treatment

Generally, people with cancer are asked to adhere to particular treatments, medication regimens, or behavioral/lifestyle changes that involve actively doing or changing something to better their outcomes. Men with very low risk prostate cancer who are eligible for active surveillance are asked to actively adhere in a very different way—to *not receive* definitive therapy such as surgery or radiation, so long as it is medically warranted (Parker, 2004). With greater awareness, improved lifestyles, and participation in preventive screening, more and more cases of low-risk prostate cancer are diagnosed each year. Although most forms follow a slow growing, indolent course, the vast majority of men who are candidates for active surveillance (e.g., 90,000) opt for immediate treatments that are associated with short- and long-term side effects such as urinary incontinence or erectile dysfunction (Ganz et al., 2011). Given the physical, psychosocial, and economic burden of overtreatment, it seems that observational management of very low risk prostate cancer could have a greater impact on more than the only 10% of eligible men who choose this approach.

To address the underutilization of this approach, a National Institutes of Health (NIH) Consensus and State-of-the-Science Statement was published on the role of Active Surveillance in the Management of Men with Localized Prostate Cancer (Ganz et al., 2011). The report highlighted three chief adherence factors that need greater attention, including (1) the offer of, (2) acceptance of, and (3) adherence to active surveillance. First, some clinicians may hold negative views of observational strategies for men with very low-risk prostate cancer. This may result in a negative presentation of the strategy to patients, perhaps framing it as "doing nothing." The fact that only 10% of men who are candidates for this approach actually choose this strategy suggests that in addition to provider factors, other considerations such as family support and perceptions of the cancer itself may play a role. Finally, upwards of 25% of men on active surveillance will leave this approach and undergo definitive treatment within 2 to 3 years, and roughly 50% will by 5 years. It is often unclear why men leave active surveillance, but it appears that the decision is frequently based on factors other than disease progression. This opens an important area for behavioral health professionals to better understand the many factors involved in acceptance and adherence to active surveillance, including the role of emotions and anxiety, influences by family and friends, and the effect of provider attitudes and communication style.

Behavioral and Lifestyle Factors During Cancer Treatment and Survivorship

For many people, a cancer diagnosis is a "wake up call," motivating them to make long-delayed lifestyle changes. Health care providers are generally in favor of this strategy, making recommendations to stop smoking, eat a balanced diet, increase the consumption of fruit and vegetables, and get regular exercise. These recommendations are thought to improve the effectiveness of cancer treatment, decrease the likelihood of relapse, or inhibit the development of other serious health conditions that share common risk factors (Demark-Wahnefried, Peterson, McBride, Lipkus, & Clipp, 2000). Indeed, Demark-Wahnefried et al. demonstrated strong interest in health promotion programs among a large sample of people who had been recently treated for early stage breast or prostate cancer. In addition, there was significant variability in the subjects' report of their current level of engagement in healthy behaviors, from a low of 45% eating the recommended daily servings of fruit and vegetables to a high of 92% who reported they did not smoke.

Higher rates of smoking have been reported among head/neck and lung cancer patients, with estimates of continuing smoking after diagnosis of 23% to 35% for the former and 13% to 20% of the latter (Schnoll et al., 2004). In a study that examined rates of participation in a smoking cessation program offered specifically for these patients, 53% of 231 eligible patients declined to participate (Schnoll et al., 2004). Most stated that they intended to quit on their own and did not need additional help to do so. Further work is needed to determine the extent to which this is possible in the midst of intensive treatment.

Behavioral recommendations that focus on physical activity and nutrition are far more popular and effective among cancer patients and survivors and are typically well supported by physicians (Doyle et al., 2006). Exercise can positively affect psychological, physical, and biological outcomes (Vallance, Courneya, Jones, & Reiman, 2006) that are related to cancer. As with similar programs in healthy populations, adherence to an exercise regimen is moderately difficult for people with cancer. In the Mock et al. (2005) trial of home-based walking exercise for women with Stage 0–III breast cancer, only 72% of the women were adherent to the prescribed exercise program. Similarly, Swenson, Nissen, and Henly (2010) reported that women with early stage breast cancer completed 67% of the 10,000 steps per day recommended in another walking intervention. The number of steps completed was significantly lower on days when chemotherapy was administered and increased significantly in the months following completion of treatment.

There is significant evidence for the positive impact of healthy behaviors on quality of life components during and after cancer treatment. For example, a meta-analysis of 14 RCTs of exercise documented small to medium effects of exercise on cancer-related fatigue, depression, and body image among breast cancer patients and survivors (Duijts et al., 2011). Evidence is also accumulating that overall and cancer-free survival may be improved by the performance of regular exercise during and after a cancer diagnosis (Barbaric, Brooks, Moore, & Cheifetz, 2010).

Interventions to improve nutrition and sleep, and to decrease/stop smoking, are also growing in popularity (Wei, Wolin, & Colditz, 2010). Women who are heavier at the time of breast cancer diagnosis have poorer long-term survival than do women who are leaner at that time and there are ongoing trials to evaluate the impact of weight loss during chemotherapy; see Chlebowski (2011) for a recent summary. An additional consideration regarding nutrition is the finding from one small, but potentially quite important, study on the relationship between the type and timing of food intake and the bioavailability of oral chemotherapy. Koch et al. (2009) determined that the fat content of a meal taken with oral capecitabine affected its bioavailability by as much as 50%, which may significantly affect the drug's safety and efficacy. Overall, it appears that the performance of routine health behaviors is at least as important in people with cancer as in the general population, if not more critical for their health and well-being.

In summary, rates of adherence to IV chemotherapy, oral chemotherapy and supportive medications, treatment appointments, behavioral changes, and follow-up visits vary widely. In some cases, such as treatment for early stage cancer, non-adherence rates are quite low. However, for most other important behaviors, non-adherence rates seem to be comparable to those found in the general medical population. This challenges the widely held notion that people will always be adherent to treatment for life-threatening illness. It also affirms the necessity of investigating potential interventions to improve adherence.

INTERVENTIONS TO IMPROVE ADHERENCE AMONG CANCER PATIENTS

Although there is a voluminous literature on interventions to improve psychosocial distress and quality of life among people with cancer, only a small fraction addresses adherence and health behavior outcomes. In addition, the literature on these behavior change interventions among people with cancer lags significantly behind that in other diseases and in the general population. However, the increasing availability of self-administered oral chemotherapies and the growing recognition of the impact of health behaviors have resulted in an increase in the number and type of such interventions since the last edition of this book. Below, we provide an overview of the current status of health behavior change interventions in oncology.

Educational Interventions

The receipt of educational materials is part of the standard of care for all cancer treatments and there are several national services that provide cancer information over the phone and via the Internet. However, there is a fairly limited body of research evaluating the impact of this education on treatment adherence and health behavior change. In one such study, breast cancer patients received either standard treatment or standard treatment plus educational materials about the importance of adherence/persistence to anastrozole, which is an adjuvant, anti-estrogen treatment for breast cancer (Hadji et al., 2013). There was no difference in adherence or persistence between the two arms across the 12-month follow-up period.

A more positive outcome was observed in a trial of education and counseling about proper nutrition for head and neck cancer patients receiving radiotherapy. The education group had superior outcomes, not only in nutritional status during and after treatment, but also less radiotherapy toxicity, better quality of life, and longer survival (Ravasco, Monteiro-Grillo, & Camilo, 2012). Similarly, Rosenzweig et al. (2011) reported that a brief intervention containing aspects of support and psychoeducation resulted in faster initiation of, and better overall adherence to, chemotherapy for breast cancer among a small sample of African American women. However, the relative importance of education versus "counseling" or support in these interventions is unknown.

Finally, a recent systematic review and meta-analysis of educational interventions for cancer pain (Bennett, Bagnall, & Closs, 2009) revealed only one study with a positive effect on pain medication adherence (Chang, Chang, Chiiou, Tsou, & Lin, 2002). The majority of the studies in this review evaluated barriers to taking pain medication and pain intensity, rather than directly measuring adherence to a prescribed regimen of pain medication.

Motivational Interventions

As in the broader health literature, Motivational Interviewing (MI) (Rollnick, Miller, & Butler, 2008) has been utilized to help people overcome resistance to performing various cancer management behaviors. While the results are generally positive, it does appear that the timing and intensity of the intervention may be important to a successful outcome. For example, a brief MI intervention delivered about a week before breast cancer surgery had only a minimal effect on rates of perioperative smoking and no effect on post-surgical complications or smoking cessation at 12-month follow-up (Thomsen et al., 2010). However, Djuric et al. (2011) published the initial results of an RCT of an MI-based telephone intervention for women receiving treatment for breast cancer, demonstrating a beneficial effect on fruit and vegetable consumption, physical activity, breast cancer specific well-being, and body fat percentage over a 12-month period. Thomas et al. (2012) found that an MI-based coaching intervention was more effective than a standard educational intervention for decreasing the interference caused by cancer pain. However, they also found that the coaching intervention did not affect actual pain levels or attitudinal barriers to pain management (e.g., fear of addiction, fear of disease progression) which were the primary outcomes of interest in this trial.

In another palliative care setting, the use of MI communication strategies has been advocated for conversations about symptom management and end-of-life decision making because of the explicit focus on addressing ambivalence and facilitating actions that are in line with patients' values (Pollak, Childers, & Arnold, 2011). To date, it does not appear that there are any empirical investigations of this. Given the importance of high quality patient–physician communication—particularly in palliative care—this seems to be a fruitful avenue of inquiry. Overall, it is also anticipated that MI approaches will continue to be evaluated in cancer-management-related interventions.

Health Care Provider Directed Interventions

The National Comprehensive Cancer Network publishes cancer care guidelines for all stages and types of cancer (NCCN, 2013). Updated annually, the guidelines are based primarily on the results of clinical trials, and adherence to guidelines is associated with better treatment outcomes (e.g., Boland et al., 2013; Schwentner et al., 2012). Interventions to improve guideline adherence include the formation of multidisciplinary treatment teams in which members of all treating disciplines (e.g., surgery, radiation therapy, medical oncology), oncology nurses, and, sometimes, support providers (e.g., psychology, speech pathology) come together to evaluate a patient and decide on a comprehensive treatment recommendation. In addition, treatment by multidisciplinary teams appears to be related to better outcomes, perhaps through adherence of guidelines (e.g., Chowdhury & Swain, 2012; Kesson, Allardice, George, Burns, & Morrison, 2012).

Technology

As is the case in medicine overall, the role of information technology (IT) is rapidly expanding in the arena of cancer care. Clauser, Wagner, Bowles, Tuzzio, and Greene (2011) provided an excellent overview of the current status of the field and promising new developments. Information technology, including electronic medical records and other electronic provider communication tools, is just beginning to be evaluated for a potential role in cancer care. Better coordination among the many providers in coordinated care for head and neck cancer was an important outcome of a database implementation project by Nouraei et al. (2007).

Another area in which IT might be useful is in electronically embedded care guidelines that prompt providers to adhere to standards for quality cancer care. Although this sort of electronic prompt has proven useful in other diseases, there is very limited data on its utility in cancer care.

E-health interventions directed toward cancer patients and survivors are increasing: for a recent review, see Ventura, Ohlen, and Koinberg (2012). Although behavior change is targeted far less frequently than psychosocial distress or cancer knowledge, two interesting examples of behavior change interventions were published recently. Ritterband et al. (2012) describes an Internet-based program to deliver the components of cognitive-behavioral therapy for insomnia (CBT-I) to people who were at least 1 month post-cancer treatment. This was a small RCT that demonstrated a significant effect on multiple self-reported sleep variables, including insomnia severity, sleep onset latency, and sleep efficiency. This is particularly interesting, since a lack of restorative sleep is a major complaint of many people undergoing chemotherapy. Second, Schover et al. (2012) found that an Internet program of brief sexual counseling was equally as effective as face-to-face counseling for improving sexual outcomes for heterosexual couples in which the male had recently been treated for localized prostate cancer.

Electronic health records, computerized decision support interventions, and e-health applications directed toward patients have the potential to vastly expand interventions to improve adherence to cancer management behaviors.

Multi-Component Interventions—Patient Navigation

As discussed throughout this chapter, the behaviors required after a cancer diagnosis are numerous and varied. Patient navigation (PN) is a comprehensive type of intervention that attempts to increase adherence to these many behaviors by reducing or removing barriers to quality cancer care (Dohan & Schrag, 2005). Flexibility is a key feature, as the type of provided service differs depending on the barriers identified.

Although barriers to cancer-related adherence are present to some degree for everyone, it is suspected that the complexity of cancer care is one important contributor to the significant disparities in cancer outcomes between non-Hispanic Whites of higher socioeconomic status and most other cultural groups in the United States. PN interventions actually commenced in 1990 in Harlem, New York, as a way to reduce systemic, provider, and patient barriers to optimal cancer treatment for people with limited financial and other resources (Freeman, 2006). In this form of individualized intervention, navigators help patients to identify possible barriers to attendance at diagnostic and treatment visits and adherence to the behaviors required for appropriate cancer care. The navigator then systematically attempts to dismantle the identified barriers so that the patient can obtain the necessary treatment. Examples of some of these barriers to treatment can be found in Table 17.1.

Until recently, evidence for the effectiveness of PN was limited to observational studies, typically with small sample sizes. However, in 2005, the National Cancer Institute and the American Cancer Society joined forces to fund a nine-site study called the Patient Navigation Research Program (PNRP), with the goal of comparing outcomes between individuals receiving PN and control groups (Freund et al., 2008). Patient navigation was defined as "the support and guidance offered to persons with abnormal cancer screening or a new cancer diagnosis in accessing the cancer care system; overcoming barriers; and facilitating timely, quality care provided in a culturally sensitive manner" (Freund et al., 2008, p. 3392). The studies focus on breast, prostate, colon, and cervical cancer care for underserved populations, with the following primary outcomes: time from abnormal cancer screening test, time to diagnostic resolution, time to initiation of primary cancer therapy when the diagnosis is positive, patient satisfaction with the PN

TABLE 17.1 Examples of Barriers to Cancer Care That May Be Addressed by Patient Navigation

PATIENT FOCUSED	PROVIDER FOCUSED	SYSTEMIC
Poor health literacy	Unwelcoming waiting areas	No, or limited, insurance
Lack of childcare or transportation	Availability of interpreters and printed information in multiple languages	Complex, fragmented oncology care
Fear, anxiety, depression	Appointment availability for patients working full time	Historical mistrust of institutions and research

intervention and the individual delivering it, psychological impact of the cancer screening and/or diagnosis, patient self-efficacy for dealing with cancer-related health care, and the cost-effectiveness of the intervention.

A recent special issue of the journal *Cancer Epidemiology, Biomarkers, & Prevention* published a number of articles on the effectiveness of some of these PNRP studies. Predicated on the assumption that a faster resolution of diagnostic uncertainty will result in better outcomes, many PN programs focus on decreasing or removing barriers to obtaining appropriate follow-up after a suspicious finding on a screening test (e.g., mammogram). Decreased time to diagnostic resolution was demonstrated for breast and cervical cancer (Battaglia et al., 2012; Markossian, Darnell, & Calhoun, 2012), as well as prostate and colorectal cancer (Raich, Whitley, Thorland, Valverde, & Fairclough, 2012) in PNRP investigations using RCT or quasi-experimental methodology. In these studies, patient navigators assisted in removing a wide variety of barriers.

There are only a few published reports of the impact of PN on cancer treatment outcomes. A retrospective chart review study did demonstrate an improvement in adherence to treatment based on breast cancer care quality indicators from 74.1% prior to a PN program to 95.5% after its implementation (Weber, Mascarenhas, Bellin, Raab, & Wong, 2012). An RCT from the PNRP network failed to demonstrate an overall advantage for their navigation intervention in time to the completion of cancer treatment, although they did find increased satisfaction with cancer care in a patient subgroup characterized by low English proficiency and a lack of insurance (Fiscella et al., 2012). Ell et al. (2009) demonstrated better than usual adherence to treatment among breast and gynecologic cancer patients, regardless of whether they were assigned to enhanced usual care with written educational materials or to PN. Follow-up focus groups indicated that the existence of funding for treatment and associated care may have been the component that most improved treatment completion rates for both groups.

There appears to be ample evidence that PN can improve adherence to diagnostic testing for cancer. However, the impact on treatment-related adherence is less clear. Hopefully, the ongoing research of PNRP investigators and others will clarify the potential benefits and associated costs of this promising type of intervention.

CONCLUSIONS

In the past decade, there has been incredible progress in the field of cancer treatment. Improved screening techniques and expanded access to them have allowed the diagnosis of many cancers while still in early, more curable stages. Novel therapies have improved effectiveness and led to fewer toxic side effects. There is real hope that many cancers can become true "chronic illnesses," rather than imminently life-threatening ones.

The true promise of such scientific discoveries can be enhanced significantly by provider and patient behaviors that support adherence, particularly adherence to oral chemotherapies. Clinicians and researchers can look for inspiration in the literature on adherence promotion in other serious illnesses, as well as to the basic cancer research demonstrating the impact of personality, treatment regimen, and patient beliefs. Thoughtfully designed research will promote the understanding of cancer-related adherence across the lifespan, since there is a real dearth of empirical information on pediatric, adolescent, and geriatric populations in this arena. It is hoped that the next 5 to 10 years will see a rapid expansion of research to evaluate the utility of PN, motivational, and educational interventions for improved patient outcomes and a harnessing of new e-health technologies to expand the delivery of successful programs.

REFERENCES

Adsay, N.V., Andea, A., Basturk, O., Kilinc, N., Nassar, H., & Cheng, J.D. (2004). Secondary tumors of the pancreas: An analysis of a surgical and autopsy database and review of the literature. *Virchows Archiv: An International Journal of Pathology*, 444, 527–535.

American Cancer Society (ACS). (2013). *Cancer facts and figures 2013*. Atlanta, Georgia: Author.

Ballantyne, J.C. (2003). Chronic pain following treatment for cancer: The role of opioids. *Oncologist*, 8, 567–575.

Barbaric, M., Brooks, E., Moore, L., & Cheifetz, O. (2010). Effects of physical activity on cancer survival: A systematic review. *Physiotherapy Canada*, 62(1), 25–34

Barofsky, I. (1984). Therapeutic compliance and the cancer patient. *Health Education Quarterly*, 10, 43–56.

Barton, D. (2011). Oral agents in cancer treatment: The context for adherence. *Seminars in Oncology Nursing*, 27(2), 104–115.

Battaglia, T. A., Bak, S. M., Heeren, T., Chen, C. A., Kalish, R., Tringale, S., … Freund, K. M. (2012). Boston Patient Navigation Research Program: The impact of navigation on time to diagnostic resolution after abnormal cancer screening. *Cancer Epidemiology, Biomarkers & Prevention*, 21(10), 1645–1654.

Bennett, M. I., Bagnall, A. M., & Closs, J. (2009). How effective are patient-based educational interventions in the management of cancer pain? A systematic review and meta-analysis. *Pain*, 143, 192–199.

Boland, G. M., Chang, G. J., Haynes, A. B., Chiang, Y.-J., Chagpar, R., Xing, Y., … Cormier, J. N. (2013). Association between adherence to National Comprehensive Cancer Network treatment guidelines and improved survival in patients with colon cancer. *Cancer*, 119(8), 1593-601. doi: 10.1002 /cncr.27935

Chang, M., Chang, Y., Chiiou, J., Tsou, T., & Lin, C. (2002). Overcoming patient-related barriers to cancer pain management for home care patients: A pilot study. *Cancer Nursing*, 25, 470–476.

Chlebowski, R.T. (2011). Obesity and breast cancer outcome: Adding to the evidence. *Journal of Clinical Oncology*, 30(2), 126–128.

Chowdhury, N., & Swain, S.M. (2012). The role of the multidisciplinary team in inflammatory breast cancer. In N. T. Ueno & T. Fink (Eds.), *Inflammatory breast cancer: An update* (pp. 121–126). New York, NY: Springer.

Clauser, S. B., Wagner, E. H., Bowles, E. J. A., Tuzzio, L., & Greene, S. M. (2011). Improving modern cancer care through information technology. *American Journal of Preventive Medicine*, 40(552), S198–S207.

De Csepel, J., Tartter, P. I., & Gajdos, C. (2002). When not to give radiation therapy after breast conservation surgery for breast cancer. *Journal of Surgical Oncology*, 74, 273–277.

Demark-Wahnefried, W., Peterson, B., McBride, C., Lipkus, I., & Clipp, E. (2000). Current health behaviors and readiness to pursue life-style changes among men and women diagnosed with early stage prostate and breast carcinomas. *Cancer*, 88, 674–684.

Desai, S. P., Ben-Josef, E., Normolle, D. P., Francis, I. R., Greenson, J. K., Simeone, D. M., … Zalupski, M. M. (2007). Phase I study of oxaliplatin, full-dose gemcitabine, and concurrent radiation therapy in pancreatic cancer. *Journal of Clinical Oncology*, 25, 4587–4592.

DiMatteo, M. R. (2004). Variations in patients' adherence to medical recommendations: A quantitative review of 30 years of research. *Medical Care*, 42, 200–209.

Djuric, Z., Ellsworth, J. S., Weldon, A. L., Ren, J., Richardson, C. R., Resnicow, K., … Sen, A. (2011). A diet and exercise intervention during chemotherapy for breast cancer. *Open Obesity Journal*, 3, 87–97.

Dohan, D., & Schrag, D. (2005). Using navigators to improve care of underserved patients. Current practices and approaches. *Cancer*, 104, 848–855.

Dowsett, M., Cuzick, J., Ingle, J., Coates, A., Forbes, J., Bliss, J., … Peto, R. (2010). Meta-analysis of breast cancer outcomes in adjuvant trials of aromatase inhibitors versus tamoxifen. *Journal of Clinical Oncology*, 28, 509–518.

Doyle, C., Kushi, L. H., Byers, T., Courneya, K. S., Demark-Wahnefried, W., Grant, B., … Andrews, K. S. (2006). Nutrition and physical activity during and after cancer treatment: An American Cancer Society guide for informed choices. *CA: A Cancer Journal for Clinicians*, 56, 323–353.

Duijts, S. F., Faber, M. M., Oldenburg, H. S., van Beurden, M., & Aaronson, N. K. (2011). Effectiveness of behavioral techniques and physical exercise on psychosocial functioning and health-related quality of life in breast cancer patients and survivors-a meta-analysis. *Psycho-Oncology*, 20(2), 115–126.

Dunbar-Jacob, J., & Mortimer-Stephens, M. K. (2001). Treatment adherence in chronic disease. *Journal of Clinical Epidemiology*, 54, S57–S60.

Early Breast Cancer Trialists' Collaborative Group. (2005). Effects of chemotherapy and hormonal therapy for early breast cancer on recurrence and 15-year survival: An overview of the randomized trials. *Lancet*, 365, 1687–1717.

Ell, K., Voulekis, B., Xie, B., Nedjat-Haiem, F. R., Lee, P.-J., Muderspach, L., ... Palinkas, L. A. (2009). Cancer treatment adherence among low-income women with breast or gynecologic cancer: A randomized controlled trial of patient navigation. *Cancer, 115*(19), 4606–4615.

Fink, A. K., Gurwitz, J., Rakowski, W., Guadagnoli, E., & Silliman, R. A. (2004). Patient beliefs and tamoxifen discontinuance in older women with estrogen receptor–positive breast cancer. *Journal of Clinical Oncology, 22*(16), 3309–3315.

Fiscella, K., Whitley, E., Hendren, S., Raich, P., Humiston, S., ... Epstein, R. (2012). Patient navigation for breast and colorectal cancer treatment: A randomized trial. *Cancer Epidemiology, Biomarkers & Prevention, 21*(10), 1673–1681.

Freeman, H.P. (2006). Patient navigation: A community based strategy to reduce cancer disparities. *Journal of Urban Health, 83*(2), 139–141.

Freund, K. M., Battaglia, T. A., Calhoun, E., Dudley, D. J., Fiscella, K., Paskett, E., ... Roetzheim, R. G. and The Patient Navigation Research Program Group. (2008). National Cancer Institute Patient Navigation Research Program. *Cancer, 113*, 3391–3399.

Furman, M. J., Lambert, L. A., Sullivan, M. E., & Whalen, G. F. (2013). Rational follow-up after curative cancer resection. *Journal of Clinical Oncology, 31*(9), 1130–1133.

Ganz, P. A., Barry, J. M., Burke, W., Col, N. F., Corso, P. S., Dodson, E., ... Wessells, H. (2011). National Institutes of Health State-of-the-Science Conference Statement: Role of active surveillance in the management of men with localized prostate cancer. *NIH Consensus State of the Science Statements, 28*(1), 1–27.

Gridelli, C., Maione, P., Illiano, A., Piantedosi, F. V., Favaretto, A., Bearz, A., ... Perrone, F. (2007). Cisplatin plus gemcitabine or vinorelbine for elderly patients with advanced non small-cell lung cancer: The MILES-2P studies. *Journal of Clinical Oncology, 25*, 4663–4669.

Hadji, P., Blettner, M., Harbeck, N., Jackisch, C., Luck, H.-J., Windemuth-Kieselbach, C., ... Kreienberg, R. (2013). The Patient's Anastrozole Compliance to Therapy (PACT) Program: A randomized, in-practice study on the impact of a standardized information program on persistence and compliance to adjuvant endocrine therapy in postmenopausal women with early breast cancer. *Annals of Oncology, 24*(6), 1505–1512.

Halfdanarson, T. R., & Jatoi, A. (2010). Oral cancer chemotherapy: The critical interplay between patient education and patient safety. *Current Oncology Reports, 12*, 247–252.

Haller, D. G., Catalano, P. J., Macdonald, J. S., O'Rourke, M. A., Frontiera, M. S., Jackson, D. V., ... Mayer, R. J. (2005). Phase III study of fluorouracil, leucovorin, and levamisole in high-risk Stage II and III colon cancer: Final report of Intergroup 0089. *Journal of Clinical Oncology, 23*, 8671–8678.

Hershman, D., & Narayanan, R. (2004). Patients' beliefs about prescribed medicines and their role in adherence to treatment in chronic physical illnesses. *Current Oncology Reports, 6*, 277–284.

Hershman, D. L., Shao, T., Kushi, L. H., Buono, D., Tsai, W. Y., Fehrenbacher, L., ... Neugut, A. I. (2011). Early discontinuation and non-adherence to adjuvant hormonal therapy are associated with increased mortality in women with breast cancer. *Breast Cancer Research and Treatment, 126*(2), 529–537.

Hohneker, J., Shah-Mehta, W., & Brandt, P. S. (2011). Perspectives on adherence and persistence with oral medications for cancer treatment. *Journal of Oncology Practice, 7*(1), 65–68.

Jeffery, M., Hickey, B. E., & Hider, P. N. (2007). Follow-up strategies for patients treated for non-metastatic colorectal cancer. *Cochrane Database of Systematic Reviews, 1* (CD002200).

Jørgensen, T. L., Teiblum, S., Paludan, M., Poulsen, L. O., Jørgensen, A. Y. S., Bruun, K. H., ... Herrstedt, J. (2012). Significance of age and comorbidity on treatment modality, treatment adherence, and prognosis in elderly ovarian cancer patients. *Gynecologic Oncology, 127*(2), 367–374.

Kahn, K. L., Schneider, E. C., Malin, J. L., Adams, J. L., & Epstein, A. M. (2007). Patient centered experiences in breast cancer: Predicting long-term adherence to tamoxifen use. *Medical Care, 45*, 431–439.

Kesson, E. M., Allardice, G. M., George, W. D., Burns, H. J. G., & Morrison, D. S. (2012). Effects of multidisciplinary team working on breast cancer survival: Retrospective, comparative, interventional cohort study of 13722 women. *British Medical Journal, 344*, e2718–e2727.

Koch, K. M., Reddy, N. J., Cohen, R. B., Lewis, N. L., Whitehead, B., Mackay, K., ... Lewis, L. D. (2009). Effects of food on the relative bioavailability of lapatinib in cancer patients. *Journal of Clinical Oncology, 27*, 1191–1196.

Lash, T. L., Fox, M. P., Westrup, J. L., Fink, A. K., & Silliman, R. A. (2006). Adherence to tamoxifen over the five-year course. *Breast Cancer Research and Treatment, 99*, 215–220.

Lewis, C. M., Hessel, A. C., Roberts, D. B., Guo, Y. Z., Holsinger, C., Ginsberg, L. E., ... Weber, R. S. (2010). Preferral head and neck cancer treatment. *Archives of Otolaryngology Head and Neck Surgery, 136*(12), 1205–1211.

Lyman, G. H., Barron, R. L., Natoli, J. L., & Miller, R. M. (2012). Systematic review of efficacy of dose-dense versus non-dose-dense chemotherapy in breast cancer, non-Hodgkin lymphoma and non-small cell lung cancer. *Critical Reviews in Oncology, 81*(3), 296–308.

Markossian, T. W., Darnell, J. S., & Calhoun, E. A. (2012). Follow-up and timeliness after an abnormal cancer screening among underserved, urban women in a patient navigation program. *Cancer Epidemiology, Biomarkers, & Prevention, 21*(10), 1691–1700.

McCready, D. R., Chapman, J. A., Hanna, W. M., Kahn, H. J., Yap, K., Fish, E. B., & Lickley, H. L. (2000). Factors associated with local breast cancer recurrence after lumpectomy alone: Postmenopausal patients. *Annals of Surgical Oncology, 7,* 562–567.

Mock, V., Frangakis, C., Davidson, N. E., Ropka, M. E., Pickett, M., Poniatowski, B., ... McCorkle, R. (2005). Exercise manages fatigue during breast cancer treatment: A randomized controlled trial. *Psycho-Oncology, 14,* 464–477.

National Comprehensive Cancer Network. (2013). Retrieved from http://www.nccn.org/index.asp

Nilsson, J. L. G., Andersson, K., Bergkvist, A., Bjorkman, I., Brismar, A., & Moen, J. (2006). Refill adherence to repeat prescriptions of cancer drugs to ambulatory patients. *European Journal of Cancer Care, 15,* 235–237.

Noens, L., van Lierde, M. A., De Bock, R., Verhoef, G., Zachée, P., Berneman, Z., ... Abraham, I. (2009). Prevalence, determinants, and outcomes of nonadherence to imatinib in patients with chronic myeloid leukemia: The ADAGIO study. *Blood, 113,* 5401–5411.

Nouraei, S., Philpott, J., Nouraei, S. M., Maude, D. C. K., Sandhu, G. S., Sandison, A., & Clarke, P. M. (2007). Reducing referral-to-treatment waiting times in cancer patients using a multidisciplinary database. *Annals of the Royal College of Surgeons England, 89*(2), 113–117.

Parker, C. (2004). Active surveillance: Towards a new paradigm in the management of early prostate cancer. *Lancet Oncology, 5*(2), 101–106.

Partridge, A. H., Wang, P. S., Winer, E. P., & Avorn, J. (2003). Nonadherence to adjuvant tamoxifen therapy in women with primary breast cancer. *Journal of Clinical Oncology, 21,* 602–606.

Pollak, K. I., Childers, J. A., & Arnold, R. M. (2011). Applying motivational interviewing techniques to palliative care communication. *Journal of Palliative Medicine, 14*(5), 587–592.

Raich, P. C., Whitley, E. M., Thorland, W., Valverde, P., & Fairclough, D. (2012). Patient navigation improves cancer diagnostic resolution: An individually randomized clinical trial in an underserved population. *Cancer Epidemiology, Biomarkers, & Prevention, 21*(10), 1629–1638.

Ravasco, P., Monteiro-Grillo, I., & Camilo, M. (2012). Individualized nutrition intervention is of major benefit to colorectal cancer patients: Long-term follow-up of a randomized controlled trial of nutritional therapy. *American Journal of Clinical Nutrition, 96*(6), 1346–1353.

Ritterband, L. M., Bailey, E. T., Thorndike, F. P., Lord, H. R., Farrell-Carnahan, L., & Baum, L. D. (2012). Initial evaluation of an internet intervention to improve the sleep of cancer survivors with insomnia. *Psycho-Oncology, 21*(7), 695–705.

Rojas, M. P., Telaro, E., Russo, A., Moschetti, I., Coe, L., Fossati, R., ... Liberati, A. (2005). Follow-up strategies for women treated for early breast cancer. *Cochrane Database of Systematic Reviews (Online),* (1), CD001768.

Rollnick, S., Miller, W. R., & Butler, C. C. (2008). *Motivational interviewing in health care: Helping patients change behavior.* New York, NY: The Guilford Press.

Rosenzweig, M., Brufsky, A., Rastogi, P., Puhalla, S., Simon, J., & Underwood, S. (2011). The attitudes, communication, treatment, and support intervention to reduce breast cancer treatment disparity. *Oncology Nursing Forum, 38*(1), 85–89.

Roth, B. J., Krilov, L., Adams, S., Aghajanian, C. A., Bach, P., Braiteh, F., ... Vogelzang, N. J. (2012). Clinical cancer advances 2012: Annual report on progress against cancer from the American Society of Clinical Oncology. *Journal of Clinical Oncology, 31*(1), 131–161.

Salloum, R. G., Hornbrook, M. C., Fishman, P. A., Ritzwoller, D. P., Rossetti, M. C., O'Keefe Rossetti, M. C., & Lafata, J. E. (2012). Adherence to surveillance care guidelines after breast and colorectal cancer treatment with curative intent. *Cancer, 118,* 5644–5651.

Sargent, D. J., Goldberg, R. M., Jacobson, S. D., Macdonald, J. S., Labianca, R., Haller, D. G., ... Francini, G. (2001). A pooled analysis of adjuvant chemotherapy for resected colon cancer in elderly patients. *New England Journal of Medicine, 345,* 1091–1097.

Schnoll, R. A., Rothman, R. L., Lerman, C., Miller, S. M., Newman, H., Movsas, B., … Cheng, J. (2004). Comparing cancer patients who enroll in a smoking cessation program at a comprehensive cancer center with those who decline enrollment. *Head Neck, 26*, 276–284.

Schover, L.R., Canada, A.L., Yuan, Y., Sui, D., Neese, L., Jenkins, R., & Rhodes, M.M. (2012). A randomized trial of internet-based versus traditional sexual counseling for couples after localized prostate cancer treatment. *Cancer, 118*(2), 500–509.

Schwentner, L., Wolters, R., Koretz, K., Wischnewsky, M. B., Kreienberg, R., Rottscholl, R., & Wockel, A. (2012). Triple-negative breast cancer: The impact of guideline-adherent adjuvant treatment on survival – a retrospective multi-centre cohort study. *Breast Cancer Research and Treatment, 132*(3), 1073–1080.

Secco, G. B., Fardelli, R., Rovida, S., Gianquinto, D., Baldi, E., Bonfante, P., & Ferraris, R. (2000). Is intensive follow-up really able to improve prognosis of patients with local recurrence after curative surgery for rectal cancer? *Annals of Surgical Oncology, 7*(1), 32–37.

Sisler, J. J., Seo, B., Katz, A., Shu, E., Chateau, D., Czaykowski, P., …. Martens, P. (2012). Concordance with ASCO guidelines for surveillance after colorectal cancer treatment: A population-based analysis. *Journal of Oncology Practice, 8*(4), e69–e79

Socinski, M. A., Schell, M. J., Bakri, K., Peterman, A., Lee, J., Unger, P., … Kies, M. S. (2002). Second-line, low-dose, weekly paclitaxel in patients with stage IIIB/IV nonsmall cell lung carcinoma who fail first-line chemotherapy with carboplatin plus paclitaxel. *Cancer, 95*, 1265–1273.

Swenson, K. K., Nissen, M. J., & Henly, S. J. (2010). Physical activity in women receiving chemotherapy for breast cancer: Adherence to a walking intervention. *Oncology Nursing Forum, 37*(3), 321–330.

Thomas, M. L., Elliott, J. E., Rao, S. M., Fahey, K. F., Paul, S. M., & Miaskowski, C. (2012). A randomized, clinical trial of education or motivational-interviewing-based coaching compared to usual care to improve cancer pain management. *Oncology Nursing Forum, 39*(1), 39–49.

Thomsen, T., Tonnesen, H., Okholm, M., Kroman, N., Maibom, A., Sauerberg, M.L., & Moller, A.M. (2010). Brief smoking cessation intervention in relation to breast cancer surgery: A randomized controlled trial. *Nicotine and Tobacco Research, 12*(11), 1118–1124.

Titu, L. V., Nicholson, A. A., Hartley, J. E., Breen, D. J., & Monson, J. R. T. (2006). Routine follow-up by magnetic resonance imaging does not improve detection of resectable local recurrences from colorectal cancer. *Annals of Surgery, 243*(3), 348–352.

Vallance, J. K. H., Courneya, K. S., Jones, L. W., & Reiman, T. (2006). Exercise preferences among a population-based sample of non-Hodgkin's lymphoma survivors. *European Journal of Cancer Care, 15*, 34–43.

Van Gerpen, R., & Mast, M. E. (2004). Thromboembolic disorders in cancer. *Clinical Journal of Oncology Nursing, 8*, 289–299.

Ventura, F., Ohlen, J., & Koinberg, I. (2013). An integrative review of supportive e-health programs in cancer care. *European Journal of Oncology Nursing, 17*(4), 498–507. Retrieved from http://dx.doi.org .librarylink.uncc.edu/10.1016/j.ejom. 2012.10.007

Verkooijen, H. M., Fioretta, G. M., Rapiti, E., Bonnefoi, H., Vlastos, G., Kurtz, J., … Bouchardy, C. (2005). Patients' refusal of surgery strongly impairs breast cancer survival. *Annals of Surgery, 242*, 276–280.

Von Minckwitz, G., Graf, E., Geberth, M., Eiermann, W., Jonat, W., Conrad, B., …. Kaufmann, M. (2006). CMF versus goserelin as adjuvant therapy for node-negative, hormone-receptor-positive breast cancer in premenopausal patients: A randomised trial (GABG trial IV-A-93). *European Journal of Cancer, 42*, 1780–1788.

Weber, J. J., Mascarenhas, D. C., Bellin, L. S., Raab, R. E., & Wong, J. H. (2012). Patient navigation and the quality of breast cancer care: An analysis of the breast cancer care quality indicators. *Annals of Surgical Oncology, 19*(10), 3251–3256.

Wei, E. K., Wolin, K. Y., & Colditz, G. A. (2010). Time course of risk factors in cancer etiology and progression. *Journal of Clinical Oncology, 28*(26), 4052–4057.

18
Obesity

LORA E. BURKE
MELANIE W. TURK

LEARNING OBJECTIVES

- Discuss the global prevalence of obesity and identify at least three associated comorbidities.
- Describe the three components of the standard behavioral approach to weight loss.
- Identify at least three behavioral strategies that are commonly used in the behavioral approach to weight loss.

EPIDEMIOLOGY AND SIGNIFICANCE OF OBESITY

PREVALENCE, COMORBIDITIES, AND SIGNIFICANCE

Overweight (a body mass index [BMI] between 25.0 and 29.9 kg/m²) and obesity (a BMI of 30 kg/m² or more; see Table 18.1) (National Heart, Lung, and Blood Institute Obesity Education Initiative Expert Panel on the Identification, Evaluation, and Treatment of Overweight and Obesity, 1998) significantly impact the health of the population (Roth, Qiang, Marban, Redelt, & Lowell, 2004). In fact, obesity has surpassed infectious disease and undernutrition as the most significant contributor to poor health and mortality globally (Obesity Canada Clinical Practice Guidelines Expert Panel, 2007). Adding to the significance of this public health problem, obesity is characterized by a pattern of weight loss and regain. In 2008, 10% of men and 14% of women over the age of 20 were obese—approximately 205 million men and 297 million women or over half a billion adults worldwide (World Health Organization Global Health Observatory, 2012). The latest prevalence statistics for the United States from 2009 to 2010 show that 69.2% of adults aged 20 and older are either overweight or obese, with 35.9% of this group considered obese (Flegal, Carroll, Kit, & Ogden, 2012). Moreover, obesity is a well-established risk factor for a myriad of chronic conditions including type 2 diabetes, hypertension, cardiovascular disease, certain cancers, sleep disorders, and arthritis (Wadden, Butryn, & Wilson, 2007).

TABLE 18.1 Classification of Overweight and Obesity (NHLBI, 1998)

OBESITY	CLASS	BMI (KG/M²)
Underweight		<18.5
Normal		18.5–24.9
Overweight		25.0–29.9
Obesity	I	30.0–34.9
	II	35.0–39.9
Extreme obesity	III	≥ 40

BEHAVIORS INCLUDED IN MANAGING OBESITY

The cornerstone of weight management today is lifestyle modification, an approach that includes reduced energy intake, increased energy expenditure, and behavioral treatment, referred to as standard behavioral treatment (SBT) (Digenio, Mancuso, Gerber, & Dvorak, 2009).

EATING HABITS AND DIETARY INTAKE

A key component of dietary therapy is a reduction in total caloric intake by 500 kcal/day. A deficit of 500 kcal/day results in a 1-pound per week weight loss (1 pound is the equivalent of 3,500 kcal). The focus of dietary change education includes the energy value of foods (e.g., fat contains 9 calories per gram compared to protein and carbohydrates, which contain 4 calories per gram), how to read food labels, the three types of fat and the recommended distribution of these in the diet, methods to reduce fat and increase fiber and complex carbohydrate intake, portion control, and how to prepare foods to reduce the addition of calories. More recently, there is a focus also on reducing beverages with added sugars. Individuals also are instructed on recipe modification, food shopping, and restaurant eating.

Addressing both fat and caloric restriction is important. The calorie goal is based on the individual's baseline body weight, for example, 1,200 kilocalories for women and 1,500 kilocalories for men (National Heart, Lung, and Blood Institute, 2007). Typically, the fat allowance is 20% to 30% of total daily calories (Wing, 2004). For example, a person who is following a 1,200 kcal/day eating plan with a 25% fat allowance would have a goal of 33 grams of fat per day.

One approach to management of energy intake is the use of meal replacements, for example, Slim Fast (Unilever, London, UK, and Rotterdam, Netherlands) or Glucerna (Abbott Laboratories, Abbott Park, IL). LOOK Ahead Trial participants were instructed to replace two meals per day with a liquid shake and one snack with a bar for the first 6 months and then replace one meal and one snack per day in the second half of the first year (Wadden et al., 2006). One year later, the number of meal replacements consumed was significantly associated with weight loss.

For several years, an intense debate occurred about the types of diets that were most effective for treating overweight, for example, high versus low carbohydrate or fat. However, few studies comparing variations of these macronutrients extended beyond

12 months and the findings were inconsistent (Dansinger, Gleason, Griffith, Selker, & Schaefer, 2005; Foster et al., 2003; Gardner et al., 2007). Sacks reported on a 2-year trial of over 800 participants and compared four diets: low fat versus high fat and average protein versus high protein and compared low and high carbohydrate content (Sacks et al., 2009). At 2 years, all diets resulted in clinically meaningful weight loss. Moreover, satiety, hunger, and satisfaction were similar across the four diet groups. Attendance at the group sessions was strongly associated with weight loss. Collectively, these studies showed that adherence to the diet declined over time indicating that adherence to the diet was more important than the diet itself (Dansinger et al., 2005).

PHYSICAL ACTIVITY

Incorporating physical activity in treatment for weight loss and maintenance is essential for successful outcomes. Recent recommendations for healthy adults from the American College of Sports Medicine (ACSM) are organized into four categories of exercise—cardiorespiratory, resistance, flexibility, and neuromotor (Garber et al., 2011). For additional information on physical activity for promoting health, please see Chapter 8. In contrast to the amount of physical activity needed for health and fitness, higher amounts of physical activity are needed to lose weight and prevent weight regain after weight loss. For a weight loss of approximately 2 to 3 kg over 4 to 6 months, moderate-intensity physical activity for at least 150 min/week is recommended; 225 to 420 minutes of moderate-intensity activity per week results in a 5 to 7.5 kg weight loss, over the same time period (Donnelly et al., 2009). Physical activity alone results in a 3% loss of body weight (Donnelly et al., 2009); therefore energy restriction is necessary for additional weight loss (Curioni & Lourenco, 2005). While the evidence does not support resistance exercise training as an effective tool for weight loss, it may help to preserve lean muscle mass and promote percentage of fat loss through increases in energy expenditure (Donnelly et al., 2009). Approximately 250 to 300 minutes per week of moderate-intensity daily activity may be necessary to maintain weight loss among persons who were formerly obese (Haskell et al., 2007). Activity may be accumulated in multiple 10-minute periods throughout the day and continues to be beneficial for weight loss (Jakicic, Winters, Lang, & Wing, 1999).

SLEEP HYGIENE

A growing body of evidence suggests that inadequate amounts and quality of sleep are associated with an increased risk of obesity (Beccutia & Pannain, 2011). In a 6-year study of 1,597 adults in Italy, decreased sleep was related to obesity such that each increased hour of total sleep time was associated with a 30% reduction in incident obesity (Bo et al., 2011). Short sleep duration has been associated with increases in BMI and abdominal adiposity, and sleeping 5 hours or less a night was associated with the largest accumulation of both subcutaneous adipose tissue and visceral adipose tissue over 5 years (Hairston et al., 2010).

The relationship between obesity and insufficient sleep might be influenced by resultant changes in appetite-regulating hormones. Ghrelin, an appetite-stimulating hormone, increases with sleep deprivation, and leptin, an appetite-suppressing hormone, decreases with sleep deprivation (Spiegel, Tasali, Penev, & Van Cauter, 2004). Inadequate sleep may affect the efficacy of dietary interventions for weight loss. A small experimental study tested the effect of 5.5 hours of sleep compared to 8.5 hours of sleep. While weight loss was the same (approximately 3 kg), the amount of fat mass lost during the 5.5-hour sleep period was smaller than during the 8.5-hour sleep period ($p = .04$) (Nedeltcheva, Kilkus, Imperial, Schoeller, & Penev, 2010).

BEHAVIORAL STRATEGIES FOR MANAGING OBESITY

The core behavioral change strategies of SBT for weight loss are based on social cognitive theory and include goal setting, self-monitoring, cognitive restructuring, self-efficacy enhancement, and social support with feedback and guidance provided by behavioral counselors to assist with development of problem-solving skills (Wing, 2004). Goal setting focuses on daily diet and weekly exercise goals; feedback on progress is provided by the counselor through written or electronic notes to the individual. Reinforcement for goals achieved and incremental increases in goals (e.g., minutes of exercise) enhances self-efficacy. Social support is provided by peers through the group sessions while problem solving is also facilitated by the counselor through the group process. A list of the behavioral strategies that are typically used in weight loss treatment is detailed in Table 18.2.

SELF-REGULATION AND SELF-MONITORING

Programs that target behavior change such as weight loss are based on strategies that promote the individual's ability to self-regulate behavior. Kanfer's theory of self-regulation, part of social cognitive theory, provides the theoretical basis for self-monitoring (Kanfer, 1991; Kanfer & Goldstein, 1991). Kanfer suggests that changing habits requires developed self-regulatory skills. He has described self-regulation as a process that includes three distinct components: self-monitoring, self-evaluation, and self-reinforcement. The behavioral strategy of self-monitoring is central to this process, and includes deliberate attention to some aspect of an individual's behavior and recording details of that behavior.

Support for the role of self-monitoring in weight control began to emerge two decades ago (Baker & Kirschenbaum, 1993). Today it is the centerpiece of weight loss treatment. Burke, Wang, and Sevick (2011) conducted a systematic review of the literature on self-monitoring in weight loss treatment programs and found consistent support for a significant association between participant self-monitoring and weight loss. Traditionally, self-monitoring includes recording one's food intake (calories and fat grams) and physical activity. More recently, self-monitoring weight has been added as an approach to increase one's awareness of weight and its relation to energy intake and expenditure, and also as an aid to prevent weight regain (VanWormer et al., 2009; Wing, Tate, Gorin, Raynor, & Fava, 2006).

MOTIVATIONAL INTERVIEWING

Motivational interviewing (MI) is a counseling strategy for behavior change that underscores the importance of a collaborative relationship between provider and patient to support behavior change. MI uses an interactive, accepting style of communication that includes reflective listening to highlight ambivalence for change and to help identify individually relevant reasons for change (Miller & Rollnick, 1991). It has been used as an adjunctive strategy in weight loss for over a decade (Armstrong et al., 2011).

Several randomized controlled trials (RCTs) in recent years have demonstrated the efficacy of incorporating MI in behavioral therapy for weight loss. Among women with

TABLE 18.2 Strategies Used in Standard Behavioral Treatment Interventions for Weight Loss

STRATEGY*	DESCRIPTION
Goal setting	Individuals are instructed to set daily and weekly goals for calorie and fat consumption, exercise time, and behavior change, e.g., to eat breakfast daily, alter the content of snacks.
Self-monitoring	Systematically observing and recording one's behavior for the purpose of increasing one's awareness of current behaviors and the settings in which they occur. Provides opportunity to make corrective action if done in a timely manner; also provides counselor material to provide feedback on progress.
Self-evaluation	Individuals compare their behavior to a desired standard. A perceived discrepancy between one's current performance and the desired standard/goal can prompt one into action. Satisfaction will occur if there is a close match between the performance criteria and feedback information.
Self-reinforcement	Occurs as the evaluation process is completed, comes from seeing personal change occur. As individuals observe their behavior change, they develop a strengthened sense of efficacy for maintaining those behaviors. Thus, self-efficacy influences maintenance and self-regulation.
Feedback	Setting specific, daily goals and evaluating one's performance in achieving these goals, as well as receiving reinforcement on performance. Individuals use the information recorded in their diaries as a source of feedback on their progress in changing their behavior. The interventionists monitor the recorded behavior and provide feedback and guidance.
Stimulus control	Refers to behavioral strategies designed to help participants alter their environment, minimize cues that might trigger undesirable behaviors related to physical activity or eating, and add cues to increase activity. Individuals rearrange their environment for this purpose, e.g., remove counterproductive items from sight.
Problem solving	Individuals learn skills to deal with situations that interfere with achieving their goals. Problem solving consists of five steps: identifying and defining the problem, brainstorming solutions, evaluating the pros and cons of the potential solution, implementing the solution plan, and evaluating its success.

(continued)

TABLE 18.2 Strategies Used in Standard Behavioral Treatment Interventions for Weight Loss (*continued*)

STRATEGY*	DESCRIPTION
Social assertion	The skill of being assertive in social situations that threaten desirable eating and physical activity behaviors is essential to behavior change in weight loss. Individuals learn three communication styles (aggressive, passive, and assertive) and how to use assertive skills in situations that may threaten their ability to meet their eating and physical activity goals.
Cognitive strategies	Individuals are taught how to recognize patterns of negative thought that can interfere with behavior change and weight control, such as perfectionism, all or none thinking, and self-doubt; to use cognitive techniques to counter these negative thoughts; and to use positive self-statements.
Relapse prevention	Marlatt and Gordon's relapse prevention model is used to teach participants to recognize situations that place them at risk for lapses from their dietary behavior change program (Marlatt & Gordon, 1980). They learn how to use behavioral and cognitive strategies for handling these situations in the future.
Portion control	Learning to recognize and control portion size is crucial to reducing food consumption. Examples of this include a group exercise in which subjects view portions of food (e.g., shredded cheese, cooked pasta, stir fried food) and estimate the amount, then are told the actual amount, having individuals serve portions of various foods, and afterward measure the exact amount.

*The strategies are based on several models of motivation and behavioral change.

type 2 diabetes who were overweight or obese, women who received MI sessions lost significantly more weight than those in the health education group at 6 months (1.6 kg, $p = .01$), and this greater weight loss was maintained at 18 months (1.8 kg, $p = .04$); MI appeared to affect weight loss through increased group meeting attendance and higher levels of self-monitoring (West, DiLillo, Bursac, Gore, & Greene, 2007). A recent meta-analysis of 11 RCTs reported that MI augments weight loss with a weighted mean difference (WMD) between MI intervention groups and controls of -1.47 kg (95% CI [-2.05, -0.88]) (Armstrong et al., 2011). However, there have been inconsistent findings. Two studies of African American women did not find a benefit of adding MI to behavioral weight loss treatment (Befort et al., 2008; West, Elaine Prewitt, Bursac, & Felix, 2008).

HEALTH CARE PROVIDER DIRECTED AND PATIENT-CENTERED INTERVENTIONS

Assessment, diagnosis, and treatment of obesity during clinical encounters in the health care practitioner setting are suboptimal. In a study of 9,827 patients, only 20% of the obese patients had that diagnosis documented in their chart (Bardia, Holtan, Slezak, & Thompson, 2007). Barriers to appropriate identification and treatment of obesity have been recognized on multiple levels—provider, patient, and health care system. Provider barriers include lack of time and insurance reimbursement along with lack of training, comfort, and useful tools for delivering weight loss treatment (Rao, 2010; Tham & Young, 2008). Patient barriers may include embarrassment, fear, or lack of motivation, while system barriers consist of limited resources and high costs (Fujioka & Bakhru, 2010). But, evidence points to strategies that practitioners may use to assist overweight and obese patients with weight loss.

In the discussion about weight management, patient preferences for communication and language must be considered. Patients have reported needing empathy and unprejudiced interaction with providers when discussing weight and prefer the use of terms such as "weight" rather than "fatness" or "obese" (Blixen, Singh, & Thacker, 2006). As a provider, being cognizant of one's speech and communication techniques can lay the foundation for a productive dialogue that is well received.

Weight loss counseling begins with a 5% to 10% weight loss goal, which has been associated with health benefits, for example, improved glycemic control (Fujioka, 2010). The U.S. Preventive Services Task Force recommends that practitioners offer obese patients intensive counseling and behavioral interventions for weight loss; intensive counseling is defined as a minimum of two visits monthly for the first 3 months (U.S. Preventive Services Task Force, 2003). Practice-based interventions that have met this intensity level resulted in significant weight losses, for example, -3.4 and -7.7 kg after 1 year for patients receiving biweekly dietician counseling with or without meal replacements (Ashley et al., 2001). Described earlier, MI for dietary counseling in a primary care setting resulted in greater weight losses among patients at risk for type 2 diabetes compared to distribution of written diet materials (Greaves et al., 2008). Patients whose physician used counseling techniques consistent with MI lost weight at 3 months while patients whose physician did not use MI-consistent counseling techniques gained weight (Pollak et al., 2010).

Recent changes to reimbursement by the Centers for Medicare and Medicaid (CMS) provide incentive for treatment of obesity by providers. CMS will reimburse primary care providers for obesity screening and intensive behavioral therapy in settings such as physicians' offices. Medicare recipients with a BMI of 30 kg/m^2 or greater are eligible to receive one weekly face-to-face counseling visit for 1 month and biweekly for 5 additional months. If the patient has achieved a weight loss of 3 kg or more after the first 6 months, he or she may then receive monthly face-to-face counseling for an additional 6 months. CMS reimbursement for this therapy is confined to primary care settings, and it must be provided by primary care physicians or primary care practitioners (defined as nurse practitioners, clinical nurse specialists, or physician assistants) (Centers for Medicare and Medicaid Services, 2011).

TECHNOLOGY-BASED INTERVENTIONS

The advent of computer-based technology, including the Internet, for use in self-monitoring spawned a new generation of studies (Tate, Jackvony, & Wing, 2006). Handheld devices such as personal digital assistants have demonstrated improved self-monitoring but not significantly greater weight loss than use of a paper diary (Burke et al., 2012). Two clinical trials have examined the use of mobile phones to deliver text messages to participants to promote behaviors for weight loss or maintenance and provided inconsistent results (Haapala, Barengo, Biggs, Surakka, & Manninen, 2009; Shapiro et al., 2012). Haapala et al. (2009) reported a significantly better weight loss in the text message versus the control group, 4.5 kg versus 1.1 kg. Shapiro et al. (2012) reported that the text message group lost 1.8% of baseline weight compared to 0.8% for the control group ($p = .394$). Participants reported moderately strong satisfaction with the program. These studies illustrate the potential of cellular-telephone-based technology in weight loss; however, the inconsistent results suggest additional study is needed to determine the best approach to using technology to enhance weight loss. It may be that the text messages are not sufficiently tailored to the person's progress in making behavior change, or possibly too focused on weight. The use of mobile technology holds great promise in reaching a larger number of individuals in need of weight loss treatment (Blackburn, 2012). However, a concern in the scientific community is the proliferation of downloadable software "apps" for weight loss that lack a theoretical or evidence base (Breton, Fuemmeler, & Abroms, 2011).

BRIEF OVERVIEW OF PHARMACOLOGY AND BARIATRIC SURGERY

PHARMACOLOGY

Although there is much interest in pharmacologic treatment, the multidimensional nature of obesity with its genetic (Loos & Bouchard, 2003), metabolic (Chitwood, Brown, Lundy, & Dupper, 1996), and behavioral contributing factors (Kayman, Bruvold, & Stem, 1990) has limited the potential for single pharmacotherapy. Pharmacotherapy is a second level of treatment that must be used in combination with lifestyle behavioral change. It is considered for individuals with no contraindications to the medication who have a BMI greater than 30 kg/m2 or a BMI less than 27 kg/m^2 with significant comorbidities (National Heart, Lung, and Blood Institute Obesity Education Initiative Expert Panel on the Identification, Evaluation, and Treatment of Overweight and Obesity, 1998). Debate exists regarding the risk/benefit ratio for pharmacologic weight loss treatment (Balkon, Balkon, & Zitkus, 2011), and few medications indicated for the treatment of obesity are U.S. Food and Drug Administration (FDA) approved (e.g., Qsymia, marketed by Vivus Inc. in Mountain View, CA, and orlistat), which result in up to 30% non-absorption of dietary fat (Sjöström et al., 1998). Medications have resulted in a 4% to 6% increase in the average amount of weight lost in 1 to 2 years (Bray, 2008; Padwal, Li, & Lau, 2003) but also undesirable or harmful side effects, some of which have necessitated removing the medication from the market, for example, cardiac valvulopathy associated with fenfluramine (Kaplan, 2010) and more recently, increased risk of stroke and heart attack with sibutramine (James et al., 2010). Response to medication therapy is also varied, and 2% to 5% experience a better than average weight loss, but a large proportion exhibit little to no weight loss (Kaplan, 2010). Medications must be combined with lifestyle modification that includes dietary planning, increased physical activity, and behavioral treatment.

BARIATRIC SURGERY

Bariatric surgery has the advantage of promoting substantial, long-term weight losses with a resultant reduction in obesity-related comorbidities, for example, type 2 diabetes mellitus, hypertension, and sleep apnea (Buchwald et al., 2004). The two most commonly performed surgeries, laparoscopic adjustable gastric banding and Roux-en-Y gastric bypass, commonly result in a loss of 20% to 25% of initial body weight, respectively, after 12 to 18 months (Buchwald et al., 2004; Maggard et al., 2005). The criteria for determining if a patient is a candidate for surgery include: Class 3 obesity (BMI 40 kg/m^2 or greater) or Class 2 obesity (BMI 35–39.9 kg/m^2) with significant obesity-related health problems (Buchwald & Consensus Conference Panel, 2005). Patients must also have failed other more conservative treatments (i.e., lifestyle intervention with dietary, exercise, and behavioral therapy) and have acceptable operative risk (i.e., physically stable for surgery) (NIH Consensus Conference Statement, 1991). Once referred for bariatric surgery, patients are assessed by members of the surgical team including a dietician and psychologist for nutritional counseling and evaluation of psychological health, capacity to make informed decisions, and motivation for actively engaging in post-operative treatment guidelines. In addition to the surgeon and anesthesiologist, a multidisciplinary team of providers (internist, nurse, dietician, cardiologist, and psychologist) is critical to the care of bariatric patients in order to achieve lasting weight loss success (Buchwald & Consensus Conference Panel, 2005). In order to promote necessary lifestyle changes for sustaining weight loss after surgery, behavioral follow-up care from a team of professionals is needed and should be maintained. There are no established guidelines or commonly accepted practices for post-operative dietary and behavioral counseling (Sarwer, Wadden, & Fabricatore, 2005), but emerging research suggests that behavioral interventions for bariatric patients may help with weight loss and maintenance (Papalazarou et al., 2010).

RELAPSE PREVENTION/MAINTENANCE OF CHANGE

Long-term maintenance of weight loss has remained a formidable challenge; approximately one third of weight lost among individuals treated with lifestyle modification is regained within 1 year (Wadden, Butryn, & Byrne, 2004); 4-year weight losses average an unremarkable 1.8 kg (Perri & Foreyt, 2004). The behaviors required for weight loss may differ from those needed in weight loss maintenance because the goal of maintenance is to undo small weight gains before the gains become large; the goal for weight loss is generally to lose sizeable amounts of weight after a prolonged period of weight gain. Weight loss treatment is temporary and often accompanied by positive comments from others, but weight loss maintenance is long-term and ongoing reinforcement usually lapses (Wadden, 1995).

A great deal of what is known about successful weight loss maintenance is a result of the National Weight Control Registry, a large registry of persons who have successfully lost 13.6 kg (30 lbs) and maintained that loss for a minimum of 1 year (Klem, Wing, McGuire, Seagle, & Hill, 1997). Much descriptive information has been reported on behavioral strategies used by these weight loss maintainers—increasing physical activity (approximately 1 hour/day of walking), consuming a diet moderate in calories (approximately 1,800 kcal/day) and low in fat (less than 30% kcal from fat), regularly self-monitoring weight and food intake, limiting the variety of foods eaten, eating breakfast and eating more frequently, restricting time spent watching television, and having a consistent dietary intake across the week (Bachman, Phelan, Wing, & Raynor, 2011; Raynor, Jeffery, Phelan, Hill, & Wing, 2005; Raynor, Phelan, Hill, & Wing, 2006; Wyatt et al., 2002). Other descriptive studies have corroborated these findings and added information related to eating low-fat, protein-rich foods and rewarding oneself for adhering to the eating and activity plan (Sciamanna et al., 2011).

Three large RCTs in recent years have examined additional maintenance methods. In the multi-site, Weight Loss Maintenance RCT, the personal contact group gained significantly less weight than the self-directed group and the interactive web-based group (Svetkey et al., 2008). The 3-group STOP Regain RCT reported significantly less weight gain in the face-to-face group compared to the control group and the Internet group participants (Wing et al., 2006). The face-to-face participants rated weighing oneself, establishing a weight loss goal, tracking calories, and maintaining a log or graph of eating and exercise as more highly important than control. The 3-group Treatment for Obesity in Underserved Rural Communities RCT found after 12 months, that the telephone-counseling and face-to-face groups gained significantly less weight than the control group. Telephone counseling and in-person counseling were equally effective, but telephone counseling was provided at half the cost (Perri et al., 2008a). Nearly 42% were able to maintain a 5% weight loss at 3.5-year follow-up (Milsom, Ross Middleton, & Perri, 2011).

Physical activity has been emphasized as a critical element of successful weight loss maintenance. The *energy gap*, which develops after weight loss, is a contributing factor to the need for physical activity (Hill, Thompson, & Wyatt, 2005). It is approximated at 8 kcal/day for each pound of body weight lost and develops because of a decrease in one's total energy expenditure due to a drop in resting metabolic rate, which occurs because less energy is needed to move a smaller body size. In the current obesogenic environment with food consumed in large portions, filling this energy gap might be more easily achieved by increasing energy expenditure through physical activity (Hill et al., 2005). While the optimal amount of physical activity for weight loss maintenance has not been identified, the most recent ACSM guidelines reinforce that weight maintenance (3% or less weight gain) likely requires approximately 60 minutes of daily, moderate-intensity physical activity, for example, brisk walking for 4 miles (Donnelly et al., 2009).

Because weight loss often peaks at 6 months after behavioral treatment begins (Jeffery et al., 2000), a plan for weight maintenance should be established at this time. Maintenance plans that include continued, regular contact with a health provider are recommended to encourage long-term weight loss maintenance (National Heart, Lung, and Blood Institute Obesity Education Initiative Expert Panel on the Identification, Evaluation, and Treatment of Overweight and Obesity, 1998). Providing contact by telephone is efficacious for promoting weight loss maintenance (Perri et al., 2008b), particularly if that contact is initiated by someone who is known to the individual (Wing, Jeffery, Hellerstedt, & Burton, 1996).

FUTURE DIRECTIONS

THE USE OF TECHNOLOGY

Mobile technology has tremendous potential in addressing the significant public health problem of obesity. Leveraging the opportunities that the new electronic communications provide could benefit many therapeutic approaches to obesity (Blackburn, 2012; Rao & Kirley, 2012; Riley, 2012). Possibly, the most promising part is the capability of mobile devices and telecommunications to reach a larger number and to deliver interventions that could augment that which is delivered by the primary care provider. Additionally, the use of technology can reduce the burden associated with self-monitoring; moreover, it could reduce the delay in providing feedback to the individual.

Rao and Kirley (2012) describe four important features of effective weight management programs that also support primary care providers' treatment of this condition: (1) convenient and accessible to the majority of people in need; (2) cost significantly less than alternatives; (3) participation should be sustainable even if it only has a modest impact on weight; and (4) it is essential that the program has the ability to retain or re-engage people over several years. Incorporating technology can facilitate the achievement of these four features.

POLICY-LEVEL INTERVENTIONS

From a public health perspective, policy-level interventions are needed to address obesity; these include policies that direct interventions to both dietary intake and physical activity at a societal level. One effective tactic could be for government to regulate foods that are non-nutritious, while urging (and perhaps incentivizing) companies to produce and sell more healthful foods, and then making available to consumers product information that facilitates their selecting healthier foods (Farley, 2012). Aspects of the built environment that limit physical activity on a population level (e.g., neighborhood design and activity facilities) must also be addressed in order to tackle obesity from an energy expenditure perspective (McCormack & Shiell, 2011).

EXPEDITE THE TRANSLATION OF RESEARCH FINDINGS INTO PRACTICE

Given the significance of the problem, it is paramount that efficacious strategies be immediately translated into practice. The Diabetes Prevention Program is an illustration of successful translation. Several investigators have demonstrated effectiveness in translating this behavioral intervention into clinical practice settings (Kramer et al., 2009) and in community-based settings (Ackermann, Finch, Brizendine, Zhou, & Marrero, 2008; Aldana et al., 2005)

CONCLUSIONS

Standard behavioral treatment focuses on lifestyle approaches augmented with counseling for behavior change. Strategies that have received the most consistent support for weight loss and maintenance include self-monitoring, use of structured meal plans or meal replacements, and ongoing contact. Other treatment approaches, such as pharmacotherapy or bariatric surgery, need to be augmented by these behavioral approaches. Given the severity and the ubiquity of this public health problem, prevention and treatment of obesity need to be incorporated into primary care settings. A recent change in CMS reimbursement is an attempt to address this issue. Recent RCTs have provided evidence for efficacious strategies to reduce the typical weight regain that occurs post-treatment. The use of technology to broaden and extend the reach of effective interventions and the implementation of policy changes at the societal level are two approaches that have potential to impact large segments of the population.

REFERENCES

Ackermann, R. T., Finch, E. A., Brizendine, E., Zhou, H., & Marrero, D. G. (2008). Translating the diabetes Prevention Program into the community. The DEPLOY Pilot Study. *American Journal of Preventive Medicine, 35*(4), 357–363. doi: S0749-3797(08)00604-1 [pii] 10.1016/j.amepre.2008.06.035 [doi]

Aldana, S. G., Barlow, M., Smith, R., Yanowitz, F. G., Adams, T., Loveday, L., ... LaMonte, M. J.(2005). The Diabetes Prevention Program: A worksite experience. *American Association of Occupational Health Nurses Journal, 53*(11), 499–505.

Armstrong, M. J., Mottershead, T. A., Ronksley, P. E., Sigal, R. J., Campbell, T. S., & Hemmelgarn, B. R. (2011). Motivational interviewing to improve weight loss in overweight and/or obese patients: A systematic review and meta-analysis of randomized controlled trials. *Obesity Reviews, 12*(9), 709–723. doi: 10.1111/j.1467-789X.2011.00892.x

Ashley, J. M., St Jeor, S. T., Schrage, J. P., Perumean-Chaney, S. E., Gilbertson, M. C., McCall, N. L., & Bovee, V. (2001). Weight control in the physician's office. *Archives of Internal Medicine, 161*(13), 1599–1604. doi: 10-1001/pubs.Arch Intern Med.-ISSN-0003-9926-161-13-ioi00661

Bachman, J. L., Phelan, S., Wing, R. R., & Raynor, H. A. (2011). Eating frequency is higher in weight loss maintainers and normal-weight individuals than in overweight individuals. *Journal of the American Dietetic Association, 111*(11), 1730–1734. doi: http://dx.doi.org/10.1016/j.jada.2011.08.006

Baker, R. C., & Kirschenbaum, D. S. (1993). Self-monitoring may be necessary for successful weight control. *Behavior Therapy, 24,* 377–394.

Balkon, N., Balkon, C., & Zitkus, B. S. (2011). Overweight and obesity: Pharmacotherapeutic considerations. *Journal of the American Academy of Nurse Practitioners, 23*(2), 61–66. doi: 10.1111/j.1745 -7599.2010.00587.x

Bardia, A., Holtan, S. G., Slezak, J. M., & Thompson, W. G. (2007). Diagnosis of obesity by primary care physicians and impact on obesity management. *Mayo Clinic Proceedings, 82*(8), 927–932. doi: http://dx.doi.org/10.4065/82.8.927

Beccutia, G., & Pannain, S. (2011). Sleep and obesity. *Current Opinion in Clinical Nutrition and Metabolic Care, 14,* 402–412.

Befort, C. A., Nollen, N., Ellerbeck, E. F., Sullivan, D. K., Thomas, J. L., & Ahluwalia, J. S. (2008). Motivational interviewing fails to improve outcomes of a behavioral weight loss program for obese African American women: A pilot randomized trial. *Journal of Behavioral Medicine, 31*(5), 367–377.

Blackburn, G. L. (2012). Weight of the nation: Moving forward, reversing the trend using medical care. *American Journal of Clinical Nutrition, 96*(5), 949–950.

Blixen, C. E., Singh, A., & Thacker, H. (2006). Values and beliefs about obesity and weight reduction among African American and Caucasian women. *Journal of Transcultural Nursing, 17*(3), 290–297.

Bo, S., Ciccone, G., Durazzo, M., Ghinamo, L., Villois, P., Canil, S., ... Cavallo-Perin, P. (2011). Contributors to the obesity and hyperglycemia epidemics. A prospective study in a population-based cohort. *International Journal of Obesity, 35,* 1442–1449.

Bray, G. A. (2008). Lifestyle and pharmacological approaches to weight loss: Efficacy and safety. *Journal of Clinical Endocrinology & Metabolism, 93*(11 Suppl. 1), s81–s88. doi: 10.1210/jc.2008-1294

Breton, E. R., Fuemmeler, B. F., & Abroms, L. C. (2011). Weight loss—there is an app for that! But does it adhere to evidence-informed practices? *Translational Behavioral Medicine, 1,* 523–529. doi: 10.1007 /s13142-011-0076-5

Buchwald, H., Avidor, Y., Braunwald, E., Jensen, M. D., Pories, W., Fahrbach, K., & Schoelles, K. (2004). Bariatric surgery: A systematic review and meta-analysis. *Journal of the American Medical Association, 292*(14), 1724–1737.

Buchwald, H., & Consensus Conference Panel. (2005). Consensus conference statement bariatric surgery for morbid obesity: Health implications for patients, health professionals, and third-party payers. *Surgery for Obesity and Related Disorders, 1,* 371–381.

Burke, L. E., Styn, M. A., Sereika, S. M., Conroy, M. B., Ye, L., Glanz, K., ... Ewing, L. J. (2012). Using mHealth technology to enhance self-monitoring for weight loss: A randomized trial. *American Journal of Preventive Medicine, 43*(1), 20–26.

Burke, L. E., Wang, J., & Sevick, M. A. (2011). Self-monitoring in weight loss: A systematic review of the literature. *J Am Diet Assoc, 111*(1), 92–102. doi: 10.1016/j.jada.2010.10.008

Centers for Medicare and Medicaid Services. (2011). *Decision memo for intensive behavioral therapy for obesity.* Retrieved from http://www.cms.gov/medicare-coverage-database/details/nca-decision -memo.aspx?&NcaName=Intensive%20Behavioral%20Therapy%20for%20Obesity&bc=ACAAA AAAIAAA&NCAId=253&

Chitwood, L. F., Brown, S. P., Lundy, M. J., & Dupper, M. A. (1996). Metabolic propensity toward obesity in black vs white females: Responses during rest, exercise and recovery. *International Journal of Obesity, 20*(5), 455–462.

Curioni, C. C., & Lourenco, P. M. (2005). Long-term weight loss after diet and exercise: A systematic review. *International Journal of Obesity, 29,* 1168–1174.

Dansinger, M. L., Gleason, J. A., Griffith, J. L., Selker, H. P., & Schaefer, E. J. (2005). Comparison of the Atkins, Ornish, Weight Watchers, and Zone diets for weight loss and heart disease risk reduction: A randomized trial. *Journal of the American Medical Association, 293*(1), 43–53.

Digenio, A. G., Mancuso, J. P., Gerber, R. A., & Dvorak, R. V. (2009). Comparison of methods for delivering a lifestyle modification program for obese patients: A randomized trial. *Annals of Internal Medicine, 150*(4), 255–262.

Donnelly, J. E., Blair, S. N., Jakicic, J. M., Manore, M. M., Rankin, J. W., & Smith, B. K. (2009). American College of Sports Medicine Position Stand. Appropriate physical activity intervention strategies for weight loss and prevention of weight regain for adults. *Medicine & Science in Sports & Exercise, 41*(2), 459–471.

Farley, T. A. (2012). The role of government in preventing excess calorie consumption: The example of New York city. *Journal of the American Medical Association, 308*(11), 1093–1094. doi: 10.1001/2012.jama.11623

Flegal, K. M., Carroll, M. D., Kit, B. K., & Ogden, C. L. (2012). Prevalence of obesity and trends in the distribution of body mass index among US adults, 1999–2010. *Journal of the American Medical Association, 307*(5), 491–497. doi: 10.1001/jama.2012.39

Foster, G. D., Wyatt, H. R., Hill, J. O., McGucki, B. G., Brill, C., Mohammed, B. S., ... Klein, S. (2003). A randomized trial of a low-carbohydrate diet for obesity [comment]. *New England Journal of Medicine, 348*(21), 2082–2090.

Fujioka, K. (2010). Benefits of moderate weight loss in patients with type 2 diabetes. *Diabetes, Obesity and Metabolism, 12*(3), 186–194. doi: 10.1111/j.1463-1326.2009.01155.x

Fujioka, K., & Bakhru, N. (2010). Office-based management of obesity. *Mount Sinai Journal of Medicine, 77,* 466–471.

Garber, C. E., Blissmer, B., Deschenes, M. R., Franklin, B. A., Lamonte, M. J., Lee, I. M., ... American College of Sports Medicine. (2011). Quantity and quality of exercise for developing and maintaining cardiorespiratory, musculoskeletal, and neuromotor fitness in apparently healthy adults: Guidance for prescribing exercise. *Medicine and Science in Sports and Exercise, 43*(7), 1334–1359.

Gardner, C. D., Kiazand, A., Alhassan, S., Kim, S., Stafford, R. S., Balise, R. R., ...King, A. C. (2007). Comparison of the Atkins, Zone, Ornish, and LEARN diets for change in weight and related risk factors among overweight premenopausal women: The A TO Z Weight Loss Study: A randomized trial. *Journal of the American Medical Association, 297*(9), 969–977.

Greaves, C. J., Middlebrooke, A., O'Loughlin, L., Holland, S., Piper, J., Steele, A., . . . Daly, M. (2008). Motivational interviewing for modifying diabetes risk: A randomised controlled trial. *The British Journal of General Practice, 58*(553), 535–540. doi: 10.3399/bjgp08X319648

Haapala, I., Barengo, N. C., Biggs, S., Surakka, L., & Manninen, P. (2009). Weight loss by mobile phone: A 1-year effectiveness study. *Public Health Nutrition, 12*(12), 2382–2391.

Hairston, K. G., Bryer-Ash, M., Norris, J. M., Haffner, S., Bowden, D. W., & Wagenknecht, L. E. (2010). Sleep duration and five-year abdominal fat accumulation in a minority cohort: The IRAS family study. *Sleep, 33,* 289–295.

Haskell, W. L., Lee, I. M., Pate, R. R., Powell, K. E., Blair, S. N., Franklin, B. A., ...American Heart Association. (2007). Physical activity and public health: Updated recommendation for adults from the American College of Sports Medicine and the American Heart Association. *Circulation, 116*(9), 1081–1093.

Hill, J. O., Thompson, H., & Wyatt, H. (2005). Weight maintenance: What's missing? *Journal of the American Dietetic Association, 105*(5), 63–66.

Jakicic, J. M., Winters, C., Lang, W., & Wing, R. R. (1999). Effects of intermittent exercise and use of home exercise equipment on adherence, weight loss, and fitness in overweight women: A randomized trial. *Journal of the American Medical Association, 282*(16), 1554–1560.

James, W. P. T., Caterson, I. D., Coutinho, W., Finer, N., Van Gaal, L. F., Maggioni, A. P., ...Renz, C. L. (2010). Effect of sibutramine on cardiovascular outcomes in overweight and obese subjects. *New England Journal of Medicine, 363*(10), 905–917. doi:10.1056/NEJMoa1003114

Jeffery, R. W., Drewnowski, A., Epstein, L. H., Stunkard, A. J., Wilson, G. T., Wing, R. R., & Hill, D. R. (2000). Long-term maintenance of weight loss: Current status. *Health Psychology, 19*(Suppl. 1), 5–16.

Kanfer, F. H. (1991). *Self-management methods* (4th ed.). New York, NY: Pergamon Press.

Kanfer, F. H., & Goldstein, A. P. (1991). *Helping people change: A textbook of methods* (4th ed.). Elmsford, NY: Pergamon Press.

Kaplan, L. M. (2010). Pharmacologic therapies for obesity. *Gastroenterology Clinics, 39*(1), 69–79.

Kayman, S., Bruvold, W., & Stem, J. S. (1990). Maintenance and relapse after weight loss in women: Behavioral aspects. *American Journal of Clinical Nutrition, 52*(5), 800–807.

Klem, M., Wing, R., McGuire, M., Seagle, H., & Hill, J. (1997). A descriptive study of individuals successful at long-term maintenance of substantial weight loss. *American Journal of Clinical Nutrition, 66*(2), 239–246.

Kramer, M. K., Kriska, A. M., Venditti, E. M., Miller, R. G., Brooks, M. M., Burke, L. E., ...Orchard, T. J. (2009). Translating the diabetes prevention program: A comprehensive model for prevention training and program delivery. *American Journal of Preventive Medicine, 37*(6), 505–511. doi: 10.1016/j.amepre.2009.07.020

Loos, R. J. F., & Bouchard, C. (2003). Obesity – Is it a genetic disorder? *Journal of Internal Medicine, 254*(5), 401–425.

Maggard, M. A., Shugarman, L. R., Suttorp, M., Maglione, M., Sugerman, H. J., Livingston, E. H., ... Shekelle, P. G. (2005). Meta-analysis: Surgical treatment of obesity. *Annals of Internal Medicine, 142*(7), 547–559.

Marlatt, G. A., & Gordon, J. R. (1980). *Determinants of relapse: Implications for the maintenance of behavior change.* New York, NY: Brunner/Mazel.

McCormack, G. R., & Shiell, A. (2011). In search of causality: A systematic review of the relationship between the built environment and physical activity among adults. *International Journal of Behavioral Nutrition and Physical Activity, 8*(125), doi:10.1186/1479-5868-1188-1125.

Miller, W. R., & Rollnick, S. (1991). *Motivational interviewing, preparing people to change addictive behavior.* New York, NY: The Guildford Press.

Milsom, V. A., Ross Middleton, K. M., & Perri, M. G. (2011). Successful long-term weight loss maintenance in a rural population. *Clinical Interventions in Aging, 6,* 303–309.

National Heart, Lung, and Blood Institute. (2007). *Guidelines on overweight and obesity: Electronic textbook – Appendix VIII. Glossary of terms.* Retrieved from http://www.nhlbi.nih.gov/guidelines/obesity/e_txtbk/appndx/apndx8.htm

National Heart, Lung, and Blood Institute Obesity Education Initiative Expert Panel on the Identification, Evaluation, and Treatment of Overweight and Obesity. (1998). Clinical guidelines on the identification, evaluation, and treatment of overweight and obesity in adults: The evidence report. *Obesity Research, 6*(Suppl. 2), 51S–209S.

Nedeltcheva, A. V., Kilkus, J. M., Imperial, J., Schoeller, D. A., & Penev, P. D. (2010). Insufficient sleep undermines dietary efforts to reduce adiposity. *Annals of Internal Medicine, 153*(7), 435–441.

NIH Consensus Conference Statement. (1991). *Gastrointestinal surgery for severe obesity.* Retrieved from http://www.ncbi.nlm.nih.gov/bookshelf/br.fcgi?book=hsnihcdc&part=A9282#A9287

Obesity Canada Clinical Practice Guidelines Expert Panel. (2007). 2006 Canadian clinical practice guidelines on the management and prevention of obesity in adults and children. *Canadian Medical Association Journal, 176*(8 Suppl), S1–S13. Retrieved from http://www.cmaj.ca/cgi/content/full/176/178/S171/DC171

Padwal, R., Li, S. K., & Lau, D. C. (2003). Long-term pharmacotherapy for overweight and obesity: A systematic review and meta-analysis of randomized controlled trials. *International Journal of Obesity & Related Metabolic Disorders, 27*(12), 1437–1446.

Papalazarou, A., Yannakoulia, M., Kavouras, S. A., Komesidou, V., Dimitriadis, G., Papakonstantinou, A., & Sidossis, L. S. (2010). Lifestyle intervention favorably affects weight loss and maintenance following obesity surgery. *Obesity, 18,* 1348–1353.

Perri, M. G., & Foreyt, J. P. (2004). Preventing weight regain after weight loss. In G. A. Bray & C. Bouchard (Eds.), *Handbook of obesity: Clinical applications* (2nd ed., pp. 185–199). New York, NY: Marcel Dekker.

Perri, M. G., Limacher, M. C., Durning, P. E., Janicke, D. M., Lutes, L. D., Bobroff, L. B., ... Martin, A. D. (2008). Extended-care programs for weight management in rural communities: The treatment of obesity in underserved rural settings (TOURS) randomized trial. *Archives of Internal Medicine, 168*(21), 2347–2354. doi: 168/21/2347 [pii]10.1001/archinte.168.21.2347

Pollak, K. I., Alexander, S. C., Coffman, C. J., Tulsky, J. A., Lyna, P., Dolor, R. J., ... Østbye, T. (2010). Physician communication techniques and weight loss in adults: Project CHAT. *American Journal of Preventive Medicine, 39*(4), 321–328. doi: http://dx.doi.org/10.1016/j.amepre.2010.06.005

Rao, G. (2010). Office-based strategies for the management of obesity. *American Family Physician, 81*(12), 1449–1456.

Rao, G., & Kirley, K. (2012). The future of obesity treatment: comment on "Integrating technology into standard weight loss treatment: A randomized controlled trial". *JAMA Intern Med, 173*(2), 111–112. doi: 10.1001/jamainternmed.2013.1232

Raynor, D. A., Phelan, S., Hill, J. O., & Wing, R. R. (2006). Television viewing and long-term weight maintenance: Results from the National Weight Control Registry. *Obesity, 14*(10), 1816–1824.

Raynor, H. A., Jeffery, R. W., Phelan, S., Hill, J. O., & Wing, R. R. (2005). Amount of food group variety consumed in the diet and long-term weight loss maintenance. *Obesity Research, 13*(5), 883–890.

Riley, W. T. (2012). Leveraging technology for multiple risk factor interventions. *Archives of Internal Medicine, 172*(10), 796–798.

Roth, J., Qiang, X., Marban, S. L., Redelt, H., & Lowell, B. C. (2004). The obesity pandemic: Where have we been and where are we going? *Obesity Research, 12*(Suppl 2), S88–S101.

Sacks, F. M., Bray, G. A., Carey, V. J., Smith, S. R., Ryan, D. H., Anton, S. D., … Williamson, D. A. (2009). Comparison of weight-loss diets with different compositions of fat, protein, and carbohydrates. *New England Journal of Medicine, 360*(9), 859–873.

Sarwer, D. B., Wadden, T. A., & Fabricatore, A. N. (2005). Psychosocial and behavioral aspects of bariatric surgery. *Obesity Research, 13*, 639–648.

Sciamanna, C. N., Kiernan, M., Rolls, B. J., Boan, J., Stuckey, H., Kephart, D., … Dellasega, C. (2011). Practices associated with weight loss versus weight-loss maintenance: Results of a national survey. *American Journal of Preventive Medicine, 41*(2), 159–166. doi: http://dx.doi.org/10.1016/j.amepre.2011.04.009

Shapiro, J. R., Koro, T., Neal Doran, N., Thompson, S., Sallis, J. F., Calfas, K., & Patrick, K. (2012). Text4Diet: A randomized controlled study using text messaging for weight loss behaviors. *Preventive Medicine, 55*, 412–417.

Sjöström, L., Rissanen, A., Andersen, T., Boldrin, M., Golay, A., Koppeschaar, H. P., & Krempf, M. (1998). Randomised placebo-controlled trial of orlistat for weight loss and prevention of weight regain in obese patients. *Lancet, 352*(9123), 167–172.

Spiegel, K., Tasali, E., Penev, P., & Van Cauter, E. (2004). Sleep curtailment in healthy young men is associated with decreased leptin levels, elevated ghrelin levels, and increased hunger and appetite. *Annals of Internal Medicine, 141*(11), 846–850.

Svetkey, L. P., Stevens, V. J., Brantley, P. J., Appel, L. J., Hollis, J. F., Loria, C. M., …. for the Weight Loss Maintenance Collaborative Research Group. (2008). Comparison of strategies for sustaining weight loss: The Weight Loss Maintenance randomized controlled trial. *Journal of the American Medical Association, 299*(10), 1139–1148.

Tate, D. F., Jackvony, E. H., & Wing, R. R. (2006). A randomized trial comparing human e-mail counseling, computer-automated tailored counseling, and no counseling in an Internet weight loss program. *Archives of Internal Medicine, 166*(15), 1620–1625. doi: 10.1001/archinte.166.15.1620

Tham, M., & Young, D. (2008). The role of the general practitioner in weight management in primary care – A cross sectional study in general practice. *BMC Family Practice, 9*(1), 66.

U.S. Preventive Services Task Force. (2003). Screening for obesity in adults: Recommendations and rationale. *Annals of Internal Medicine, 139*, 930–932.

VanWormer, J. J., Martinez, A. M., Martinson, B. C., Crain, A. L., Benson, G. A., Cosentino, D. L., & Pronk, N. P. (2009). Self-weighing promotes weight loss for obese adults. *American Journal of Preventive Medicine, 36*(1), 70–73.

Wadden, T. A. (1995). What characterizes successful weight maintainers? In D. B. Allison & F. Pi-Sunyer (Eds.), *Obesity treatment: Establishing goals, improving outcomes, and reviewing the research agenda* (pp. 103–111). New York, NY: Plenum Publishing.

Wadden, T. A., Butryn, M. L., & Byrne, K. J. (2004). Efficacy of lifestyle modification for long-term weight control. *Obesity Research, 12*(Suppl.), S151–S162.

Wadden, T. A., Butryn, M. L., & Wilson, C. (2007). Lifestyle modification for the management of obesity. *Gastroenterology, 132*(6), 2226–2238. doi: 10.1053/j.gastro.2007.03.051

Wadden, T. A., West, D. S., Delahanty, L., Jakicic, J., Rejeski, J., Williamson, D., …. Kumanyika, S. (2006). The Look AHEAD study: A description of the lifestyle intervention and the evidence supporting it. *Obesity, 14*(5), 737–752. doi: 14/5/737 [pii]10.1038/oby.2006.84

West, D. S., DiLillo, V., Bursac, Z., Gore, S. A., & Greene, P. G. (2007). Motivational interviewing improves weight loss in women with type 2 diabetes. *Diabetes Care, 30*(5), 1081–1087. doi: 10.2337/dc06-1966

West, D. S., Elaine Prewitt, T., Bursac, Z., & Felix, H. C. (2008). Weight loss of black, white, and Hispanic men and women in the Diabetes Prevention Program. *Obesity (Silver Spring), 16*(6), 1413–1420. doi: 10.1038/oby.2008.224

Wing, R. R. (2004). Behavioral approaches to the treatment of obesity. In G. A. Bray, C. Bourchard, & W. P. T. James (Eds.), *Handbook of obesity: Clinical applications* (2nd ed., pp. 147–167). New York, NY: Marcel Dekker.

Wing, R. R., Jeffery, R. W., Hellerstedt, W. L., & Burton, L. R. (1996). Effect of frequent phone contacts and optional food provision on maintenance of weight loss. *Annals of Behavioral Medicine, 18*(3), 172–176.

Wing, R. R., Tate, D. F., Gorin, A. A., Raynor, H. A., & Fava, J. L. (2006). A self-regulation program for maintenance of weight loss. *New England Journal of Medicine, 355*(15), 1563–1571.

World Health Organization Global Health Observatory. (2012). *Obesity: Situation and trends.*Retrieved from http://www.who.int/gho/ncd/risk_factors/obesity_text/en/index.html

Wyatt, H. R., Grunwald, G. K., Mosca, C. L., Klem, M. L., Wing, R. R., & Hill, J. O. (2002). Long-term weight loss and breakfast in subjects in the National Weight Control Registry. *Obesity Research, 10*(2), 78–82.

V

Community, System, and Provider Interventions to Support Health Behavior Change

Section V is new to this edition of the handbook and reflects the growing recognition of the role of community settings such as schools and worksites as well as the built environment and health care systems to health behavior change. These chapters describe the implementation of health behavior change through a range of different contexts. A consistent theme that emerges across the chapters in this section is that multicomponent or comprehensive programs have the greatest likelihood of success in changing health behaviors, regardless of the context in which health behavior change approaches are applied.

In Chapter 19, "School Interventions to Support Health Behavior Change," Lee and Gortmaker provide a strong rationale for the potential public health impact of promoting health behavior change through the school setting. They acknowledge the challenges faced in using schools for health promotion and the need to find cost-effective, easily adaptable strategies that align with the mission of schools. The authors describe the different types of school-based health behavior change interventions, providing illustrative examples of each. These include the delivery of individualized clinical services such as body mass index (BMI) screening and mental health services, educational interventions laying the foundation for lifelong healthy behaviors, and behavioral interventions to improve social skills and executive function. The authors tackle the issue of technology, both from the perspective of delivering health behavior change interventions through electronic devices commonly used by youth, as well as strategies designed to reduce the potential negative effects of excessive technology use such as television viewing and cell phone usage. They discuss the importance of policies at the national, state, district, and school level such as state laws mandating minimum physical activity time in schools and school policies on tobacco and food services, noting how such policies can have a significant impact on health behaviors. The most significant improvements in targeted behaviors have been found with multicomponent school-based interventions combining two or more intervention types, such as those used in Planet Health and Coordinated Approaches to Child Health (CATCH) for preventing childhood obesity. Lastly, Lee and Gortmaker recommend that researchers use a community-based participatory research (CBPR) approach involving key stakeholders including students, parents, teachers, and other school personnel to ensure that relevant questions are being asked and interventions are designed that can be best integrated and sustained in the school setting.

Lemon and Estabrook make a compelling argument for health promotion programs and policies within the worksite setting in Chapter 20, "Prevention and Management of Chronic Disease Through Worksite Health Promotion." They note that the majority of adults in the United States are in the workforce and the worksite environment provides access to resources and social support that can reduce barriers to health behavior change. Based on a review of the scientific evidence, the authors conclude that worksite health promotion programs have demonstrated modest effects on health behaviors such as smoking cessation, nutrition, physical activity, and weight, and on clinical outcomes in chronic disease management and are cost-effective, decreasing medical care costs over the cost of the programs. Of interest is that current evidence does not support the use of environmental and policy strategies alone in the worksite setting; these population-based strategies show greater promise when part of multicomponent or comprehensive programs. The authors describe key components of successful programs, which include integration into the worksite culture, combining health risk assessments with referral to evidence-based interventions, targeting high-risk individuals, and tailoring programs to the individual's risk level, readiness to change, and preferences. Yet they found that current practice is not consistent with best evidence. While many worksites offer some form of health promotion programming, strategies most commonly used are information focused, not comprehensive, and do not involve evidence-based approaches considered the best practice. In addition, employee participation in worksite programs is low. Lemon and Estabrook note the tremendous potential for the Patient Protection and Affordable Care Act (ACA) to support and strengthen worksite health promotion, as it provides an opportunity to evaluate real-world implementation of worksite health promotion programs that are based on current evidence of best practices. The authors make a number of recommendations for research and practice, including the use of more rigorous study designs and measurement protocols to address methodological challenges to evaluating the impact of worksite health promotion interventions, better understanding of how to promote employer buy-in and employee participation, and exploring the use of technology-based interventions for greater reach.

In Chapter 21, Dobmeyer, Goodie, and Hunter draw our attention to the primary care setting as an important venue for implementing system interventions to support health behavior change in "Health Care Provider and System Interventions Promoting Health Behavior Change." A challenge to targeting health care systems has been the inadequate teaching of health behavior change during medical school and residency, resulting in a recent call for better integration of behavioral and social science training in undergraduate and graduate medical education. Research has shown that training alone, however, is not sufficient; structured office support and health care system-wide changes are needed for primary care providers to deliver health behavior change interventions, including systems to prompt assessment and brief intervention with linkage of patients with more intensive services, and the use of a team approach in the clinic to deliver counseling interventions. The authors lay out two models of integrated-collaborative care for primary care settings. The first are care management models, in which providers refer patients with specific clinical problems to a care manager who assists the patient in adhering to the provider's recommended behavioral treatment plan. While effective, Dobmeyer, Goodie, and Hunter note that this model has limited reach and impact beyond the one or two areas of clinical focus. In the second model, the Primary Care Behavioral Health (PCBH) model, behavioral health consultants (BHCs) embedded and integrated into the primary care clinic deliver targeted, evidence-based interventions for a wide range of problem behaviors, and model health behavior change skills for providers to improve their own skills. The authors make a convincing argument that existing fee-for-service models and mental health carve-outs do not allow for financial sustainability of integrating behavioral health into primary care, and recommend alternative funding strategies such as reimbursement for bundled services or higher payments for services involving collaborative team-based care. Consistent with the other chapters in this section, the authors note the need for multicomponent interventions; this could include exposure to behavior change principles and interventions early in medical school training and continued through continuing education, health care systems to support providers in delivering health behavior change interventions, and financial incentives for integrated-collaborative care models.

This section concludes with Chapter 22 by Cradock and Duncan on "The Role of the Built Environment in Supporting Health Behavior Change." This is an exciting and relatively new topic with tremendous potential to impact health behavior at the population level. The authors describe the benefits and limitations of existing tools by which the built environment is measured, recommending the use of multiple methods to provide the most comprehensive understanding of the built environment. Connecting to earlier chapters in this section, they note that context is an important factor on the impact of the built environment. For example, when designing interventions to improve nutrition and physical activity, the school environment is important for children and adolescents, while adult interventions may be best focused on the work environment. The authors note mixed findings regarding associations between the built environment and a variety of health behaviors, reflecting the challenges in conducting research in this burgeoning area (e.g., lack of feasibility in using random assignment). Cradock and Duncan provide a rich set of examples illustrating how built environment interventions can influence health behaviors. For instance, new technologies such as geographic information systems can identify areas needing environmental intervention or assist in tailoring individual interventions. School environments can influence both student and teacher/employee behaviors by making the "healthy choice the easy choice" through direct modification of the physical infrastructure (e.g., healthier options in the cafeteria and changes to the school playgrounds) along with education. The authors note that multicomponent interventions to the built environment that include both changes to the environment and informational strategies and behavior modification are most promising in having an impact on behavior. In a nice tie-in to the chapter on culture, behavior, and health in Section II of this book, the authors note how in the future, built environment interventions may be used to reduce health inequities by eliminating differential exposure to either health-promoting or health-harming environments.

19

School Interventions to Support Health Behavior Change

REBEKKA M. LEE
STEVEN L. GORTMAKER

LEARNING OBJECTIVES

- Explain the benefits of situating health behavior change interventions in schools.
- Name at least two challenges to implementing school-based health behavior change interventions and discuss strategies for overcoming these barriers.
- Describe and give examples of seven types of school-based health behavior change interventions.

WHY TARGET SCHOOLS?

Promoting health behavior change within the school setting is an excellent approach for impacting population health. Because people spend most their youth in the classroom, schools are a natural choice as settings to situate interventions that establish healthy habits early in life for the prevention of disease across the life course. Elementary, middle, and high schools as well as preschools and afterschool programs have the potential for tremendous reach. Particularly in the United States where public education has been mandated since the early 1900s but the right to health care is still up for debate, schools can promote healthy behaviors and deliver services to a broad population in a way that other settings cannot. Children spend roughly 1,260 hours (180 days, 7 hours per day) at school each year, while they will likely only spend about a half hour with a primary care provider during a yearly physical exam. Although doctors and other health care providers play a vital role in promoting health behaviors, schools can be critical supports to reinforce health messages via educational programming, provide more constant individualized services, and model healthy environments that can shift norms throughout a child's formative years of life (Lee & Gortmaker, 2012).

Developing strategies to promote health within schools could also help to address health disparities by influencing rural, low-income teens or city-dwelling children of color just as they would reach suburban White youth of higher income. However, while the impact of school-based health behavior change strategies may be great, public health professionals should keep in mind that the resources and quality of public schools, particularly in the United States, vary greatly. With about half of funding coming from local sources (Kenyon, 2007), initiatives within public schools must be carefully planned and implemented in order to serve populations that are most in need.

CHALLENGES IN WORKING WITH SCHOOLS

The first, and probably most evident, challenge for those hoping to promote health behaviors within schools is the fact that a school's primary mission is teaching (Lee & Gortmaker, 2012). All patient-centered health initiatives, health education, behavioral health interventions, technology-based strategies, system and environmental change efforts, and health policies should be designed to align with current school practices and mission to be most effective and sustainable over time. Interventions that explicitly aim to promote academic objectives such as building skills in reading, writing, and math as well as working to meet health goals will likely achieve the most support from teachers and school administrators (Gortmaker et al., 1999).

It is also important that school-based interventions are designed to be easily adaptable across a range of school norms and cultures (Lee & Gortmaker, 2012). This flexibility allows for local relevance that is also essential for buy-in from teachers, parents, students, and administrators. For example, nutrition interventions should allow for adaptation based on differences in the types of whole grains and produce that have the best cultural fit with the diets of the school population. Emphasizing the healthy choices available in people's regular diet such as serving corn tortillas over refined grain options in a school that is predominately Latino may have more acceptability than introducing unfamiliar whole grains such as quinoa or bulgur to a school menu.

Finding cost-effective strategies is particularly important for making health promotion appealing to education leaders, teachers, policy makers, and tax payers. Promoting health in public schools where budgets are tight and resources must be allocated carefully is particularly challenging. While cost-effectiveness research was first undertaken in the education field in the 1970s, only a few studies have compared the relative costs and effect of interventions in schools (Hummel-Rossi & Ashdown, 2002; Levin, 2001; Levin, Glass, & Meister, 1987). Interventions that have a broad reach and make use of existing personnel and infrastructure can be particularly cost-effective and may even be cost saving in the long run (Vos et al., 2010). One example of this type of cost-effectiveness strategy is the middle school nutrition and physical activity curriculum Planet Health, which weaves grade and subject specific lessons into existing class time, is led by classroom teachers, and requires minimal materials to implement (Franks et al., 2007; Gortmaker et al., 1999; Wang, Yang, Lowry, & Wechsler, 2003). While cost is a major challenge for creating change in educational settings, thoughtful planning and prioritization can help ensure that the right interventions are implemented for optimal impact on the health of all students.

INTERVENTIONS TO CHANGE HEALTH BEHAVIORS

EDUCATION AS HEALTH INTERVENTION

Before detailing the multitude of interventions shown to be effective in schools, it is important to highlight that education, in its own right, is a predictor of better health and should be acknowledged as an important strategy to promote healthy behaviors (Pincus, Callahan, & Burkhauser, 1987; Sander, 1995). Recognizing the profound influence of education on health, the United Nations has named the achievement of universal primary education as one of its eight Millennium Development Goals for 2015, and the World Health Organization (WHO) named schools as key settings to promote health in the 2008 *European Strategy for Child and Adolescent Health and Development* (United Nations, 2012; WHO, 2008).

GUIDELINES FOR HEALTH BEHAVIOR CHANGE IN SCHOOLS

Both the Centers for Disease Control and Prevention (CDC) and Schools for Health in Europe (SHE) have set forth guidance for how healthy behaviors can be promoted in schools. In the United States, the CDC's Coordinated School Health is meant to be a "systematic approach to improving the health and well-being of students so they can fully participate and be successful in school" (CDC, 2011). It names eight components for promoting health in the school setting: health education, physical education, health services, nutrition services, counseling and psychological services, healthy and safe school environment, staff health promotion, and family/community involvement (CDC, 2011). Its four overarching goals are to increase students' health-related knowledge, attitudes, and skills; improve students' health behaviors and health outcomes; improve student achievement; and improve social outcomes (Kolbe, 2002). In addition to laying out the Coordinated School Health framework, the CDC supports schools with guidance documents based on the latest science and works to monitor health in schools via tools such as the Youth Risk Behavior Survey, the School Health Profiles, the School Health Policies and Practices Study, and the Physical Education Curriculum Analysis Tool (CDC, 2011).

SHE takes a different, more holistic approach to promoting health in schools by emphasizing educational and health equity, sustainability, inclusion, empowerment, and democracy (www.schoolsforhealth.eu). Rather than addressing topics individually, their objective is to focus on achieving healthy, supportive school environments. Strategies to promote health include enhancing schools' physical spaces, strengthening programs on health-related topics, building democracy in schools through more student input, developing policies and materials for training teachers on health education, and improving teachers' communication and active teaching skills. SHE takes a multi-sectorial approach by encouraging coordination across educational, medical, and social service providers.

TYPES OF SCHOOL-BASED HEALTH BEHAVIOR CHANGE INTERVENTIONS

Promoting healthy behaviors in schools can take many forms. As a means of organizing these different approaches, we have developed a typology of school-based health behavior change interventions (Table 19.1) that displays seven category types, as well as a working definition and bulleted examples for each type. This typology and the summary of evidence-based interventions below present health behavior strategies from those focused most on the individual at the top to those that take the broadest population approach at the bottom. It is important to understand the impact of these levels for targeting behavior change when taking up health initiatives in schools (Stokols, 1996). For example, interventions that rely on nurses or specialized professionals like therapists may be time-consuming and costly to deliver. They might only be available to a small part of the school population; however, the benefits to individuals most in need will likely be quite high. Conversely, policy interventions at the national, state, and schools level are usually relatively low in cost and easy to disseminate resulting in a small impact

TABLE 19.1 Typology of School-Based Health Behavior Change Interventions

TYPE	DEFINITION	EXAMPLES
Patient-centered	Delivery of individualized clinical services	Body mass index screening Mental health assessments & counseling
Education	Health lessons and messages designed to lay the foundation for lifelong health	Sexual health education Classroom-based nutrition & physical activity curricula Substance use prevention interventions Healthy messaging directed toward students, staff, and parents on posters, newsletters, etc.
Behavioral	Strategies to improve children's social or emotional development	Classroom-based social skills development Executive functioning
Technology	Health interventions delivered by electronic devices and strategies designed to limit the damaging effects of excessive technology use	Computer-based learning Policies limiting smartphones or Channel 1 television in schools
System	School practices or environments that are intended to promote health for children	School food service Physical education Afterschool sports Healthy options in vending machines on school grounds
Policy	Regulations implemented at the national, state, district, or school level intended to promote children's health in schools	District wellness policies State law mandating physical activity time National policy mandating access to potable drinking water during lunch
Multicomponent	Strategies intervene at multiple levels to affect behavior change	Planet Health CATCH Safer Choices

to a broad population of students. Schools should seek to match the level of intervention they choose with the scope of the health problem they aim to address. Often a mixture of individualized and population approaches, highlighted in the multicomponent type, are appropriate for meetings the needs of a given student body.

Patient-Centered Interventions

Patient-centered interventions are those that deliver individualized clinical services to children within the school setting. According to the latest data from the School Health Policies and Programs (SHPPS) assessment, 86% of U.S. schools have a part or full time nurse to deliver health services (Kann, Brener, & Wechsler, 2007). Packaging behavior change interventions with traditional school-based health services like first aid and CPR, medication administration, vaccination, and vision and hearing screenings can be an effective way to address child health needs. In the case of childhood obesity, school-based nutrition counseling has been successful in changing the eating behaviors among overweight youth (Story, 1999). More recently, schools have attempted (with limited evidence of success) to charge nurses with tackling the prevention of the disease—measuring body mass index that becomes part of a "report card" with tailored information and advice for behavior change delivered to all parents with the weight status of their children (Chomitz, Collins, Kim, Kramer, & McGowan, 2003; Nihiser et al., 2007).

Another example of patient-centered care in the school setting is the work of school-based speech–language pathologists, who work with children to improve communication behaviors and outcomes. These practitioners use a variety of strategies to address the various needs identified, from social communication to literacy to sound production and intelligibility, in students' individualized education plans (IEPs) (Cirrin et al., 2010). While research on the effectiveness of these interventions in schools is limited, a recent review found that speech and language interventions delivered in the classroom may be similarly effective to traditional pullout approaches that work with students one on one (Cirrin et al., 2010).

In just over 6% of U.S. schools, the nurse's office has transformed into a full service school-based health clinic (Kann et al., 2007). These clinics have been particularly important for serving as a "medical home" to teenagers in urban and rural areas who often do not receive primary care services and, in some cases, provide improved access to care for the entire family. They take an integrated approach to care—focusing on both physical and mental health—and encourage behavior change by emphasizing the modifiable risk factors (e.g., smoking, drug use, inactivity, unsafe sexual activity, and poor diet) that most contribute to health problems in youth (Brindis & Sanghvi, 1997). Studies of school-based health clinics have found higher utilization of primary clinical care, improved educational outcomes, and increased contraceptive use among students (Brindis & Sanghvi, 1997).

Education

Educational interventions are health lessons and messages designed to lay the foundation for lifelong health. Health education in schools has been implemented across grade levels and can be delivered by classroom teachers or specialists such as physical education teachers, school social workers or psychologists, or full time health teachers. Data from 2006 indicate that about 75% of U.S. states have a policy requiring schools to follow national or state health education standards (Kann et al., 2007).

School-based education interventions have been shown to increase such health-promoting behaviors as bicycle helmet wearing (Owen, Kendrick, Mulvaney, Coleman, & Royal, 2011), physical activity (Dobbins, De Corby, Robeson, Husson, & Tirilis, 2009), fruit and vegetable consumption (Gortmaker et al., 1999), as well as decrease television watching (Dobbins et al., 2009; Gortmaker et al., 1999). Research also demonstrates evidence for decreases in risk taking behaviors such as smoking (Thomas & Perera, 2008), early drug use (Faggiano et al., 2008), and unprotected sex for the prevention of unintended pregnancies (Oringanje et al., 2010) if educational interventions include components on social influences and skill building in addition to the delivery of information. On the other hand, there is no strong evidence in support of classroom interventions for the prevention of child sexual abuse (Zwi et al., 2009) or driver education in schools for the prevention of traffic accident involvement (Roberts & Kwan, 2008), and results are mixed on the effectiveness of school-based interventions to prevent alcohol misuse (Foxcroft & Tsertsvadze, 2011).

Behavioral Interventions

For the purposes of this chapter, behavioral interventions refer to school-based strategies aimed at addressing children's social and emotional development. It is estimated that about 78% of U.S. schools have a counselor employed full or part time for the delivery of mental health and social services (Kann et al., 2007). Research has shown a range of behavioral interventions to be effective in schools. Programs for preventing or reducing aggressive behavior have proven successful, particularly among high-risk youth (Wilson, Lipsey, & Derzon, 2003). Similarly, studies have shown reductions in symptoms of anxiety among participants in prevention and early intervention programs targeting these outcomes (Neil & Christensen, 2009). To date, most of these anxiety prevention programs have been conducted among high school age youth employing cognitive behavioral therapy (Neil & Christensen, 2009). A range of interventions that aim to improve young children's executive functioning including cognitive flexibility, inhibition, and working memory have proven effective (Diamond & Lee, 2011). Children with attention deficit hyperactivity disorder, those with lower working memory spans, and those from low-income families have shown particularly high gains. While these interventions can be delivered by specialists individually, children have also shown significant improvements in executive functioning via curriculum delivery by classroom teachers (Diamond & Lee, 2011).

Technology

The category of technological health behavior change interventions is twofold in meaning: it refers both to health interventions delivered by electronic devices such as computers, iPads, and smartphone apps as well as interventions designed to limit the harmful effects of excessive technology use. Research on health behavior interventions that utilize a computer-based platform is relatively sparse; those that have evidence for effectiveness have the commonality of delivering tailored change strategies that other modes cannot do as easily. For instance, the Cogmed working memory training uses computer games that become progressively more difficult to improve young children's skills for better executive functioning (Diamond & Lee, 2011). Highly interactive computerized cognitive behavioral therapy has also been tested in schools to meet the emotional health needs of students, showing success at reducing anxiety as both a targeted intervention delivered to high-risk individuals and a more general population-based approach (Attwood, Meadows, Stallard, & Richardson, 2012). New technologies like iPad and smartphone apps are quickly emerging as useful tools to help promote the health behaviors of students. For instance, researchers have developed a web app to help afterschool providers validly assess the practices of their programs for supporting children's physical activity and healthy eating; and the eSchoolCare iPad app delivers step-by-step evidence-based guidance to school nurses for the management of children's common chronic conditions like asthma, attention deficit disorder, diabetes, and allergies (Anderson, 2012; Lee, Mozaffarian, Gortmaker, Burchard, & Gortmaker, 2012). In addition, there are a host of apps to support lessons for the promotion of physical activity and healthy eating behaviors designed specifically for physical education teachers (www.sparkpe.org/blog/physical-education-pe-apps-for-teachers). These interventions demonstrate the influence that technology can have on health behavior change in the school setting; in particular, they highlight the potential to increase access to therapeutic strategies that are typically high cost and the ways new app technology is being developed to make school-based health promotion simpler.

Conversely, research across a wide variety of health fields has inquired about the possible harmful effect of technology—cell phone usage, television viewing, and excessive computer use—in the school setting. For instance, toxicologists are concerned with the harmful effects of radiation on teenagers and have studied the implementation of school policies to ban cell phone use in schools (Redmayne, Smith, & Abramson, 2011). They found that in New Zealand 87% of schools ban cell phone use, yet 42% of students reported texting daily at a median of 5 times each day (Redmayne et al., 2011), indicating that school policies are not very effective at eliminating cell phone use behaviors. As laptop computers are rapidly becoming used as part of regular daily classroom instruction, occupational health researchers are interested in developing ergonomic interventions for healthy computer usage (Ciccarelli, Portsmouth, Harris, & Jacobs, 2012). Meanwhile, researchers concerned with the harmful impacts of Internet usage, such as exposure to violent and sexual images, have investigated the acceptability of Internet filtering in schools (Subrahmanyam & Greenfield, 2008).

Researchers are also concerned with the harmful effects of television viewing within school walls on children's dietary and physical activity behaviors. Channel 1, the school-based news program operated by Alloy Media and Marketing that is delivered to students in over a quarter of U.S. schools, is the ultimate example of this risk—as teenagers are exposed daily in the classroom setting to advertisements geared specifically for them (Austin, Chen, Pinkleton, & Johnson, 2006). In fact, a survey indicated that students have significantly better recall of the advertisements they viewed on Channel 1 than the news stories; they also reported purchasing an average of 2.5 of the 11 advertised products on the survey, indicating the effectiveness of the marketing to teens (Austin et al., 2006). The American Academy of Pediatrics has expressed concern over this commercialization in the school setting, but the only intervention to address Channel 1 viewing has been to provide media literacy training alongside the programming (Austin et al., 2006).

This preliminary research demonstrates that initiatives aimed at reducing the potentially harmful effects of technology usage in schools are disparate and siloed; investigators should consider working together to develop studies that are meaningful across disciplines. As technology usage among children continues to increase, it will become imperative to maximize the benefits of using technology to support health behavior change while understanding any negative health impacts and developing school-based solutions to minimize these risks.

System

School practices or environments that are intended to promote health for children fall under the system category of health behavior change interventions. Two major facets of the school systems that influence child health are the meals and snacks delivered via school food services and the activity provided via physical education classes. School feeding programs have been developed primarily as a strategy for addressing hunger among disadvantaged youth (Kristjansson et al., 2009). Poor dietary intake can lead to such serious health outcomes as lower disease immunity, underweight, and poor cognition and attention (Kristjansson et al., 2009). In lower income countries where inadequate dietary intake is a common health behavior challenge, school feeding interventions have shown small positive effects on growth and cognition (Kristjansson et al., 2009). In higher income countries, as obesity and cardiovascular disease have increased, the aim of school feeding programs has shifted from providing students adequate caloric intake to promoting specific components of healthy eating in the school setting. Interventions designed to improve the healthfulness of foods and beverages served and available in schools have been successful (Goldberg et al., 2009; Osganian et al., 1996). Increases in water access have also been a recent and promising success. A group randomized control trial among afterschool programs that serve school-provided snacks was able to increase servings of water to children (Giles et al., 2012), and a study of water fountain installation in German public schools showed positive effects on risk of overweight at follow-up (Muckelbauer et al., 2009).

Physical education is another keystone of the school system that promotes healthy behaviors among students. While 78% of U.S. schools require some physical education for students, only 4% of elementary schools, 8% of middle schools, and 2% of high schools offer daily physical education for all students (Kann et al., 2007). Interventions to improve physical education have found some increases in child activity levels and fitness (Manios, Kafatos, & Mamalakis, 1998; McKenzie et al., 2004; Sallis et al., 2003) and afterschool sports have also been shown to contribute positively to students' physical activity in youth and adulthood (Bailey 2006). Other practice and environmental changes that have been effective at creating health behavior change in schools include making pricing and product changes to vending machines to improve healthy eating (Kocken et al., 2012) and delaying school start times to improve adolescents' sleep (Owens, Belon, & Moss, 2010).

Policy

Any regulations implemented at the national, state, district, or school level intended to promote children's health in schools are considered policies. At the local school and district level, research has shown that tobacco policies that are comprehensive and strictly enforced can decrease smoking behavior (Evans-Whipp et al., 2004), while school policies mandating nutrition guidelines can increase fruit and vegetable consumption, among other healthy eating behaviors (Jaime & Lock, 2009). Research on policies banning junk food from vending machines and school stores, found that state policies for elementary and middle schools corresponded to less junk food offered by schools, but this policy relationship was not found at the district level (Kubik et al., 2010). Policies to promote health behaviors even reach to the level of national policy. The recent passage of the Healthy, Hunger-Free Kids Act (www.fns.usda.gov/cnd/Governance/Legislation/CNR_2010.htm), which strengthens the health requirements for foods and beverages served as school meals, is one example of such policy.

Multicomponent Interventions

Multicomponent health behavior interventions are any strategies that contain two or more of the intervention types detailed above—this could include a curriculum that is implemented in conjunction with changes to the practices and environment within a school or a state policy that mandates implementation of clinical services for a high-risk population of students in the school setting. Planet Health and CATCH are two successful examples of multicomponent school-based interventions designed to improve child physical activity and nutrition behaviors for the prevention of child obesity (Gortmaker et al., 1999; Luepker et al., 1996). In Planet Health, educational and skill-building lessons promoting healthy changes in nutrition and physical activity behaviors were accompanied by changes to the physical education lessons and practices delivered in the school. Results showed that these two strategies reduced television viewing and increased fruit and vegetable consumption among middle school students; the prevalence of obesity among girls also decreased (Gortmaker et al., 1999). The CATCH elementary school intervention included a nutrition and physical activity classroom component and changes to physical education, and also consisted of changes to the meals delivered via school food service and a strategy to engage families. Studies of its effectiveness found that children in the intervention program reported significantly more minutes of vigorous activity than those in the control program (Luepker et al., 1996). Similar multicomponent obesity-prevention efforts have been successful at creating behavior change in afterschool settings as well (Gortmaker et al., 2012; Kelder et al., 2005). The YMCA-Harvard Food and Fitness Project, which utilized a combination of learning collaborative trainings with program staff to change practices at their programs and an evidence-based education curriculum (available at www.foodandfun.org), yielded increases in daily physical activity among elementary age children (Gortmaker et al., 2012). Safer Choices is an excellent demonstration of a multicomponent intervention designed to address students' sexual health risk behaviors (Coyle et al., 1999). Results indicate that this intervention that uses five components—school health promotion councils at the school organization level, curriculum and staff development, peer leadership, parent education, and activities to connect students to services within their community—increased condom and contraceptive usage (Coyle et al., 1999). Finally, a multicomponent asthma intervention that provided individual education to students, support for linking parents and students to physicians and nurses, and a school action committee has proven effective at improving young children's self-management behaviors (Bartholomew et al., 2006).

CONCLUSIONS

Although this overview demonstrates that there are numerous effective strategies for promoting healthy behaviors in schools, there is still much room to advance the field and make the most out of the school setting. As researchers are developing new school-based health interventions, they should look to the community-based participatory research (CBPR) approach for strategies to involve students, teachers, parents, administrators, and other school personnel (Israel, Schulz, Parker, & Becker, 1998; Leung, Yen, & Minkler, 2004). In CBPR, key stakeholders are included in all stages of the research process. They use their real world experience to help researchers determine if they are asking the right questions, designing and testing suitable interventions, and interpreting results appropriately. School-based health interventions developed via CBPR are likely to meet the needs of teachers and fit into the daily practices of schools with this attention to context. Furthermore, health behavior change strategies designed with early feedback from stakeholders have promise for making a sustained impact on child health over time.

Because health is not the first priority in schools and funds and staff time must first go toward academic subjects, finding cost-effective strategies for supporting health behavior change is an important area for future research that will gain long-term buy-in among school administrators and policy makers. To date, only a handful of cost-effectiveness research studies on school-based health behavior change strategies have been conducted. Obesity-prevention programs like Planet Health (Wang et al., 2003) and the afterschool Georgia Fit Kid Project (Wang et al., 2008) have shown evidence of cost-effectiveness, as have the Project Toward No Tobacco Use (Wang, Crossett, Lowry, Sussman, & Dent, 2001) and the Safer Choices sexual health intervention (Wang et al., 2000).

The science of dissemination and implementation is an emerging field of research that needs further application in the study of school-based health initiatives. Studying dissemination and implementation shifts the focus from determining the efficacy of school-based interventions to investigating whether (and how) intervention can be implemented as intended by school personnel and maintained over time (Lee & Gortmaker, 2012). Researchers looking specifically at school-based interventions have determined that factors related to the intervention design, such as its cost and time, the quality and amount of training required, and how well the intervention is standardized and incorporated into typical school practices, influence its effectiveness (Payne & Eckert, 2010; Rohrbach, D'Onofrio, Backer, & Montgomery, 1996). Factors beyond the intervention, such as characteristics of the teacher or other school personnel (e.g., years of experience, motivation, and education level), may also influence effectiveness in schools (Klimes-Dougan et al., 2009; Payne & Eckert, 2010; Ransford, Greenberg, Domitrovich, Small, & Jacobson, 2009). Looking beyond the classroom, researchers have also investigated how school and external community factors influence the success of health behavior interventions in schools (Klimes-Dougan et al., 2009; Payne & Eckert, 2010; Ransford et al., 2009). The field of dissemination and implementation science is new and growing; future research is needed to understand the degree to which each of these types of factors influences health behavior change intervention success.

REFERENCES

Anderson, L. S. (2012). *The eSchoolCare project: School nurses improving care for children with chronic illness.* Paper presented at the International Nursing Research Congress, Madison, Wisconsin.

Attwood, M., Meadows, S., Stallard, P., & Richardson, T. (2012). Universal and targeted computerised cognitive behavioural therapy (Think, Feel, Do) for emotional health in schools: Results from two exploratory studies. *Child and Adolescent Mental Health, 17*(3), 173–178.

Austin, E. W., Chen, Y. C., Pinkleton, B. E., & Johnson, J. Q. (2006). Benefits and costs of Channel One in a middle school setting and the role of media-literacy training. *Pediatrics, 117*(3), E423–E433.

Bailey, R. (2006). Physical education and sport in schools: A review of benefits and outcomes. *Journal of School Health, 76,* 397–401.

Bartholomew, L. K., Sockrider, M. M., Abramson, S. L., Swank, P. R., Czyzewski, D. I., Tortolero, S. R., ... Tyrrell, S. (2006). Partners in school asthma management: Evaluation of a self-management program for children with asthma. *Journal of School Health, 76*(6), 283–290.

Brindis, C. D., & Sanghvi, R. V. (1997). School-based health clinics: Remaining viable in a changing health care delivery system. *Annual Review of Public Health, 18,* 567–587.

Centers for Disease Control and Prevention. (2011). *School health programs: Improving the health of our nation's youth—At a glance.* From http://www.cdc.gov/chronicdisease/resources/publications/aag/dash.htm

Chomitz, V. R., Collins, J., Kim, J., Kramer, E., & McGowan, R. (2003). Promoting healthy weight among elementary school children via a health report card approach. *Archives of Pediatrics & Adolescent Medicine, 157*(8), 765–772.

Ciccarelli, M., Portsmouth, L., Harris, C., & Jacobs, K. (2012). Promoting healthy computer use among middle school students: A pilot school-based health promotion program. *Work: A Journal of Prevention, Assessment & Rehabilitation, 41*, 851–856.

Cirrin, F. M., Schooling, T. L., Nelson, N. W., Diehl, S. F., Flynn, P. F., Staskowski, M., ... Adamczyk, D. F. (2010). Evidence-based systematic review: Effects of different service delivery models on communication outcomes for elementary school-age children. *Language Speech and Hearing Services in Schools, 41*(3), 233–264.

Coyle, K., Basen-Engquist, K., Kirby, D., Parcel, G., Banspach, S., Harrist, R., ... Weil, M. (1999). Short-term impact of safer choices: A multicomponent, school-based HIV, other STD, and pregnancy prevention program. *Journal of School Health, 69*(5), 181–188.

Diamond, A., & Lee, K. (2011). Interventions shown to aid executive function development in children 4 to 12 years old. *Science, 333*(6045), 959–964.

Dobbins, M., De Corby, K., Robeson, P., Husson, H., & Tirilis, D. (2009). School-based physical activity programs for promoting physical activity and fitness in children and adolescents aged 6-18 (Review). *The Cochrane Library* (3).

Evans-Whipp, T., Beyers, J. M., Lloyd, S., Lafazia, A. N., Toumbourou, J. W., Arthur, M. W., & Catalano, R. F. (2004). A review of school drug policies and their impact on youth substance use. *Health Promotion International, 19*(2), 227–234.

Faggiano, F., Vigna-Taglianti, F., Versino, E., Zambon, A., Borraccino, A., & Lemma, P. (2008). School-based prevention for illicit drugs' use (Review). *The Cochrane Library* (3).

Foxcroft, D. R., & Tsertsvadze, A. (2011). Universal school-based prevention programs for alcohol misuse in young people. *Cochrane Database of Systematic Reviews* (5).

Franks, A., Kelder, S. H., Dino, G. A., Horn, K. A., Gortmaker, S. L., Wiecha, J. L., & Simoes, E. J. (2007). School-based programs: Lessons learned from CATCH, Planet Health, and Not-On-Tobacco. *Preventing Chronic Disease, 4*(2), A33.

Giles, C. M., Kenney, E. L., Gortmaker, S. L., Lee, R. M., Thayer, J. C., Mont-Ferguson, H., & Cradock, A. L. (2012). Increasing water availability during afterschool snack: Evidence, strategies, and partnerships from a group randomized trial. *American Journal of Preventive Medicine, 43*(3), S136–S142.

Goldberg, J. P., Collins, J. J., Folta, S. C., McLarney, M. J., Kozower, C., Kuder, J., ... Economos, C.D. (2009). Retooling food service for early elementary school students in Somerville, Massachusetts: The shape up Somerville experience. *Preventing Chronic Disease, 6*(3).

Gortmaker, S., Lee, R. M., Mozaffarian, R. S., Sobol, A. M., Nelson, T. F., Roth, B. A., & Wiecha, J. L. (2012). Impact of an after-school intervention on increases in children's physical activity. *Medicine and Science in Sports and Exercise, 44*(3), 450–457.

Gortmaker, S. L., Peterson, K., Wiecha, J., Sobol, A. M., Dixit, S., Fox, M. K., & Laird, N. (1999). Reducing obesity via a school-based interdisciplinary intervention among youth: Planet Health. *Archives of Pediatrics & Adolescent Medicine, 153*(4), 409–418.

Hummel-Rossi, B., & Ashdown, J. (2002). The state of cost-benefit and cost-effectiveness analyses in education. *Review of Educational Research, 72*(1), 1–30.

Israel, B. A., Schulz, A. J., Parker, E. A., & Becker, A. B. (1998). Review of community-based research: Assessing partnership approaches to improve public health. *Annual Review of Public Health, 19*, 173–202.

Jaime, P. C., & Lock, K. (2009). Do school based food and nutrition policies improve diet and reduce obesity? *Preventive Medicine, 48*(1), 45–53.

Kann, L., Brener, N. D., & Wechsler, H. (2007). Overview and summary: School Health Policies and Programs Study 2006. *Journal of School Health, 77*(8), 385–397.

Kelder, S., Hoelscher, D. M., Barroso, C. S., Walker, J. L., Cribb, P., & Hu, S. (2005). The CATCH Kids Club: A pilot after-school study for improving elementary students' nutrition and physical activity. *Public Health Nutrition, 8*(02), 133–140.

Kenyon, D. A. (2007). *The property tax-school funding dilemma.* Cambridge, MA: Lincoln Institute of Land Policy.

Klimes-Dougan, B., August, G. J., Lee, C. Y. S., Realmuto, G. M., Bloomquist, M. L., Horowitz, J. L., & Eisenberg, T. L. (2009). Practitioner and site characteristics that relate to fidelity of implementation: The early risers prevention program in a going-to-scale intervention trial. *Professional Psychology: Research and Practice, 40*(5), 467–475.

Kocken, P. L., Eeuwijk, J., van Kesteren, N. M. C., Dusseldorp, E., Buijs, G., Bassa-Dafesh, Z., & Snel, J. (2012). Promoting the purchase of low-calorie foods from school vending machines: A cluster-randomized controlled study. *Journal of School Health, 82*(3), 115–122.

Kolbe, L. (2002). Education reform and the goals of modern school health programs. *State Education Standard, 3*(4), 4–11.

Kristjansson, B., MacDonald, B., Krasevec, J., Janzen, L., Greenhalgh, T., Wells, G. A., ... Welch, V. (2009). School feeding for improving the physical and psychosocial health of disadvantaged students (Review). *The Cochrane Library* (1).

Kubik, M. Y., Wall, M., Shen, L., Nanney, M. S., Nelson, T. F., Laska, M. N., & Story, M. (2010). State but not district nutrition policies are associated with less junk food in vending machines and school stores in US public schools. *Journal of the American Dietetic Association, 110*(7), 1043–1048.

Lee, R. M., & Gortmaker, S. L. (2012). Health dissemination and implementation within schools. In R. C. Brownson, G. A. Colditz, & Proctor, E. K. (Eds.), *Dissemination and implementation research in health: Translating science to practice.* New York, NY: Oxford University Press.

Lee, R. M., Mozaffarian, R., Gortmaker, J., Burchard, J., & Gortmaker, S. (2012). *Apps for nutrition and physical activity education and environmental change in out-of-school time programs.* Paper presented at the American Public Health Association Annual Meeting, San Francisco, CA.

Leung, M. W., Yen, I. H., & Minkler, M. (2004). Community based participatory research: A promising approach for increasing epidemiology's relevance in the 21st century. *International Journal of Epidemiology, 33*(3), 499–506.

Levin, H. M. (2001). Waiting for Godot: Cost-effectiveness analysis in education. *New Directions for Evaluation, 90,* 55–68.

Levin, H. M., Glass, G. V., & Meister, G. R. (1987). Cost-effectiveness of computer-assisted instruction. *Evaluation Review, 11,* 50–72.

Luepker, R. V., Perry, C. L., McKinlay, S. M., Nader, P. R., Parcel, G. S., Stone, E. J., ... Johnson, C. C. (1996). Outcomes of a field trial to improve children's dietary patterns and physical activity. The Child and Adolescent Trial for Cardiovascular Health. CATCH collaborative group. *Journal of the American Medical Association, 275*(10), 768–776.

Manios, Y., Kafatos, A., & Mamalakis, G. (1998). The effects of a health education intervention initiated at first grade over a 3 year period: Physical activity and fitness indices. *Health Education Research, 13*(4), 593–606.

McKenzie, T. L., Sallis, J. F., Prochaska, J. J., Conway, T. L., Marshall, S. J., & Rosengard, P. (2004). Evaluation of a two-year middle-school physical education intervention: M-SPAN. *Medicine and Science in Sports and Exercise, 36*(8), 1382–1388.

Muckelbauer, R., Libuda, L., Clausen, K., Toschke, A. M., Reinehr, T., & Kersting, M. (2009). Promotion and provision of drinking water in schools for overweight prevention: Randomized, controlled cluster trial. *Pediatrics, 123*(4), e661–e667.

Neil, A. L., & Christensen, H. (2009). Efficacy and effectiveness of school-based prevention and early intervention programs for anxiety. *Clinical Psychology Review, 29*(3), 208–215.

Nihiser, A. J., Lee, S. M., Wechsler, H., McKenna, M., Odom, E., Reinold, C., ... Grummer-Strawn, L. (2007). Body mass index measurement in schools. *Journal of School Health, 77*(10), 651–671; quiz 722–654.

Oringanje, C., Meremikwu, M. M., Eko, H., Esu, E., Meremikwu, A., & Ehir, J. E. (2010). Interventions for preventing unintended pregnancies among adolescents (Review). *The Cochrane Library* (1).

Osganian, S. K., Ebzery, M. K., Montgomery, D. H., Nicklas, T. A., Evans, M. K., Mitchell, P. D., ... Parcel, G. S. (1996). Changes in the nutrient content of school lunches: Results from the CATCH eat smart food service intervention. *Preventive Medicine, 25*(4), 400–412.

Owen, R., Kendrick, D., Mulvaney, C., Coleman, T., & Royal, S. (2011). Non-legislative interventions for the promotion of cycle helmet wearing by children. *Cochrane Database of Systematic Reviews* (11).

Owens, J. A., Belon, K., & Moss, P. (2010). Impact of delaying school start time on adolescent sleep, mood, and behavior. *Archives of Pediatrics & Adolescent Medicine, 164*(7), 608–614.

Payne, A. A., & Eckert, R. (2010). The relative importance of provider, program, school, and community predictors of the implementation quality of school-based prevention programs. *Prevention Science : The Official Journal of the Society for Prevention Research, 11*(2), 126-141.

Pincus, T., Callahan, L. F., & Burkhauser, R. V. (1987). Most chronic diseases are reported more frequently by individuals with fewer than 12 years of formal education in the age 19–64 United States population. *Journal of Chronic Diseases, 40*(9), 865–874.

Ransford, C. R., Greenberg, M. T., Domitrovich, C. E., Small, M., & Jacobson, L. (2009). The role of teachers' psychological experiences and perceptions of curriculum supports on the implementation of a social and emotional learning curriculum. *School Psychology Review, 38*(4), 510–532.

Redmayne, M., Smith, E., & Abramson, M. J. (2011). Adolescent in-school cellphone habits: A census of rules, survey of their effectiveness, and fertility implications. *Reproductive Toxicology, 32*(3), 354–359.

Roberts, I., & Kwan, I. (2008). School-based driver education for the prevention of traffic crashes (Review). *The Cochrane Library* (4).

Rohrbach, L. A., D'Onofrio, C. N., Backer, T. E., & Montgomery, S. B. (1996). Diffusion of school-based substance abuse prevention programs. *American Behavioral Scientist, 39*, 919–934.

Sallis, J. F., McKenzie, T. L., Conway, T. L., Elder, J. P., Prochaska, J. J., Brown, M., ... Alcaraz, J. E. (2003). Environmental interventions for eating and physical activity: A randomized controlled trial in middle schools. *American Journal of Preventive Medicine, 24*(3), 209–217.

Sander, W. (1995). Schools and smoking. *Economics of Education Review, 14*(1), 23–33.

Stokols, D. (1996). Translating social ecological theory into guidelines for community health promotion. *American Journal of Health Promotion, 10*(4), 282–298.

Story, M. (1999). School-based approaches for preventing and treating obesity. *International Journal of Obesity, 23*, S43–S51.

Subrahmanyam, K., & Greenfield, P. (2008). Online communication and adolescent relationships. *Future of Children, 18*(1), 119–146.

Thomas, R. E., & Perera, R. (2008). School-based programmes for preventing smoking (Review). *The Cochrane Library* (4).

United Nations. Millennium Project. (2012). Retrieved from http://www.unmillenniumproject.org

Vos, T., Carter, R., Barendregt, J., Mihalopoulos, C., Veerman, J., Magnus, A., ...Wallace, A. (2010). *Assessing cost-effectiveness in prevention (ACE–Prevention): Final Report.* University of Queensland, Brisbane and Deakin University, Melbourne.

Wang, L. Y., Crossett, L. S., Lowry, R., Sussman, S., & Dent, C. W. (2001). Cost-effectiveness of a school-based tobacco-use prevention program. *Archives of Pediatrics & Adolescent Medicine, 155*(9), 1043–1050.

Wang, L. Y., Davis, M., Robin, L., Collins, J., Coyle, K., & Baumler, E. (2000). Economic evaluation of Safer Choices: A school-based human immunodeficiency virus, other sexually transmitted diseases, and pregnancy prevention program. *Archives of Pediatrics & Adolescent Medicine, 154*(10), 1017–1024.

Wang, L. Y., Gutin, B., Barbeau, P., Moore, J. B., Hanes, J., Johnson, M. H., ... Yin, Z. (2008). Cost-effectiveness of a school-based obesity prevention program. *Journal of School Health, 78*(12), 619–624.

Wang, L. Y., Yang, Q., Lowry, R., & Wechsler, H. (2003). Economic analysis of a school-based obesity prevention program. *Obesity Research, 11*(11), 1313–1324.

Wilson, S. J., Lipsey, M. W., & Derzon, J. H. (2003). The effects of school-based intervention programs on aggressive behavior: A meta-analysis. *Journal of Consulting and Clinical Psychology, 71*(1), 136–149.

World Health Organization (WHO). (2008). *European strategy for child and adolescent health and development.* Copenhagen, Denmark: WHO Regional Office for Europe.

Zwi, K., Woolfenden, S., Wheeler, D. M., O'Brien, T., Tait, P., & Williams, K. J. (2009). School-based education programmes for the prevention of child sexual abuse. *The Cochrane Library* (1).

20

Prevention and Management of Chronic Disease Through Worksite Health Promotion

STEPHENIE C. LEMON
BARBARA ESTABROOK

LEARNING OBJECTIVES

- Summarize the rationale and scientific evidence for providing health promotion programs at worksites.
- Describe the current state of worksite health promotion programs in practice, the current and predicted characteristics of the workforce, and the worksite environment.
- Identify challenges and gaps in the research literature of worksite health promotion, and make recommendations for future research and practice.

Worksite health promotion consists of employer-sponsored coordinated initiatives to improve employee health through programs and policies designed to facilitate healthy lifestyles and improve health and well-being (Centers for Disease Control and Prevention, Office on Smoking and Health, 2012). Worksite health promotion programs and policies (WHPPP) are offered with the intention of not only improving employee health, but also decreasing the financial burden that employers incur because of poor employee health and its impact on performance. Worksite health promotion is recognized as an important opportunity for improving the population's health. Healthy People 2020 includes objectives related to worksite health promotion, such as increasing the proportion of U.S. employers who offer worksite health promotion programs, and specific objectives related to worksite weight and nutrition counseling programs, opportunities for physical activity, tobacco-free policies, and stress reduction programs (U.S. Department of Health and Human Services, 2013). Several additional national organizations and initiatives, such as the Centers for Disease Control and Prevention (Centers for Disease Control and Prevention, Division of Population Health/Workplace Health Promotion, 2012), the Community Guide (Community Prevention Services Taskforce, 2011), and the U.S. National Physical Activity Action Plan (National Physical Activity Plan for the United States, 2009) also include WHPPP recommendations. The purpose of this chapter is to describe the rationale for offering WHPPP, to evaluate the current state of the scientific evidence in support of WHPPP, to describe the current state of WHPPP in practice, and to describe challenges and make future recommendations for research and practice specific to WHPPP.

RATIONALE FOR WORKSITE HEALTH PROMOTION PROGRAMS AND POLICIES

THE U.S. WORKING POPULATION

Worksites are an important venue for promoting health among adults, as worksites provide important opportunities to reach a substantial proportion of the U.S. adult population. Nearly two-thirds of the U.S. civilian adult population is in the labor force, and many employed persons spend a significant amount of their time at work. The American workforce includes a broad representation of sectors and occupations, which has changed significantly over time (Table 20.1) (U.S. Department of Labor, 2011). Occupational groups differ vastly in the demographic profiles of their employees. Adults in the workforce are diverse with respect to socio-demographic characteristics and industry and occupation (Bureau of Labor Statistics, 2011) (Table 20.2). In 2011, the median age of all employed persons was 42 years. The number of men employed outnumbered women by more than 8 million. The majority of the labor force in 2011 was made up of White workers (81%), with 15% being of Hispanic or Latino ethnicity, 12% Black or African American, and 5% Asians.

TABLE 20.1 Changes in U.S. Employment by Industry, 1972 and 2012

INDUSTRY	PERCENTAGE OF ALL U.S. WORKERS EMPLOYED, 1972	PERCENTAGE OF ALL U.S. WORKERS EMPLOYED, 2012
Government (federal, state, and local, public schools, military, etc.)	18.3%	16.6%
Wholesale and retail trade	15.7%	15.3%
Education and health services (private education, health care, nursing care, day care, etc.)	6.6%	15.2%
Professional and business services (accounting, administrative services, IT, legal services, etc.)	7.4%	13.4%
Leisure and hospitality (restaurants, hotels, the arts, museums, etc.)	6.9%	10.2%
Manufacturing	23.9%	9.0%
Financial activities (banking, real estate, insurance, etc.)	5.3%	5.8%
Construction	5.4%	4.2%
Other services	2.6%	4.0%
Transport and utilities	4.4%	3.4%
Media and telecommunications	2.8%	2.0%
Mining and logging	0.9%	0.6%

From Bureau of Labor Statistics (2011).

TABLE 20.2 Demographic Characteristics of Employed Persons by Occupational Group, 2011

	TOTAL	EMPLOYED MEN					EMPLOYED WOMEN				
		ALL	WHITE	BLACK	ASIAN	HISPANIC	ALL	WHITE	BLACK	ASIAN	HISPANIC
Total of employed persons (in thousands)	139,869	74,290	61,920	6,953	3,703	12,049	65,579	52,770	8,096	3,165	8,220
% participating in the labor force	64.1%	70.5%	71.3%	64.2%	73.2%	76.5%	58.1%	58.0%	59.1%	56.8%	55.9%
By occupational group											
Management, professional, and related	37.6%	34.4%	34.9%	23.5%	49.1%	15.6%	41.2%	42.3%	34.1%	44.4%	25.2%
Service	17.7%	14.7%	13.8%	22.3%	14.2%	21.9%	21.1%	19.9%	28.0%	21.8%	31.2%
Sales and office	23.6%	16.8%	16.6%	18.0%	17.1%	14.6%	31.4%	31.8%	30.8%	26.3%	31.8%
Natural resources, construction, and maintenance	9.3%	16.8%	17.9%	11.6%	6.5%	26.1%	0.8%	0.9%	0.5%	0.6%	1.8%
Production, transportation, and material moving	11.8%	17.4%	7.8%	24.6%	13.0%	21.8%	5.4%	5.1%	6.7%	6.9%	10.1%

From Bureau of Labor Statistics (2011).

WORKSITE AND OCCUPATIONAL RISK FACTORS FOR CHRONIC DISEASE

There are worksite and occupational factors that influence an individual's risk for behaviors associated with chronic conditions and that act as independent risk factors for chronic conditions. For example, worksites may constitute *obesogenic* environments. More and more jobs worldwide are sedentary in nature. A recent analysis of how Americans spend their time showed that from 1965 to 2009, energy expenditure in the United States dropped 32%, led by declining occupational activity (Ng & Popkin, 2012). Similar changes were seen in the United Kingdom, China, and Brazil. The large amount of time spent at work indicates that a substantial amount of calories is typically consumed while working. Occupational factors, including long hours, shift work, and high-demand, low-control work environments, have also been shown to be independent risk factors for obesity (Schulte et al., 2007).

EMPLOYER BENEFITS OF WORKSITE HEALTH PROMOTION PROGRAMS AND POLICIES

From the employers' perspective, there is a strong rationale to seeking opportunities to reduce health-related costs. As worksites commonly provide health insurance benefits to employees (Blumenthal, 2006), there is a direct economic benefit to offering programs that can reduce costs. Costs of employee illness to employers and the U.S. economy are enormous and unsustainable. Costs incurred by employers include direct medical costs and costs related to decreased productivity, such as absenteeism, lost productivity while on the job (*presenteeism*), and lost productivity of caretakers (Goetzel & Ozminkowski, 2008).

In 2012, the average cost of employer-sponsored health insurance premiums was $15,745 for family coverage, of which employees paid 73%. This represents a total premium increase of 97% since 2002 (Kaiser Family Foundation & Health Research & Educational Trust [HRET], 2012). A 2012 study of 92,486 employees at seven organizations over an average 3-year period assessed the impact of 10 modifiable chronic disease risk factors on employer and employee health care costs. Overall, this analysis found that the 10 risk factors accounted for 22.4% of all costs, with clinical indicators (high blood glucose, obesity, and high blood pressure), health behaviors (smoking and physical inactivity), and depressive symptoms and high stress levels all important contributors (Goetzel et al., 2012). Disparities in health care costs within the worksite setting are similar to those that occur overall within the U.S. population, with risk of chronic disease inversely associated with income and education level, and persons of racial/ethnic minority backgrounds and those in the South experiencing highest rates of lifestyle risk behaviors and chronic disease diagnosis (Mendes, 2010).

In addition to direct medical costs, absenteeism due to illness or injury is higher among persons with poor health indicators. For example, a meta-analysis found that smokers have a 33% increased risk of absenteeism, compared to non-smokers, equivalent to an average of 2.7 days per year (Weng, Ali, & Leonardi-Bee, 2013). A multi-site study of 10,026 employees in diverse worksites observed that annual absenteeism costs were $872 for normal weight employees compared to $1,180 for obese employees (Goetzel et al., 2010).

EMPLOYEE BENEFITS OF WORKSITE HEALTH PROMOTION PROGRAMS AND POLICIES

WHPPP provide potential benefits through opportunities for employees to improve health and quality of life. WHPPP offer employees access to resources that might otherwise be unavailable (Goetzel & Ozminkowski, 2008) while potentially alleviating the additional barriers of cost, limited time, and inconvenience (Cahill, Moher, & Lancaster, 2008). The contained worksite environment and existence of ongoing relationships allow potential social support and positive peer pressure. At the institutional level, organizational support and a culture of health can support positive social norms and healthy environments and policies. Each of these factors is a key facilitator of health behavior change (Lemon, Liu, Magner, Schneider, & Pbert, 2013; Lemon et al., 2009). There are also potential financial benefits to employees through incentive-based programs and reductions in health insurance premiums, which are increasingly recommended.

WORKSITES AS A VENUE FOR HEALTH PROMOTION

From an intervention implementation perspective, worksites offer several advantages (Fabius & Frazee, 2009). Worksites have access to concentrated, large, and relatively stable populations of people who share geographic proximity and often have common characteristics and goals (Goetzel & Ozminkowski, 2008). In addition, worksites provide access to populations that exhibit high levels of risk, but otherwise may not seek out or have access to health promotion programs (Cahill et al., 2008). Workplaces typically have an organizational structure, shared physical spaces including work space and places to consume meals or beverages, and internal communication mechanisms, all of which can be used in support of WHPPP. Other common features that can be utilized, if available, to facilitate employee health include health insurance and other employee benefits, occupational health and safety departments, human resource departments with an employee health mission, interior and exterior physical plant attributes, and cafeterias and vending options, among others. In addition, worksites have the ability to implement organizational policies supporting health and wellness.

SOCIAL ECOLOGICAL MODEL OF WORKSITE HEALTH PROMOTION

Social ecological models (Green, Richard, & Potvin, 1996; Sallis, Owen, & Fisher, 2008) provide a useful framework for understanding how the worksite can affect individual health and well-being, and in turn, how worksite wellness interventions can be designed. The social ecological model is described in detail in Chapter 2. In the context of the worksite environment, levels of influence that affect worker health include organizational factors such as interpersonal environments, physical environments, worksite systems, and worksite policies, each of which impacts the larger organizational culture and climate, as well as individual factors. These levels are depicted in Figure 20.1.

The Organizational Health Environment Model (OHEM) provides a helpful framework from which to conceptualize organizational factors that impact employee health and health behaviors (Golaszewski, Allen, & Edington, 2008). The OHEM posits that three domains within an organization impact health: work factors, physical structural factors, and organizational cultural factors, represented as the three outer layers of the social ecological model shown in Figure 20.1. *Work factors* relate to the primary business of the organization and include organizational size, industry type, management style, the economic climate of the organization and industry and associated job security, job design, performance demands, and employee control. *Physical structural factors* are organizational characteristics and resources that provide opportunities for health

FIGURE 20.1 Social ecological model for worksite health promotion interventions.

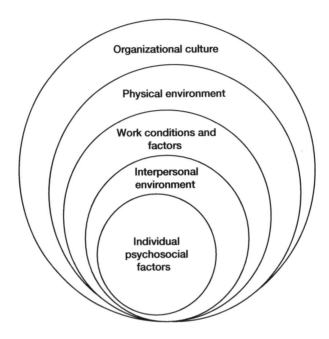

promotion activities such as facilities, benefits plans, and policies that are directly intended to influence health.

The OHEM posits that *organizational culture* influences employee health behaviors through five dimensions: norms, values, touch points, peer support, and overall cultural climate. *Organizational norms* are implicitly or explicitly defined acceptable and expected ways of behaving. *Values* refer to collective beliefs about health and health behaviors within an organization. *Touch points* include formal and informal mechanisms by which culture is reinforced. Such mechanisms are diverse and specific to a given organization. Some examples include communication systems, leadership and peer behavioral modeling, recognition and reward programs, and participation in symbolic initiatives (e.g., sponsoring an employee sports team) that reflect a message of supporting health. *Peer support* includes the quality and quantity of assistance offered and received for health promotion activities. Interpersonal relationships within a worksite are unique to an individual employee and can include professional and personal relationships. Consistent with broader conceptualizations of social support in other venues, peer support within the worksite context can include tangible, emotional, and instrumental support. *Overall cultural climate* includes the cohesiveness of those within an organization which is influenced by having a common purpose, trust of the organization, and an overall sense of community.

Individually targeted intervention approaches to worksite health promotion activities are often based on constructs that form the basis of common health behavior change theories, such as the Health Belief Model, Social Cognitive Theory, the Theory of Reasoned Action, and stage-based models, such as the Transtheoretical Model of Change (Glanz, Rimer, & Viswanath, 2008) described in Chapter 2. Likewise, individually targeted intervention strategies can be aimed at improving knowledge, attitudes, beliefs, and skills, which can ultimately lead to improvements in health behaviors.

SCIENTIFIC EVIDENCE IN SUPPORT OF WORKSITE HEALTH PROMOTION

A growing body of research has examined the effectiveness of interventions that incorporate a range of programs and policies designed to improve health behaviors and health outcomes within the worksite setting. Such interventions have addressed a range of disease risk factors, such as nutrition, physical activity, obesity, and tobacco, as well as chronic disease management. A variety of strategies have been tested, consistent with the social ecological model described above. Broadly, interventions fall into two categories: population-based strategies that target all employees regardless of risk factors or health status, and strategies that are targeted specifically at high-risk employees with specific risk factors or conditions. Outcomes assessed in these studies have included health and disease outcomes, health behavior changes, and economic indicators that are important to employers, namely absenteeism, presenteeism, disability, and health care utilization, with a focus on return on investment analysis.

The sections below describe the current state of the scientific literature in four of the most commonly assessed areas of worksite health promotion: health risk assessments (HRAs); tobacco and smoking prevention and cessation; nutrition, physical activity, and obesity; and chronic disease management. Occupational safety and work-related stress reduction programs and policies are beyond the scope of this chapter.

HEALTH RISK ASSESSMENTS

Health risk assessments (HRAs) can be described as programs in which individual employee health data are collected and used to establish a personal disease risk profile. Employers collect data using methods such as electronic and written questionnaires, medical record abstraction, and in-person clinical assessments with interviews. A range of information can be collected in HRAs, such as lifestyle behaviors (e.g., tobacco use and alcohol use), family history of specific diseases, and biometric screenings (e.g., body mass index and blood pressure). Feedback from this data can be provided to employees in the form of a qualitative assessment of risk status overall or for specific conditions, quantitative results from the tests given, or a summarized risk profile or score. Feedback can be provided in a variety of verbal, print, and electronic formats.

HRAs often function as a "gateway" intervention (Soler et al., 2010), with results and feedback used as the basis for referrals and linkages to interventions aimed at reducing risk. A variety of referral interventions have been examined. These generally reflect the types of individually targeted strategies tested and offered in other settings and can include health education, counseling, pharmacologic treatments, and financial incentives.

A recent systematic review performed by Soler and colleagues (Soler et al., 2010) on behalf of the Task Force on Community Preventive Services assessed published intervention studies that evaluated the effectiveness of HRAs with feedback across a range of health and risk indicators, including diet, physical activity, tobacco, alcohol, seatbelt use, blood pressure, body composition, cholesterol, and fitness. This included 32 studies that evaluated HRAs with feedback alone and 59 studies that evaluated HRAs with feedback and referral to additional interventions. This review concluded that HRAs can be effective when coupled with referrals to evidence-based individually targeted intervention strategies, such as those described in the subsequent sections. Based on these reviews, the Guide to Community Preventive Services (Community Prevention Services Taskforce, 2011a) recommends HRAs with feedback and referrals as an evidence-based worksite health promotion strategy. The evidence in support of HRAs standing alone or providing feedback without referral was deemed to be insufficient.

TOBACCO AND SMOKING PREVENTION AND CESSATION

Consistent with research conducted in other settings, worksite-based interventions targeting tobacco use include those directed at the entire workplace, including bans and restrictions on smoking and those designed to help individuals quit smoking.

A recent systematic review of smoke-free policies was conducted for the Task Force on Community Preventive Services (Hopkins et al., 2010), examining policies that prohibit smoking and evidence regarding the impact of these policies on smoking. The review found that smoke-free policies result in decreased smoking, increased quit attempts, increased cessation rates, and decreased smoking prevalence. The studies cover a wide range of populations, communities, and individual worksites, suggesting that findings are applicable to almost all workplaces in the United States and elsewhere. Economic studies included in this review found that smoke-free policies are nine times more cost-effective than free nicotine replacement programs, and estimated a net benefit of smoke-free policies of $48 billion to $89 billion annually in the United States.

Banning or restricting smoking in the workplace has become very common. Restrictions range from smoking allowed in designated outdoor areas to complete bans. Smoking restrictions have been enacted by employers as well as by local and state governments. As of 2012, 48 states had some form of smoking restrictions in government workplaces and 42 states restricted smoking to some extent in private workplaces (Centers for Disease Control and Prevention). Such bans reduce rates of smoking and incidence of heart attack (Hurt et al., 2012) as well as reduce exposure to secondhand smoke.

A 2008 systematic review of workplace-based interventions to help individual smokers quit or cut down, identified 51 randomized or quasi-randomized trials covering 53 interventions (Cahill et al., 2008). Thirty-seven studies assessed interventions aimed at individual workers, including group therapy, individual counseling, self-help materials, nicotine replacement therapy, and social support. Group programs, individual counseling, and nicotine replacement increased cessation rates, as has been found in reviews of smoking cessation interventions in other settings. Self-help materials were less effective. Combining several smoking cessation reviews, Cahill and colleagues (2008) found no evidence that intensive counseling is more effective than brief counseling, nor that either group counseling or individual counseling is more effective. They also note the historically low rate of recruitment into counseling as a limitation of the method. The workplace review included 16 studies testing multi-faceted comprehensive programs, which did not reduce the prevalence of smoking. The authors conclude that despite a strong theoretical foundation for approaches that integrate smoking cessation with comprehensive worksite health promotion programs, studies testing such approaches have not decreased overall prevalence of smoking (Cahill et al., 2008).

Competitions and incentives for smoking cessation as solitary interventions are not supported by sufficient evidence, but the Community Prevention Services Task Force (2011) does recommend their use when combined with other interventions to increase individual smoking cessation. Studies providing the evidence for this recommendation evaluated additional interventions that included client education, smoking cessation groups, self-help cessation materials, telephone cessation support, workplace smoke-free policies, and social support networks. These findings are echoed in a more recent and broader review of incentives for smoking cessation across intervention settings. Nineteen randomized controlled trials were identified. Only one of the 19 had significantly higher quit rates beyond the 6-month follow-up for the group receiving incentives, and that trial offered large cash payments for abstinence from smoking (up to $750), relying on referrals to local smoking cessation providers instead of offering cessation programs (Volpp et al., 2009). There was no clear evidence of effectiveness in the remaining trials and early success dropped off when incentives were discontinued.

Availability of incentives may increase quit attempts but does not seem to enhance cessation rates (Cahill & Perera, 2011).

NUTRITION, PHYSICAL ACTIVITY, AND OBESITY INTERVENTIONS

A growing body of research has assessed WHPPP focused on improving dietary quality, increasing physical activity, and weight control through dietary and physical activity strategies. We describe this literature together because a substantial proportion of this literature examined a combination of weight and behavioral outcomes.

In general, effective individually targeted interventions focused on behavior change are similar to those that have demonstrated success in other settings. Individual and group-based weight loss interventions (Aldana et al., 2005, 2006; Dallam & Foust, 2013; Dejoy, Padilla, Wilson, Vandenberg, & Davis, 2012) that have incorporated state-of-the-art behavioral strategies focused on building knowledge and skills for goal setting, self-monitoring, and problem solving have successfully achieved modest weight loss when delivered in the worksite setting. Such interventions have typically involved multiple sessions over an extended period of time. Less intensive educational and information strategies have typically proven ineffective in promoting meaningful weight loss outcomes (Benedict & Arterburn, 2008). Like effective strategies for weight loss, effective dietary and physical activity strategies targeting individuals largely build from a strong theoretical base such as cognitive-behavioral, education, motivational enhancement, or social influence (Hutchinson & Wilson, 2012). Individual and group-based programs that teach behavioral skills through strategies such as modeling and goal setting and/or that provide social support can be effective. Programs based on motivational enhancement showed the largest short- and long-term change (Hutchinson & Wilson, 2012). These behaviorally focused programs have been tested with and without financial incentives, and both conditions appear to hold promise for weight management, raising the question of whether incentives are needed (Archer et al., 2011). Educational programs to improve dietary behaviors, particularly fruit and vegetable consumption and fat consumption, have demonstrated small improvements both when offered alone and as part of multicomponent programs. A common limitation of this body of work is lack of long-term effectiveness (Ni Mhurchu, Aston, & Jebb, 2010).

Incentives and competitions have demonstrated modest effectiveness in improving behaviors and outcomes in worksite settings, particularly for physical activity and weight loss (Archer et al., 2011). Competition-based interventions include individual and group-based programs in which employees try to maximize performance or outcomes over a defined period of time, and are often combined with rewards or incentives. Rewards or incentives are provided for achieving milestones or for winning. Incentives tested have included financial incentives for participation in programs, insurance benefits, such as lower co-pays and premiums, and non-monetary incentives, such as prizes or merchandise.

Environmental and policy targeted interventions have aimed to increase access to opportunities for making healthy choices at the worksite. Examples of physical-activity-focused interventions include building walking trails and having onsite fitness centers. Diet-focused interventions have included initiatives focused on food availability and providing information to improve behavioral choices. For example, cafeteria and vending modifications have been implemented to increase availability of healthy foods and beverages, decrease availability of unhealthy foods, reduce costs for healthier foods, decrease portion sizes, and provide point-of-selection nutritional information. Collectively, studies that have evaluated the implementation of environmental and policy strategies alone have generally produced null or inconclusive results, and two recent systematic reviews concluded that the available scientific evidence does not support stand-alone environmental and policy strategies in the worksite setting (Archer et al., 2011; Kahn-Marshall & Gallant, 2012). However, studies that have incorporated these population-based strategies as part of multicomponent interventions that include, for example, strategies targeting employee awareness, knowledge, and skills demonstrate considerably more promise for impacting behaviors and weight outcomes (Archer et al., 2011).

DISEASE MANAGEMENT

Disease management is an increasing focus of workplace health promotion programs (Pelletier, 1991). Although health care plans provide coverage for and often services for management of chronic diseases, employers many times capitalize on access to employees by providing workplace-based disease management programs. Employer-based plans can achieve a level of consistency of approach and services for workers which may be lacking across various health plans that cover employees (Musich, Schultz, Burton, & Edington, 2004).

Over recent decades, a large body of literature has assessed the impact of worksite disease management programs on clinical and/or cost outcomes (Pelletier, 1991, 1993, 1996, 1999, 2001, 2005, 2011). The vast majority of these studies were conducted in corporate settings; many were demonstration projects and showed positive outcomes. Worksite-based disease management programs have addressed a broad range of health conditions that impact employee health and productivity and cost, including cardiovascular disease, diabetes, depression, asthma, arthritis, and cancer screening (Musich et al., 2004).

Programmatic strategies have largely focused on education and self-care (Serxner & Anderson, 2002) and include disease screening, education, and behavioral skill development components (Musich et al., 2004). More recent WHPPP have incorporated technology-based delivery such as personal health records, electronic medical records, web-based health improvement programs, and handheld information portals for various purposes including tracking, reminders, oversight, reporting, and communication components (Pelletier, 1991, 1993, 1996, 1999, 2001, 2005, 2011). Multicomponent or comprehensive programs have resulted in the greatest impact on clinical outcomes and are more cost-beneficial than single-focus or intermittent programs. The crucial element is individualized risk reduction, targeting high-risk persons, within a context of multicomponent or comprehensive programming as distinct from single-component programs (Whitmer, Pelletier, Anderson, Baase, & Frost, 2003). Stratification of persons with disease by level of risk and individual tailoring of disease management interventions improve a program's cost-effectiveness. Tailoring of materials, frequency, and method of contact to the individual's risk level, self-efficacy, readiness to change, and preferences is an important element of successful worksite disease management programs. Others are the development of multiple points of contact (managers, peers, health promotion, and occupational health staff) and incorporating access to external resources that can be organized to reinforce messages and support individual efforts (Serxner & Anderson, 2002).

SUMMARY OF EVIDENCE

A range of approaches to WHPPP conducted to date have demonstrated modest effects on health behaviors and outcomes and meaningful return on investment with both reduced direct medical care costs and reduced costs associated with absenteeism. For example, a meta-analysis of effectiveness of smoking cessation, physical activity, healthy nutrition, and/or obesity programs conducted by Rongen and colleagues showed small effect sizes overall, with greater effectiveness in younger populations, and with weekly intervention contacts (Rongen, Robroek, van Lenthe, & Burdorf, 2013). Another meta-analysis by Baicker and colleagues of wellness programs conducted primarily in large worksites observed a decrease of $3.27 in direct medical care costs for every dollar spent on worksite wellness programs focused on weight loss and fitness, smoking cessation, and multiple risk factors (Baicker, Cutler, & Song, 2010). This study also found a return on investment of $2.73 for absenteeism. Multicomponent programs typically demonstrate greater impact on both health and financial outcomes. Comprehensive WHPPP have been described as having several critical components: programs that are well integrated into the worksite culture and climate, multiple approaches to reaching and engaging numerous people, a variety of programs that meet the needs of diverse employees, health screenings that identify at-risk individuals, health programs that foster awareness, motivation and skills, supportive social and physical environments, linkages to evidence-based programs and treatments that have a foundation in behavioral theory, and visible support from organizational leadership (Goetzel & Ozminkowski, 2008; O'Donnell, 2009; Sparling, 2010; U.S. Department of Health and Human Services, 2000).

CURRENT STATE OF WORKSITE HEALTH PROMOTION PROGRAMS AND POLICIES IN PRACTICE

EMPLOYER PARTICIPATION IN WORKSITE HEALTH PROMOTION PROGRAMS AND POLICIES

The 2012 annual survey of employer benefits conducted by the Kaiser Family Foundation and Health Research and Educational Trust provides the best available information on the state of WHPPP in practice (Kaiser Family Foundation & Health Research & Educational Trust [HRET], 2012). This nationally representative telephone survey of human resource and benefits managers of 2,121 worksites found that 63% of companies with three or more employees that offered health insurance benefits also offered at least one of eight types of health promotion programs assessed. This varied by company size, with 63% of small companies (3 to 199 employees) offering at least one program compared to 94% of large companies (300 or more employees). WHPPP was primarily offered through health insurance benefits in 80% of small companies and 60% of large companies. Eighteen percent of worksites surveyed asked their employees to complete HRAs. The most commonly offered programs were health-education based (45% offered newsletters and 45% offered web-based resources), followed by smoking cessation programs (30%), onsite gyms or gym memberships (29%), weight loss programs (27%), nutrition classes (24%), and lifestyle coaching (22%). Incentive programs were not common, with 8% offering cash, gift card, or merchandise for participation, 3% lowering health insurance premium contributions, and 1% cost sharing. Large employers were substantially more likely to offer all program types than were small employers. While a sizeable proportion of companies offer some form of wellness program, the strategies provided are most commonly information focused (e.g., newsletters and web resources), with intensive behavioral change approaches much less common, and strategies offered are not routinely comprehensive nor aligned with evidence-based best practices.

The available evidence points to key barriers to employer adoption of evidence-based WHPPP. Perceptions of the high cost and the types of resources needed are critical. Despite scientific evidence supporting a return on investment of WHPPP, the considerable start-up costs required to initiate comprehensive WHPPP may be prohibitive. Small and mid-sized employers in particular may not have immediate access to resources, such as human resources or benefits departments, that could assume leadership on such initiatives (Hannon et al., 2012). Even when such departments are available, WHPPP may be an add-on to existing responsibilities. The addition of responsibilities to implement WHPPP initiatives without modification of job responsibilities has been shown to negatively impact implementation (Estabrook, Zapka, & Lemon, 2012). Employer perceptions that WHPPP can decrease costs and improve productivity are critical to worksite adoption. In addition, worksites with leadership that values employee health and well-being and supports healthy cultures are more likely to offer WHPPP (Emmons et al., 2000). Without sufficient resources, knowledge of the potential financial benefits, and recognition that improved employee health is consistent with the core organizational mission, employers are not likely to prioritize WHPPPs.

EMPLOYEE PARTICIPATION IN WORKSITE HEALTH PROMOTION PROGRAMS

A key rationale for implementing health promotion programs in worksites is the potential to reach large numbers of people. However, in practice high levels of participation are not often achieved. Most published reports indicate that employee participation and engagement in worksite-based programs are low. Robroek and colleagues (2009), for example, conducted a systematic review of determinants of employee participation in WHPPP addressing nutrition and/or physical activity. This review of 22 individual studies found that the median rate of participation was only 33%. The studies primarily assessed socio-demographic factors in relation to program participation. Females had higher rates of participation than males in most types of interventions, with the exception of use of exercise facilities. Otherwise, no clear patterns emerged by factors such as age, income level, and race/ethnicity (Robroek, van Lenthe, van Empelen, & Burdorf, 2009). This pattern is similar to a systematic assessment of factors associated with worksite smoking cessation programs, in which younger men in particular had low rates of participation (Cahill et al., 2008).

The available literature sheds some light on barriers to participation and how participation can be increased. Barriers commonly reported include insufficient time for participating, inconvenient schedules, and lack of interest in the topic or the program (Kim et al., 2012; Kruger, Yore, Bauer, & Kohl, 2007; Person, Colby, Bulova, & Eubanks, 2010). The implementation of interventions without modifying job expectations or allowing protected time for participation will not result in high participation rates. Expecting a one-size-fits-all approach to WHPPP, similarly cannot be expected to yield numbers of participants; multicomponent WHPPP have been shown to increase participation rates.

Facilitators of participation in WHPPP have also been identified. *Financial incentives* have been shown to increase WHPPP participation (Seaverson, Grossmeier, Miller, & Anderson, 2009; Serxner, Anderson, & Gold, 2004; Taitel, Haufle, Heck, Loeppke, & Fetterolf, 2008; Volpp et al., 2008). However, financial incentives do not necessarily result in health behavior or health outcome improvements, and must be incorporated as part of an evidence-based program to achieve such results (Gingerich, Anderson, & Koland, 2012). The likelihood of worksites offering financial incentives likely is directly linked to the ability to demonstrate return on investment. Research has demonstrated that employee perception of organizational commitment to employee health and a *culture of health* within the worksite are associated with improved health behaviors and participation in WHPPP (Aldana et al., 2012). Strong, comprehensive, and integrated *communication strategies* to promote HRAs, including multiple communication tools and channels of delivery appropriate to the employee population, appear to be linked to a strong climate of health and highest participation in HRAs (Seaverson et al., 2009). To maximize employer investment in WHPPP, development of new and better strategies to enhance employee participation is warranted.

THE AFFORDABLE CARE ACT AND WORKSITE HEALTH PROMOTION

The provisions of the Patient Protection and Affordable Care Act (ACA) of 2010 will provide support and strengthen opportunities for worksite health promotion efforts beginning in 2014 (*Patient Protection and Affordable Care Act*, 2010; Robert Wood Johnson Foundation, 2012). The existing system of employer-based health care coverage is the basis for many of the reforms in the Act. Small businesses that have not offered health insurance to employees will be eligible for tax credits for insurance purchase, and eventually will have access to health insurance exchanges that are intended to provide cost savings.

Specific provisions within the ACA build directly from the current scientific base. Recognizing the potential of financial incentives, the ACA expands non-discrimination provisions enacted initially through Health Insurance Portability and Accountability Act (HIPAA). The maximum value of incentives that employers can offer to employees for achieving specific health-related goals increases from 20% of health insurance coverage costs to 30% and allows the Secretary of Health and Human Services to increase the maximum limit to 50%. Recognizing the specific challenges experienced by small businesses, the ACA establishes a Department of Health and Human Services grant program for small businesses to implement worksite health promotion initiatives, with the initial appropriation of $200 million. Businesses that employ fewer than 100 people are eligible and must implement comprehensive programs based on the currently available scientific evidence of best of practices for health promotion programs. Recommended programs will include health risk assessments or screening programs, such as HRAs; provide access to programs that offer education and/or counseling for health behavior change, such as counseling and self-directed interventions; develop environmental and policy strategies; and include health communication strategies, such as newsletters and websites. The Act requires the U.S. Centers for Disease Control and Prevention to study and evaluate best practices in employer-sponsored wellness programs and to provide technical assistance to promote the benefits of such programs to employers, as well as submit a report to Congress indicating best practices for WHPPP. The provisions in the ACA bring worksite health promotion initiatives to the forefront and will greatly increase the number of worksite health promotion initiatives that are offered and the number of employees who have access to them.

RECOMMENDATIONS FOR RESEARCH AND PRACTICE: FUTURE PRIORITIES

WHPPP are likely to continue to expand across the United States. Without significant investments in prevention and disease management, the impact of chronic disease on U.S. worker health and productivity is likely to worsen. Employment projections for 2020 anticipate that the proportion of workers aged 55 and older will increase to include more than one-quarter of all workers, an increasing proportion of whom say they intend to continue working beyond age 65 (Lopez, 2005). With the aging of the workforce comes greater financial burden to employers and likely greater demand for WHPPP. Workforce diversity is expected to increase, reflecting the changing demographic profile of the country as a whole, which will require a greater variety of program delivery methods and materials. As previously described, the ACA dictates that WHPPP will

TABLE 20.3 Summary of Future Research and Evaluation Recommendations to Advance Worksite Health Promotion

- Expanded focus on financial outcomes
- Rigorous designs that take into consideration "real world" implementation, with an emphasis on both internal and external validity and appropriate measurement tools
- Dissemination and implementation research that will maximize employer buy-in and employee participation
- Incorporation of lessons learned from the ongoing CDC evaluation on the impact of the Affordable Care Act on the quantity and quality of worksite health promotion efforts to inform new research questions and implementation of evidence-based programs
- Establishment of best practices for worksite health promotion initiatives within small businesses
- Development of interventions for telecommuters
- Integration of technology and social media in interventions

expand vastly in coming years, assuming it is implemented as intended. Given the tense political climate in which this Act will be implemented, the impact of worksite health promotion efforts will likely be closely scrutinized.

Given this context, continued focus is needed on strengthening the evidence base and the associated financial case of WHPPP and disseminating this information broadly to the private and public work sectors. There is a growing body of scientific evidence to support worksite health promotion initiatives, and numerous recommendations and initiatives from a range of stakeholders recognize and promote the value of such programs for improving population health. Despite this, the benefits of worksite health promotion initiatives have yet to reach their full potential. There are several priority areas for future inquiry that stem from gaps in the scientific literature and from the current political and social context of the United States. These are described below and summarized in Table 20.3.

IMPROVEMENTS IN STUDY DESIGN AND MEASUREMENT

From a scientific perspective, there have been methodological challenges to evaluating the impact of worksite health promotion interventions. Randomized controlled clinical trials, although traditionally considered the gold standard, may not be of high quality. Rongen et al. (2013) found that effect size was more than twice as high in studies of poor methodological quality as in those of high quality. Furthermore, RCTs often are not feasible, and much of the published literature has used cluster-randomized trials and pre-post designs with no comparison or control condition (Kahn-Marshall & Gallant, 2012; Soler et al., 2010). Such design selections reflect the reality in which WHPPP have been implemented. The evidence for effective WHPPP has been generated by a range of stakeholders. Consistent with other types of health promotion research, a substantial proportion of worksite health promotion research has been funded by the Department of Health and Human Services to academic institutions in partnership with specific worksites. However, a sizeable amount of this evidence has been generated by businesses, particularly the corporate world. The latter has typically evaluated the impact of health promotion programs as implemented in practice, rather than using controlled research designs. As such, comparison conditions are not feasible. Similarly, health and behavioral measurement tools often rely on what can readily be administered in the context of day-to-day worksite operations, such as self-report surveys, in lieu of expensive and time-intensive gold standard clinical metrics.

The next generation of research needs to incorporate rigorous designs and measurement protocols that are appropriate to the goals of the research, while recognizing the real world circumstances under which WHPPP are implemented (Sorensen et al., 2011). Evaluating multilevel interventions with appropriate cluster-randomized designs and hierarchical statistical methodologies is one priority. In addition, rigorous observational and single-condition designs appropriate for natural experiments, such as panel studies and time series analyses, are important and must be implemented with methodological diligence. While expensive, timely measurement strategies are often not feasible in worksite contexts, attention must be paid to using high-quality measures that are consistent across studies whenever possible. For example, WHPPP researchers and companies that implement HRAs can learn from initiatives that aim to include brief, standardized patient-reported behavioral measures of demonstrated validity (National Institutes of Health & Society of Behavioral Medicine, 2011).

FOCUSING ON IMPLEMENTATION

The majority of intervention research on worksite health promotion to date has focused on determining the impact of WHPPP on health and financial outcomes. Despite the recognized difficulties in achieving employer buy-in and employee participation, there has been limited research focused on identifying approaches to improving these factors. Assessment of factors associated with implementation is crucial to the success of worksite wellness programs and policies in practice (Estabrook et al., 2012). A key component of this may be a focus on promoting organizational culture change and leadership support. The impact of organizational climate on worksite health promotion participation and strategies to improve organizational climate are not well understood, despite being considered critical elements of effective worksite health promotion. Approaches to improving stakeholder engagement are needed to maximize WHPPP implementation (Sorensen et al., 2011).

EVALUATION OF TIME-SENSITIVE REAL WORLD APPLICATIONS

Given that worksite health promotion has the potential to expand substantially under the provisions of the ACA, there are incredible opportunities to strengthen the evidence base for best practices. The CDC will evaluate the impact of the ACA on the quality and quantity of worksite health promotion programs. Collaborations among public health practitioners, scientists, and worksites will allow the incorporation of lessons learned to inform new research questions and the implementation of evidence-based programs. Research must proceed along a continuum in order to encourage the development and implementation of effective programs that are sustainable, and then encourage the broad adoption of sustainable programs. Best practices for technical assistance models that provide support to worksites for adoption of WHPPP need to be empirically established.

Small businesses are considerably less likely to offer health promotion programs and have experienced considerable financial barriers to doing so. The ACA specifically prioritizes small businesses by offering grant programs and technical assistance to implementing such programs. Despite these provisions, there is a dearth of knowledge related to implementation of evidence-based practices within diverse small businesses. Effective implementation approaches need to be established. In addition, the majority of evidence on WHPPP return on investment has been generated among large worksites. Despite the potential financial assistance provided by ACA, making a financial case to small businesses will be critical.

NEW INTERVENTION APPROACHES: LEVERAGING TECHNOLOGY

WHPPPs must adapt to changing times to maximize effectiveness. Technology-based interventions that utilize the web, M-health, social media, and emerging technologies are critical. In 2010, 3 million people, about 2.5% of the workforce not including the self-employed or unpaid volunteers, reported home as their primary place of work. Employees primarily based onsite but working from home multiple days per week increased 66% from 2005 to 2010 (Global Workplace Analytics and the Telework Research Network, 2011). Many experts expect the trend of telecommuting to continue to grow. To be effective in the future, WHPPP must include ways of reaching employees remotely. In addition, technology-based interventions offer the advantages of being able to reach large numbers of employees, and allowing access at the employee's convenience, including after work hours. Technology-based interventions also hold potential within traditional worksites, as they can leverage the widespread use of technology-focused aspects of job design as well as social networks and support within the worksite context.

The current scientific literature focusing on technology-based interventions within worksites is in development. While computer-based HRAs are increasing, a small body of literature has examined the effectiveness of technology-delivered behavior change interventions within the worksite setting. Challenges to this work include heterogeneity across studies and the rapid pace of technological change. These types of interventions may be integrated as virtual support for other interventions or as stand-alone interventions and can be informed by emerging evidence on technology-based health promotion (Baker et al., 2010; Burke, Wang, & Sevick, 2011; Cole-Lewis & Kershaw, 2010; Hall, Chavarria, Maneeratana, & Bernhardt, 2012; Korda & Itani, 2013; Krebs, Prochaska, & Rossi, 2010; Murray, Burns, See, Lai, & Nazareth, 2005; Peng, Crouse, & Lin, 2013; Portnoy, Scott-Sheldon, Johnson, & Carey, 2008; Samoocha, Bruinvels, Elbers, Anema, & van der Beek, 2010). A key factor of likely importance to employers is the potential cost-effectiveness of technology-based interventions (Chen et al., 2012), and future research is needed to establish best practices and the business case for such interventions within worksites.

CONCLUSIONS

There is a large body of evidence supporting the effectiveness of WHPPPs. Staggering health care costs and provisions within the Affordable Care Act are bringing wide scale implementation of WHPPPs to the forefront. To achieve the full potential of WHPPPs in the United States, concerted effort is needed to identify and ensure that evidence-based programs and policies are adopted and sustained across diverse worksites. The next generation of research should address emerging issues related to the political and health care context and technology-based delivery approaches.

REFERENCES

Aldana, S., Barlow, M., Smith, R., Yanowitz, F., Adams, T., Loveday, L., & Merrill, R.M. (2006). A worksite diabetes prevention program: Two-year impact on employee health. *AAOHN Journal, 54*(9), 389–395.

Aldana, S. G., Anderson, D. R., Adams, T. B., Whitmer, R. W., Merrill, R. M., George, V., & Noyce, J. (2012). A review of the knowledge base on healthy worksite culture. *Journal of Occupational and Environmental Medicine, 54*(4), 414–419.

Aldana, S. G., Barlow, M., Smith, R., Yanowitz, F. G., Adams, T., Loveday, L., & LaMonte, M. J. (2005). The diabetes prevention program: A worksite experience. *AAOHN Journal, 53*(11), 499–505; quiz 506-497.

Archer, W. R., Batan, M. C., Buchanan, L. R., Soler, R. E., Ramsey, D. C., Kirchhofer, A., & Reyes, M. (2011). Promising practices for the prevention and control of obesity in the worksite. *American Journal of Health Promotion, 25*(3), e12–e26.

Baicker, K., Cutler, D., & Song, Z. (2010). Workplace wellness programs can generate savings. *Health Affairs, 29*(2), 304–311.

Baker, R., Camosso-Stefinovic, J., Gillies, C., Shaw, E. J., Cheater, F., Flottorp, S., & Robertson, N. (2010). Tailored interventions to overcome identified barriers to change: Effects on professional practice and health care outcomes. *Cochrane Database of Systematic Reviews*, (3), CD005470.

Benedict, M. A., & Arterburn, D. (2008). Worksite-based weight loss programs: A systematic review of recent literature. *American Journal of Health Promotion, 22*(6), 408–416.

Blumenthal, D. (2006). Employer-sponsored health insurance in the United States—origins and implications. *New England Journal of Medicine, 355*(1), 82–88.

Bureau of Labor Statistics. (2011). *Labor force statistics from the current population survey. Household data annual averages. Employed persons by occupation, race, Hispanic or Latino ethnicity, and sex.* Retrieved from http://www.bls.gov/cps/cpsaat14.pdf

Burke, L. E., Wang, J., & Sevick, M. A. (2011). Self-monitoring in weight loss: A systematic review of the literature. *Journal of the American Dietetic Association, 111*(1), 92–102.

Cahill, K., Moher, M., & Lancaster, T. (2008). Workplace interventions for smoking cessation. *Cochrane Database System Review* (4), CD003440.

Cahill, K., & Perera, R. (2011). Competitions and incentives for smoking cessation. *Cochrane Database System Review* (4), CD004307.

Centers for Disease Control and Prevention, Office on Smoking and Health. (2012). *State tobacco activities tracking and evaluation (STATE) system.* Retrieved from http://apps.nccd.cdc.gov/statesystem/Default/Default.aspx

Centers for Disease Control and Prevention, Division of Population Health/Workplace Health Promotion. (2012, August). *Workplace health model.* Retrieved from http://www.cdc.gov/workplacehealthpromotion/model/index.html

Chen, Y. F., Madan, J., Welton, N., Yahaya, I., Aveyard, P., Bauld, L., …Munafò, M. R. (2012). Effectiveness and cost-effectiveness of computer and other electronic aids for smoking cessation: A systematic review and network meta-analysis. *Health Technology Assessment, 16*(38), 1–205, iii-v.

Cole-Lewis, H., & Kershaw, T. (2010). Text messaging as a tool for behavior change in disease prevention and management. *Epidemiologic Reviews, 32*(1), 56–69.

Community Prevention Services Taskforce. (2011). *Guide to community prevention services. Assessment of health risks with feedback to change employees' health.* Retrieved from http://www.thecommunityguide.org/worksite/ahrf.html

Dallam, G. M., & Foust, C. (2013). A comparative approach to using the Diabetes Prevention Program to reduce diabetes risk in a worksite setting. *Health Promotion Practice, 14*(2), 199–204.

Dejoy, D. M., Padilla, H. M., Wilson, M. G., Vandenberg, R. J., & Davis, M. A. (2012). Worksite translation of the Diabetes Prevention Program: Formative research and pilot study results from FUEL your life. *Health Promotion Practice, 14*(4), 506-13.

Emmons, K. M., Thompson, B., McLerran, D., Sorensen, G., Linnan, L., Basen-Enquist, K., & Biener, L. (2000). The relationship between organizational characteristics and the adoption of workplace smoking policies. *Health Education and Behavior, 27*(4), 483–501.

Estabrook, B., Zapka, J., & Lemon, S. C. (2012). Evaluating the implementation of a hospital work-site obesity prevention intervention: Applying the RE-AIM framework. *Health Promotion Practice, 13*(2), 190–197.

Fabius, R. J., & Frazee, S. G. (2009). Workplace-based health and wellness services. In N. P. Pronk (Ed.), *ACSM's worksite health handbook: A guide to building healthy and productive companies*. Champaign, IL: Human Kinetics.

Gingerich, S. B., Anderson, D. R., & Koland, H. (2012). Impact of financial incentives on behavior change program participation and risk reduction in worksite health promotion. *American Journal of Health Promotion, 27*(2), 119–122.

Glanz, K., Rimer, B. K., & Viswanath, K. (Eds.). (2008). *Health behavior and health education: Theory, research and practice* (4th ed.). San Francisco, CA: Jossey-Bass.

Global Workplace Analytics and the Telework Research Network. (2011). Retrieved from http://www.TeleworkResearchNetwork.com

Goetzel, R. Z., Gibson, T. B., Short, M. E., Chu, B. C., Waddell, J., Bowen, J., ...DeJoy, D. M. (2010). A multi-worksite analysis of the relationships among body mass index, medical utilization, and worker productivity. *Journal of Occupational and Environmental Medicine, 52*(Suppl. 1), S52–S58.

Goetzel, R. Z., & Ozminkowski, R. J. (2008). The health and cost benefits of work site health-promotion programs. *Annual Review of Public Health, 29*, 303–323.

Goetzel, R. Z., Pei, X., Tabrizi, M. J., Henke, R. M., Kowlessar, N., Nelson, C. F., & Metz, R. D. (2012). Ten modifiable health risk factors are linked to more than one-fifth of employer-employee health care spending. *Health Affairs, 31*(11), 2474–2484.

Golaszewski, T., Allen, J., & Edington, D. (2008). Working together to create supportive environments in worksite health promotion. *American Journal of Health Promotion, 22*(4), 1–10, iii.

Green, L. W., Richard, L., & Potvin, L. (1996). Ecological foundations of health promotion. *American Journal of Health Promotion, 10*(4), 270–281.

Hall, A. K., Chavarria, E., Maneeratana, V., & Bernhardt, J. M. (2012). Health benefits of digital video-games for older adults: A systematic review of the literature. *Games for Health Journal, 1*, 402-410.

Hannon, P. A., Garson, G., Harris, J. R., Hammerback, K., Sopher, C. J., & Clegg-Thorp, C. (2012). Work-place health promotion implementation, readiness, and capacity among midsize employers in low-wage industries: A national survey. *Journal of Occupational and Environmental Medicine, 54*(11), 1337-1343.

Hopkins, D. P., Razi, S., Leeks, K. D., Priya Kalra, G., Chattopadhyay, S. K., & Soler, R. E. (2010). Smoke-free policies to reduce tobacco use. A systematic review. *American Journal of Preventive Medicine, 38*(2 Suppl.), S275–289.

Hurt, R. D., Weston, S. A., Ebbert, J. O., McNallan, S. M., Croghan, I. T., Schroeder, D. R., Roger, V. L. (2012). Myocardial infarction and sudden cardiac death in Olmsted County, Minnesota, before and after smoke-free workplace laws. *Archives of Internal Medicine, 172*(21), 1635–1641.

Hutchinson, A. D., & Wilson, C. (2012). Improving nutrition and physical activity in the workplace: A meta-analysis of intervention studies. *Health Promotion International, 27*(2), 238–249.

Kahn-Marshall, J. L., & Gallant, M. P. (2012). Making healthy behaviors the easy choice for employees: A review of the literature on environmental and policy changes in worksite health promotion. *Health Education and Behavior, 39*(6), 752–776.

Kaiser Family Foundation & Health Research & Educational Trust (HRET). (2012). *Employer health benefits 2012 annual survey*. Retrieved from http://ehbs.kff.org/pdf/2012/8345.pdf

Kim, A. E., Towers, A., Renaud, J., Zhu, J., Shea, J. A., Galvin, R., & Volpp, K. G. (2012). Application of the RE-AIM framework to evaluate the impact of a worksite-based financial incentive intervention for smoking cessation. *Journal of Occupational and Environmental Medicine, 54*(5), 610–614.

Korda, H., & Itani, Z. (2013). Harnessing social media for health promotion and behavior change. *Health Promotion Practice, 14*(1), 15–23.

Krebs, P., Prochaska, J. O., & Rossi, J. S. (2010). A meta-analysis of computer-tailored interventions for health behavior change. *Preventive Medicine, 51*(3-4), 214–221.

Kruger, J., Yore, M. M., Bauer, D. R., & Kohl, H. W. (2007). Selected barriers and incentives for worksite health promotion services and policies. *American Journal of Health Promotion, 21*(5), 439–447.

Lemon, S. C., Liu, Q., Magner, R., Schneider, K. L., & Pbert, L. (2013). Development and validation of work-site weight-related social norms surveys. *American Journal of Health Behavior, 37*(1), 122–129.

Lemon, S. C., Zapka, J., Li, W., Estabrook, B., Magner, R., & Rosal, M. C. (2009). Perceptions of worksite support and employee obesity, activity, and diet. *American Journal of Health Behavior, 33*(3), 299–308.

Lopez, K. (2005). The three changing faces of the US workforce. *Occupational health & safety*. Retrieved from http://ohsonline.com/articles/2005/01/the-three-changing-faces-of-the-us-workforce.aspx

Mendes, E. (2010). *In U.S., health disparities across incomes are wide-ranging*. Washington, DC: Gallup-Healthways: Retrieved from http://www.gallup.com/poll/143696/Health-Disparities-Across-Income-Wide-Ranging.aspx

Murray, E., Burns, J., See, T. S., Lai, R., & Nazareth, I. (2005). Interactive health communication applications for people with chronic disease. *Cochrane Database of Systematic Reviews* (4), CD004274.

Musich, S. A., Schultz, A. B., Burton, W. N., & Edington, D. W. (2004). Overview of disease-management approaches: Implications for corporate sponsored programs. *Disease Management and Health Outcomes, 12*(5), 299–326.

National Institutes of Health & Society of Behavioral Medicine. (2011). *Identifying core behavioral and psychosocial data elements for the electronic health record. Executive summary.* Retrieved from http://www.sbm.org/UserFiles/file/EHR_Meeting_May_2-3-2011—Executive_Summary.pdf

National Physical Activity Plan for the United States. (2009). Retrieved from http://www.physicalactivityplan.org/theplan.php

Ng, S. W., & Popkin, B. M. (2012). Time use and physical activity: A shift away from movement across the globe. *Obesity Reviews, 13*(8), 659–680.

Ni Mhurchu, C., Aston, L. M., & Jebb, S. A. (2010). Effects of worksite health promotion interventions on employee diets: A systematic review. *BMC Public Health, 10*, 62.

O'Donnell, M. P. (2009). Definition of health promotion 2.0: Embracing passion, enhancing motivation, recognizing dynamic balance, and creating opportunities. *American Journal of Health Promotion, 24*(1), iv.

Patient Protection and Affordable Care Act. (2010). Public Law No. 111-148, page 124 Stat 119. Washington, DC: US Government Printing Office.

Pelletier, K. R. (1991). A review and analysis of the health and cost-effective outcome studies of comprehensive health promotion and disease prevention programs. *American Journal of Health Promotion, 5*(4), 311–313.

Pelletier, K. R. (1993). A review and analysis of the health and cost-effective outcome studies of comprehensive health promotion and disease prevention programs at the worksite: 1991-1993 update. *American Journal of Health Promotion, 8*(1), 50–62.

Pelletier, K. R. (1996). A review and analysis of the health and cost-effective outcome studies of comprehensive health promotion and disease prevention programs at the worksite: 1993-1995 update. *American Journal of Health Promotion, 10*(5), 380–388.

Pelletier, K. R. (1999). A review and analysis of the clinical and cost-effectiveness studies of comprehensive health promotion and disease management programs at the worksite: 1995-1998 update (IV). *American Journal of Health Promotion, 13*(6), 333–345, iii.

Pelletier, K. R. (2001). A review and analysis of the clinical- and cost-effectiveness studies of comprehensive health promotion and disease management programs at the worksite: 1998-2000 update. *American Journal of Health Promotion, 16*(2), 107–116.

Pelletier, K. R. (2005). A review and analysis of the clinical and cost-effectiveness studies of comprehensive health promotion and disease management programs at the worksite: Update VI 2000-2004. *Journal of Occupational and Environmental Medicine, 47*(10), 1051–1058.

Pelletier, K. R. (2011). A review and analysis of the clinical and cost-effectiveness studies of comprehensive health promotion and disease management programs at the worksite: Update VIII 2008 to 2010. *Journal of Occupational and Environmental Medicine, 53*(11), 1310–1331.

Peng, W., Crouse, J. C., & Lin, J. H. (2013). Using active video games for physical activity promotion: A systematic review of the current state of research. *Health Education and Behavior, 40*(2), 171–192.

Person, A. L., Colby, S. E., Bulova, J. A., & Eubanks, J. W. (2010). Barriers to participation in a worksite wellness program. *Nutrition Research and Practice, 4*(2), 149–154.

Portnoy, D. B., Scott-Sheldon, L. A., Johnson, B. T., & Carey, M. P. (2008). Computer-delivered interventions for health promotion and behavioral risk reduction: A meta-analysis of 75 randomized controlled trials, 1988-2007. *Preventive Medicine, 47*(1), 3–16.

Robroek, S. J., van Lenthe, F. J., van Empelen, P., & Burdorf, A. (2009). Determinants of participation in worksite health promotion programmes: A systematic review. *International Journal of Behavioral Nutrition and Physical Activity, 6*, 26.

Robert Wood Johnson Foundation. (2012). *Health affairs: Health policy brief. Workplace wellness programs.* Retrieved from http://www.healthaffairs.org/healthpolicybriefs/brief.php?brief_id=69

Rongen, A., Robroek, S. J., van Lenthe, F. J., & Burdorf, A. (2013). Workplace health promotion: A meta-analysis of effectiveness. *American Journal of Preventive Medicine, 44*(4), 406–415.

Sallis, J. F., Owen, N., & Fisher, E. B. (2008). Ecological models of health behavior. In K. Glanz, B. K. Rimer, & K. Viswanath (Eds.), *Health behavior and health education. Theory, research, and practice* (4th ed.). San Francisco, CA: Jossey-Bass.

Samoocha, D., Bruinvels, D. J., Elbers, N. A., Anema, J. R., & van der Beek, A. J. (2010). Effectiveness of web-based interventions on patient empowerment: A systematic review and meta-analysis. *Journal of Medical Internet Research, 12*(2), e23.

Schulte, P. A., Wagner, G. R., Ostry, A., Blanciforti, L. A., Cutlip, R. G., Krajnak, K. M., ... Miller, D. B. (2007). Work, obesity, and occupational safety and health. *American Journal of Public Health, 97*(3), 428–436.

Seaverson, E. L., Grossmeier, J., Miller, T. M., & Anderson, D. R. (2009). The role of incentive design, incentive value, communications strategy, and worksite culture on health risk assessment participation. *American Journal of Health Promotion, 23*(5), 343–352.

Serxner, S., & Anderson, D. (2002). Practical considerations for the design and evaluation of disease education and management programs in the workplace. *Disease Management and Health Outcomes, 10*(2), 109–115.

Serxner, S., Anderson, D. R., & Gold, D. (2004). Building program participation: Strategies for recruitment and retention in worksite health promotion programs. *American Journal of Health Promotion, 18*(4), 1–6, iii.

Soler, R. E., Leeks, K. D., Razi, S., Hopkins, D. P., Griffith, M., Aten, A., ... Walker, A. M. (2010). A systematic review of selected interventions for worksite health promotion. The assessment of health risks with feedback. *American Journal of Preventive Medicine, 38*(2 Suppl.), S237–S262.

Sorensen, G., Landsbergis, P., Hammer, L., Amick, B. C., 3rd, Linnan, L., Yancey, A., ... Pratt, C. (2011). Preventing chronic disease in the workplace: A workshop report and recommendations. *American Journal of Public Health, 101*(Suppl. 1), S196–S207.

Sparling, P. B. (2010). Worksite health promotion: Principles, resources, and challenges. *Preventing Chronic Disease, 7*(1), A25.

Taitel, M. S., Haufle, V., Heck, D., Loeppke, R., & Fetterolf, D. (2008). Incentives and other factors associated with employee participation in health risk assessments. *Journal of Occupational and Environmental Medicine, 50*(8), 863–872.

U.S. Department of Health and Human Services. (2000). *Healthy People 2010: Understanding and improving health.* Publication No. 017-001-001-00-550-9. Washington, DC: U.S. Government Printing Office.

U.S. Department of Health and Human Services. (2010). *Healthy People 2020 – Improving the health of Americans.* Retrieved from http://www.healthypeople.gov/2020/default.aspx

U.S. Department of Labor. Bureau of Labor Statistics. (2011). Retrieved from http://www.bls.gov

Volpp, K. G., John, L. K., Troxel, A. B., Norton, L., Fassbender, J., & Loewenstein, G. (2008). Financial incentive-based approaches for weight loss: A randomized trial. *Journal of the American Medical Association, 300*(22), 2631–2637.

Volpp, K. G., Troxel, A. B., Pauly, M. V., Glick, H. A., Puig, A., Asch, D. A., ...McGovern, J. A. (2009). A randomized, controlled trial of financial incentives for smoking cessation. *New England Journal of Medicine, 360*(7), 699–709.

Weng, S. F., Ali, S., & Leonardi-Bee, J. (2013). Smoking and absence from work: Systematic review and meta-analysis of occupational studies. *Addiction, 108*(2), 307–319.

Whitmer, R. W., Pelletier, K. R., Anderson, D. R., Baase, C. M., & Frost, G. J. (2003). A wake-up call for corporate America. *Journal of Occupational and Environmental Medicine, 45*(9), 916–925.

21

Health Care Provider and System Interventions Promoting Health Behavior Change

ANNE C. DOBMEYER
JEFFREY L. GOODIE
CHRISTOPHER L. HUNTER

LEARNING OBJECTIVES

- Summarize two benefits of targeting health care providers and health care systems to effect health behavior change.
- Identify three challenges in targeting health care systems for health behavior change.
- Describe an example of how system supports or practice redesign could improve health behavior change interventions in primary care settings.

As highlighted in this book, effective interventions for modifying a wide range of health behaviors exist. To be maximally effective, strategies for promoting healthier behaviors need to address not just the individual patient, but also health care providers and systems. Expanding beyond individual approaches results in a broader impact on the population in a shorter period of time. For example, system interventions targeting the assessment of tobacco use by implementing a tobacco use status identification system in the primary care clinic improve identification of tobacco use and increase frequency of physician interventions for tobacco and subsequent cessation rates (Fiore, Bailey, & Cohen, et al., 2000).

The primary care setting is a particularly important arena for implementing system interventions. Because the majority of health care occurs in primary care and up to 70% to 75% of primary care visits involve some form of psychosocial or behavioral health component (Fries et al., 1993; Kessler et al., 2005), primary care is an important venue for delivering health behavior interventions that have the potential for significant population health impact. This chapter focuses on interventions targeting primary care staff, providers, and health care systems of service delivery. We identify challenges in targeting health care systems for health behavior change. To overcome these challenges we focus on provider- and system-centered needs for educational changes, integrated-collaborative care approaches of health care service delivery, the use of technology, and other clinic process changes. We conclude with a review of the policy and reimbursement barriers and implications and discuss areas for future research.

CHALLENGES IN HEALTH CARE SYSTEMS

Despite the ubiquitous need for evidence-based health behavior interventions in primary care settings, multiple barriers interfere with the widespread adoption of these approaches. These barriers result from how medical providers are trained, providers' attitudes and beliefs about health behavior change, and the health care system itself.

MEDICAL EDUCATION

The opening of the Johns Hopkins Medical School in 1893 and the publication of the "Flexner Report" in 1910 guided the redesign of the American medical education system between the 1870s and 1920s (Cuff & Vanselow, 2004; Ludmerer, 1999). Until recently, this fundamental training model remained largely unchanged, with the first two years of medical education focused on preclinical basic science and the last two years on clinical studies, leaving little room for formal instruction about how to counsel patients to improve unhealthy behaviors (Moser & Stagnaro-Green, 2009). After evaluating medical education, the Institute of Medicine (IOM) (Cuff & Vanselow, 2004) concluded that medical schools inadequately teach methods for targeting problem health behaviors (e.g., tobacco use, diet, and inactivity). Limited exposure to health behavior change skills during medical school decreases the likelihood that these future physicians will value and apply these skills.

BELIEFS AND ATTITUDES

Health behavior change is often not discussed during patient encounters (Ellerbeck, Ahluwalia, Jolicoeur, Gladden, & Mosier, 2001; Heywood, Firman, Sanson-Fisher, Mudge, & Ring, 1996; Stafford, Farhat, Misra, & Schoenfeld, 2000). Using tobacco cessation counseling as an example, many physicians believe that patients are not motivated to quit, that patients usually fail to quit, that there is not enough appointment time to target quitting, and that there are other priorities besides tobacco cessation during the appointment (Association of American Medical Colleges [AAMC], 2007; Vogt, Hall, & Marteau, 2005). Additionally, most physicians report low confidence in their ability to motivate patients to stop smoking (AAMC, 2007). Physicians believe that patients would find discussions about diet, weight, and physical activity more embarrassing than smoking cessation counseling and would be unlikely to follow their advice (Dolor et al., 2010), suggesting even more significant barriers to targeting these behaviors.

LIMITED RESOURCES SUPPORTING HEALTH BEHAVIOR INTERVENTIONS

Primary care physicians typically rely on their colleagues and textbooks when they need information (Coumou & Meijman, 2006). Multiple electronic databases (e.g., Up-To-Date, Essential Evidence Plus Patient-Oriented Evidence that Matters [POEMs]) exist to provide evidence-based answers to clinical questions; however, these databases may not provide the specific answers needed for point-of-care questions regarding health behavior change interventions (Coumou & Meijman, 2007). Additionally, most physicians are unlikely to attend the professional conferences or read the professional journals focusing on health behavior change. Unless physicians have quick, easy access to colleagues or resources that provide guidance on how to target health behaviors, they are less likely to learn how to apply health behavior change interventions in practice.

In addition, often the health care system fails to support primary care providers (PCPs) and their efforts to promote health behavior change interventions. Health care systems have developed to respond to acute needs, with a limited focus on prevention and effective management of chronic problems. The "tyranny of the urgent" consistently interferes with providers' opportunities to target health behavior change (Bodenheimer, Wagner, & Grumbach, 2002).

LACK OF TEAM-BASED APPROACHES

Often in medical settings, including primary care, there are limited team-based approaches to medical care. The lack of team-based care places the burden for health behavior change on individual medical providers. Although it is essential for physicians to discuss and initiate conversations about behavior change, they are not working at their peak scope of practice if they bear complete responsibility for the assessment, initiation, and maintenance of behavior change counseling. Team-based care integrates other primary care staff, such as nurses, behavior specialists, and medical technicians, who could assist with behavior change counseling across the population served in the clinic.

LACK OF SYSTEMS TO SUPPORT PCP INTERVENTION

In primary care it is essential that there are systems to support quick assessments, decision making, and referrals. Often algorithms derived from clinical guidelines and evidence-based reviews serve to inform decision making. Pairing these algorithms with electronic medical records and other integrated systems can help to quickly identify patients who may benefit from more intensive treatment and facilitate referrals to specialty care. The absence of these algorithms and systems to support health behavior change serves as another barrier to promoting behavior change.

INADEQUATE INTENSIVE TREATMENT OPTIONS

The referral process to specialty mental health services and options for intensive behavioral change treatment are often limited and difficult to access. For PCPs this means that even if they identify the need to target health-related behaviors and determine that a patient needs specialty or more intensive care, there are significant barriers and limited options. It becomes easier to focus on the aspects of care for which they have treatment options available and that they believe they can affect.

REIMBURSEMENT AND FINANCIAL BARRIERS

Health care organizations that do not value or view chronic care management as important are unlikely to reimburse and reward efforts to reduce chronic disease through health behavior change (Bodenheimer et al., 2002). Relative to other interventions, preventive interventions have lower reimbursement rates. Most physicians described the limited coverage for tobacco cessation and limited reimbursement for physician's time as significant barriers for targeting tobacco use (AAMC, 2007). In environments where financial reimbursement must be considered, there is less incentive to prioritize behavior change counseling.

LACK OF ELECTRONIC PATIENT REGISTRIES

Patient registries provide a health care system an easy way of identifying and targeting patients diagnosed with particular conditions. Registries list patients with particular conditions. This information can then be paired with a reminder system and evidence-based clinical practice guidelines to signal providers and staff to conduct assessments or interventions on a schedule (Bodenheimer et al., 2002). Many systems do not invest in the technical and human resources to establish and maintain these registries.

LACK OF INTEGRATION OF MEDICAL AND BEHAVIORAL HEALTH PROVIDERS

In many health care systems, behavioral health providers are not a direct part of the system, with offices separated from where individuals receive their medical care. Even systemic efforts to integrate behavioral health specialty assets into primary care do not necessarily improve the PCP's ability to implement health behavior change. Placing behavioral health providers near the PCP's point of care may ease the referral process and increase communication between the PCP and behavioral health provider, but as long as separate standards of care are maintained and each provider is separately responsible for the care provided, there is limited opportunity for medical providers to learn how they could change their practice using health behavior change methods.

These individual and systemic barriers to health behavior change interventions are long-standing and have stifled the integration of behavior change counseling into routine health care. A broad range of changes are needed to affect the practice of physicians and the health care systems in which they provide care.

TRAINING FOR THE 21ST CENTURY

The medical education system and the health care system are undergoing radical changes presenting opportunities for improving how health behavior change is taught. Many medical schools are undertaking curriculum reform and reconsidering the Flexner model of education. A Carnegie Foundation study and subsequent recommendations made by Cook, Irby, and O'Brien (2010), which have been called "Flexner II," are guiding the process of curriculum reform. The authors use the four goals of medical education introduced by Flexner (i.e., standardization, integration, habits of inquiry and improvement, and professional formation) to identify challenges and make recommendations for improvement. To achieve the goal of integration, the authors specifically encourage the integration of basic, clinical, and social sciences as well as interprofessional education and teamwork. To promote habits of inquiry and improvement, the authors encourage participation in initiatives focusing on population health and quality improvement. These recommendations along with the awareness of the impact of health behaviors on morbidity and mortality (Mokdad, Marks, Stroup, & Gerberding, 2004) provide the rationale and opportunities to integrate health behavior change training into medical education.

Increasingly more emphasis is being placed on behavioral and social science in undergraduate medical education. The IOM (Cuff & Vanselow, 2004) argued:

> To make measurable improvements in the health of Americans, physicians must be equipped with the knowledge and skills from the behavioral and social sciences needed to recognize, understand, and effectively respond to patients as individuals, not just their symptoms (p. 3)

Given the state of training, the IOM developed five recommendations for improving the integration of behavioral and social science training, summarized in Table 21.1 (Cuff & Vanselow, 2004). The IOM also identified important behavioral and social science curriculum content organized across five domains: biological, psychological, social, behavioral, and economic. In the psychological and behavioral domains, the IOM encouraged teaching the transtheoretical model of change and maladaptive behavior patterns of patients, including health risk behaviors.

In 2011, the AAMC published a report on the behavioral and social science foundations for future physicians. The authors stated, "A complete medical education must include, alongside physical and biological science, the perspectives and findings that flow from the behavioral and social sciences" (p. 5). The report adopted the recommendations of the IOM report (Cuff & Vanselow, 2004) along with recommendations of the Royal College of Physicians and Surgeons of Canada to create a framework for how to teach and apply the behavioral and social sciences across clinical, educational, and curriculum applications (Frank, 2005). The framework is presented in Table 21.2.

TABLE 21.1 Institute of Medicine Recommendations for Integrating Behavioral and Social Science into Medical School Curricula

RECOMMENDATION
1. Develop and maintain a database on behavioral and social science curricular content, teaching techniques, and assessment methodologies in U.S. medical schools.
2. Provide an integrated 4-year curriculum in the behavioral and social sciences. Medical students should demonstrate competency in the following domains: • Mind–body interactions in health and disease • Patient behavior • Physician role and behavior • Physician–patient interactions • Social and cultural issues in health care • Health policy and economics
3. Establish a career development award strategy to produce leaders in the behavioral and social sciences in medical schools.
4. Establish curriculum development demonstration project awards that fund demonstration projects in behavioral and social science curriculum development at U.S. medical schools.
5. Increase behavioral and social science content on the U.S. Medical Licensing Examination.

TABLE 21.2 AAMC Behavioral and Social Science Matrix

IOM Behavioral & Social Science Knowledge Domains	CanMEDS PHYSICIAN ROLES*					
	PROFESSIONAL	COMMUNICATOR	COLLABORATOR	MANAGER AND SYSTEM THINKER	HEALTH ADVOCATE	SCHOLAR
Patient Behavior						
Mind–Body Interaction						
Physician Role & Behavior						
Physician–Patient Interaction						
Health Policy, Economics, and Systems						
Social and Cultural Context						

Adapted from Association of American Medical Colleges (2011).

* CanMEDS is a framework developed by the Royal College of Physicians and Surgeons of Canada that describes the physician roles leading to optimal health and health care outcomes. Additional information is available at www.royalcollege.ca

Knowledge of behavioral sciences will begin to impact who is selected for medical training. Starting in 2015, the Medical College Admission Test (MCAT), the prerequisite standardized exam used to guide decisions about medical school acceptance, will include a section on the psychological, social, and biological foundations of behavior, requiring applicants to medical school to have a basic understanding of the social and behavioral sciences (Kaplan, Satterfield, & Kington, 2012).

The increased emphasis on behavioral and social sciences is also growing in graduate medical education. Although family medicine has required residents to be exposed to the behavioral sciences, the Accreditation Council for Graduate Medical Education (ACGME) has proposed that family medicine residencies have faculty dedicated to the integration of behavioral health for at least 10 hours per week, that residents are able to diagnose, manage, and coordinate the care for common behavioral issues in patients of all ages, and that behavioral health is integrated into the residents' total educational experience (Accreditation Council for Graduate Medical Education [ACGME], 2012). The ACGME requires exposure to behavioral science for other primary care specialties (i.e., internal medicine and pediatrics); however, the requirements are not nearly as specific as those proposed for family medicine. In the context of all of these recommendations for changes, there is a growing body of evidence that teaching health behavior change to medical students can change their knowledge, attitudes, and skills related to health behavior change counseling (Bell & Cole, 2008; Martino, Haeseler, Belitsky, Pantalon, & Fortin, 2007; Moser & Stagnaro-Green, 2009; Spollen et al., 2010).

MEDICAL SCHOOL/INTERNSHIP/RESIDENCY

A systematic review of efforts to teach health behavior change interventions during medical school and residency demonstrated that these efforts can be successful (Hauer, Carney, Chang, & Satterfield, 2012). Effective interventions were based on existing frameworks such as the National Cancer Institute's 5 As (Ask, Advise, Assess, Assist, and Arrange) and/or motivational interviewing within a stages-of-change framework. These educators used active learning strategies, structured practice with feedback to learners, and/or opportunities to practice after receiving feedback. Many of these efforts emphasize training brief, effective behavior change interventions, which could be used in primary care settings. Some researchers (Goodie, Williams, Kurzweil, & Marcellas, 2011) are examining how to couple classroom learning experiences with distributed learning methods, which use a range of technologies and media (e.g., electronic text, pictures, files, video, and discussion boards) to allow students to engage with course content from anywhere, anytime, and at their own pace (Simonson, Smaldino, Albright, & Zvacek, 2008). Distributed learning methods may use the electronically based, bidirectional communication methods of distance learning, but distributed learning is a broader educational model that includes teaching methods that can be incorporated into traditional face-to-face classroom experiences (Fleming & Hiple, 2004).

TRAINING FOR ESTABLISHING OFFICE SYSTEMS SUPPORTING PCP INTERVENTIONS AND REFERRAL

Medical providers may benefit from specific training in the availability and procedures for establishing electronic systems for helping to guide evidence-based care and identifying criteria for making referrals to specialty providers. Even if the PCPs are not the ones implementing these programs they can be the ones insisting on the systems to ensure quality care.

EXPOSURE TO EFFECTIVE INTEGRATED-COLLABORATIVE CARE MODELS DURING TRAINING

As we highlight later, integrating behavioral health providers into primary care settings provides an important opportunity for not only delivering behavior change counseling, but also teaching other providers and team members how to implement behavior change counseling. Current ACGME Program requirements for graduate medical education in family medicine require that there are behavioral specialists on faculty, familiar with evidence-based health behavior change assessments and interventions, who are specifically designated to teach modern behavioral and psychiatric principles to residents.

INCREASED EXPOSURE TO RESOURCES TO SUPPORT HEALTH BEHAVIOR CHANGE INTERVENTIONS

Although there are multidisciplinary organizations (e.g., American Psychosomatic Society, Collaborative Family Healthcare Association, and Society of Behavioral Medicine) and journals (e.g., *Families, Systems, and Health; Psychosomatic Medicine; Translational Behavioral Medicine*) where the science regarding health behavior change is presented and discussed, the vast majority of PCPs will not be exposed to these conferences and articles. It is important for health behavior change experts to present at and write for the venues where PCPs attend and to translate the science into clinically relevant and meaningful concepts. For example, the most widely circulated medical journal is the *American Family Physician*. Articles in this journal are required to use existing literature to guide practice in primary care clinical settings. Behavior change counseling experts should collaborate with medical colleagues to prepare appropriate manuscripts for journals like *American Family Physician* to translate the health behavior change science for the broader medical community. Taking the science to the PCPs and other medical providers, rather than expecting them to seek out that science and those resources, may help to shape current PCP behavior.

CHANGING THE HEALTH CARE SYSTEM

Improving the education of physicians about health behavior interventions is an important start, but unless the health care system supports the promotion of health behavior change, it will be difficult to sustain these changes. Beyond changes in the training of medical providers, health care system-wide changes in the way behavioral health care is delivered offer another method of improving health behavior change efforts.

CHRONIC CARE MODEL

In an effort to broaden the focus of health care from acute to more chronic problems, the Chronic Care Model was developed to guide quality improvement efforts (Bodenheimer et al., 2002; Wagner et al., 2001). The Chronic Care Model recommends that a patient with a chronic medical condition has a primary care team organizing and coordinating their care. The team reviews data and collaborates with the patient, sets goals and promotes self-management, applies behavioral interventions intended to maximize health, and ensures continuous follow-up. In the Chronic Care Model, the health system is assumed to be part of a community. There are six primary elements of the Chronic Care Model as shown in Table 21.3. Improving these six elements fundamentally assists providers

TABLE 21.3 Components of the Chronic Care Model

CHRONIC CARE MODEL COMPONENT	DESCRIPTION
1. Health systems	Create a culture and practice of promoting safe and high quality care
2. Community resources and policies	Mobilize community programming, counseling, support groups to meet patient needs
3. Self-management support	Empower and prepare patients to manage their health
4. Delivery system design	Ensure delivery of effective and efficient clinical care and self-management support
5. Decision support	Promote evidence-based clinical care consistent with patient preferences
6. Clinical information system	Organize patient and population data to facilitate efficient and effective care

Adapted from Wagner, Austin, & Von Korff (1996) and www.improvingchroniccare.org

in their ability to target health behaviors contributing to disease. Evidence suggests that care redesigned around the Chronic Care Model results in improved patient care and health outcomes (Coleman, Austin, Brach, & Wagner, 2009). Recent information regarding the Chronic Care Model and tools for applying the Chronic Care Model to practice are available at www.improvingchroniccare.org. The Chronic Care Model promotes changing the focus from the "tyranny of the urgent" to a broader and life course perspective on health care.

SYSTEM SUPPORTS AND PRACTICE LEVEL REDESIGNS

As suggested by the Chronic Care Model, there is a growing body of research suggesting that system support/practice level redesign for the delivery of health behavior change interventions by PCPs can be effective. Data from the Worcester Area Trial for Counseling in Hyperlipidemia (WATCH; Ockene et al., 1996) demonstrated that PCPs trained to deliver nutritional counseling with structured office support from prompts and standardized forms to assist with dietary assessment and counseling intervention, engaged in significantly greater implementation of protocols than PCPs in usual care and education-only groups. In fact, PCPs in the education-only group provided no more counseling to their patients than the untrained physicians in the usual care group. An extension of the WATCH study (Ockene et al., 1999) demonstrated that only when PCPs have the training and structured office support can they effectively assist their patients in producing significant decreases in energy consumed from saturated fat, decreased weight, and low-density lipoprotein cholesterol level. Similar outcomes for physician intervention for tobacco use have also been demonstrated (Goldstein et al., 2003). This practice redesign included academic detailing for physician tobacco cessation intervention around a 4 As (Ask, Advise, Assist, and Arrange) conceptual framework. A menu of resources including patient education materials, identification and tracking tools, local smoking cessation programs, office staff training, and environmental prompts (e.g., posters) were used to achieve superior quit rates over controls.

Intensive counseling can enhance behavior change, but may be out of the range of many ordinary primary care practices (Woolf et al., 2005). However, most practices do have the capability to ensure that patients receive high-quality behavior change counseling through practice redesign. Having PCPs and staff spend a few minutes identifying behavior change opportunities and the importance of making those changes can have an impact. These steps can be integrated with other interventions/programs within or outside of the primary care office for more extensive follow-up in concert with a primary care team approach.

In 2002, the Robert Wood Johnson Foundation (RWJF) launched the *Prescription for Health: Promoting Healthy Behaviors in Primary Care Research Networks*. This program consisted of 22 practice-based research networks that were targeting at least two of the following four behaviors: smoking, unhealthy diet, physical inactivity, and risky alcohol use. The results of the various projects are summarized in two journal supplements in the *Annals of Family Medicine (2005)* and *American Journal of Preventive Medicine (2008)*. Key points in program redesign include:

1. To assess and modify patient health behaviors, practices had to undergo substantial practice redesign of staff roles, workflow, office systems, and creating a "bridge" to connect the clinic to community resources.
2. Practices benefitted from the use of the 5 As (Assess, Advise, Agree, Assist, and Arrange) and the Chronic Care Model as vital platforms for addressing health-related behaviors.
3. Effective interventions included the use of:
   a. New technological tools like a personal digital assistant to screen for unhealthy behaviors;
   b. Patient web-based information tools;
   c. Reminder systems, prompts, and care delivery processes to facilitate work of the team, including the provider, during daily clinical practice;
   d. Links to get patients to appropriate services within and outside of the primary care practice;
   e. Training and modified roles for staff to assist with functioning at peak scope of practice.
4. Effectiveness of clinicians in promoting health behaviors appeared to be maximized when a system change supported the entire 5 As' counseling sequence, rather than just the components of the process.
5. Because of limited physician time, successful practices often relied on a team approach, with the physician reinforcing the health behavior change message and front-office staff and nurses screening patients for health behavior problems and delivering counseling interventions prior to or after the patient appointment.

INTEGRATED-COLLABORATIVE BEHAVIORAL HEALTH CARE

Integrating behavioral health providers into health care settings, particularly primary care, offers opportunities for patients and medical providers to be exposed to evidence-based behavioral health interventions. However, the model of care used for integrated-collaborative care influences how much of the practice population is exposed to evidence-based interventions.

As described by Hunter and Goodie (2010), the terminology associated with integrated and collaborative care is inconsistent and poorly defined. There is a continuum of models for integrating behavioral health into primary care (Collins et al., 2010);

however, what constitutes a model of care and what serves as a descriptor of care is confusing. There are two models of integrated-collaborative care commonly implemented in primary care settings, the care management model and the primary care behavioral health model (PCBH). In some cases, these two models are both introduced to produce a blended model of care management and PCBH to maximize the strengths and minimize the weaknesses of each model.

Care Management Models

In care management models (Nutting et al., 2008; Williams et al., 2007), specific pathways for providing enhanced identification and treatment of discrete clinical problems, such as depression or obesity, are developed. Medical providers refer patients to a care manager (e.g., registered nurse or provider with a master's degree in a behavioral health field, typically embedded within the primary care clinic) who assists the patient in adhering to the PCP's recommended behavioral health treatment plan through several processes. The care manager initiates planned, periodic contacts with patients over time, either in person or via telephone. During these contacts, the care manager assesses clinical progress (e.g., for depression, might administer a brief, standardized measure of depression at each contact) to determine whether symptoms are improving. Information regarding patient progress is provided to the PCP, who can then make determinations regarding modifying the treatment plan, if needed. The care manager also monitors and reinforces patients' adherence to the treatment plan. For example, if the PCP prescribed a medication, the care manager might assess whether the patient has filled the prescription and begun taking the medication. The care manager might also ask about any barriers to following the plan (e.g., side effects, cost) and work with the patient on problem solving to overcome barriers. If the PCP recommended a behavior change such as increasing physical activity, the care manager could assist the patient with effective goal setting, increasing motivation for behavior change, and overcoming barriers to adherence.

In some care management models, additional behavioral health resources may also be utilized to enhance behavioral health treatment in primary care. For example, in the Three-Component Model (Oxman, Dietrich, Williams, & Kroenke, 2002), a consulting psychiatrist (external to primary care) routinely staffs cases with the care manager and provides consultative feedback on recommended treatment changes (e.g., change in medication, recommended referrals) to the PCP. In other settings, the presence of an embedded primary care behavioral health consultant (BHC) in addition to a care manager provides the opportunity for a "blended" model, in which the care manager assists with tracking progress and reinforcing the behavior change plan for patients seen by the PCP and/or a BHC for a variety of concerns.

Care management models have been shown to improve treatment of depression (e.g., Gilbody, Bower, Fletcher, Richards, & Sutton, 2006), and have been used extensively in civilian primary care clinics as well as the Department of Defense (Engel et al., 2008), which has implemented programs targeting both depression and post-traumatic stress disorder (PTSD) in active duty members. The care management model enhances the likelihood that patients are exposed to evidence-based treatments. However, this model has limited reach into the population and limited health impact beyond the one or two areas of clinical focus. Only those demonstrating the discrete clinical problem are targeted for enhanced care. Fundamentally, the health care system remains the same, with medical care being provided in the primary care clinic and the majority of behavioral health interventions provided in specialty care clinics.

Primary Care Behavioral Health Model

The primary care behavioral health (PCBH) model is a fundamentally different model of targeting health behaviors (Robinson & Reiter, 2007; Strosahl, 1998). In the PCBH model, behavioral health providers, who function as behavioral health consultants (BHCs), are embedded into the primary care clinic and follow the standards of care within that clinic. These standards of care are different than those in specialty care as we summarize in Table 21.4. Patients are referred to the BHC and are typically seen one to four times in 15- to 30-minute appointment slots. The focus is on targeted, evidence-based interventions for problem behaviors. Patients can book future appointments to see the BHC or may be taken directly from the medical provider to the BHC on the same day for a "warm hand-off." When managing a chronic medical problem (e.g., chronic pain and obesity), patients may be seen periodically over time (e.g., one appointment per month) by the BHC alone or in conjunction with the PCP or other team members to target complex health behaviors. All of these adaptations allow the BHC to seamlessly operate within the context of the primary care clinic and interact with a broad swath of the population.

Embedding and integrating BHCs into the primary care environment is a health care system intervention for changing how health behavior change counseling occurs. Like their PCP counterparts, the embedded BHC can conduct assessments, interventions, and/or consultation for anyone served by the clinic. The PCBH model has the potential to be applied to a broad range of health behavior and behavioral health concerns (Hunter, Goodie, Oordt, & Dobmeyer, 2009; Robinson & Reiter, 2007), and has been shown to be effective for improving outcomes for patients presenting with heterogeneous problems (Bryan et al., 2012), insomnia (Goodie, Isler, Hunter, & Peterson, 2009), and PTSD (Cigrang et al., 2011). However, this model of care needs far more research and rigorous testing to determine its overall efficacy and effectiveness.

The PCBH model has the potential to improve the skills of the PCPs in implementing health behavior change interventions with patients. The BHCs directly interact with PCPs around specific patient needs and provide focused BHC interventions as well as consultative recommendations on what the PCP might target and how they might

TABLE 21.4 Comparison of Behavioral Health Standards of Care in Specialty Mental Health and Primary Care Settings

	SPECIALTY MENTAL HEALTH CARE	PRIMARY CARE BEHAVIORAL HEALTH
Appointment time	50–120 minutes	15–30 minutes
Initiation of care	Self-referral or formal referral from clinic	Patient walked directly to appointment or makes appointment in same clinic
Responsibility of care	Behavioral health provider	Primary care provider
Assessments	Extensive interviews and psychological testing	Targeted functional analyses, brief assessment measures
Interventions	6–12 weeks	1–4 contacts
Documentation	Comprehensive, multipage reports, separate record keeping	Brief, integrated part of the medical record
Follow-up	1–2 week follow-ups	Not at all, next day, 1 week, 1 month, 3–6 months

deliver focused interventions in their follow-up appointments. BHC recommendations are evidence based/informed and can be delivered by the PCP in 1 to 3 minutes. When PCPs see the skills used by the BHC and the positive outcomes on patient behavior, then the PCP's comfort level and willingness to develop their own skills for implementing health behavior change interventions may improve. PCPs see more directly how health behavior change counseling can work, even in the fast-paced environment of primary care. As discussed earlier, if PCPs rely heavily on consultations with colleagues to guide their own clinical interventions, working side by side with a behavioral expert allows for easy access to a collegial voice for health behavior interventions. When BHCs are integrated into primary care settings, patients and PCPs report high levels of satisfaction with the delivery of behavioral health services and PCPs report improved recognition and treatment of behavioral health concerns (Runyan, Fonseca, & Hunter, 2003). Whether the PCBH model improves PCP skills for intervening with behavioral health problems remains untested.

The widespread implementation of the PCBH model has been limited by many of the same barriers discussed for the health care system. In a system where a patient visit cannot be reimbursed if seen for smoking on the same day by a physician and a behavioral specialist, then the opportunities for warm handoffs are eliminated.

The ongoing changes associated with health care reform such as the passing of the Patient Protection and Affordable Care Act, the formation of Accountable Care Organizations, and the continued development of the Patient-Centered Medical Home (PCMH) create an uncertain future for integrated-collaborative care efforts, as behavioral health has been excluded from health care reform (Levey, Miller, & deGruy, 2012). Although medicine is increasingly valuing the contributions of behavioral science for improving the health of the nation, the health care financial system to support the necessary changes to implement this science has been inadequate.

PERSON-CENTERED PROVIDER AND SYSTEM INTERVENTIONS

It is well known that patients' level of readiness for behavior change constitutes an important variable in treatment success. Interventions tailored to match the patients' level of readiness have been widely promoted in effective health behavior change efforts. A similar focus can be taken when the health care provider or health care system is the target of behavior change interventions. Medical students, PCPs, staff, and health care systems (like the patients they serve) will fall along a continuum of readiness to embrace health behavior change interventions. Some will not have substantial awareness of the need to change their practice approach for health behavior change. Others may be aware of a need to alter their approach but may believe they do not have the resources, time, or skills to do so. Still others may be highly motivated and ready to actively implement health behavior change strategies with their patients. Therefore, adopting a person- or system-centered, supportive approach to behavior change may be just as important when working with medical providers, staff, and systems as it is when assisting individual patients in changing health behaviors.

An initial step in moving toward a person- or system-centered approach to promoting adoption of health behavior change strategies involves assessing readiness for change. This assessment can be accomplished through informal or formal means. Informal discussions regarding proposals for changing a PCP's (or clinic's) approach to trying out a different approach toward health behavior change promotion may yield fruitful and rich information. Hallway or break room discussions about a topic such as implementing a reminder system within the electronic medical record to prompt providers to ask tobacco users if they would consider a quit attempt within the next month are likely to engender some debate, and yield good information regarding readiness to approach such an endeavor. Additionally, formal assessment of PCPs or clinic staff and leadership can be conducted to determine levels of readiness to change specific aspects of provider or system behavior. The U.S. Air Force, for example, developed a questionnaire to gauge PCPs' readiness (as well as barriers) to altering their referral and consultation behaviors with integrated BHCs in their clinics (Air Force Medical Operations Agency, 2011). Results assist in understanding sources of low utilization of embedded BHCs. Such information can then be used to develop a tailored intervention plan to increase desired PCP behavior. In this example, results of the assessment might reveal the following three barriers to PCP use of BHCs: (1) unsure how to refer; (2) discomfort in discussing referral to BHC with patients; (3) belief that behavioral health consultation is unlikely to benefit patients. A plan to increase the PCPs' use of the BHC, therefore, might need to include educational components as well as skill- and efficacy-building elements.

Thus, provider and system interventions can be tailored to match levels of readiness to change practices related to promoting health behavior change in patients. This involves meeting PCPs at their level of readiness, and working with them to gradually build their skills and confidence to increase their readiness to take even small steps at change. A PCP may not be ready, for example, to work with depressed patients on increasing their social or enjoyable activities, but might be able to learn and implement a brief intervention to increase adherence to taking prescribed antidepressants. Similarly, on a broader system level, a primary care clinic might not be ready to implement a full clinical pathway for managing obesity in primary care, but might be ready to start a patient registry of obese patients and implement a clinical reminder to cue PCPs to develop small, feasible behavior change plans with patients (e.g., related to eating or physical activity) and to refer patients for more intensive treatment when necessary.

FINANCE AND POLICY SYSTEM INTERVENTIONS

The broad system changes required to implement and sustain integrated primary care models described above face substantial barriers from multiple sources. Of primary concern are policies related to funding of behavioral health and primary care treatment. Financial sustainability of integrated care programs has been cited as the largest challenge facing these models of care (Kathol, Butler, McAlpine, & Kane, 2010). Broadly, fee-for-service models and mental health carve-outs perpetuate the problems with financial sustainability. Examples of specific barriers include policies prohibiting reimbursement for physical health and behavioral health visits on the same day in the same primary care clinic, and inconsistent policies across various payors for reimbursement of the "Health and Behavior" assessment and intervention series of Current Procedural Terminology (CPT) codes.

Various recommendations to improve financial sustainability have been proposed. Some have described approaches to enhance revenue generation through billing of BHC services (Monson, Sheldon, Ivey, Kinman, & Beacham, 2012), while acknowledging that alternate approaches are needed, since direct billing did not fully cover the BHC salary. Miller and colleagues (2011) report that primary care physicians spend 3 to 4 more minutes per appointment with patients who have comorbid medical and mental health conditions, compared to those without comorbidity. They argue that better integration of physical and behavioral health care through PCMH redesign affords the possibility to better meet patient needs while at the same time constraining overall health care spending. They also note that "mental health services must be considered part of primary care and included as an essential health benefit and necessary expense in healthcare redesign ... The new payment must cover the cost of time and teamwork in primary care to realize the national clinical and financial benefits now possible" (p. 145).

Monson et al. (2012) also argue that the current, prevalent fee-for-service approach may never sustain integrated primary care approaches. They suggest use of alternative funding strategies, including reimbursement strategies allowing for payment of bundled services, and higher payments for services that involve collaborative team-based care. They also recommend exploring use of financial incentives for improved health outcomes, posited to occur with integrated care models. Dickinson and Miller (2010) advocate, at a minimum, for adoption of the payment model described in the PCMH Joint Principles (American Academy of Family Physicians, American Academy of Pediatrics, American College of Physicians, and American Osteopathic Association, 2007). One such payment principle is the reimbursement for "services associated with coordination of care both within a given practice and between consultants, ancillary providers, and community resources" (p. 2). The Joint Principles also recommend (similar to Monson et al., 2012) a payment system in which practices are financially rewarded for making measurable improvements in quality of care.

Dickinson and Miller (2010) argue that financial reform must go beyond these Joint Principles recommendations for the PCMH, and that ultimately the behavioral health carve-out system must be replaced through health care reform. This echoes a conclusion of the Agency for Healthcare Research and Quality (AHRQ) Evidence Report on Integration of Mental Health/Substance Abuse and Primary Care (Butler et al., 2008), which notes that integrated care approaches are "fundamentally inconsistent with the dominant fee-for-service payment system. Health plans must be convinced of the subsequent savings ... and thus be willing to underwrite the additional cost, or some other approach to payment must be created" (p. 173).

Thus, the system approaches described here to promote health behavior change in primary care settings are currently limited by significant financial barriers. Numerous authors (Dickinson and Miller, 2010; Miller, Teevan, Phillips, Petterson, & Bazemore, 2011; Monson et al., 2012) have advocated for policy reform to allow for sustainable integration of behavioral health and primary care. There is some optimism that the shift toward adoption of the PCMH concept holds promise, but recognition that further health care policy reform is needed.

ADDRESSING ONE COMPONENT IS NOT ENOUGH

For system changes to be maximally effective in leading to positive health behavior change, there is a need for multicomponent interventions. A "cradle to grave" approach, with multiple factors or contingencies in place, would allow distinct interventions to complement and potentially augment each other.

At a foundational level, there is a need to expose medical students early in training to behavior change principles and interventions. This exposure should expand and continue throughout their training and lifelong continuing education of PCPs. Health care systems need to be changed in order to support provider interventions for health behavior change. Financial factors need to be addressed, either with a financial incentive for integrated-collaborative care models, or at minimum with finance-neutral programs, to promote uptake of changing the service delivery system from separate primary care and behavioral health systems, to integrated models of care. When integrated-collaborative care models are feasible, efforts need to be made to ensure they fit into primary care clinic workflow, and that the behavioral health components can be supported by multiple primary care team members. Contingencies in integrated-collaborative care clinics need to support and reinforce behavior change (e.g., consequences tied to screening rate targets, etc.). When integrated-collaborative care models are not feasible (for financial, personnel availability, or other reasons), clinics should be encouraged to use alternative system approaches incorporating screening and treatment algorithms, technology assistance, and automated referral processes to increase the primary care team's ability to deliver effective health behavior change interventions.

CONCLUSIONS

Health care provider and system interventions are crucial for expanding the impact of health behavior change interventions. Moving forward requires innovation and effort at multiple levels, most importantly in the areas of training, health care policy reform, and research. Future directions for training efforts need to expand the available training for behavioral health providers seeking to work in primary care environments. Some psychology training programs and internships now include coursework and/or clinical supervision in primary care settings. Certificate programs in integrated primary care, ranging from 36 to 80 hours of continuing education and training, have also been developed for those who would like to specialize in this area (e.g., Massachusetts Medical School Certificate Program in Primary Care Behavioral Health, www.integrat edprimarycare.com; Fairleigh Dickinson Certificate Program in Integrated Primary Care, http://integratedcare.fdu.edu). Nevertheless, the growing demand for behavioral health providers with training in integrated care models underscores the need for additional training opportunities and models.

The AAMC Behavioral and Social Science Matrix is a useful guide for conceptualizing when and where to integrate health behavior change education. Experts in health behavior change should collaborate with medical school administrators and faculty to capitalize on current curriculum reform efforts to inject the fundamentals of health behavior change into the earliest medical school classes. As students move from medical school clerkships to internships and residencies, health behavior change experts should promote teaching and evaluation of health behavior change skills, across all medical specialties.

As described earlier, health care policy reform, particularly related to funding and reimbursement for models involving system approaches for health behavior change (e.g., integrated-collaborative care models such as PCBH or care management), is sorely needed. Even expertly trained BHCs and prepared primary care practices and providers will not result in sustainable implementation of integrated care approaches without the financial business plan to support it. To this end, research focused on identifying effective, key components of these system approaches, with a focus on addressing the costs and benefits of such approaches, is needed. Additionally, studies demonstrating that provider and system approaches can effectively lead to behavior change in patients, with subsequent impact on symptoms, functioning, quality of life, and health care utilization patterns, are warranted. Although evidence is strong in some problem areas (e.g., care management for depression; systematic screening for tobacco), other problem areas, behaviors, and outcomes are understudied. Bolstering the evidence that provider and system interventions effectively lead to improved patient outcomes in a cost-effective manner will help drive the case for much needed health care policy reform.

REFERENCES

Accreditation Council for Graduate Medical Education (ACGME). (2012). *ACGME program requirements for graduate medical education in family medicine.* Retrieved from ACGME website http://www .acgme-nas.org/assets/pdf/120_family_medicine_PRs_RC.pdf

Air Force Medical Operations Agency. (2011). *Primary behavioral health care services practice manual* (2nd ed). Lackland AFB, TX: Author.

American Academy of Family Physicians, American Academy of Pediatrics, American College of Physicians, & American Osteopathic Association. (2007). *Joint principles of the patient-centered medical home.* Retrieved from http://www.medicalhomeinfo.org/Joint%20Statement.pdf

Association of American Medical Colleges. (2007). *Physician behavior and practice patterns related to smoking cessation.* Washington, DC: Author.

Association of American Medical Colleges. (2011). *Behavioral and social science foundations for future physicians.* Washington, DC: Author. Retrieved from https://www.aamc.org/download/271020 /data/behavioralandsocialsciencefoundationsforfuturephysicians.pdf.

Bell, K., & Cole, B. A. (2008). Improving medical students' success in promoting health behavior change: A curriculum evaluation. *Journal of General Internal Medicine, 23,* 1503–1506. doi: 10.1007/s11606-008-0678

Bodenheimer, T., Wagner, E. H., & Grumbach, K. (2002). Improving primary care for patients with chronic illness. *Journal of the American Medical Association, 288,* 1775–1779. doi: 10.1001/jama.288.14.1775

Bryan, C. J., Corso, M. L., Corso, K. A., Morrow, C. E., Kanzler, K. E., & Ray-Sannerud, B. (2012). Severity of mental health impairment and trajectories of improvement in an integrated primary care clinic. *Journal of Consulting and Clinical Psychology, 80,* 396–403. doi: 10.1037/a0027726

Butler, M., Kane, R. L., McAlpine, D., Kathol, R. G., Fu, S. S., Hagedorn, H., & Wilt, T. J. (2008). *Integration of Mental Health/Substance Abuse and Primary Care No. 173* (Prepared by the Minnesota Evidence-based Practice Center under Contract No. 290-02-0009.) AHRQ Publication No. 09-E003. Rockville, MD: Agency for Healthcare Research and Quality.

Cigrang, J. A., Rauch, S. A. M., Avila, L. L., Bryan, C. J., Goodie, J. L., Hryshko-Mullen, A., Peterson, A. L., & the STRONG STAR Consortium. (2011). Treatment of active-duty military with PTSD in primary care: Early findings. *Psychological Services, 8,* 104–113. doi:10.1037/a0022740

Coleman, K., Austin, B. T., Brach, C., & Wagner, E. H. (2009). Evidence on the chronic care model in the new millennium. *Health Affairs, 28,* 75–85.

Cook, M., Irby, D. M., & O'Brien, B. C. (2010). *Educating physicians: A call for reform of medical school and residency.* Stanford, CA: Jossey-Bass.

Collins, C., Hewson, D. L., Munger, R., & Wade, T. (2010). *Evolving models of behavioral health integration in primary care.* New York: The Milbank Memorial Fund.

Coumou, H. C. H., & Meijman, F. J. (2006). How do primary care physicians seek answers to clinical questions. A literature review. *Journal of the Medical Library Association, 94,* 55–60.

Cuff, P. A., & Vanselow, N. A. (Eds.). (2004). *Improving medical education: Enhancing the behavioral and social science content of medical school curricula.* Washington, DC: National Academies Press.

Dickinson, W. P., & Miller, B. F. (2010). Comprehensiveness and continuity of care and the inseparability of mental and behavioral health from the patient-centered medical home. *Families, Systems, and Health, 28,* 348–355.

Dolor, R. J., Østbye, T., Lyna, P., Coffman, C. J., Alexander, S. C., Tulsky, J. A., … Pollak, K. I. (2010). What are physicians' and patients' beliefs about diet, weight, exercise, and smoking cessation counseling? *Preventive Medicine, 51,* 440–442. doi: 10.1016/j.ypmed.2010.07.023

Ellerbeck, E. F., Ahluwalia, J. S., Jolicoeur, D. G., Gladden, J., & Mosier, M. C. (2001). Direct observation of smoking cessation activities in primary care practice. *Journal of Family Practice, 50,* 688–693.

Engel, C. C., Oxman, T., Yamamoto, C., Gould, D., Barry, S., Stewart, P., … Dietrich, A. J. (2008). RESPECT-Mil: Feasibility of a systems-level collaborative care approach to depression and post-traumatic stress disorder in military primary care. *Military Medicine, 173,* 935–940.

Fiore, M. C., Bailey, W. C., Cohen, S. J., Dorfman, S. F., Goldstein, M. G., Gritz, E. R., … Wewers, M. E. (2000). *Treating tobacco use and dependence. Clinical practice guideline.* Rockville, MD: U.S. Department of Health and Human Services. Public Health Service.

Fleming, S., & Hiple, D. (2004). Distance education to distributed learning: Multiple formats and technologies in language instruction. *CALICO Journal, 22,* 63–82.

Frank, J. R. (2005). *The CanMEDS 2005 Physician Competency Framework.* The Royal College of Physicians and Surgeons of Canada. Retrieved from http://meds.queensu.ca/medicine/obgyn/pdf /CanMEDS2005.booklet.pdf

Fries, J. F., Koop, C. E., Beadle, C. E., Cooper, P. P., England, M. J., Greaves, R. F., Sokolov, J. J., Wright, D., & the Health Project Consortium. (1993). Reducing health care costs by reducing the need and demand for medical services. *New England Journal of Medicine, 329,* 321–325.

Gilbody, S., Bower, P., Fletcher, J., Richards, D., & Sutton, A. J. (2006). Collaborative care for depression: A cumulative meta-analysis and review of longer-term outcomes. *Archives of Internal Medicine, 166,* 2314–2321.

Goldstein, M. G., Niaura, R., Willey, C., Kazura, A., Rakowski, W., DePue, J., & Park, E. (2003). An academic detailing intervention to disseminate physician-delivered smoking cessation counseling: Smoking cessation outcomes of the Physicians Counseling Smokers Project. *Preventive Medicine, 36,* 185–196.

Goodie, J. L., Isler, W., Hunter, C. L., & Peterson, A. L. (2009). Using behavioral health consultants to treat insomnia in primary care: A clinical case series. *Journal of Clinical Psychology, 65,* 294–304.

Goodie, J. L., Williams, P. W., Kurzweil, D., & Marcellas, K. B. (2011). Can blended classroom and distributed learning approaches be used to teach medical students how to initiate behavior change counseling during a clinical clerkship? *Journal of Clinical Psychology in Medical Settings, 18,* 353–360.

Hauer, K. E., Carney, P. A., Chang, A., & Satterfield, J. (2012). Behavior change counseling curricula for medical trainees: A systematic review. *Academic Medicine, 87,* 956–968.

Heywood, A., Firman, D., Sanson-Fisher, R., Mudge, P., & Ring, I. (1996). Correlates of physician counseling associated with obesity and smoking. *Preventive Medicine, 25,* 268–276. doi: 10.1006/pmed.1996.0056

Hunter, C. L., & Goodie, J. L. (2010). Operational and clinical components for integrated-collaborative behavioral health care in the patient centered medical home. *Families, Systems, and Health, 28,* 308–321.

Hunter, C. L., Goodie, J. L., Oordt, M. S., & Dobmeyer, A. (2009). *Integrated behavioral health in primary care; step-by-step guidance for assessment and intervention.* Washington, DC: American Psychological Association.

Kaplan, R. M., Satterfield, J. M., & Kington, R. S. (2012). Building a better physician—The case for the new MCAT. *New England Journal of Medicine, 366,* 1265–1268. doi: doi:10.1056/NEJMp1113274

Kathol, R. G., Butler, M., McAlpine, D. D., & Kane, R. L. (2010). Barriers to physical and mental condition integrated service delivery. *Psychosomatic Medicine, 72,* 511–518.

Kessler, R. C., Demler, O., Frank, R. G., Olfson, M., Pincus, H. A., Walters, E. E., … Zaslavsky, A. M. (2005). Prevalence and treatment of mental disorders, 1990 to 2003. *New England Journal of Medicine, 352,* 2515–2523.

Levey, S. M. B., Miller, B. F., & deGruy, F. V. (2012). Behavioral health integration: An essential element of population-based healthcare redesign. *Translational Behavioral Medicine, 2,* 364–371.

Ludmerer, K. M. (1999). *Time to heal: American medical education from the turn of the century to the era of managed care.* New York, NY: Oxford University Press.

Martino, S., Haeseler, F., Belitsky, R., Pantalon, M., & Fortin, A. H. (2007). Teaching brief motivational interviewing to year three medical students. *Medical Education, 41,* 160–167.

Miller, B. F., Teevan, B., Phillips, R. L., Petterson, S. M., & Bazemore, A. W. (2011). The importance of time in treating mental health in primary care. *Families, Systems, and Health, 29,* 144–145.

Mokdad, A. H., Marks, J. S., Stroup, D. F., & Gerberding, J. L. (2004). Actual causes of death in the United States, 2000. *Journal of the American Medical Association, 291,* 1238–1245. doi: 10.1001/jama.291.10.1238.

Monson, S. P., Sheldon, J. C., Ivey, L. C., Kinman, C. R., & Beacham, A. O. (2012). Working toward financial sustainability of integrated behavioral health services in a public health care system. *Families, Systems, and Health, 30,* 181–186.

Moser, E. M., & Stagnaro-Green, A. (2009). Teaching behavior change concepts and skills during the third-year medicine clerkship. *Academic Medicine, 84,* 851–858. doi: 10.1097/ACM.0b013e3181a856f8

Nutting, P. A., Gallagher, K., Riley, K., White, S., Dickinson, W. P., Korsen, N., & Dietrich, A. (2008). Care management for depression in primary care practice: Findings from the RESPECT-Depression trial. *Annals of Family Medicine, 6,* 30–37.

Ockene, I. S., Hebert, J. R., Ockene, J. K., Merrikam, P. A., Hurley, T. G., & Saperia, G. M. (1996). Effect of training and a structured office practice on physician-delivered nutrition counseling: The Worcester-Area Trial for Counseling in Hyperlipidemia (WATCH). *American Journal of Preventive Medicine, 12,* 252–258.

Ockene, I. S., Hebert, J. R., Ockene, J. K., Saperia, G. M., Stanek, E., Nicolosi, R., Merriam, P. A., Hurley, T. G. (1999). Effect of physician-delivered nutrition counseling training and an office-support program on saturated fat intake, weight, and serum lipid measurements in a hyperlipidemic population: Worcester Area Trial for Counseling in Hyperlipidemia (Watch). *Archives of Internal Medicine, 159*, 725–731.

Oxman, T. E., Dietrich, A. J., Williams, J. W., & Kroenke, K. (2002). A three-component model for reengineering systems for the treatment of depression in primary care. *Psychosomatics, 43*, 441–450.

Prescription for Health: Changing Primary Care Practice to Foster Healthy Behaviors. (2005). *Annals of Family Medicine, 3*(Suppl.).

Prescription for Health: Reshaping Practice to Support Health Behavior Change in Primary Care. (2008). *American Journal of Preventive Medicine, 35*,(5 Suppl.).

Robinson, P. J., & Reiter, J. T. (2007). *Behavioral consultation and primary care: A guide to integrating services.* New York, NY: Springer.

Runyan, C. N., Fonseca, V. P., & Hunter, C. (2003). Integrating consultative behavioral healthcare into the Air Force medical system. In N. A. Cummings, W. T. O'Donohue, & K. E. Ferguson (Eds.), *Behavioral health as primary care: Beyond efficacy to effectiveness* (pp. 145–163). Reno, NV: Context Press.

Simonson, M., Smaldino, S. E., Albright, M., & Zvacek, S. (2008). *Teaching and learning at a distance: Foundations of distance education* (4th ed.). Upper Saddle River, NJ: Prentice Hall.

Spollen, J. J., Thrush, C. R., Dan-Vy, M., Woods, M. B., Tariq, S. G., & Hicks, E. (2010). A randomized controlled trial of behavior change counseling education for medical students. *Medical Teacher, 32*, e170–e177. doi: 10.3109/01421590903514614

Stafford, R. S., Farhat, J. H., Misra, B., & Schoenfeld, D. A. (2000). National patterns of physician activities related to obesity management. *Archives of Family Medicine, 9*, 631–638.

Strosahl, K. (1998). Integrating behavioral health and primary care services: The primary mental health care model. In A. Blount (Ed.), *Integrated primary care: The future of medical and mental health collaboration* (pp. 139–166). New York, NY: Norton.

Vogt, F., Hall, S., & Marteau, T. M. (2005). General practitioners' and family physicians' negative beliefs and attitudes towards discussing smoking cessation with patients: A systematic review. *Addiction, 100*, 1423–1431.

Wagner, E. H., Austin, B. T., Davis, C., Hindmarsh, M., Schaefer, J., & Bonomi, A. (2001). Improving chronic illness care: Translating evidence into action. *Health Affairs, 20*, 64–78.

Wagner, E. H., Austin, B. T., & Von Korff, M. (1996). Organizing care for patients with chronic illness. *Milbank Quarterly, 74*, 511–544.

Williams, J. W., Gerrity, M., Holsinger, T., Dobscha, S., Gaynes, B., & Dietrich, A. (2007). Systematic review of multifaceted interventions to improve depression care. *General Hospital Psychiatry, 29*, 91–116.

Woolf, S. H., Glasgow, R. E., Krist, A., Bartz, C., Flocke, S. A., Summers-Holtrop, J., … Wald, E. R. (2005). Finding success in behavior change through integration of services. *Annals of Family Medicine, 3*, S20–S27.

22

The Role of the Built Environment in Supporting Health Behavior Change

ANGIE L. CRADOCK
DUSTIN T. DUNCAN

LEARNING OBJECTIVES

- To define the built environment and identify ways in which the built environment is measured including advantages and disadvantages of using different built environment metrics.
- To describe how the built environment can impact health behaviors and interventions to promote behavior change.
- To identify examples of built environment interventions that have been used to influence health-related behaviors.

WHY TARGET THE BUILT ENVIRONMENT FOR HEALTH BEHAVIOR CHANGE?

The notion that the environment can influence our health is not new. Historically, urban planning and public health have had strong links through interventions implemented to address and alleviate communicable diseases (Corburn, 2004). More recently, these links have been rekindled via interdisciplinary research addressing health disparities and chronic diseases, and the health-related behaviors associated with them. Theoretically, features of the built environment can influence health behaviors directly via differential access or exposure to health-promoting or damaging environments or they may enhance or inhibit impact of health behavior change interventions. Therefore, interventions directed at physical surroundings—the environments that we create and within which we live, work, play, socialize, and shop—may serve to initiate and sustain meaningful health-related behavior change.

This chapter reviews research on various aspects of the built environment in relation to health behaviors and health behavior change including the various ways in which it is measured in research and practice. Examples of built environment interventions and related research illustrate the variety of relevant contexts and mechanisms by which the built environment may shape and define health and health-related behaviors. Finally, novel directions and technologies for research and practice provide ideas for innovation in both understanding the links between the built environment and health behavior and in the design and evaluation of health behavior change interventions.

FIGURE 22.1 Determinants of health and well-being in local neighborhoods. (Reprinted from Rao, Prasad, Adshead, & Tissera, 2007. Copyright 2007, with permission from Elsevier)

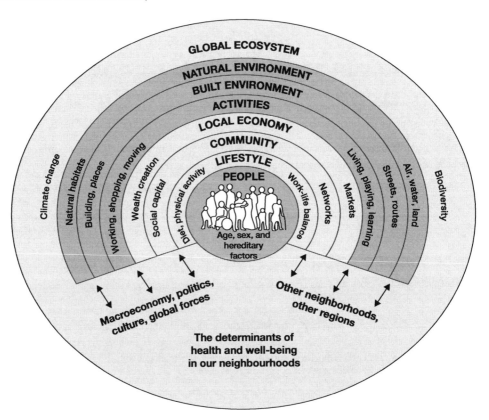

DEFINING THE BUILT ENVIRONMENT

The "built environment" comprises human-made structures and systems that physically define regions, communities, and neighborhoods, including the buildings, houses, streets, and physical systems that serve them (Figure 22.1). The domains, definitions, and measures of the built environment used in research vary considerably in the scientific literature, in part because of the large number of features or characteristics that researchers have studied and measured (Brownson, Hoehner, Day, Forsyth, & Sallis, 2009; Thornton, Pearce, & Kavanagh, 2011). Broadly defined as separate from the natural environment (e.g., air quality and water quality) and the social environment (e.g., social support and social capital), the built environment is often characterized by domains such as access (e.g., proximity, density) and attributes of amenities (e.g., quality) including transportation systems, stores, libraries, and sidewalks. The built environment can be conceptualized and measured at specific geographic scales and is frequently defined for research and intervention at multiple nested levels (Figure 22.2). These levels can include community or neighborhood design features (e.g., regional bicycle networks and community zoning), building site selection and design (e.g., the location and siting of new school buildings), building/facility design (e.g., square footage for physical activity), and element design (e.g., width and lighting of stairwell) (Zimring, Joseph, Nicoll, & Tsepas, 2005).

FIGURE 22.2 Geographic scale of built environment.

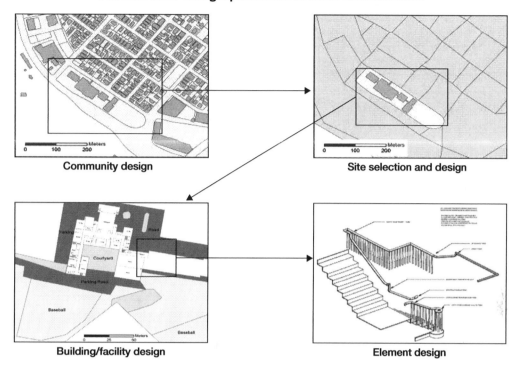

MEASUREMENT OF THE BUILT ENVIRONMENT

Various metrics can be used to measure the built environment (Table 22.1) and measures of the built environment vary enormously from study to study. Researchers frequently measure the built environment via a *self-reported questionnaire* (Brownson et al., 2009). This type of survey data measures the respondents' perceptions of characteristics of the built environment such as their access to neighborhood parks or recreational facilities. One such survey measure of the built environment is the Neighborhood Environment Walkability Survey (NEWS) (Cerin, Saelens, Sallis, & Frank, 2006; Rosenberg et al., 2009) which can be used to characterize perceptions of access via questions such as "About how long would it take you to walk from your home to the nearest basketball court?" While self-reported assessment of the built environment may have several benefits, it can be difficult for study participants to disentangle the perception of their environment from their usual health-related behavior practices (Diez Roux, 2007). For example, independent of actual measured distance, regular walkers may report their local grocery as quite accessible via walking more often than those who are less inclined or able to walk longer distances.

Systematic social observations (SSOs) or environmental audits (Brownson et al., 2009) have increased in popularity as a tool to measure the built environment. Traditional SSOs are in-person assessments of neighborhoods or physical spaces such as stores or building features. When conducting SSOs, researchers can assess various built environment features via walking or driving, using handheld computers or simply documenting features using a paper-and-pencil tool. Usually these observations are based on an existing tool such as the Environmental Assessment of Public Recreation Spaces (EAPRS) tool (Saelens et al., 2006). This method of assessing the built environment can be particularly time intensive and requires well-trained data collectors to ensure reliable and valid assessments. To overcome these limitations, researchers now increasingly use Google Street View, an online resource with visual assessments of neighborhood streets made from traveling vehicle-mounted cameras.

Geographic Information System (GIS) methods are commonly used to measure features and characteristics of the built environment (Matthews, Moudon, & Daniel, 2009). GIS technology facilitates storing, managing, analyzing, and presenting data that is linked with a specific geographic location. Although complete GIS data layers are not always readily accessible for all geographic regions, researchers and practitioners can obtain or create GIS data layers and then perform various functions in a GIS package (e.g., ArcGIS) to assess and define measures such as geographic proximity or density measures (e.g., distance to grocery store and park density). Some studies have coupled GIS analysis with Global Positioning System (GPS) technology to track people's movements in order to link behaviors or exposures with characteristics of the built environments as study participants move through space and time.

Wearable sensing methods and web-based geospatial data are more recently developed tools for measuring the built environment. *Wearable sensing methods* including cameras or other sensing and recording systems can be used to measure one's built environment. For example, the SenseCam is a small lightweight wearable camera worn via a lanyard around the neck that can capture up to 3,000 first-person point-of-view images per day (Doherty et al., 2011; Hodges et al., 2006). The ability to collect this measurement data in real time in conjunction with behavioral data and to capture aspects of the built environment that other methods cannot (e.g., physical obstructions such as construction work and parked cars in cycle lanes) are unique features of these tools and techniques. However, these methods currently are not able to capture images in dark environments, management of the large amounts of data retrieved can be difficult (Doherty et al., 2011; Kelly et al., 2011), and the device and its use in research can be costly.

Web-based geospatial technologies are emerging tools to measure the built environment. For example, the web-based Walk Score tool (freely available at www.walkscore .com) is a popular tool due to its accessibility, international scale, and use of timely data. Walk Score allows a user to enter any query location into the online interface on its website and receive the Walk Score assigned to that location that is calculated based on distance to various categories of "walkable" amenities (e.g., schools, stores, parks, and libraries). Walk Score can accurately characterize several aspects of the built environment (e.g., density of retail destinations, density of recreational open space, intersection density, and residential density) across geographies and spatial scales (Carr, Dunsiger, & Marcus, 2010, 2011; Duncan, Aldstadt, Whalen, Melly, & Gortmaker, 2011), but only provides an overall assessment of neighborhood walkability rather than characterizing specific features that may be of interest for certain purposes.

Each of these built environment measurement tools has strengths and limitations for characterizing important aspects of the built environment. The use of multiple methods of measuring the built environment may provide a fuller picture of environmental conditions. A particular method (or methods) may be used because of cost or implementation concerns or its utility in characterizing the specific features or geographic scale of the environment that is the point for understanding and intervention.

TABLE 22.1 Built Environment Measurement Metrics

TYPE OF ASSESSMENT	KEY FEATURES	RELEVANT SCALE OF MEASURE
Self-Reported Questionnaire *Questionnaires that are designed to characterize personal perceptions of local built environment features*	+ Ease of administration + Individualized information − Perception may be related to behavior of interest	Community Design Site Selection and Design Building/Facility Design Element Design
Traditional Systematic Social Observation (SSO) *In-person assessments of the neighborhood, including assessing various built environment features via walking or driving, using handheld computers or simply with a paper and pencil*	+ Objective assessment − Can be time/resource intensive − Required level of training to conduct assessments	Community Design Site Selection and Design Building/Facility Design Element Design
Geographic Information Systems (GIS) *GIS technology, which facilitates storing, managing, analyzing, and presenting data that is linked to a location, can measure the built environment*	+ Can manage and store many types of data + Visual display − Not always available in all areas	Community Design Site Selection and Design Building/Facility Design
Wearable Sensing Data *Wearable cameras with multiple sensors that are worn via a lanyard around the neck to measure the built environment*	+ Collects data in real time with relevant behaviors + Captures features/ elements of personal environment − Costly equipment − Limited to daytime collection	Site Selection and Design Building/Facility Design Element Design
Web-Based Geospatial Data *Web-based data that can be used to measure the built environment*	+ Accessibility + Often timely data + Geographic coverage − Sometimes cannot characterize specific features/elements	Community Design Site Selection and Design

LIFE-COURSE PERSPECTIVE AND CONTEXT-SPECIFIC BEHAVIORS

The impact and importance of the built environment in health behavior change interventions will differ according to the behaviors, context and population of interest. For example, features within the built environment of the street setting such as a sidewalk or crossing signal may be particularly relevant to interventions promoting walking behaviors among children, the elderly, and other vulnerable populations with different visual or mobility levels. In many cases, context is a key consideration. School environments are relevant contexts in the lives of children and adolescents and may be particularly pertinent for interventions influencing both nutrition and physical activity while the work environment is likely central to many adult behavioral interventions. Other built environment contexts, for example, community parks where people "play" and socialize may be important to interventions focused on overall leisure-time physical activities. Therefore, successful research and intervention studies must use measurement strategies that are relevant to the specific behavior being studied, the context in which the behavior occurs, and capture and assess the built environment at an appropriate geographic scale to quantify its potential impact. The following provides some examples of the associations between features of the built environment and behaviors including physical activity, healthy eating, tobacco and alcohol use, as well as association with mental health outcomes, injury prevention, and traffic safety.

Physical Activity

Built environments can promote physical activity via physical activity promoting facilities and environments (Figure 22.3). Physical activity behaviors and built environment characteristics that influence them have been studied extensively, albeit primarily in observational studies. Physical activity, measured objectively via monitoring devices or via self-report from study participants, is often segmented into various domains (e.g., transport and recreational) or activity types (e.g., walking and cycling) in studies of the built environment–physical activity link. Among adults, cycling for transportation has been associated with amenities such as dedicated cycle routes or other road structures enhancing separation of cycling from other traffic as well as with factors such as high population density and distance. Among children, bicycling for transport is also associated with projects promoting safe routes to school (Fraser & Lock, 2011). Similarly, attributes of destinations (e.g., presence and proximity) and route (e.g., sidewalks and street connectivity) are frequent correlates of both utilitarian and recreational walking among adults (Sugiyama, Neuhaus, Cole, Giles-Corti, & Owen, 2012). Among children and adolescents, research suggests walkability, traffic speed/volume, access/proximity to recreational facilities, and the urban form characteristics of land-use mix and residential density are some important correlates of physical activity participation (Ding, Sallis, Kerr, Lee, & Rosenberg, 2011).

Nutrition-Related Behaviors

Local stores, supermarkets, and fast food restaurants can influence nutrition-related behaviors via access and marketing of foods and beverages. The built environment for food access broadly shaped by policy and organizational factors (Story, Kaphingst, Robinson-O'Brien, & Glanz, 2008) is often characterized according to measures of availability (e.g., shelf-space placement of healthy items) or access (e.g., distance to supermarket and density of fast food establishments) (Charreire et al., 2010; Gustafson, Hankins, & Jilcott, 2012).

Research that has evaluated a variety of different dietary patterns, foods, or nutrients suggests evidence for association with nutrition built environments. However, studies have examined associations between the built environment and nutrition-related behaviors using perceived availability and objectively measured accessibility to different effect. In many cases, measures of perceived availability are linked to healthy nutritional behaviors while objective accessibility measures receive less support from the literature. Researchers suggest this may be because the distance-based accessibility measures fail to capture other relevant measures of the food environment that influence purchasing including affordability, acceptability, and accommodation (Caspi, Sorensen, Subramanian, & Kawachi, 2012). Also, within the same geographic context perception- and objective GIS-based characterizations of the food environment are associated but are not identical (Moore, Roux, & Franco, 2012). As measures of nutritional behaviors are complex and varied, the inconsistent importance of the built environment may have something to do with the quality and type of nutritional outcome measure studied and the context of assessment. There is a need for more attention to the measurement of food access and food environments (Caspi et al., 2012). Furthermore, it is recognized that access to healthy foods is not uniform across all settings including low-income, minority, and rural areas (Larson, Story, & Nelson, 2009).

FIGURE 22.3 An ecological model of physical activity behaviors (Salis, Floyd, Rodriquez, & Saelens, 2009, by permission of Wolters Kluwer Health).

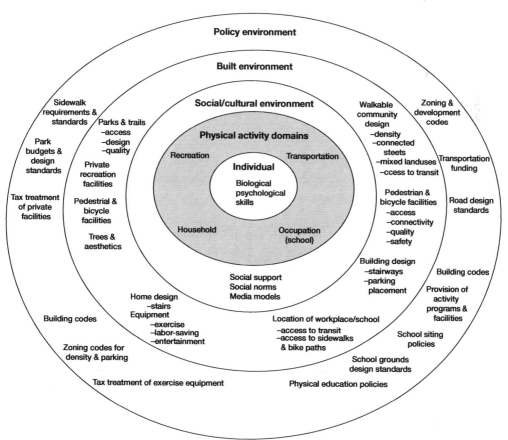

Tobacco and Alcohol Use

Some research has evaluated associations between the built environment and substance use (e.g., tobacco and alcohol use), positing that access can influence use. A growing body of research demonstrates that accessibility to tobacco retailers is associated with increased tobacco use. For example, several studies show that access to tobacco retailers in the residential and school neighborhood environments of youth is associated with their increased tobacco use (Chan & Leatherdale, 2011; Henriksen et al., 2008; Leatherdale & Strath, 2007; McCarthy et al., 2007; Novak, Reardon, Raudenbush, & Buka, 2006). While some research has found a positive association between alcohol availability and alcohol use (Halonen et al., 2012; Kypri, Bell, Hay, & Baxter, 2008), several studies have found no association between availability of alcohol outlets and alcohol use (Connor, Kypri, Bell, & Cousins, 2011; McKinney, Chartier, Caetano, & Harris, 2012; Pasch, Hearst, Nelson, Forsyth, & Lytle, 2009; Waller et al., 2012). Further research is needed to understand relationships between the built environment and substance use outcomes.

Mental Health

Research on built environments and depression outcomes suggests that the built environment can be associated with depression and depressive symptoms (Kim, 2008; Mair, Roux, & Galea, 2008) through a variety of pathways (Figure 22.4). Potentially, greater access to destinations and community design features in the built environment may promote socialization (Cohen, Inagami, & Finch, 2008; de Toit, Cerin, Leslie, & Owen, 2007; Leyden, 2003; Rogers, Halstead, Gardner, & Carlson, 2011) and physical activity (Davison & Lawson, 2006; Ding et al., 2011; Giles-Corti, Kelty, Zubrick, & Villanueva, 2009; Rosso, Auchincloss, & Michael, 2011; Saelens & Handy, 2008; Saelens & Papadopoulos, 2008; Saelens, Sallis, & Frank, 2003), both of which may contribute to improved mental health (Kawachi & Berkman, 2001; Kim, 2008; Mair et al., 2008; Teychenne, Ball, & Salmon, 2008). Studies assessing the association between measures of neighborhood walkability and depression have shown mixed results, perhaps due to differences in measurement, study population or design. Some evidence supports pathways linking the built environment to decreased depression (Berke, Gottlieb, Moudon, & Larson, 2008; Galea, Ahern, Rudenstine, Walllace, & Vlahove, 2005; Stockdale et al. 2007) while other studies suggested a null association (Kubzansky et al., 2005; Schootman et al., 2007).

Injury Prevention and Traffic Safety

As programs and public health campaigns promote physically active transportation, the safety of pedestrians and bicyclists becomes an important concern. Disparities exist in pedestrian injuries by neighborhood and by socioeconomic status with greater numbers of traffic injuries occurring among young people, children from lower social positions, and in more deprived socioeconomic areas, perhaps due to differential hazard exposures (Laflamme & Diderichsen, 2000). Targeted investments in infrastructure and physical improvements may serve to prevent injury and decrease potential barriers to active transport. Research suggests that environmental traffic-calming measures such as speed bumps can contribute to a reduction in vehicle operating speeds, while safe crossing strategies such as provision of marked crosswalks and wide, raised medians result in more pedestrians crossing at identified crossing locations and fewer pedestrian crashes, respectively (Dumbaugh & Frank, 2007).

FIGURE 22.4 Relationships between neighborhood characteristics and adult depression (Kim, 2008, by permission of Oxford University Press).

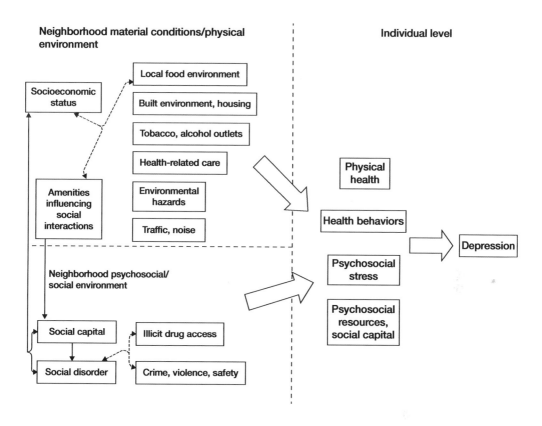

CHALLENGES WITH INTERVENTIONS IN THE BUILT ENVIRONMENT

Interventions within the built environment to influence health behaviors have the capacity to reach populations of individuals defined by geographic context and the potential for sustainability over time. However, there are several challenges related to the identification and dissemination of effective built environment interventions. These include the early phase of research documenting the impact of built environment interventions, the potential long time course and cost associated with large-scale built environment interventions and the need for development of cross-sector or cross-organizational partners to implement multi-sector or multi-system interventions.

IDENTIFYING EFFECTIVE BUILT ENVIRONMENT INTERVENTIONS

Most research on the role of the built environment in health behavior change has been correlational research, a first step to identify promising areas for interventional research. However, it is now a rapidly evolving area of research for both implementation and evaluation as communities and organizations undertake to implement and evaluate new evidence-based or evidence-informed built environment initiatives (Table 22.2). As with the built environment itself, built environment interventions vary considerably with regard to their scale, from smaller scale efforts in changing specific design features inside a

TABLE 22.2 Resources for Identifying and Implementing Built Environment Interventions

RESOURCE	HEALTH BEHAVIOR AREA(S)	SOURCE
Active Living Research	Physical activity	www.activelivingresearch.org
The Community Guide: Environmental and Policy Approaches to Increase Physical Activity: Street-Scale Urban Design Land Use Policies	Physical activity	www.thecommunityguide.org/pa/environmental-policy/streetscale.html
Active Design Guidelines: Promoting Physical Activity and Health in Design	Physical activity	www.nyc.gov/html/ddc/html/design/active_design.shtml
Healthy Eating Design Guidelines for School Architecture	Healthy eating	www.cdc.gov/pcd/issues/2013/12_0084.htm
Active Design Supplement: Promoting Safety	Safety-related behaviors	http://centerforactivedesign.org/promotingsafety
The Center for Training and Research Translation (Center TRT)	Multiple	www.centertrt.org
Built Environment + Public Health Curriculum	Multiple	www.bephc.com/resources/web-resources

building to larger scale efforts such as the design and construction of a network of bicycling pathways. In many cases, random assignment to intervention condition is not an option due to the nature of these changes. Oftentimes, research opportunity comes through evaluation of natural experiments, interventions already under way for which evaluation can be conducted. Research using experimental and quasi-experimental studies has expanded in recent decades.

TIME COURSE, COST, AND SUSTAINABILITY OF INTERVENTIONS IN THE BUILT ENVIRONMENT

Generally, built environmental interventions could be considered sustainable interventions in that they influence the structure and function of the physical environment in which health behaviors occur but do not require repeated introduction in order to be maintained. Depending on the intervention strategy and the scale at which it is implemented, the cost and the time frame for execution may be important considerations in both intervention evaluation study design and the replication or dissemination of effective built environment interventions. Increasingly, studies have sought to evaluate or report intervention implementation costs (Hannon & Brown, 2008; Ridgers, Stratton, Fairclough, & Twisk, 2007); however, cost effectiveness studies of built environment interventions are a nascent area of research (Roux et al., 2008; Wu, Cohen, Shi, Pearson, & Sturm, 2011).

DEVELOPING NECESSARY PARTNERSHIPS ACROSS SECTORS

Many interventional strategies necessitate the development of partnerships to ensure appropriate implementation and effectiveness. However, interventions within the built environment can require new or cross-sector partnerships, particularly for interventions using a system perspective that require changes across multiple sectors within a system to implement (Kohl et al., 2012). Such collaborations can include urban planners, parks/recreation officials, transportation engineers, and public health officials. Transport system intervention, such as the implementation of a light rail system, or citywide planning and zoning changes mandating a certain percentage of neighborhoods dedicated to parks or open space are examples of system interventions that may require partnerships across sectors for appropriate implementation.

INTERVENTIONS TO CHANGE BEHAVIORS ACROSS SECTORS

Intervention within the built environment can be instrumental in helping to influence health behavior in at least three ways. First, through modification of the built environment directly, interventions may create prompts or structure the built environment to *make the desired health behavior easier or even automatic* while less desirable health behaviors are made more difficult. This interventional strategy is often included as a component of multicomponent health behavior change interventions. Second, the built environment may also serve to modify interventional impact by *moderating the effects of a behavioral intervention* that has been introduced. Third, characteristics of the built environment may *require that existing health behavior change interventions be modified (or adapted) prior to implementation* in order to achieve fidelity of the interventional implementation and maximum intervention effectiveness. The following sections provide examples of these types of influence across a number of sectors (Figure 22.5) that impact health behavior (Chaix, 2009).

FIGURE 22.5 Sectors and environments that influence health behavior and health outcomes (Chaix, 2009, with permission).

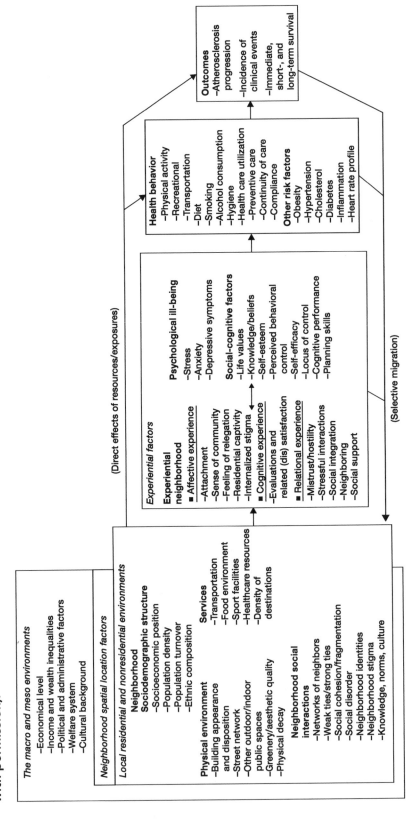

NEW TECHNOLOGY AND THE BUILT ENVIRONMENT

New technologies, particularly geo-referencing technology and associated spatial analysis techniques, have altered the potential for place-specific targeted intervention strategies focused on promoting health-related behaviors and environments that are conducive to positive health outcomes. Geographic information system based methods can be used to identify and characterize areas in need of environmental intervention to increase safety and reduce injury among bicyclists and pedestrians (Poulos, Hatfield, Rissel, Grzebieta, & McIntosh, 2012; Rodgers, Jones, Macey, & Lyons, 2010) or to tailor individually focused behavioral interventions (e.g., identifying neighborhood facilities and dispensing walking prescriptions by health care providers) (Carr et al., 2010; Duncan et al., 2011).

EDUCATION, TOOLS, AND TRAINING TO FACILITATE BUILT ENVIRONMENT INTERVENTIONS

Training programs, community assessment tools, and educational settings each provide opportunities for educating students, professionals, and the public regarding the roles of the built environment in influencing health behaviors and other health-related outcomes. Training programs for transportation professionals address topics including pedestrian safety, pedestrian and bicycle planning, and pedestrian and bicycle facility design (Dill & Weigand, 2010) building on interdisciplinary model curricula that have been outlined (Botchwey et al., 2009). Additionally tools for transport and planning practitioners (Forsyth, Slotterback, & Krizek, 2010) and initiatives that include training public health practitioners and community members on methods for measuring and assessing the built environment is an approach to promote and enhance health and health-related behaviors used increasingly in interventions by public health agencies and health departments (Bias, Leyden, Abildso, Reger-Nash, & Bauman, 2010; Reger-Nash, Bauman, Cooper, Chey, & Simon, 2006).

SCHOOL ENVIRONMENTS AND PHYSICAL SPACES TO PROMOTE HEALTH BEHAVIORS

Schools are important environments for influencing the health-related behaviors of both the students and teachers and other employees for whom the school itself is a worksite. Interventions within the built environments of schools have been developed to address dietary behaviors as well as physical activity and tobacco use. Often making the "healthy choice the easy choice" in school-based interventions has included a *mix of a physical infrastructure change intervention as well as awareness and education.*

Many students consume foods and beverages while on school property making the built environment of schools a popular setting for interventions to promote healthy eating and drinking behaviors. Adequate fruit and vegetable intake is recommended to promote health and reduce chronic disease risk and may help with maintaining a healthy weight when consumed in place of more calorically dense foods (U.S. Department of Agriculture, 2010). In the Los Angeles Unified School District, school building infrastructure changes including the addition of salad bars to the cafeteria and the promotion of the salad bar as an option for reimbursable school lunch program were accompanied by an increase in reported fruit and vegetable consumption among students (Slusser, Cumberland, Browdy, Lange, & Neumann, 2007). In some instances, the school built environment may serve as a barrier. For example, promoting adequate water intake among students may produce health benefits as water provides a calorie-free source of hydration. However, in some schools drinking water access is poor due to inadequate plumbing or contaminated drinking water sources. In order to implement an intervention to promote tap water as a primary beverage during after-school snack periods, participants had to modify the intervention activities and provide alternate drinking water sources due to the lack of potable tap water in some schools (Giles et al. 2012).

School playgrounds are a common context for play and physical activity among students. Several studies have evaluated the impact on physical activity of interventions that include modification to the playground built environment. Among preschool aged students, physical activity friendly equipment appropriate for younger children was added to the outdoor play area in a childcare center in order to promote active play. The young attendees significantly decreased the percentage of outdoor playtime spent in sedentary behavior and increased light, moderate, and vigorous physical activity over 5 days of measurement following the intervention (Hannon & Brown, 2008). Among older children, researchers found that direct modification of the built environment, including setting up painted playground markings identifying appropriate activity-specific play areas and installing physical structures including goal posts and basketball hoops, fencing, and seating areas, led to increased time that students attending these schools spent in moderate and vigorous physical activity over 6 months compared with students attending schools that did not receive the environmental intervention (Ridgers et al., 2007). The newness and level of physically active play promoting *attributes of built environment interventions may also be important considerations* for physical activity. Researchers found that although playground utilization was greater, physical activity levels did not increase in a playground intervention study incorporating art, shade structures, and garden elements into playground environments (Anthamatten et al., 2011) and that over longer periods even effective renovation intervention impacts may diminish (Ridgers, Fairclough, & Stratton, 2010).

PROMPTING HEALTHY BEHAVIORS IN OTHER EVERYDAY ENVIRONMENTS

The built environment may be used to promote and prompt healthy behaviors in everyday activities and environments beyond schools as well. For example, taking the stairs is one way to be more physically active in everyday environments and has been associated with improvements in fitness over short intervention periods (Boreham et al., 2005). Examples of interventions promoting stair use in place of elevators and escalators have generally relied on point-of-decision signage frequently demonstrating statistically significant increases in stair use with potential for longer-term sustainability (Soler et al., 2010). However, research suggests that building feature design characteristics can impede or promote stair use. Relevant features include the number of floors in a building (Bungum, Meacham, & Truax, 2007), the visibility (Bungum et al., 2007; Grimstvedt et al., 2010), width (Nicoll, 2007), and the relative time costs of using the stairs versus other methods based on location and accessibility within a setting (Lewis & Eves, 2012). Stairwell lighting, restrictions or key access, and the number of stairs between floors are additional factors associated with stair use (Titze, Martin, Seiler, & Marti, 2001). For example, researchers conducted an innovative natural experiment in an office setting that was designed to promote stair use. In one study group, the workers' offices clustered around the skip-stop elevator, an elevator that was designed not to stop at every floor but located adjacent to an open stairway, whereas other workers' offices accessed an elevator that stopped at each floor with nearby enclosed fire exit stairs. Researchers measured stair use with infrared monitors and card-reader activity logs and found that the skip-stop stair design was used 33 times more than the enclosed stair of the traditional elevator core (Nicoll & Zimring, 2009).

Other examples of interventions to prompt and improve health-related behaviors occur outside of buildings on the streets of cities and towns. Transportation planning professionals use several *design features* for streets and street crossings to prompt and encourage appropriate driving speeds and traffic safety behaviors among pedestrians to reduce potential for injury and make these environments more walkable and safe for all users (Dumbaugh & Frank, 2007). For example, installations of marked crosswalks identify for pedestrians and drivers the expected and appropriate locations for pedestrian road crossings. Accessible pedestrian crossing countdown signals, visual signals that provide information on the amount of time remaining on signalized intersections as well as auditory information for pedestrians with visual can prompt safe street-crossing behaviors, thereby decreasing the potential for pedestrian injury. Installation of traffic-calming measures including speed feedback signs, speed bumps to reduce traffic speed, and designing streets with special features such as chicanes (mid-block bump outs on alternate sides of the street) are strategies used to reduce traffic speed and cut-through on residential streets (Bunn et al., 2009). These types of interventions are often employed together in areas with heightened pedestrian and vehicle conflict or in places where improved walkability is desired to promote physically active transportation modes.

PATIENT-CENTERED SUPPORTIVE ENVIRONMENTS: NEW DIRECTIONS IN HEALTH FACILITY DESIGN

The purpose of innovative health facility design is not only to provide adequate functionality for performance of services (*Guidelines for Design and Construction of Health Care Facilities*, 2010) but also to underscore the ways in which the facility itself can help promote appropriate health behaviors, remove exposures to environmental stressors, and promote positive distraction and emotion that may influence health outcomes directly. Studies have looked at ways in which built environment features of health care settings such as access to natural views and gardens and decreased exposure to noise through facility element design features may help alleviate stress and promote recovery (Drahota et al., 2012; Ulrich et al., 2008). Public health and design professionals have jointly developed evidence-based guiding principles for health care facility design for intensive care units including outlining access to hand hygiene facilities (Thompson et al., 2012). Hand washing behaviors are a key component to infection control and public health. Both hygienic soap and alcohol solutions can be used to beneficial effect (Zaragoza, Salles, Gomez, Bayas, & Trilla, 1999) and are considered as important features of adequate health facility design for infection control. Appropriate access to hand washing facilities through environmental design and implementation of easily accessible dispensers, both in proper placement of facilities and density of dispensers per hospital bed, result in better compliance with accepted hand hygiene protocols (Bischoff, Reynolds, Sessler, Edmond, & Wenzel, 2000).

USING PLANNING, DESIGN, AND TRANSPORTATION TO INFLUENCE AND MODIFY COMMUNITY SPACES: SYSTEM PERSPECTIVES

Planning, design, and transportation are three key systems used to promote health-related behaviors while simultaneously preventing or reducing injury or unwanted environmental exposures (Rydin, Bleahu, & Davis, 2012). Using system perspectives, built environment interventions can be implemented across entire communities as they are being developed, or redeveloped. For example, the Smart Growth movement often

TABLE 22.3 Smart Growth Principles

1. Mix land uses
2. Take advantage of compact building design
3. Create a range of housing opportunities and choices
4. Create walkable neighborhoods
5. Foster distinctive, attractive communities with a strong sense of place
6. Preserve open space, farmland, natural beauty, and critical environmental areas
7. Strengthen and direct development toward existing communities
8. Provide a variety of transportation choices
9. Make development decisions predictable, fair, and cost-effective
10. Encourage community and stakeholder collaboration in development decisions

Smart Growth Online (2013).

involves multi-disciplinary partners from planning, design, transportation, the environment, and health as well as safety sectors, among others (Geller, 2003). It is based on 10 principles (Table 22.3) that can be followed in development and redevelopment policies and practices at the local, state, and federal levels to support communities that promote health and well-being (Geller, 2003).

In other cases, communities may work locally within a single system. Domestically and internationally, bicycling planning, policy, and infrastructure development have led to variations in bicycling across communities of various sizes (Pucher, Dill, & Handy, 2010). Interventions within the transportation system to increase the share of road users who travel via bicycle and foster safe travel focus on provision of bikeway facilities that may include on-street bike lanes, on-street bike paths (or cycle tracks), and off-street bike paths. Minneapolis, Minnesota, and Portland, Oregon, are examples of two cities that have substantially increased per capita bicycling infrastructure such as bike lanes and paths over the past decade. These infrastructure improvements have come with complementary features including bicycle parking and improved integration with transit or local bicycle sharing programs. In these communities of Minneapolis and Portland, the comprehensive transportation interventions accompanied twofold to fivefold increases in bicycling rates among commuters (Pucher, Buehler, & Seinen, 2011).

Community and transportation planners have also undertaken initiatives to improve access and promote safety across entire neighborhoods. Area-specific traffic-calming interventions appear to contribute to injury reduction and safety improvements (Bunn et al., 2009; Elvik, 2001), and improved reported physical health, increased local pedestrian activity, and decreased traffic nuisance (Morrison, Thomson, & Petticrew, 2004). These types of "complete streets" initiatives are becoming more commonly integrated transportation system strategies to enhance walkability and mobility in communities (Shinkle, Rall & Wheet, 2012).

USING LOCAL, STATE, AND NATIONAL POLICY TO INFLUENCE THE BUILT ENVIRONMENT

Policy change can be an important component and contributor to intervention in the built environment. Relevant policy may exist within organizations or at various levels of government including federal, state, or local authority levels and include administrative policy enacted and implemented in counties, cities, and through other legal entities. Policy-focused interventions may begin with the identification of relevant policies followed by efforts to identify the relevant policy-making body with legal authority to change or implement specific policy. Relevant policy may be assistive policies that enable modifications to the built environment to promote certain types of health behaviors (e.g., federal policy requiring water access in meal service areas for schools participating in the National School Lunch Program) whereas other types of policy may be restrictive, thereby inhibiting changes to the built environment in order to decrease exposure to unhealthy built environments (Perdue, Stone, & Gostin, 2003).

Some local policies can *determine how and where physical infrastructure is developed*. Local zoning policies can influence developments in the structure of locales including the land-use mix, connectivity of streets, the planned infrastructure for pedestrians, and other neighborhood aesthetics (Lopez, 2012) often associated with neighborhood walkability and physical activity (Mozaffarian et al., 2012). Because local zoning and building ordinances also define appropriate land uses, they may be used to restrict certain unwanted uses or types of development. For example, several studies suggest links between the density of tobacco retail outlets around schools or homes and smoking prevalence (Mozaffarian et al., 2012). In some communities in California, zoning ordinances, conditional use permits, and direct regulation have restricted location of tobacco retail establishments within a certain distance of schools and other community resources including parks and playgrounds (Center for Tobacco Policy & Organizing, 2011).

Policy can also serve to *facilitate access to existing built environment infrastructure*. For example, shared-use arrangements, or creating sharing agreements that facilitate public use of community resources such as schools or recreation facilities, are recommended by several leading public health authorities (Council on Sports Medicine and Fitness 2006; Institute of Medicine [IOM], 2013) and are one of the strategies included in the National Physical Activity Plan (www.physicalactivity plan.org). In many cases, the sharing of these community resources is facilitated by written contracts or legal arrangements. These shared or joint-use agreements specify liability, use, maintenance, and responsibilities of the parties engaged in the facility sharing arrangements (Public Health Law & Policy 2010a). Community-use policy strategies may be one way to alleviate the lack of available recreational facilities in some communities, particularly in those areas with populations at high risk for disease or lower income communities or neighborhoods with higher proportions of residents of color, where studies have documented disparities in physical activity promoting amenities (Powell, Slater, Chaloupka, & Harper, 2006) and recreational open space (Duncan, Kawachi, White, & Williams, 2013). An intervention focused on community use of an existing renovated school playground was associated with a measureable increase in the numbers of children who were physically active on the school grounds and in the local neighborhoods when compared with a similar sized neighborhood and school that had not been renovated nor opened for community use (Farley et al., 2007). Model community-use agreement templates may be important facilitators in the dissemination of these policies to local communities and school districts (Eyler & Swaller, 2012) and many states now have laws addressing use of school property by community members (Public Health Law & Policy, 2010b).

CREATING A HEALTHY COMMUNITY THROUGH MULTICOMPONENT BUILT ENVIRONMENT INTERVENTIONS

Multicomponent built environment interventions include changes to the built environment in addition to other behavior change intervention components including informational strategies and behavior modification. For example, as walking and bicy-cling to school can help kids be more physically active (Faulkner, Buliung, Flora, & Fusco, 2009), Safe Routes to School (SRTS) programs in the United States were created as part of federal transportation policy that provided funding to support local pro-grams in each state. These programs work to create safe and convenient opportunities for children to walk and bicycle to school via changes in the built environment and use education, promotion, and enforcement strategies at the school and community levels (Cradock, Fields, Barrett, & Melly, 2012). Evaluation of the local implementation of safe routes programs suggests that interventions have varied on the spectrum from focus-ing primarily on making built environment improvements (Boarnet, Anderson, Day, McMillan, & Alfonzo, 2005; Boarnet, Day, Anderson, McMillan, & Alfonzo, 2005) to providing information to families on how to safely and effectively navigate obstacles within the built environment (Rowland, DiGuiseppi, Gross, Afolabi, & Roberts, 2003). However, the most promising examples include multicomponent intervention strate-gies. These include involving schools in implementation and providing parents with materials specific to their local built environment to encourage them to walk (Chillon, Evenson, Vaughn, & Ward, 2011).

Multicomponent interventions can also support healthy eating behaviors. In a recent collaboration in design and health promotion in Virginia, partners outlined plans for school designs that promote procurement, preparation, and storage of foods to preserve nutritional value, teaching kitchen areas for student educational activities and extracurricular use, serving zones designed to promote display of healthy foods and minimize visibility of less healthy options, water access, and on-site food produc-tion facilities. This application of evidence and theory-based behavioral science prin-ciples is intended to facilitate the implementation of multi-faceted and multicomponent education, communication, and marketing activities to prompt teachers and students toward more healthy nutrition behaviors through their daily interactions with the built environment of the school itself (Huang et al., 2013).

FUTURE DIRECTIONS FOR INTERVENTIONS IN THE BUILT ENVIRONMENT

Future iterations of interventional research will benefit from advances in tools and tech-nology to assess and interact with the built environment as well as by identifying new ways to implement these tools to address environmental sustainability and inequities in access to health-promoting built environments.

HEALTH DISPARITIES, INEQUITIES, AND THE BUILT ENVIRONMENT

Health disparities or health inequalities are differences in health outcomes (or their determinants) among populations based on categories of social, geographic, demo-graphic, or environmental attributes. Health inequities, a subset of disparities, are modifiable, often occur among disadvantaged groups, and are considered to be unjust (Truman et al., 2011) . An emerging field of inquiry identifies how interventions within the built environment can be used to promote social and environmental justice and reduce health inequities by eliminating the differential exposures to health-promoting or health-harming environments that are found among particular populations defined by social, demographic, or geographic attributes. For example, several reviews have shown that racial/ethnic minority and low-income populations are exposed to features of the built environment that may contribute to obesity (e.g., fewer parks and recre-ational facilities as well as fewer supermarkets) (Larson et al., 2009; Lovasi et al., 2009;

Powell et al., 2006; Walker et al., 2010). In one community, when inequities in access to quality playgrounds and programmatic opportunities for physical activity were observed via a community-wide assessment, city officials and partners took action through a participatory process (Cradock et al., 2005; Hannon et al., 2006). The type of built environment assessments conducted in this example illustrates the importance of consideration of both the metric and scale of assessment of the built environment that is used in research and intervention (Duncan et al., 2012). This illustration also points to the important role of community input and collaboration in interventions to address inequalities (Hannon et al., 2006). In this case, these community collaborations led to more equity in access to quality facilities over time (Barrett, Hannon, Keefe, Gortmaker, & Cradock, 2011).

ADVANCES IN PLANNING AND DEVELOPMENT TO PROMOTE HEALTH AND ENVIRONMENTAL SUSTAINABILITY

Increasingly, city agencies are working together in ways that synergistically serve to promote health, environmental sustainability, and other design principles simultaneously. For example, in 2010, the New York City Departments of Design and Construction (DDC), Health and Mental Hygiene, Transportation (DOT), and City Planning jointly released *Active Design Guidelines: Promoting Physical Activity and Health in Design* (City of New York, 2010). As part of a mayoral initiative to promote excellence in design, these guidelines were directed at those responsible for street, neighborhood, and building planning and construction. Strategies cover each scale of the built environment from urban land-use planning to the specifics of stairway construction and are applicable to a variety of different project types, locations, and settings (e.g., public and private, urban and suburban). The developers also incorporated information to help users of the guidelines understand the strength of the research evidence behind the strategies and as an educational tool for students and the public. These planning guidelines also serve to address sustainability and promote environmental health through strategies that encourage healthy and sustainable behaviors such as physically active transportation and decreased energy consumption. Such tools and guidance plans are also developed and promoted specifically to address sustainable building design and neighborhood development through the U.S. Green Building Council. A variety of LEED (Leadership in Energy and Environmental Design) voluntary, consensus-based standards and guidance documents are available to promote sustainable construction and design practices for buildings and communities (https://new.usgbc.org/leed).

ADVANCES IN TOOLS AND TECHNIQUES

Health Impact Assessment (HIA) is a tool and organizing framework to help define for planners, developers, and other stakeholders the potential impacts on health of various interventions. HIAs include several steps from the screening and scoping of the intervention to the reporting and evaluation of the processes of the HIA or the outcomes of intervention (Wernham, 2011). HIAs seek to promote public awareness and involvement in decision making and improve communication among stakeholders while allowing mitigation of potential negative impacts of planned development or change (Forsyth et al., 2010). HIAs have been used in the United States to define the impacts of various policies and developments and internationally as well (Dannenberg et al., 2008). The focus of recent developments and discussion has addressed the tools necessary to help planners and public health professionals evaluate and examine the impact of HIA interventions in order to facilitate greater use of HIAs (Forsyth et al, 2010).

CONCLUSIONS

Researchers and practitioners use various strategies and metrics to measure the built environment that can also be used to design and evaluate interventions within the built environment that influence health and health behavior change. Interventions to promote healthy behaviors have been implemented in contexts including school settings, worksites, and across communities. The built environment may influence health behaviors directly or indirectly. Novel tools, technologies, and directions in research and practice for interventional research suggest potential for innovation in engaging multi-disciplinary partners and educating professionals to advance and design built environment interventions to promote health and equitable health outcomes.

REFERENCES

Anthamatten, P., Brink, L., Lampe, S., Greenwood, E., Kingston, B., & Nigg, C. (2011). An assessment of schoolyard renovation strategies to encourage children's physical activity. *International Journal of Behavioral Nutrition and Physical Activity, 8*. doi: 2710.1186/1479-5868-8-27

Barrett, J. L., Hannon, C., Keefe, L., Gortmaker, S. L., & Cradock, A. L. (2011). Playground renovations and quality at public parks in Boston, Massachusetts, 1996–2007. *Preventing Chronic Disease, 8*(4).

Berke, E. M., Gottlieb, L. M., Moudon, A. V., & Larson, E. B. (2007). Protective association between neighborhood walkability and depression in older men. *Journal of the American Geriatrics Society, 55*(4), 526–533. doi: 10.1111/j.1532-5415.2007.01108.x

Bias, T. K., Leyden, K. M., Abildso, C. G., Reger-Nash, B., & Bauman, A. (2010). The importance of being parsimonious: Reliability of a brief community walkability assessment instrument. *Health & Place, 16*(4), 755–758. doi: 10.1016/j.healthplace.2010.01.008

Bischoff, W. E., Reynolds, T. M., Sessler, C. N., Edmond, M. B., & Wenzel, R. P. (2000). Handwashing compliance by health care workers - The impact of introducing an accessible, alcohol-based hand antiseptic. *Archives of Internal Medicine, 160*(7), 1017–1021. doi: 10.1001/archinte.160.7.1017

Boarnet, M. G., Anderson, C. L., Day, K., McMillan, T., & Alfonzo, M. (2005). Evaluation of the California Safe Routes to School legislation—Urban form changes and children's active transportation to school. *American Journal of Preventive Medicine, 28*(2), 134–140. doi: 10.1016/j.amepre.2004.10.026

Boarnet, M. G., Day, K., Anderson, C., McMillan, T., & Alfonzo, M. (2005). California's safe routes to school program - Impacts on walking, bicycling, and pedestrian safety. *Journal of the American Planning Association, 71*(3), 301–317. doi: 10.1080/01944360508976700

Boreham, C. A. G., Kennedy, R. A., Murphy, M. H., Tully, M., Wallace, W. F. M., & Young, I. (2005). Training effects of short bouts of stair climbing on cardiorespiratory fitness, blood lipids, and homocysteine in sedentary young women. *British Journal of Sports Medicine, 39*(9), 590–593. doi: 10.1136/bjsm.2002.001131

Botchwey, N. D., Hobson, S. E., Dannenberg, A. L., Mumford, K. G., Contant, C. K., McMillan, T. E., ... Winkle, C. (2009). A model curriculum for a course on the built environment and public health training for an interdisciplinary workforce. *American Journal of Preventive Medicine, 36*(2 Suppl), S63–S71. doi: 10.1016/j.amepre.2008.10.003

Brownson, R., Hoehner, C., Day, K., Forsyth, A., & Sallis, J. (2009). Measuring the food and physical activity environments: State of the science. *American Journal of Preventive Medicine, 36*(4S), 25.

Bungum, T., Meacham, M., & Truax, N. (2007). The effects of signage and the physical environment on stair usage. *Journal of Physical Activity & Health, 4*(3), 237–244.

Bunn F., Collier T., Frost C., Ker K., Steinback R., Roberts I., & Wentz, R. (2009). Area wide traffic calming for preventing traffic related injuries. *Cochrane Database of Systematic Reviews* 2003; Issue 1. Art. No: CD003110, doi: 10.1002/14651858.CD003110

Carr, L. J., Dunsiger, S. I., & Marcus, B. H. (2010). Walk Score (TM) as a global estimate of neighbor-hood walkability. *American Journal of Preventive Medicine, 39*(5), 460–463. doi: 10.1016/j.amepre .2010.07.007

Carr, L. J., Dunsiger, S. I., & Marcus, B. H. (2011). Validation of Walk Score for estimating access to walkable amenities. *British Journal of Sports Medicine, 45*(14), 1144–1148. doi: 10.1136/bjsm.2009 .069609

Caspi, C. E., Sorensen, G., Subramanian, S. V., & Kawachi, I. (2012). The local food environment and diet: A systematic review. *Health & Place, 18*(5), 1172–1187. doi: 10.1016/j.healthplace.2012.05.00

Cerin, E., Saelens, B. E., Sallis, J. F., & Frank, L. D. (2006). Neighborhood environment walkability scale: Validity and development of a short form. *Medicine and Science in Sports and Exercise, 38*(9), 10, 1682–1691.

Center for Tobacco Policy & Organizing. (2011). *Matrix of local ordinances restricting tobacco retailers wit hin a certain distance of schools.* Retrieved from http://www.center4tobaccopolicy.org

Chaix, B. (2009). Geographic life environments and coronary heart disease: A literature review, theoreti-cal contributions, methodological updates, and a research agenda. *Annual Review of Public Health, 30*, 81–105. doi: 10.1146/annurev.publhealth.031308.100158

Chan, W. C., & Leatherdale, S. T. (2011). Tobacco retailer density surrounding schools and youth smoking behaviour: A multi-level analysis. *Tobacco Induced Diseases, 9*(1), 9.

Charreire, H., Casey, R., Salze, P., Simon, C., Chaix, B., Banos, A., ... Oppert, J. M. (2010). Measuring the food environment using geographical information systems: A methodological review. *Public Health Nutrition, 13*(11), 1773–1785. doi: 10.1017/S1368980010000753

Chillon, P., Evenson, K. R., Vaughn, A., & Ward, D. S. (2011). A systematic review of interventions for promoting active transportation to school. *International Journal of Behavioral Nutrition and Physical Activity, 8*, 10. doi: 10.1186/1479-5868-8-10

The City of New York. (2010). *The active design guidelines: Promoting physical activity through design.* The City of New York, New York. Retrieved from www.nyc.gov/adg

Cohen, D. A., Inagami, S., & Finch, B. (2008). The built environment and collective efficacy. *Health & Place, 14*(2), 198–208. doi: 10.1016/j.healthplace.2007.06.001

Connor, J., Kypri, K., Bell, M., & Cousins, K. (2011). Alcohol outlet density, levels of drinking and alcohol-related harm in New Zealand: A national study. *Journal of Epidemiology and Community Health, 65*(10), 841–846. doi: 10.1136/jech.2009.104935

Corburn, J. (2004). Confronting the challenges in reconnecting urban planning and public health. *American Journal of Public Health, 94*(4), 541–546. doi: 10.2105/ajph.94.4.541

Council on Sports Medicine and Fitness; Council on School Health. (2006). Active healthy living: Pre-vention of childhood obesity through increased physical activity. *Pediatrics, 117*(5), 1834-1842. PubMed PMID: 16651347.

Cradock, A. L., Fields, B., Barrett, J. L., & Melly, S. (2012). Program practices and demographic factors associated with federal funding for the Safe Routes to School program in the United States. *Health & Place, 18*(1), 16–23. doi: 10.1016/j.healthplace.2011.08.015

Cradock, A. L., Kawachi, I., Colditz, G. A., Hannon, C., Melly, S. J., Wiecha, J. L., & Gortmaker, S. L. (2005). Playground safety and access in Boston neighborhoods. *American Journal of Preventive Medicine, 28*(4), 357–363. doi: 10.1016/j.amepre.2005.01.012

Dannenberg, A. L., Bhatia, R., Cole, B. L., Heaton, S. K., Feldman, J. D., & Rutt, C. D. (2008). Use of health impact assessment in the US - 27 case studies, 1999–2007. *American Journal of Preventive Medicine, 34*(3), 241–256. doi: 10.1016/j.amepre.2007.11.015

Davison, K. K., & Lawson, C. T. (2006). Do attributes in the physical environment influence children's physical activity? A review of the literature. *International Journal of Behavioral Nutrition and Physical Activity, 3*. doi: 10.1186/1479-5868-3-19

Diez Roux, A. V. (2007). Neighborhoods and health: Where are we and where do we go from here? *Revue d'epidemiologie et de sante publique, 55*(1), 13–21.

Dill, J., & Weigand, L. (2010). Incorporating bicycle and pedestrian topics in university transportation courses: A national scan. *Transportation Research Record* (2198), 1–7. doi: 10.3141/2198-01

Ding, D., Sallis, J. F., Kerr, J., Lee, S., & Rosenberg, D. E. (2011). Neighborhood environment and physi-cal activity among youth: A review. *American Journal of Preventive Medicine, 41*(4). doi: 10.1016/j .amepre.2011.06.036

Doherty, A. R., Caprani, N., Conaire, C. O., Kalnikaite, V., Gurrin, C., Smeaton, A. F., & O'Connor, N. E. (2011). Passively recognising human activities through lifelogging. *Computers in Human Behavior, 27*(5), 1948–1958. doi: 10.1016/j.chb.2011.05.002

Drahota, A., Ward, D., Mackenzie, H., Stores, R., Higgins, B., Gal, D., & Dean, T. P. (2012). Sensory environment on health-related outcomes of hospital patients. *Cochrane Database of Systematic Reviews* (3), 362. doi: 10.1002/14651858.CD005315.pub2

du Toit, L., Cerin, E., Leslie, E., & Owen, N. (2007). Does walking in the neighborhood enhance local sociability? *Urban Studies, 44*(9), 1677–1695. doi: 10.1080/00420980701426665

Dumbaugh, E., & Frank, L. (2007). Traffic safety and Safe Routes to Schools - Synthesizing the empirical evidence. *Transportation Research Record* (2009), 89–97. doi: 10.3141/2009-12

Duncan, D. T., Kawachi, I., White, K., & Williams, D. R. (2013). The geography of recreational open space: Influence of neighborhood racial composition and neighborhood poverty. *Journal of Urban Health, 90*(4), 618–631. doi: 10.1007/s11524-012-9770-y

Duncan, D. T., Aldstadt, J., Whalen, J., Melly, S. J., & Gortmaker, S. L. (2011). Validation of Walk Score (R) for estimating neighborhood walkability: An analysis of four US metropolitan areas. *International Journal of Environmental Research and Public Health, 8*(11). doi: 10.3390/ijerph8114160

Duncan, D. T., Aldstadt, J., Whalen, J., White, K., Castro, M. C., & Williams, D. R. (2012). Space, race, and poverty: Spatial inequalities in walkable neighborhood amenities? *Demographic Research, 26.* doi: 10.4054/DemRes.2012.26.17

Elvik, R. (2001). Area-wide urban trafficcalming schemes: A meta-analysis of safety effects. *Accident Analysis and Prevention, 33*(3), 327–336. doi: 10.1016/s0001-4575(00)00046-4

Eyler, A. A., & Swaller, E. M. (2012). An analysis of community use policies in Missouri school districts. *Journal of School Health, 82*(4), 157–179. doi: 10.1111/j.1746-1561.2011.00683.x

Farley, T. A., Meriwether, R. A., Baker, E. T., Watkins, L. T., Johnson, C. C., & Webber, L. S. (2007). Safe play spaces to promote physical activity in inner-city children: Results from a pilot study of an environmental intervention. *American Journal of Public Health, 97*(9), 1625–1631. doi: 10.2105/ajph.2006.092692

Faulkner, G. E. J., Buliung, R. N., Flora, P. K., & Fusco, C. (2009). Active school transport, physical activity levels and body weight of children and youth: A systematic review. *Preventive Medicine, 48*(1), 3–8. doi: 10.1016/j.ypmed.2008.10.017

Forsyth, A., Slotterback, C. S., & Krizek, K. (2010). Health impact assessment (HIA) for planners: What tools are useful? *Journal of Planning Literature, 24*(3), 1–15. doi: 10.1177/0885412209358047

Fraser, S. D. S., & Lock, K. (2011). Cycling for transport and public health: A systematic review of the effect of the environment on cycling. *European Journal of Public Health, 21*(6), 738–743. doi: 10.1093/eurpub/ckq145

Galea, S., Ahern, J., Rudenstine, S., Wallace, Z., & Vlahov, D. (2005). Urban built environment and depression: A multilevel analysis. *Journal of Epidemiology and Community Health, 59*(10), 822–827. doi: 10.1136/jech.2005.033084

Geller, A. L. (2003). Smart growth: A prescription for livable cities. *American Journal of Public Health, 93*(9), 1410–1415. doi: 10.2105/ajph.93.9.1410

Giles, C. M., Kenney, E. L., Gortmaker, S. L., Lee, R. M., Thayer, J. C., Mont-Ferguson, H., & Cradock, A. L. (2012). Increasing water availability during afterschool: Evidence, strategies and partnerships from the OSNAP Group Randomized Trial. *American Journal of Preventive Medicine, 43*(3S2), S136. doi: 10.1016/j.amepre.2012.05.013

Giles-Corti, B., Kelty, S. F., Zubrick, S. R., & Villanueva, K. P. (2009). Encouraging walking for transport and physical activity in children and adolescents: How important is the built environment? *Sports Medicine, 39*(12), 995–1009.

Grimstvedt, M. E., Kerr, J., Oswalt, S. B., Fogt, D. L., Vargas-Tonsing, T. M., & Yin, Z. N. (2010). Using signage to promote stair use on a university campus in hidden and visible stairwells. *Journal of Physical Activity & Health, 7*(2), 232–238.

Guidelines for Design and Construction of Health Care Facilities. (2010). Chicago, IL: American Society for Healthcare Engineering of the American Hospital Association.

Gustafson, A., Hankins, S., & Jilcott, S. (2012). Measures of the consumer food store environment: A systematic review of the evidence 2000–2011. *Journal of Community Health, 37*(4), 897–911. doi: 10.1007/s10900-011-9524-x

Halonen, J., Kiyimaki, M., Virtanen, M., Pentti, J., Subramanian, S., Kawachi, I., & Vahtera, J. (2013). Living in proximity of a bar and risky alcohol behaviors: A longitudinal study. *Addiction, 108*(2), 320–328. doi: 10.1111/j.1360-0443.2012.04053

Hannon, C., Cradock, A., Gortmaker, S. L., Wiecha, J., El Ayadi, A., Keefe, L., & Harris, A. (2006). Play across Boston: A community initiative to reduce disparities in access to after-school physical activity programs for inner-city youths. *Preventing Chronic Disease, 3*(3), A100–A100.

Hannon, J. C., & Brown, B. B. (2008). Increasing preschoolers' physical activity intensities: An activity friendly preschool playground intervention. *Preventive Medicine, 46*(6), 532–536. doi: 10.1016/j.ypmed.2008.01.006

Henriksen, L., Feighery, E. C., Schleicher, N. C., Cowling, D. W., Kline, R. S., & Fortmann, S. P. (2008). Is adolescent smoking related to the density and proximity of tobacco outlets and retail cigarette advertising near schools? *Preventive Medicine, 47*(2), 210–214. doi: 10.1016/j.ypmed.2008.04.008

Hodges, S., Williams, L., Berry, E., Izadi, S., Srinivansan, J., & Butler, A. (2006). *SenseCam: A 226 Retrospective Memory Aid.* Paper presented at the UbiComp: 8th International Conference on Ubiquitous 227 Computering, Berlin, Heidelberg.

Huang, T. T. K., Sorensen, D., Davis, S., Frerichs, L., Brittin, J., & Celentano, J. (2013). Healthy eating design guidelines for school architecture. *Preventing Chronic Disease, 10*, E27. doi: 10.5888/pcd10.120084

IOM (Institute of Medicine). (2013). *Educating the student body: Taking physical activity and physical education to school.* Washington, DC: The National Academies Press.

Kawachi, I., & Berkman, L. F. (2001). Social ties and mental health. *Journal of Urban Health-Bulletin of the New York Academy of Medicine, 78*(3), 458–467. doi: 10.1093/jurban/78.3.458

Kelly, P., Doherty, A., Berry, E., Hodges, S., Batterham, A. M., & Foster, C. (2011). Can we use digital life-log images to investigate active and sedentary travel behaviour? Results from a pilot study. *International Journal of Behavioral Nutrition and Physical Activity, 8*(44), 1–9. doi: 10.1186/1479-5868-8-44

Kim, D. (2008). Blues from the neighborhood? Neighborhood characteristics and depression. *Epidemiologic Reviews, 30*(1), 101–117. doi: 10.1093/epirev/mxn009

Kohl, H. W., Craig, C. L., Lambert, E. V., Inoue, S., Alkandari, J. R., Leetongin, G., … Lancet Physical Activity Series Working Group. (2012). The pandemic of physical inactivity: Global action for public health. *Lancet, 380*(9838), 294–305. doi: 10.1016/s0140-6736(12)60898-8

Kubzansky, L. D., Subramanian, S. V., Kawachi, I., Fay, M. E., Soobader, M. J., & Berkman, L. F. (2005). Neighborhood contextual inf uences on depressive symptoms in the elderly. *American Journal of Epidemiology, 162*(3), 253–260. doi: 10.1093/aje/kwi185

Kypri, K., Bell, M., Hay, G., & Baxter, J. (2008). Alcohol outlet density and university student drinking:A national study. *Addiction, 103*(7), 1131–1138. doi: 10.1111/j.1360-0443.2008.02239.x

Laflamme, L., & Diderichsen, F. (2000). Social differences in traffic injury risks in childhood and youth—A literature review and a research agenda. *Injury Prevention: Journal of the International Society for Child and Adolescent Injury Prevention, 6*(4). doi: 10.1136/ip.6.4.293

Larson, N. I., Story, M. T., & Nelson, M. C. (2009). Neighborhood environments disparities in access to healthy foods in the US. *American Journal of Preventive Medicine, 36*(1), 74–81. doi:10.1016/j.amepre.2008.09.025

Leatherdale, S., & Strath, J. (2007). Tobacco retailer density surrounding schools and cigarette access behaviors among underage smoking students. *Annals of Behavior Medicine, 33*(1), 105–111.

Lewis, A., & Eves, F. (2012). Testing the theory underlying the success of point-of-choice prompts: A multi-component stair climbing intervention. *Psychology of Sport and Exercise, 13*(2), 126–132. From http://dx.doi.org/10.1016/j.psychsport.2011.10.001

Leyden, K. M. (2003). Social capital and the built environment: The importance of walkable neighborhoods. *American Journal of Public Health, 93*(9), 1546–1551. doi: 10.2105/ajph.93.9.1546

Lopez, R. P. (2012). *The built environment and public health* (1st ed.). San Francisco, CA: Jossey-Bass.

Lovasi, G. S., Hutson, M. A., Guerra, M., & Neckerman, K. M. (2009). Built environments and obesity in disadvantaged populations. *Epidemiological Review, 31*, 7–20.

Mair, C., Roux, A. V. D., & Galea, S. (2008). Are neighbourhood characteristics associated with depressive symptoms? A review of evidence. *Journal of Epidemiology and Community Health, 62*(11), 940–946. doi: 10.1136/jech.2007.066605

Matthews, S. A., Moudon, A. V., & Daniel, M. (2009). Work group II: Using geographic information systems for enhancing research relevant to policy on diet, physical activity, and weight. *American Journal of Preventive Medicine, 36*(4), S171–S176. doi: 10.1016/j.amepre.2009.01.011

McCarthy, W. J., Mistry, R., Lu, Y., Patel, M., Zheng, H., & Dietsch, B. (2009). Density of tobacco retailers near schools: Effects on tobacco use among students. *American Journal of Public Health, 99*(11), 2006–2013. doi: 10.2105/AJPH.2008.145128

McKinney, C., Chartier, K., Caetano, R., & Harris, T. (2012). Alcohol availability and neighborhood poverty and their relationship to binge drinking and related problems among drinkers in committed relationships. *Journal of Interpersonal Violence, 27*(13), 2703–2727. doi: 10.1177/0886260512436396

Moore, L. V., Roux, A. V. D., & Franco, M. (2012). Measuring availability of healthy foods: Agreement between directly measured and self-reported data. *American Journal of Epidemiology, 175*(10), 1037–1044. doi: 10.1093/aje/kwr445

Morrison, D. S., Thomson, H., & Petticrew, M. (2004). Evaluation of the health effects of a neighbourhood traffic calming scheme. *Journal of Epidemiology and Community Health, 58*(10), 837–840. doi: 10.1136/jech.2003.017509

Mozaffarian, D., Afshin, A., Benowitz, N. L., Bittner, V., Daniels, S. R., Franch, H. A., ... Zakai, N. A.; on behalf of the American Heart Association Council on Epidemiology and Prevention, Council on Nutrition, Physical Activity and Metabolism, Council on Clinical Cardiology, Council on Cardiovascular Disease in the Young, Council on the Kidney in Cardiovascular Disease, Council on Peripheral Vascular Disease, and the Advocacy Coordinating Committee. (2012). Population approaches to improve diet, physical activity, and smoking habits: A scientific statement from the American Heart Association. *Circulation, 126*, 1514–1563. doi: 0.1161/CIR.0b013e318260a20b

Nicoll, G. (2007). Spatial measures associated with stair use. *American Journal of Health Promotion, 21*(4S), 346–352, doi: 10.4278/0890-1171-21.4s.346

Nicoll, G., & Zimring, C. (2009). Effect of innovative building design on physical activity. *Journal of Public Health Policy, 30*, S111–S123. doi: 10.1057/jphp.2008.55

Novak, S., Reardon, S., Raudenbush, S., & Buka, S. (2006). Retail tobacco outlet density and youth cigarette smoking: A propensity-modeling approach. *American Journal of Public Health, 96*(4), 670–676. doi: 10.2105/AJPH.2004.061622

Pasch, K., Hearst, M., Nelson, M., Forsyth, A., & Lytle, L. (2009). Alcohol outlets and youth alcohol use: Exposure in suburban areas. *Health Place, 15*(2), 642–646. doi: 10.1016/j.healthplace.2008.10.002

Perdue, W. C., Stone, L. A., & Gostin, L. O. (2003). The built environment and its relationship to the public's health: The legal framework. *American Journal of Public Health, 93*(9), 1390–1394. doi: 10.2105/ajph.93.9.1390

Poulos, R. G., Hatfield, J., Rissel, C., Grzebieta, R., & McIntosh, A. S. (2012). Exposure-based cycling crash, near miss and injury rates: The Safer Cycling Prospective Cohort Study protocol. *Injury Prevention, 18*, e1. doi: 10.1136/injuryprev-2011-040160

Powell, L. M., Slater, S., Chaloupka, F. J., & Harper, D. (2006). Availability of physical activity-related facilities and neighborhood demographic and socioeconomic characteristics: A national study. *American Journal of Public Health, 96*(9), 1676–1680. doi: 10.2105/ajph.2005.065573

Public Health Law & Policy. (2010a). Summary of legal rules governing liability for recreational use of school facilities public health law and policy. Retrieved from http://changelabsolutions.org/sites/phlpnet.org/files/Liability_RecUse_JU_FINAL_2010.03.19_revised_20111213.pdf

Public Health Law & Policy. (2010b). Fifty-state scan of laws addressing community use of schools. Retrieved from http://changelabsolutions.org/sites/phlpnet.org/files/JU_StateSurvey_FINAL_2010.03.19.pdf

Pucher, J., Buehler, R., & Seinen, M. (2011). Bicycling renaissance in North America? An update and re-appraisal of cycling trends and policies. *Transportation Research Part A-Policy and Practice, 45*(6). 443–453. doi: 10.1016/j.tra.2011.03.001

Pucher, J., Dill, J., & Handy, S. (2010). Infrastructure, programs, and policies to increase bicycling: An international review. *Preventive Medicine, 50*, S106–S125. doi: 10.1016/j.ypmed.2009.07.028

Rao, M., Prasad, S., Adshead, F., & Tissera, H. (2007). The built environment and health. *Lancet, 370*(9593), 1111–1113. PubMed PMID: 17868821

Reger-Nash, B., Bauman, A., Cooper, L., Chey, T., & Simon, K. J. (2006). Evaluating communitywide walking interventions. *Evaluation and Program Planning, 29*(3), 251–259. doi: 10.1016/j.evalprogplan.2005.12.005

Ridgers, N. D., Fairclough, S. J., & Stratton, G. (2010). Twelve-month effects of a playground intervention on children's morning and lunchtime recess physical activity levels. *Journal of Physical Activity & Health, 7*(2), 167–175.

Ridgers, N. D., Stratton, G., Fairclough, S. J., & Twisk, J. W. R. (2007). Long-term effects of a playground markings and physical structures on children's recess physical activity levels. *Preventive Medicine, 44*(5), 393–397. doi: 10.1016/j.ypmed.2007.01.009

Rodgers, S. E., Jones, S. J., Macey, S. M., & Lyons, R. A. (2010). Using geographical information system to assess the equitable distribution of traffic-calming measures: Translational research. *Injury Prevention, 16*(1), 7–11. doi: 10.1136/ip.2009.022426

Rogers, S. H., Halstead, J. M., Gardner, K. H., & Carlson, C. H. (2011). Examining walkability and social capital as indicators of quality of life at the municipal and neighborhood scales. *Applied Research in Quality of Life, 6*(2), 215–216. doi: 10.1007/s11482-010-9132-4

Rosenberg, D., Ding, D., Sallis, J. F., Kerr, J., Norman, G.J., Durant, N., ... Saelens, B. E. (2009). Neighborhood environment walkability scale for youth (NEWS-Y): Reliability and relationship with physical activity. *Preventive Medicine, 49*, 213–218.

Rosso, A. L., Auchincloss, A. H., & Michael, Y. L. (2011). The urban built environment and mobility in olderadults: A comprehensive review. *Journal of Aging Research, 2011*, 1–10. doi: 10.4061/2011/816106

Roux, L., Pratt, M., Tengs, T. O., Yore, M. M., Yanagawa, T. L., Van Den Bos, J., ... Buchner, D. M. (2008). Cost effectiveness of community-based physical activity interventions. *American Journal of Preventive Medicine, 35*(6), 578–588. doi: 10.1016/j.amepre.2008.06.040

Rowland, D., DiGuiseppi, C., Gross, M., Afolabi, E., & Roberts, I. (2003). Randomised controlled trial of site specific advice on school travel patterns. *Archives of Disease in Childhood, 88*(1), 8–11. doi: 10.1136/adc.88.1.8

Rydin, Y., Bleahu, A., Davies, M., Dávila, J. D., Friel, S., De Grandis, G., ... Wilson, J. (2012). Shaping cities for health: Complexity and the planning of urban environments in the 21st century. *Lancet, 379*(9831), 2079–2108. doi: 10.1016/S0140-6736(12)60435-8

Saarloos, D., Alfonso, H., Giles-Corti, B., Middleton, N., & Almeida, O. P. (2011). The built environment and depression in later life: The Health in Men Study. *American Journal of Geriatric Psychiatry, 19*(5), 461–471. doi: 10.1097/JGP.0b013e3181e9b9bf

Saelens, B. E., Frank, L. D., Auffrey, C., Whitaker, R. C., Burdette, H. L., & Colabianchi, N. (2006). Measuring physical environments of parks and playgrounds: EAPRS instrument of development and inter-rater reliability. *Journal of Physical Activity and Health, 3*(1S), S190–S207.

Saelens, B. E., & Handy, S. L. (2008). Built environment correlates of walking: A review. *Medicine and Science in Sports and Exercise, 40*(7), S550–S566. doi: 10.1249/MSS.0b013e31817e67a4

Saelens, B. E., & Papadopoulos, C. (2008). The importance of the built environment in older adults' physical activity: A review of the literature. *Washington State Journal of Public Health Practice, 1*(1), 13–21.

Saelens, B. E., Sallis, J. F., & Frank, L. D. (2003). Environmental correlates of walking and cycling: Findings from the transportation, urban design, and planning literatures. *Annals of Behavioral Medicine, 25*(2), 80–91. doi: 10.1207/s15324796abm2502_03

Sallis, J. F., Floyd, M. F., Rodriquez, D. A., & Saelens, B. E. (2012). Role of built environments in physical activity, obesity, and cardiovascular disease. *Circulation, 125*, 729–737. doi: 10.1161/CIRCULATIONAHA.110.969022

Sallis, J. F., Saelens, B. E., Frank, L. D., Conway, T. L., Slymen, D. J., Cain, K. L., ... Kerr, J. (2009). Neighborhood built environment and income: Examining multiple health outcomes. *Social Science & Medicine, 68*(7), 1285–1293. doi: 10.1016/j.socscimed.2009.01.017

Schootman, M., Andresen, E. M., Wolinsky, F. D., Malmstrom, T. K., Miller, J. P., & Miller, D. K. (2007). Neighbourhood environment and the incidence of depressive symptoms among middle-aged African Americans. *Journal of Epidemiology and Community Health, 61*(6), 527–532. doi: 10.1136/jech.2006.050088

Shinkle, D., Rall, J., Wheet, A., Rockefeller Foundation, & National Conference of State Legislatures. (2012). *On the move: State strategies for 21st century transportation solutions*. Denver, CO: National Conference of State Legislatures.

Slusser, W. M., Cumberland, W. G., Browdy, B. L., Lange, L., & Neumann, C. (2007). A school salad bar increases frequency of fruit and vegetable consumption among children living in low-income households. *Public Health Nutrition, 10*(12), 1490–1496. doi: 10.1017/s1368980007000444

Smart Growth Online. (2013). Retrieved from http://www.smartgrowth.org/

Soler, R. E., Leeks, K. D., Buchanan, L. R., Brownson, R. C., Heath, G. W., Hopkins, D. H., & Task Force Community Preventive Services. (2010). Point-of-decision prompts to increase stair use. A systematic review update. *American Journal of Preventive Medicine, 38*(2), S292–S300. doi: 10.1016/j.amepre.2009.10.028

Stockdale, S. E., Wells, K. B., Tang, L., Belin, T. R., Zhang, L., & Sherbourne, C. D. (2007). The importance of social context: Neighborhood stressors, stress-buffering mechanisms, and alcohol, drug, and mental health disorders. *Social Science & Medicine, 65*(9), 1867–1868. doi: 10.1016/j.socscimed.2007.05.045

Story, M., Kaphingst, K. M., Robinson-O'Brien, R., & Glanz, K. (2008). Creating healthy food and eating environments: Policy and environmental approaches. *Annual Review of Public Health, 29*, 253–272. doi: 10.1146/annurev.publhealth.29.020907.090926

Sugiyama, T., Neuhaus, M., Cole, R., Giles-Corti, B., & Owen, N. (2012). Destination and route attributes associated with adults' walking: A review. *Medicine and Science in Sports and Exercise, 44*(7), 1275–1286. doi: 10.1249/MSS.0b013e318247d286

Teychenne, M., Ball, K., & Salmon, J. (2008). Physical activity and likelihood of depression in adults: A review. *Preventive Medicine, 46*(5), 397–411. doi: 10.1016/j.ypmed.2008.01.009

Thompson, D. R., Hamilton, D. K., Cadenhead, C. D., Swoboda, S. M., Schwindel, S. M., ... Petersen, C. (2012). Guidelines for intensive care unit design. *Critical Care Medicine, 40*(5), 1486–1600. doi: 10.1097/CCM.0b013e3182413bb2

Thornton, L. E., Pearce, J. R., & Kavanagh, A. M. (2011). Using Geographic Information Systems (GIS) to assess the role of the built environment in influencing obesity: A glossary. *International Journal of Behavioral Nutrition and Physical Activity, 8*, 71. doi: 10.1186/1479-5868-8-71

Titze, S., Martin, B. W., Seiler, R., & Marti, B. (2001). A worksite intervention module encouraging the use of stairs: Results and evaluation. *Sozial-Und Praventivmedizin, 46*(1), 13–19. doi: 10.1007/bf01318794

Truman, B. I., Smith, C. K., Roy, K., Chen, Z., Moonesinghe, R., Zhu, J., Crawford, C. G., & Zaza, S. (2011). Rationale for regular reporting on health disparities and inequalities—United States. *Morbidity and Mortality Weekly Report (MMWR), 60*(01), 3–10.

U.S. Department of Agriculture. (2010). *Dietary Guidelines for Americans.* Washington, DC: U.S. Government Printing Office Retrieved from http://www.health.gov/dietaryguidelines/dga2010/dietaryguidelines2010.pdf

Ulrich, R. S., Zimring, C., Zhu, X., DuBose, J., Seo, H.-B., Choi, Y.-S., Quan X., & Joseph, A. (2008). A review of the research literature on evidence-based healthcare design. *Herd-Health Environments Research & Design Journal, 1*(3), 61–125.

Waller, M., Iritani, B., Christ, S., Clark, H., Moracco, K., Halpern, C., & Flewelling, R. (2012). Relationships among alcohol outlet density, alcohol use, and intimate partner violence victimization among young women in the United States. *Journal of Interpersonal Violence, 27*(10), 2062–2086.

Walker, R. E., Keane, C. R., & Burke, J. G. (2010). Disparities and access to healthy food in the United States: A review of food deserts literature. *Health Place, 16*(5), 876–884.

Wernham, A. (2011). Health impact assessments are needed in decision making about environmental and land-use policy. *Health Affairs, 30*(5), 947–956. doi: 10.1377/hlthaff.2011.0050

Wu, S. Y., Cohen, D., Shi, Y. Y., Pearson, M., & Sturm, R. (2011). Economic analysis of physical activity interventions. *American Journal of Preventive Medicine, 40*(2), 149–158. doi: 10.1016/j.amepre.2010.10.029

Zaragoza, M., Salles, M., Gomez, J., Bayas, J. M., & Trilla, A. (1999). Handwashing with soap or alcoholic solutions? A randomized clinical trial of its effectiveness. *American Journal of Infection Control, 27*(3), 258–261. doi: 10.1053/ic.1999.v27.a97622

Zimring, C., Joseph, A., Nicoll, G. L., & Tsepas, S. (2005). Influences of building design and site design on physical activity—Research and intervention opportunities. *American Journal of Preventive Medicine, 28*(2), 186–193. doi: 10.1016/j.amepre.2004.10.025

VI
Health Behavior Change Research Methodology

High-quality research is needed to understand which intervention approaches will provide the best health outcomes from an individual and public health perspective and is therefore the topic of Section VI. Using reliable and valid measures of behavior is essential to understand how interventions affect behavior change and how behavior change affects health outcomes. Moreover choosing the right study design for the research question and ensuring that research is conducted at all translational phases (e.g., from the basic mechanistic level through dissemination into communities) are important to ensure that efficacious interventions are not only developed, but are adopted by health care and other settings to have population-level benefit.

In Chapter 23, "Principles of Health Behavior Measurement," Hilliard takes on the task of describing and evaluating assessment strategies for three domains of health behaviors: eating behaviors, physical activity, and medical regimen adherence. These behaviors have cross-cutting applicability and are used here to illustrate how best to select the appropriate measurement for assessment, whether objective or subjective, for the intended purpose. Newer technologies, such as biochemical analysis and ecological momentary assessment, are discussed, as well as more traditional methods such as diaries and pill counters. Hilliard gives particular attention to the needs of special populations, including young children and the elderly, and covers advances in the field, including the implementation of electronic medical records. While technology, including the widespread adoption of electronic medical records, offers health care providers the opportunity to incorporate valid protocols for assessing regimen adherence into their clinic practice, its use is still far from routine.

New to this edition is a chapter on translational research in health behavior change. Lemon and colleagues address the subject in Chapter 24, "Translational Research Phases in the Behavioral and Social Sciences: Adaptations From the Biomedical Sciences," using as their template the biomedical focus that has been the mainstay of translational research since its original 2003 inclusion in the NIH Roadmap. As the authors note, adopting this framework for health behavior change research will help establish a common language among researchers from different disciplines while highlighting the unique contributions of the behavioral and social sciences to improving health outcomes. Moving through the phases of translational research, they discuss its implication for health behavior change research and present a case study—the 5 As model for treating tobacco use and dependence—for illustration. They present clear steps for the advancement of translational research in the field of behavioral research, starting with the establishment of common definitions and ending with the importance of integrating behavioral and social research into a larger biomedical context for the purpose of improving population health.

23

Principles of Health Behavior Measurement

MARISA E. HILLIARD

LEARNING OBJECTIVES

- Distinguish between objective and subjective measures of health behavior and discuss benefits and downsides of each.
- Describe psychometric and measurement design characteristics of health behavior instruments, including validity, reliability, and sensitivity.
- Identify strategies to adapt measures for special populations such as children or the elderly.

PRINCIPLES OF HEALTH BEHAVIOR MEASUREMENT

Accurate behavioral measurement is an essential part of many clinical and research activities related to health behavior change. First, public health efforts by agencies such as the Centers for Disease Control and Prevention rely on health surveillance, or tracking changes in a population's health and behaviors over time. Second, health behavior screening is used to identify or classify individuals for research or care delivery. For example, people who report sedentary lifestyles may be targeted for an exercise-promotion intervention. Third, health behavior researchers often study associations among individual or environmental characteristics, health behaviors, and clinical outcomes. For example, a dietician may wish to investigate how emotional distress influences eating behaviors and weight gain over the first year of college. Fourth, monitoring health behaviors and providing feedback may be integrated as a component of behavior change interventions. For example, a physician may ask a patient to track his or her food intake and physical activity for a month, then review those data together to identify patterns, and discuss strategies to make improvements. Finally, clinicians and researchers use health behavior assessments to determine the impact of clinical interventions on key health behaviors and outcomes. For example, to evaluate a nursing intervention designed to improve glycemic control in individuals with type 2 diabetes, precise measurement of both blood glucose values and medication adherence rates would be necessary. Within the domain of medication adherence, the conclusions drawn in drug trials can be compromised or skewed without a careful assessment of whether and to what degree the drug was actually delivered to study participants.

This chapter focuses on assessment strategies for three domains of health behaviors that have cross-cutting applicability for common health concerns: eating behaviors, physical activity, and medical regimen adherence. Assessment of eating includes the frequency, amount, and nutritional characteristics of foods ingested.[1] Physical activity assessment encompasses the frequency, duration, intensity, and types of energy expending activities in which individuals engage. Measurement of medical regimen adherence comprises assessing the frequency, quantity, timing, persistence, and duration of activities required for disease management, including taking prescribed medications and completing therapies. In treatment adherence assessment, it is critical to determine the specific regimen that has been prescribed or recommended (Quittner, Modi, Lemanek, Ievers-Landis, & Rapoff, 2008). The most basic approach to calculate an adherence rate is to divide the quantity of completed tasks by the quantity of prescribed tasks, although other calculation methods are available and suitable to different assessment approaches (for a detailed explanation, see Hess, Raebel, Conner, & Malone, 2006). Across methods, however, it is critical to note that without knowledge of the prescribed regimen, one can only provide data on the amount of therapy executed but cannot provide a percentage or rate of adherence.

CONSIDERATIONS FOR ASSESSMENT SELECTION

When selecting assessment measures for clinical research or practice, there are multiple considerations related to instrument development and study design. The ability of an instrument to make accurate and consistent measurements is referred to as psychometric properties. A summary of the key psychometric issues to be aware of when selecting health behavior measures is provided in Table 23.1. Readers interested in learning more or who plan to develop measures are directed to Streiner and Norman's guide on psychometrics in assessment development (2008). In addition to psychometrics, health behavior clinicians and researchers must consider other properties of measurement tools. For example, one challenge is to identify assessment methods that are less vulnerable to demand characteristics (Streiner & Norman, 2008). Demand characteristics occur when responses are influenced by the rater's perceptions about or awareness of being involved in research. Health behavior measures often have high demand characteristics in that it can be difficult to elicit honest endorsements of socially undesirable behaviors including sedentary behavior, unhealthy eating, and medication non-adherence. Measurement reactivity occurs when one changes his or her behavior (e.g., eating healthier or taking medication more frequently) and when one knows his or her behaviors are being measured or observed. Another important consideration is balancing the wish to collect maximally informative, comprehensive data versus the need to minimize participant burden and burnout. Collecting longitudinal or repeated assessments using a multi-method, multi-informant assessment approach is often recommended and can increase the validity of conclusions that are drawn from the data (Garvie, Wilkins, & Young, 2010; Schafer-Keller, Steiger, Bock, Denhaerynck, & De Geest, 2008; Rapoff, 2010). However, overburdening participants with multiple assessments can lead to fatigue and irritation and may discourage participants from completing all measures or returning for follow-up, resulting in missing data and potentially biased results. Sternfeld and Goldman-Rosas (2012) suggest carefully evaluating the essential purpose of the study to help limit the assessment battery to the maximally informative and minimally burdensome combination of measures. Constructs directly related to the study's primary

---

[1] Although not discussed in detail here, diagnostic measures of disordered eating behaviors are also available (Anderson, Lundgren, Shapiro, & Paulosky, 2004).

TABLE 23.1 Key Concepts in Psychometrics and Measurement Design

PROPERTY	DEFINITION	EXAMPLE
Validity	The degree to which an instrument measures what it aims to measure	
Construct validity	The degree to which an instrument captures or represents a specific underlying concept	An interview about diabetes treatment adherence that assesses a broad range of related diabetes self-management practices
Face validity	The degree to which an instrument's item content appears to represent the construct. Face validity does not necessarily indicate accuracy	A questionnaire about fresh produce consumption frequency in which all items query how often the respondent eats different types of fruits and vegetables
Concurrent validity	The degree to which scores on one instrument correlate with scores on another, validated instrument assessing a similar or associated construct	A self-report measure of exercise intensity that correlates with a validated exercise observation coding scheme
Criterion validity	The degree to which scores on one instrument are associated with an outcome measure that is known to relate to the construct	A physician-rated measure of anti-hypertensive medication adherence that correlates with lower blood pressure
Reliability	Production of consistent results when instrument is completed in similar conditions; necessary but not sufficient to determine reliability	
Internal consistency	How well the items in a measure correlate with one another, ranges between 0 and 1, represented by the Greek letter α	Associations among items assessing adherence to different components of a cystic fibrosis treatment regimen, including medications, chest physiotherapy, and nutritional intake
Test–retest reliability	The degree to which a measure produces similar scores when completed under similar conditions at two points in time	A self-report measure of beliefs about the importance of physical activity, administered 2 weeks apart, with no intervention between administrations

(continued)

467

TABLE 23.1 Key Concepts in Psychometrics and Measurement Design (continued)

PROPERTY	DEFINITION	EXAMPLE
Inter-rater reliability	The degree to which different raters obtain similar scores when completing the measure under similar conditions about the same target person	Agreement between two dieticians coding the nutritional characteristics of a participant's report of a meal
Sensitivity	**The degree to which an instrument detects meaningful information**	
Sensitivity to change	The ability to detect when a change in a measure's score crosses a meaningful threshold	A measure that identifies a person having 80% adherence to a particular medication, if 80% is considered clinically meaningful
Sensitivity	Ability to detect "true positives"	Person with high levels of inactivity correctly identified as "sedentary" based on observation measure of physical activity
Specificity	Ability to detect "true negatives"	Endorsement of low medication adherence on a self-report adherence questionnaire

aims may require multiple or more intensive measures to ensure precise assessment, as compared to constructs that are peripherally related. Additionally, large epidemiologic studies may be logistically constrained from resource- or time-intensive measures, while smaller scale studies may have the ability to spend more time or resources conducting comprehensive assessments with each participant.

MEASUREMENT METHODOLOGIES

Health behavior assessment strategies can be subjective or objective, and can be measured in a number of ways, including by paper-and-pencil rating forms, in vivo observations, biomarker assays, or electronically collected objective measures. The benefits and drawbacks of various methods that are currently in use for assessment of eating, physical activity, and medication adherence are described below and summarized in Table 23.2. Examples of instruments from the three health behavior domains are provided in text.

OBJECTIVE METHODS

Objective measures of health behaviors can take two forms: direct observation and indirect inference of a behavior based on concrete outcomes of the behavior (e.g., blood assays, body weight, and pharmacy refill records).

Direct Measures

Direct measures of behavior monitor the occurrence of behaviors as they happen. In behavioral observation methods, a trained observer watches an individual, either live or via recording, and keeps count of each target behavior as it happens. Observation can occur in a naturalistic setting (e.g., at home or school) or in a staged scenario (e.g., eating a meal in a research lab), and is used to track the frequency and duration of specific behaviors over a set period of time. Observers may keep track of behaviors with simple counts, rating scales, or coding systems. Behavioral observation has evolved to include electronic monitoring, in which technologies such as electronic pill bottles, medical devices, accelerometers, electronic scales, or wearable cameras record the occurrence of specific health behaviors. Examples of direct assessment methods for each health behavior domain are described below.

DIET

Compared to other health behavior domains, technological assessment development has been relatively slower for dietary behavior assessment (Thompson et al., 2010) and is used primarily to facilitate direct observation of eating. The remote food photography method (RFPM) (Martin et al., 2009) represents one important technological advance in this area. Using a mobile phone based camera, individuals send researchers photographs and detailed descriptions of their food prior to and following meals. Researchers train study participants to standardize the distance and angle of the photograph to facilitate serving size calculations. Dieticians then analyze the information and images for food type, quantity, and energy (calories) with comparisons to archived photographs of common foods, when available. The RFPM approach has demonstrated inter-rater reliability and validity compared with other food intake measures such as self-report and weighted plates (Martin et al., 2009).

TABLE 23.2 Summary of Assessment Methods

METHOD	DESCRIPTION	BENEFITS	DRAWBACKS
Objective (Direct)	Measurement of behavior as it occurs	• Measures behavior itself rather than byproduct or report of behavior • Higher validity than subjective data	• Long observation period needed to capture sufficient behavior sample • Behavioral reactivity potential
Behavioral observation	Live or recorded activity is watched and coded for frequency/length of target behaviors	• Greatest certainty of data's validity • Minimal risk for rater bias	• Time, resources to train observers to reliability • Risk of human error in coding
Electronic monitoring	Technologies capture and document the occurrence of target behaviors	• Low burden, integrates easily into regular activities • Ability to collect data remotely • Large amount of data collected • Reduced risk of human error	• Medication ingestion not necessarily certain • Expense of devices and software • Risk of device malfunction, damage, or loss • Resources needed for data management
Objective (indirect)	Measurement of the byproducts of previous behavior	• Often more feasible to collect than observation data • Higher validity than subjective data	• Infers rather than measures behavior • May be influenced by other factors aside from health behavior
Biochemical analysis	Measurement of physiological markers associated with health behaviors	• Often collected in routine clinical care • High reliability and validity (for recent/short-term behaviors)	• Expense, resources needed to collect data • Influence of individual metabolism • Potential participant discomfort (e.g., blood draws)
Manual measurements	Counts of physical products of health behaviors	• Minimal risk for rater bias • Straightforward data collection	• Risk of human error in counting • Time intensive • Potential for behavioral reactivity or manipulation of data (e.g., "pill dumping")

Subjective (indirect)	Reports of health behaviors by individuals (self or others)	• Ease of data collection • Wide range of constructs can be assessed	• Do not measure behavior itself • Susceptible to reporter bias or fabricated/inaccurate data
Rating forms (self)	Individual reports on own behavior in the past using a questionnaire or rating form	• Ease of data collection • Low resource needs • Can survey large samples • Can assess large periods of time	• Requires literacy, fluency in survey language • Difficult/impossible to request clarification, can lead to missing or inaccurate responses • Risk of rater bias or memory errors with longer recall period
24-hour recall interviews (self)	Individual reports on specific health behaviors that occurred during previous day	• Short recall period—reduced risk of bias or memory errors	• Time intensive • May be biased by unique circumstances of previous day
Daily diaries/logs (self)	Individual tracks specific health behaviors that occurred each day	• Short recall period • Brief/easy to complete • Useful for behaviors that typically occur daily	• Rely on participant remembering to complete daily • Risk for retrospective completion
Ecological momentary assessment (self)	Individual is prompted throughout the day to track or report on specific behaviors that are currently occurring or occurred in the immediate past	• Very short recall period • Assessment of behaviors in context of natural events/settings • Ease/convenience of data collection	• Risk for missing data due to non-responses to prompts • May disrupt activities • Behavioral reactivity potential
Clinical judgment	Medical professionals rate their patients' health status or behaviors	• Can provide global rating of patient • Inexpensive, easy to collect	• Not useful for specific behavior ratings • Subject to rater bias • Questionable accuracy
Others' reports	Parents, spouses, or other caregivers rate an individual's health behaviors	• Can be used to support/compare validity of self-report • May be beneficial in conjunction with self-report	• May have incomplete knowledge of target individual's behaviors • Social desirability and other rater biases may apply

PHYSICAL ACTIVITY

Pedometers, accelerometers, and actigraphs worn on the body during everyday activities measure the acceleration of physical movements. Devices calculate and track amount, types, intensity, and duration of activity. Because day-to-day variation can occur, such devices are typically worn for several days to identify patterns (Warren et al., 2010). Newer devices such as FitBit (FitBit Inc, San Francisco, CA) are parts of larger health behavior monitoring programs that not only document fitness activities but also link with data about other health behaviors (e.g., weight from electronic scales, sleep quality from actigraph, and user-inputted data about food intake) to a centralized individual profile. Such devices have the potential to capture multiple measures of health behaviors in a single system and to verify self-reported data with electronically captured data. Electronic devices such as accelerometers have been validated against other measures such as heart rate telemetry (Puyau, Adolph, Vohra, & Butte, 2002) and the gold standard measure doubly labeled water (described below; Plasqui & Westerterp, 2007), and have demonstrated better psychometric and predictive properties than subjective assessments of physical activity (Bonomi, Plasqui, Goris, & Westerterp, 2009). Of note, depending on where the device is worn on the body (e.g., hip or lower back), sensitivity may be low for smaller movements in other parts of the body (e.g., upper body) and thus underestimates can occur (Schutz, Weinsier, & Hunter, 2012; Warren et al., 2010).

TREATMENT ADHERENCE

Behavioral observation of medication adherence is known as "directly observed therapy" (DOT). Due to the inherent behavioral impact of being observed, DOT is often considered an intervention more than an assessment (Hart et al., 2010). Medication electronic monitoring devices capture and timestamp the opening or actuation of medication packages. Examples include MEMS™ (Medication Event Monitoring System) caps for pill bottles (Aardex Group Ltd., Switzerland), Med-eMonitor™ "smart pillboxes" (InforMedix, Rockville, MD), and Smartinhaler devices for inhaled medications (Nexus6 Ltd., New Zealand). Medical devices such as blood glucose meters track the occurrence of health behaviors such as checking one's blood sugar in people with diabetes. Associated software programs typically compile frequency and timing data into lists or calendars. Growing research in this field supports the reliability and validity of electronic monitors for adherence assessment and documents a strong association with health outcomes across diseases and age groups (Christensen, Osterberg, & Hansen, 2009; Haberer et al., 2012; Quittner et al., 2008; Riekert & Rand, 2002). The potential for impacting adherence behavior by providing feedback of electronic monitoring makes this a promising avenue for behavior change interventions (Herzer, Ramey, Rohan, & Cortina, 2012; Spaulding, Devine, Duncan, Wilson, & Hogan, 2012).

Indirect Objective Measures

Indirect measures result from a behavior after it has occurred. Objective indirect measures include analysis of biochemical markers that are produced from a behavior or manual counts of behavior byproducts such as leftover food or medications. Manual measurements include counts of the physical products of health behaviors, and biochemical analysis tracks physiological markers associated with health behaviors. Examples from each method follow.

DIET

Using weighed food inventory methods, a meal is weighed before eating and the remaining food is weighed after the individual is done eating. Food samples may be analyzed in conjunction with the weighing to determine nutritional content. Benefits include low cost and precise measurements. Downsides include intrusiveness and burden for participants, as well as the potential for repeated measurements to impact eating behavior (Wolper, Heshka, & Heymsfield, 1995).

PHYSICAL ACTIVITY

Doubly labeled water is a biochemical analysis that is considered a premier assessment of energy expenditure, and is a reliable proxy for overall physical activity over the previous 1 to 2 weeks (Westerterp, 2009; Wolper et al., 1995). Using this approach, body fluid samples are obtained from an individual who has drunk enriched water to determine the rates at which enriched oxygen and hydrogen isotopes are being expelled from the body. After considering body height, weight, and fat composition, the difference in slopes between rates of hydrogen and oxygen expulsion serves as a precise measurement of energy expenditure (i.e., physical activity). Doubly labeled water is the gold standard criterion against which other measures of physical activity are commonly validated (Plasqui & Westerterp, 2007).

TREATMENT ADHERENCE

Medication adherence assessment often uses biochemical analysis to quantify the concentration of a drug's metabolic byproducts in the body by analyzing blood, saliva, or urine (Hommel, Davis, & Baldassano, 2008; Kalichman et al., 2008; Schafer-Keller et al., 2008). This estimates how much of the medication was administered prior to the assay. While this strategy provides an objective value representing the amount of medication in the body, it is difficult to account for individual (e.g., metabolism) or drug-specific factors (e.g., half-life, dose or form of medication, and timing of administration) that can impact the drug's bioavailability (Rapoff, 2010). For example, biomarkers cannot identify white coat compliance which is a marked increase in adherence in the days before a clinic visit. As such, drug assays are typically recommended as screeners for recent non-adherence, but not as sole or definitive measures of overall adherence rates (Hommel et al., 2008).

Pill counting is a common manual measurement approach to adherence assessment. Counting pills at two time points allows the inference of how many doses were used during the interval. However, this method does not confirm that medications were administered or ingested by the individual to whom they were prescribed. Particularly in the case where pills are counted at clinic visits or scheduled home visits, it is possible that individuals could dispose of medications in other ways prior to counting. Despite this potential problem, pill counts are easy to conduct in clinic or research settings, have good psychometric properties, and are associated with health outcomes (Kalichman et al., 2008). Unannounced phone-based pill counts may alleviate some of these challenges and are associated with health outcomes, such as viral load in youth with HIV, although missing data due to unanswered telephone calls can occur (Farley et al., 2008; Kalichman et al., 2008).

Pharmacy refill records represent another form of indirect measurement of remaining medication doses. Basic calculation of adherence rates from pharmacy administrative data (e.g., medication possession ratio) entails comparing the amount of medication prescribed with the days' supply of medication dispensed from the pharmacy over a set period of time to determine the rate at which the individual uses up their existing supply (Hess et al., 2006). For example, if a prescription designed to last 30 days is not refilled for 60 days, an estimate of 50% adherence can be inferred. This method does not confirm medication ingestion and is subject to inaccurate or incomplete data from pharmacies. This method also does not provide insight about day-to-day patterns of medication administration, such as timing or missed days. Obtaining and processing data from pharmacy records can be time and resource intensive, and making nuanced decisions about how to calculate the data can be quite complicated (Hess et al., 2006).

SUBJECTIVE METHODS

Subjective measures of health behaviors rely on individuals to report on the occurrence of health behaviors, and are thus indirect in nature. Reporters can include oneself, clinicians, and others (e.g., parent and spouse). Self-report measures ask people to provide data on their own engagement in health behaviors and may be administered in a range of formats. On rating forms, respondents are asked to rate the frequency of a behavior or other aspects of the behavior (e.g., duration, difficulty completing, or attitudes about the behavior) over a specific period of time. The length of the recall period can impact the accuracy of reports, as retrospective accounts can be impacted by memory lapses, intervening events, attitudes about the behavior, social desirability bias, and current emotional states (Jones & Johnston, 2011). Although shorter recall periods tend to have higher validity, there is no optimal recall range for all behaviors or all measures (Stull, Leidy, Parasuraman, & Chassany, 2009). Across a range of health behaviors, measures with longer recall periods compare poorly with objective or real-time measures (Jones & Johnston, 2011; Shiffman, 2009).

To address this challenge, strategies that use shorter recall periods have been developed. For example, 24-hour recall interviews assess health behaviors over the 24 hours immediately prior to the interview. Variants of the recall interview assess single behaviors (e.g., physical activities; Foley, Maddison, Olds, & Ridley, 2012), all behaviors associated with a theme (e.g., adherence to diet, exercise, and medical treatment components of a treatment regimen; Baeyens et al., 2009), or even more broadly, all daily activities (Wiener, Riekert, Ryder, & Wood, 2004). Using logs or diaries, participants track target behaviors daily. Detailed questions can accompany these log entries; however because this method is repeated over a number of days, the greater the amount of information collected at each entry, the greater the burden for participants and the higher the likelihood of missing data. With technological advances, daily behavior tracking may be completed more conveniently online or with mobile devices (Foley et al., 2012). Using ecological momentary assessment (EMA), participants receive prompts (e.g., by alarm or text message) to report or track targeted behaviors throughout the day, occurring randomly, at set intervals, or following particular events such as meals (Shiffman, Stone, & Hufford, 2008). Tracking may be completed on paper forms, online, or using a mobile device application or text message (Jones & Johnston, 2011). Examples of self-report methods across the three health behavior domains follow.

Diet

Given numerous challenges in attending to, quantifying, and accurately recalling food intake over extended periods of time, self-report measurements of diet and eating behaviors tend to emphasize short-term recall periods (e.g., daily diaries and 24-hour recall interviews) or real-time reports. Food frequency questionnaires and diet history interviews are commonly used to assess an individual's average amounts and types of food eaten over a long period (i.e., several months–years), and can be adapted for specific study aims (McPherson, Hoelscher, Alexander, Scanlon, & Serdula, 2000; Thompson, Subar, Loria, Reedy, & Baranowsky, 2010; Wolper et al., 1995). Self-report measures of eating behavior are typically recommended for studies that aim to capture large-scale population-level eating trends, rather than those that aim to assess very specific data about individual food intake (McPherson et al., 2000; Wolper et al., 1995). The tendency to under-report food intake is an important validity consideration (Wolper et al., 1995).

Physical Activity

Self-report activity measures assess global trends in one's activity level, historical patterns (e.g., spanning more than 1 year to lifetime), or specific activities over a particular period (Sternfeld & Goldman-Rosas, 2012). While global measures of a "typical day" or "typical week" tend to be useful for population-level surveillance they may not detect incremental change, and recall methods that span a specific and relatively brief period of time (e.g., the previous week) are commonly used to assess short-term variations in behavior, impact of intervention, or to rank individuals with different levels of physical activity (Haskell, 2012; Mâsse & de Niet, 2012; Shelton & Klesges, 1995). In comparison with direct, objective measures of physical activity, self-report measures can either over- or underestimate activity levels, raising questions about reliability and validity, and making it difficult to correct for measurement error (Prince et al., 2008; Warren et al., 2010).

Treatment Adherence

Self-report measures of adherence may ask for global adherence ratings or assess specific disease management behaviors, including medication administration, special diet, and engagement in various therapies. A number of self-report measures of treatment adherence exist (Garber, Nau, Erickson, Aikens, & Lawrence, 2004; Quittner et al., 2008), and data from questionnaires and diaries often are significantly correlated with other measures of adherence and health status (Garber et al., 2004; Kichler, Kaugars, Maglio, & Alemzadeh, 2010). However, many measures have insufficient psychometric properties including poor sensitivity and specificity (Koschack, Marx, Schnakenberg, Kochen, & Himmel, 2010), and over-reporting adherence is common in comparison to objective measures (Garber et al., 2004; Shi et al., 2010). In addition to the impact of social desirability on responses (Nieuwkerk, de Boer-van der Kolk, Prins, Locadia, & Sprangers, 2010), a major challenge of self-reports of adherence is the difficulty of providing average estimates of adherence when one adheres differently to the various components of a regimen or when one's adherence varies over time (Garfield, Clifford, Eliasson, Barber, & Willson, 2011). It is therefore recommended that self-report adherence measures, particularly single-item global ratings, be used to screen and identify individuals who endorse non-adherence, but not for the purpose of ruling out non-adherence in those who endorse being adherent. That is, individuals who "admit" to low or no adherence likely have low to no adherence (although their self-reported adherence rates may still be overestimates). On the other hand, people who report high to perfect adherence have more variable rates of objectively measured adherence.

Although it is well established that self-reported adherence rates are subject to bias, demand characteristics, and inflation, individuals are noted to be the best reporters of their personal and cultural experiences, beliefs, and attitudes that influence adherence. While clinicians and researchers interested in adherence are advised to use direct, objective measures of adherence rates, self-reports are recommended to assess the barriers to adherence (Rand, 2000). The Brief Medication Questionnaire (Svarstad, Chewning, Sleath, & Claesson, 1999) and the Illness Management Survey (Logan, Zelikovsky, Labay, & Spergel, 2003) are examples of such measures.

Clinical Judgment

Medical providers are often asked to provide global ratings of their patients' overall health status or behaviors. This is particularly common as a proxy assessment of treatment adherence, based on the presumptions that doctors and patients have candid conversations about adherence and that accurate conclusions about adherence can be drawn from a patient's health status, neither of which is necessarily true. Compared to objective adherence measures, physician ratings tend to be overestimates (Copher et al., 2010; Miller et al., 2002) and in some cases are no better than chance (Daniels et al., 2011). Moreover, they rarely coincide with patients' self-reports (Murri et al., 2004; Shemesh et al., 2004).

Clinicians often make judgments about patients' adherence or health behaviors based on health outcomes measured by biomarkers. For example, glycosylated hemoglobin A1c represents an individual's average blood glucose level over the previous 2 to 3 months and is a key indicator of overall glycemic control. It is not uncommon for diabetes clinicians and clinical researchers to rely on A1c values to serve as a proxy indicator of adherence. Although adherence is strongly correlated with overall glycemic control, and it can be argued that adherence influences or leads to glycemic control, the A1c value is impacted by many other factors and is not a valid direct measure of adherence (Hood, Peterson, Rohan, & Drotar, 2009). Similar arguments can be made for using outcomes such as nutritional biomarkers (e.g., toenail selenium and serum folate), body mass index, or heart rate as direct assessments of diet or physical activity, as these physiological indices are also highly impacted by genetics and other factors unrelated to diet or activity (Schutz et al., 2012; Thompson et al., 2010; Westerterp, 2009), and thus are not definitively informative about specific health behaviors.

In addition to their knowledge of health status, clinical judgments can also be influenced by factors including perceptions of personal and family characteristics (e.g., intelligence and responsibility), patient or family reports of engaging in the behavior, and demographic factors (e.g., race, age, and education) all of which are subject to bias and may or may not directly reflect actual engagement in health behaviors (Lutfey & Ketcham, 2005). Thus, except in cases where direct, objective measures of adherence behaviors are obtained during the medical visit (e.g., medication blood assays and electronic monitor downloads), relying solely on clinical judgment as a measure of health behaviors is considered too susceptible to bias to be recommended.

Reports From Others

Like self-reports, reports from parents, caregivers, spouses, or others can take the form of retrospective ratings or daily diaries or logs, can be completed by questionnaire or interview, and can be specific or global. Parent ratings are commonly used as an adjunct or proxy for self-report for young children or those with limited cognitive capacity (Quittner et al., 2008). From a multi-method, multi-source assessment perspective, using parent reports in combination with children's self-reports has been recommended as a way to improve reliability and validity (Burrows, Martin, & Collins, 2010; McPherson et al., 2000). However, potential pitfalls of reports from parents or others include limited knowledge of a child's daily activities, particularly during adolescence when teens begin to spend less time at home and may not disclose to their parents the details of their activities, diet, or medical regimen adherence as well as the general biases of self-report.

MEASUREMENT CONSIDERATIONS IN SPECIAL POPULATIONS

Measurement methods used with younger and older people often require special considerations to account for developmentally expected differences in cognitive or physical functioning. Given limited ability to self-report about health behaviors in early childhood (e.g., under 6–7 years of age), parents are typically consulted as the primary reporters about their children's engagement in specific behaviors (Babbitt, Elden-Nazin, Manikam, Summers, & Murphy, 1995; Quittner et al., 2008). Direct measures, such as behavioral observation, electronic monitors, pill counts, or weighing food, may be best for children, especially very young children (Burrows et al., 2010; Farley et al., 2008; Puyau et al., 2002). Simplified questionnaires may be used for older children and adolescents, such as focusing on very concrete tasks, recording events in a diary, or using recall interviews rather than self-reported rating scales, or limiting recall periods to shorter intervals (Burrows et al., 2010; McPherson et al., 2000). Due to questionable psychometrics of self-report rating scales completed by children, recall interviews have been identified as particularly useful in childhood (Quittner et al., 2008; Warren et al., 2010). For 24-hour recall interviews, breaking the day into short, meaningful chunks (e.g., after waking up and before leaving for school) can help prompt children's memory (Foley et al., 2012). Language may be simplified and simple line drawings may be used on written materials to help illustrate complex concepts and facilitate comprehension. Results from children's self-reports are typically not used in isolation but rather in coordination with reports from parents or others, such as school personnel who observe food intake or exercise or who assist with administering medical treatments (Babbitt et al., 1995; Burrows et al., 2010; McPherson et al., 2000).

Health behavior assessment with elderly individuals may be impacted by declines in memory, comprehension, and visual or hearing abilities. Unlike assessment for children, many older people are able to self-report. However, obtaining data from additional reporters or observation is recommended for validation and verification (Babbitt et al., 1995; Prince et al., 2008). De Vries and colleagues (2009) note that a primary challenge among older individuals is distinguishing between those who are able to self-report and those whose age-related cognitive declines make self-report untenable and thus are better assessed with direct or observational measures. When assessing participants with a wide range of cognitive abilities the challenge is to select assessments that are appropriate across the full range of ability levels. Adaptations to meet the needs of elderly research participants and patients can include using larger fonts and/or reading questionnaires aloud or by interview, and using pictures to help clarify abstract or complex concepts, such as food serving sizes (Smith, Mitchell, Reay, Webb, & Harvey, 1998). Because physical functioning and mobility may decline with age, the content of measures of physical activity has been adapted to reflect common types and ranges of activity in older people (Babbitt et al., 1995). While problems with declarative memory may pose a challenge for elders in recalling specific behaviors (e.g., whether one has taken a particular medication at a particular time), open-ended interviews and tasks that tap procedural memory, such as describing daily medication routines, may be more appropriate and valid in this population (MacLaughlin et al., 2005).

CONCLUSIONS

As our knowledge of health behaviors and scientific pursuits become increasingly nuanced and complex, the need for precise, accurate measurement also grows. Technological advances over the past several years have helped make significant progress in this area. Electronic monitors have become more sophisticated and now allow for a great deal of valid and reliable remote data collection (e.g., RFPM methods for photography-based food assessment) and "smart" integration of multiple assessment methods (e.g., self-report with physical measurements with accelerometer data).

New, integrated technologies like these continue to be developed that expand, extend, and strengthen existing self-report and observational instruments. For example, physical activity monitors are being developed that not only identify behavioral patterns and recognize specific activities, but also that can combine measures of physical acceleration and heart rate to rate overall fitness and ability (Warren et al., 2010; Westerterp et al., 2009). Electronic medication monitors are being developed that integrate social networking features that track one's location with the use of GPS software, and that communicate directly with researcher or medical teams about the behavior being assessed (e.g., taking a specific medication). Currently, researchers at the University of Pittsburgh are developing new technology called e-Button that integrates many of the technologies described in this chapter for comprehensive evaluation of a range of health behaviors. E-Buttons are discrete video cameras worn on the body that can document and timestamp one's daily activities, provide high-resolution images of food, track location and speed of movement with accelerometers and GPS software, and calculate information including activity intensity, caloric intake, and time spent in different postures or locations.

Innovative, mobile programs like these that combine measurement strategies and that blend into users' day-to-day lives hold incredible potential. As the technology, especially software for mobile applications, continues to evolve, health behaviors may be more easily linked with remotely collected biological data such as blood glucose readings and lung function. Together, these data can be used to evaluate concurrent links between behavioral processes and health outcomes. This may open the door for greater coordination between assessment and real-time feedback and intervention to promote healthy behaviors.

Finally, the movement toward widespread use of electronic health records (EHRs) brings great potential to systematically collect and evaluate health and health behavior data in research and clinical practice (Estabrooks et al., 2012). As calls for patient-reported data gain momentum, health care systems will have the opportunity to integrate patient questionnaires and other instruments into the EHR (e.g., via patient access portals, at kiosks or tablets during medical visits) to collect these data in an efficient, systematic, and consistent manner (Glasgow & Emmons, 2011). Although these data will likely make clinician and researcher access to behavioral health data easier, a number of risks and challenges accompany this (as every) technological advance. A primary concern is the likelihood of having inconsistent, slightly different measures administered at different institutions or even by different providers within the same health care system, thus limiting our ability to compare data across large groups of people. There will also be a need to ensure that questions are well validated and reliable, cost-efficient, and feasible for administration to diverse populations. Given the risk of making clinical decisions based on information in the EHR, care will need to be taken to not inappropriately reduce nuanced behavioral measures to simple numbers that could be misinterpreted out of context. For example, EHR notation of behavioral health data will need to clearly indicate whether scores reported in the EHR represent a full, diagnostic measure or a brief screener, whether the data were provided by patients or by clinician assessment, and the frequency of assessments. As a first step to address these concerns, the Society of Behavioral Medicine has proposed a "harmonized set" of brief behavioral measures that can be used across providers and health care systems (Estabrooks et al., 2012; Glasgow & Emmons, 2011), with items including physical activity, eating patterns, and medication taking among others. As this movement proceeds, research is under way to evaluate the feasibility and usefulness of EHR-based assessment of patient-reported behavioral health data for research, clinical practice, and ultimately individuals' health and well-being.

REFERENCES

Anderson, D. A., Lundgren, J. D., Shapiro, J. R., & Paulosky, C. A. (2004). Assessment of eating disorders: Review and recommendations for clinical use. *Behavior Modification, 28,* 763–782.

Babbitt, R. L., Elden-Nazin, L., Manikam, R., Summers, J. A., & Murphy, C. M. (1995). Assessment of eating and weight-related problems in children and special populations. In D. B. Allison (Ed.), *Handbook of assessment methods for eating behaviors and weight related problems: Measures, theory and research.* Thousand Oaks, CA: Sage Publications.

Baeyens, D., Lierman, A., Roeyers, H., Hoebeke, P., & Vande Walle, J. (2009). Adherence in children with nocturnal enuresis. *Journal of Pediatric Urology, 5,* 105–109.

Bonomi, A. G., Plasqui, G., Goris, A. H., & Westerterp, K. R. (2009). Improving assessment of daily energy expenditure by identifying types of physical activity with a single accelerometer. *Journal of Applied Physiology, 107,* 655–661.

Burrows, T. L., Martin, R. J., & Collins, C. E. (2010). A systematic review of the validity of dietary assessment methods in children when compared with the method of doubly labeled water. *Journal of the American Dietetic Association,* 1501–1510.

Christensen, A., Osterberg, L., & Hansen, E. H. (2009). Electronic monitoring of patient adherence to oral antihypertensive medical treatment: A systematic review. *Journal of Hypertension,* 1540–1551.

Copher, R., Buzinec, P., Zarotsky, V., Kazis, L., Iqbal, S. U., & Macarios D. (2010). Physician perception of patient adherence compared to patient adherence of osteoporosis medications from pharmacy claims. *Current Medical Research Opinion,* 777–785.

Daniels, T., Goodacre, L., Sutton, C., Pollard, K., Conway, S., & Peckham, D. (2011). Accurate assessment of adherence: Self-report and clinician report vs. Electronic monitoring of nebulizers. *Chest, 140,* 425–432.

De Vries, J. H. M., de Groot, L. C., & van Staveren, W. A. (2009). Dietary assessment in elderly people: Experiences gained from studies in the Netherlands. *European Journal of Clinical Nutrition,* S69–S74.

Estabrooks, P. A., Boyle, M., Emmons, K. M., Glasgow, R. E., Hesse, B. W., Kaplan, R. M., ... Taylor, M. V. (2012). Harmonized patient-reported data elements in the electronic health record: Supporting meaningful use by primary care action on health behaviors and key psychosocial factors. *Journal of the American Medical Informatics Association: JAMIA,* 575–582.

Farley, J. J., Montepiedra, G., Storm, D., Sirois, P. A., Malee, K., Garvie, P., ... Nichols, S. (2008). Assessment of adherence to antiretroviral therapy in perinatally HIV-infected children and youth using self-report measures and pill count. *Journal of Developmental and Behavioral Pediatrics,* 377–384.

Foley, L., Maddison, R., Olds, T., & Ridley, K. (2012). Self-report use-of-time tools for the assessment of physical activity and sedentary behavior in young people: A systematic review. *Obesity Review,* 711–722.

Garber, M. C., Nau, D. P., Erickson, S. R., Aikens, J. E., & Lawrence, J. B. (2004). The concordance of self-report with other measures of medication adherence: A summary of the literature. *Medical Care,* 649–652.

Garfield, S., Clifford, S., Eliasson, L., Barber, N., & Willson, A. (2011). Suitability of measures of self-reported medication adherence for clinical use: A systematic review. *BMC Medical Research Methodology,* 149–157.

Garvie, P. A., Wilkins, M. L., & Young, J. C. (2010). Medication adherence in adolescents with behaviorally-acquired HIV: Evidence for using a multimethod assessment protocol. *Journal of Adolescent Health,* 504–511.

Glasgow, R., & Emmons, K. M. (2011). The public health need for patient-reported measures and health behaviors in electronic health records: A policy statement of the Society of Behavioral Medicine. *Translational Behavioral Medicine,* 108–109.

Haberer, J. E., Robbins, G. K., Ybarra, M., Monk, A., Ragland, K., Weiser, S. D., & Bangsberg, D. R. (2012). Real-time electronic monitoring is feasible, comparable to unannounced pill counts, and acceptable. *AIDS and Behavior*, 375–382.

Hart, J. E., Jeon, C. Y., Ivers, L. C., Behforouz, H. L., Caldas, A., Drobac, P. C., ... Shin, S. S. (2010). Effect of directly observed therapy for highly active antiretroviral therapy on virologic, immunologic, and adherence outcomes: A meta-analysis and systematic review. *Journal of Acquired Immune Deficiency Syndrome*, 54, 167–179.

Haskell, W. L. (2012). Physical activity by self-report: A brief history and future issues. *Journal of Physical Activity & Health*, S5–S10.

Hess, L. M., Raebel, M. A., Conner, D. A., & Malone, D. C. (2006). Measurement of adherence in pharmacy administrative databases: A proposal for standard definitions and preferred measures. *Annals of Pharmacotherapy*, 1280–1288.

Herzer, M., Ramey, C., Rohan, J., & Cortina, C. (2012). Incorporating electronic monitoring feedback into clinical care: A novel and promising adherence promotion approach. *Clinical Child Psychology and Psychiatry*, 505–518.

Hommel, K. A., Davis, C. M., & Baldassano, R. N. (2008). Objective versus subjective assessment of oral medication adherence in pediatric inflammatory bowel disease. *Inflammatory Bowel Diseases*, 589–593.

Hood, K. K., Peterson, C. M., Rohan, J. S., & Drotar, D. (2009). Association between adherence and glycemic control in pediatric type 1 diabetes: A meta-analysis. *Pediatrics*, e1171–e1179.

Jones, M., & Johnston, D. (2011). Understanding phenomena in the real world: The case for real time data collection in health services research. *Journal of Health Services Research & Policy*, 172–176.

Kalichman, S. C., Amaral, C. M., Cherry, C., Flanagan, J., Pope, H., Eaton, L., ... Schinazi, R. F. (2008). Monitoring medication adherence by unannounced pill counts conducted by telephone: Reliability and criterion-related validity. *HIV Clinical Trials*, 298–308.

Kichler, J. C., Kaugars, A. S., Maglio, K., & Alemzadeh, R. (2010). Exploratory analysis among different methods of assessing adherence and glycemic control in youth with type 1 diabetes mellitus. *Health Psychology*, 35–42.

Koschack, J., Marx, G., Schnakenberg, J., Kochen, M. M., & Himmel, W. (2010). Comparison of two self-rating instruments for medication adherence assessment in hypertension revealed insufficient psychometric properties. *Journal of Clinical Epidemiology*, 299–306.

Logan, D., Zelikovsky, N., Labay, L., & Spergel, J. (2003). The illness management survey: Identifying adolescents' perceptions of barriers to adherence. *Journal of Pediatric Psychology*, 383–392.

Lutfey, K. E., & Ketcham, J. D. (2005). Patient and provider assessments of adherence and the sources of disparities: Evidence from diabetes care. *Health Services Research*, 1803–1817.

MacLaughlin, E. J., Raehl, C. L., Treadway, A. K., Sterling, T. L., Zoller, D. P., & Bond, C. A. (2005). Assessing medication adherence in the elderly: Which tools to use in clinical practice? *Drugs & Aging*, 231–255.

Martin, C. K., Han, H., Coulon, S. M., Allen, H. R., Champagne, C. M., & Anton, S. D. (2009). A novel method to remotely measure food intake of free-living individuals in real time: The remote food photography method. *British Journal of Nutrition*, 101, 446–456.

Mâsse, L. C., & de Niet, J. E. (2012). Sources of validity evidence needed with self-report measures of physical activity. *Journal of Physical Activity & Health*, S44–S55.

McPherson, R. S., Hoelscher, D. M., Alexander, M., Scanlon, K. S., & Serdula, M. K. (2000). Dietary assessment methods among school-age children: Validity and reliability. *Preventive Medicine*, S11–S33.

Miller, L. G., Liu, H., Hays, R. D., Golin, C. E., Beck, C. K., Asch, S. M., ... Wenger, N. S. (2002). How well do clinicians estimate patients' adherence to combination antiretroviral therapy? *Journal of General Internal Medicine*, 17, 1–11.

Murri, R., Ammassari, A., Trotta, M. P., De Luca, A., Melzi, S., Minardi, C., ... Wu, A. W. (2004). Patient-reported and physician-estimated adherence to HAART. *Journal of General Internal Medicine*, 1104–1110.

Nieuwkerk, P. T., de Boer-van der Kolk, I. M., Prins, J. M., Locadia, M., & Sprangers, M. A. (2010). Self-reported adherence is more predictive of virological treatment response among patients with a lower tendency toward socially desirable responding. *Antiviral Therapy*, 913–916.

Plasqui, G., & Westerterp, K. R. (2007). Physical activity assessment with accelerometers: An evaluation against doubly labeled water. *Obesity*, 2371–2379.

Prince, S. A., Adamo, K. B., Hamel, M. E., Hardt, J., Gorber, S. C., & Tremblay, M. (2008). A comparison of direct versus self-report measures for assessing physical activity in adults: A systematic review. *International Journal of Behavioral Nutrition and Physical Activity*, 56–80.

Puyau, M. R., Adolph, A. L., Vohra, F. A., & Butte, N. F. (2002). Validation and calibration of physical activity monitors in children. *Obesity Research*, 150–157.

Quittner, A. L., Modi, A. C., Lemanek, K. L., Ievers-Landis, C. E., & Rapoff, M. A. (2008). Evidence-based assessment of adherence to medical treatments in pediatric psychology. *Journal of Pediatric Psychology*, 916–936.

Rand, C. S. (2000). "I took the medication like you told me, doctor": Self-report of adherence with medical regimens. In A. A. Stone, C. A. Bachrach, J. B. Jobe, H. S. Kurtzman, & V. S. Cain (Eds.), *The science of self-report: Implications for research and practice*. Mahwah, NJ: Lawrence Earlbaum.

Rapoff, M. A. (2010). *Adherence to pediatric medical regimens* (2nd ed.). New York, NY: Springer.

Riekert, K. A., & Rand, C. S. (2002). Electronic monitoring of medication adherence: When is high-tech best? *Journal of Clinical Psychology in Medical Settings, 9*, 25–34.

Schafer-Keller, P., Steiger, J., Bock, A., Denhaerynck, K., & De Geest, S. (2008). Diagnostic accuracy of measurement methods to assess non-adherence to immunosuppressive drugs in kidney transplant recipients. *American Journal of Transplantation*, 616–626.

Schutz, Y., Weinsier, R. L., & Hunter, G. R. (2012). Assessment of free-living physical activity in humans: An overview of currently available and proposed new measures. *Obesity Research*, 368–379.

Shelton, M. L., & Klesges, R. C. (1995). Measures of physical activity and exercise. In D. B. Allison (Ed.), *Handbook of assessment methods for eating behaviors and weight-related problems: Measures, theory, and research*. Thousand Oaks, CA: Sage Publications.

Shemesh, E., Shneider, B. L., Savitzky, J. K., Arnott, L., Gondolesi, G. E., Krieger, N. R., ... Emre, S. (2004). Medication adherence in pediatric and adolescent liver transplant recipients. *Pediatrics*, 825–832.

Shi, L., Liu, J., Koleva, Y., Fonseca, V., Kalsekar, A., & Pawaskar, M. (2010). Concordance of adherence measurement using self-reported adherence questionnaires and medication monitoring devices. *Pharmacoeconomics*, 1097–1107.

Shiffman, S. (2009). How many cigarettes did you smoke? Assessing cigarette consumption by global report, time-line follow-back, and ecological momentary assessment. *Health Psychology*, 519–526.

Shiffman, S., Stone, A. A., & Hufford, M. R. (2008). Ecological momentary assessment. *Annual Review of Clinical Psychology*, 1–32.

Smith, W., Mitchell, P., Reay, E. M., Webb, K., & Harvey, P. W. J. (1998). Validity and reproducibility of a self-administered food frequency questionnaire in older people. *Australian and New Zealand Journal of Public Health*, 456–463.

Spaulding, S. A., Devine, K. A., Duncan, C. L., Wilson, N. W., & Hogan, M. B. (2012). Electronic monitoring and feedback to improve adherence in pediatric asthma. *Journal of Pediatric Psychology*, 64–74.

Sternfeld, B., & Goldman-Rosas, L. (2012). A systematic approach to selecting an appropriate measure of self-reported physical activity or sedentary behavior. *Journal of Physical Activity & Health*, S19–S28.

Streiner, D. L., & Norman, G. R. (2008). *Health measurement scales: A practical guide to their development and use* (4th ed.). New York, NY: Oxford University Press.

Stull, D. E., Leidy, N. K., Parasuraman, B., & Chassany, O. (2009). Optimal recall periods for patient-reported outcomes: Challenge and potential solutions. *Current Medical Research Opinion*, 929–942.

Svarstad, B. L., Chewning, B. A., Sleath, B. L., & Claesson, C. (1999). The brief medication questionnaire: A tool for screening patient adherence and barriers to adherence. *Patient Education and Counseling*, 113–124.

Thompson, F. E., Subar, A. F., Loria, C. M., Reedy, J. L., & Baranowsky, T. (2010). Need for technological innovation in dietary assessment. *Journal of the American Dietetic Association*, 48–51.

Warren, J. M., Ekelund, U., Besson, H., Mazzani, A., Geladas, N., & Vanhees, L. (2010). Assessment of physical activity – A review of methodologies with reference to epidemiological research: A report of the exercise physiology section of the European Association of Cardiovascular Prevention and Rehabilitation. *European Journal of Preventive Cardiology*, 127–139.

Westerterp, K. R. (2009). Assessment of physical activity: A critical appraisal. *European Journal of Applied Physiology*, 823–828.

Wiener, L., Riekert, K., Ryder, C., & Wood, L. V. (2004). Assessing medication adherence in adolescents with HIV when electronic monitoring is not feasible. *AIDS Patient Care and STDs*, 31–42.

Wolper, C., Heshka, S., & Heymsfield, S. B. (1995). Measuring food intake: An overview. In D. B. Allison (Ed.), *Handbook of assessment methods for eating behaviors and weight-related problems: Measures, theory, and research*. Thousand Oaks, CA: Sage Publications.

24

Translational Research Phases in the Behavioral and Social Sciences: Adaptations From the Biomedical Sciences

STEPHENIE C. LEMON

DEBORAH J. BOWEN

MILAGROS C. ROSAL

SHERRY L. PAGOTO

KRISTIN L. SCHNEIDER

LORI PBERT

MONICA L. WANG

JENNIFER D. ALLEN

JUDITH K. OCKENE

LEARNING OBJECTIVES

- Define translational research and understand its importance to improve population health.
- Compare and contrast translational research phases in biomedical research with behavioral and social science research.
- Identify strategies to improve translational research in health behavior change interventions.

Health-related research may be defined as "a systematic investigation, including research development, testing and evaluation, designed to develop or contribute to generalizable knowledge" related to health behaviors and/or outcomes (Centers for Disease Control and Prevention [CDC], 2010). While the majority of health-related research, funding, and organizations in the United States have been historically, biomedically and basic science oriented, health behaviors and factors influencing those behaviors play an important role in shaping population patterns in health, particularly as preventable and/or chronic diseases increasingly contribute to the overall population morbidity and mortality in the 21st century. The development, application, and advancement of health behavior change research methodology are therefore essential in informing behavioral and social health interventions in an effort to promote population health.

Translational research, included in 2003 in the National Institutes of Health (NIH) Roadmap (Zerhouni, 2003), has been part of a paradigm shift in health-related research over the past decade. The catalyst behind this shift has been a call to action to address the documented lag from basic research discoveries, to application and dissemination, leading to an eventual population health benefit. The median time from the initial publication of a basic scientific discovery to the publication of its use for health benefit is 24 years (Contopoulos-Ioannidis, Alexiou, Gouvias, & Ioannidis, 2008). Timely implementation and dissemination of successful, evidence-based health interventions, informed by health behavior change research methods, are necessary to effectively address changing population health patterns.

As described by Woolf (2008), there is general consensus that translational research is essential to improving population health, but there is less agreement on how to define it. Initial definitions of translational research made a distinction between "T1" research, which focuses on translation from basic science discovery to human studies, and "T2" research, which focuses on translation from scientific discovery to adoption of best clinical practices that result in human benefit (Sung et al., 2003). This distinction is important because it highlights the different disciplines, tools, skill sets, and infrastructure required to achieve the goals of lab-based and human-focused research.

Since its original conceptualization, definitions of translational research have evolved to further differentiate phases of "T2" research to reflect the continuum from evidence generated through clinical trials to widespread population surveillance research (Khoury, Gwinn, & Ioannidis, 2010; Waldman & Terzic, 2010). However, to date, the phases of human-focused translational research have primarily been illustrated using a biomedical focus (Khoury et al., 2010) with research products that include treatments such as drugs and devices, usually delivered within health care settings by health care professionals. To achieve population health benefit, the conceptualization and application of translational research must extend beyond treatment-focused biomedical research and include a wide spectrum of research disciplines, in particular recognizing the essential role of health behavior change research methods in guiding behavioral and social interventions that lead to improved health behaviors and/or health outcomes.

The behavioral and social phases of the research continuum in the area of cancer prevention and control were first articulated 30 years ago (Greenwalk & Cullen, 1985) and were updated in the 1990s (Best, Hiatt, Cameron, Rimer, & Abrams, 2003). Adapting these frameworks to integrate current biomedical perspectives on translational research will help establish a common language while emphasizing the unique contributions of the behavioral and social sciences and the importance of health behavior change research: the focus is both prevention and treatment, and research products include programs, policies, and other interventions aimed at achieving behavior change and health outcomes. The types of behavioral and social interventions vary widely and include educational interventions to increase knowledge and awareness related to a health behavior or outcome, programs targeting specific health behaviors, and environmental and policy changes that influence health behaviors and access to health-related resources. These interventions can be single- or multi-level designs and can be delivered across numerous settings, including health care settings (e.g., hospitals and clinics) and community settings (e.g., schools, worksites, homes, and community organizations). The delivery agents, target populations, and intensity and duration of the interventions also widely vary. The purpose of this chapter is to provide and illustrate a current framework for translational research specific to the health behavior change research methods, and to compare these methods to a translational research framework developed from a biomedical perspective (Khoury et al., 2010).

PHASES OF TRANSLATIONAL RESEARCH: APPLICATION TO THE BEHAVIORAL AND SOCIAL SCIENCES

Figure 24.1 presents the stages of translational research, as identified and defined by current thought pieces and position papers (Khoury et al., 2010; Waldman & Terzic, 2010). These definitions were developed with respect to biomedical fields. Behavioral and social science research follows the same translational trajectory as biomedical research, but with different types of research questions and methodologies. Here we describe each phase of translational research and provide two realms of application, biomedical and behavioral/social, and compare them to illustrate the similarities and differences in the application of the translational model to these different areas.

T1: FROM SCIENTIFIC DISCOVERY TO HEALTH APPLICATION

Broadly, T1 research consists of applying scientific discovery of human processes to health-related interventions.

Biomedical Sciences

T1 research is the identification and characterization of basic processes of human functioning. It is the largest research area funded by NIH (Collins, 2012). In the biomedical sciences, T1 research could be the discovery of a molecule known to play a role in the cycle of a cell that is changing from the normal to the cancerous stage, or the identification of a genetic mutation in individuals who are at high risk for developing a chronic disease. T1 research

FIGURE 24.1 **Phases of translational research (Khoury et al., 2010).**

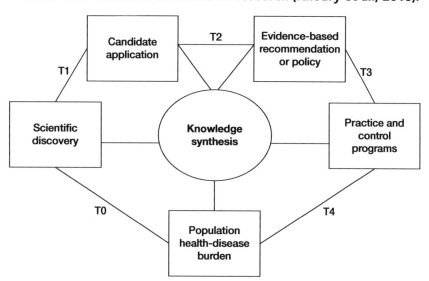

is critical to understanding the basic mechanisms of biological function and dysfunction. The major challenge for T1 research is to identify efficiently which basic discoveries can lead to meaningful clinical products in later stages of translation. In the translational process from T1 to T2, candidate findings are selected from the vast array of basic findings, to use when designing a specific clinical or public health tool for use in practice.

Behavioral and Social Sciences

In the behavioral and social sciences, T1 research consists of the identification and characterization of basic processes of human social and psychological functioning. The Office of Behavioral and Social Science Research defines basic social and behavioral research as "...designed to further our understanding of fundamental mechanisms and patterns of behavioral and social functioning relevant to the Nation's health and well-being, and as they interact with each other, with biology and the environment" (Office of Behavioral and Social Sciences Research & National Institutes of Health, 2013). The essential questions posed by T1 behavioral research are ones of why: Why do people make (or not make) certain types of health-related decisions? Why do social groups behave in certain ways? Why do people make choices to improve or not improve health? Within this context, this type of research seeks to identify and characterize essential processes related to health behavior change, such as human knowledge acquisition, affect management, coping, human interactions, social processes, group and organizational functioning, culture formation and maintenance, and social movement changes. Examples of products from T1 behavioral and social science research include behavioral theories, specific methods, measures, and understanding of behavioral and social mechanisms. The health behavior change research methodologies used at the T1 stage in the behavioral and social sciences are diverse (Creswell, Klassen, Plano Clark, Smith, for the Office of Behavioral and Social Sciences Research, 2011; National Institutes of Health, Office of Behavioral and Social Sciences Research, 2001; Weathington, Cunningham, & Pittenger, 2010). They include retrospective and prospective longitudinal designs, and basic behavioral laboratory designs, which often use covert methods such as confederates and bogus pipelines, and cross-sectional assessments. One challenge for the movement of T1 behavioral and social research into the next stage is the same as for biomedical research: knowing which of the vast number of findings will be relevant to clinical or public health practice, and can be developed into specific interventions for use by the general public. A unique methodological challenge to social and behavioral research and a threat to construct validity is the reactivity to the experimental situation; unlike cells, people may intentionally or unintentionally change their behavior or responses as a result of being part of the experiment situation, rather than or in addition to the responses reflective of the treatments or interventions being delivered (Shadish, Cook, & Campbell, 2002).

T2: FROM APPLICATION TO GUIDELINES

The T2 phase consists of applying scientific knowledge of human health processes to guide the development of evidence-based guidelines to improve health and prevent disease.

Biomedical Sciences

T2 research is the study of the efficacy of potential applications to clinical or public health practice. In the biomedical sciences, examples of T2 research include the identification of the usefulness and harms of a genetic test, a medical application, or a vaccine to prevent a disease of public health importance. Methodologies to address this stage of translation often involve the assessment of a broad array of health outcomes in controlled settings. Very often this involves a randomized controlled trial in a defined population.

Challenges during the T2 stage include identification of potential harms as well as benefits, comparisons of sensitivity and specificity in practice settings, expense of trials, and considerations of cost relative to the positive effects of the test or procedure. The outcome of T2 research is to formulate guidelines for the use of the new test or practice that are based in empirical evidence of benefit and lack of harm, such as the U.S. Guide to Clinical Preventive Services (U.S. Preventive Services Task Force, 2012).

Behavioral and Social Sciences

In the behavioral and social sciences, efficacy research is defined as the testing of interventions in controlled situations with defined populations to determine its effects on key outcomes linked to health behaviors. Efficacy research asks the question "Did "X" intervention, program, policy, or practice work in a highly controlled setting?" The strongest evidence in efficacy research comes from randomized trials, but quasi-experimental designs are often used in health behavior change research studies. Often internal validity, defined as the rigor of study design, measurement, and control with respect to establishing causal inference, is paramount to external validity, or the relevance of the study to real life settings. External validity is often maximized in studies that follow efficacy testing. Thus, the goals of efficacy research are to establish a proof of concept and the products include evidence-based interventions and strategies.

Efficacy research in the behavioral and social sciences often uses randomized controlled trial research designs, as in the biomedical sciences. There are multiple challenges in efficacy research that are common to both biomedical research and social and behavioral science research. Large-scale randomized controlled trials are often expensive, requiring large sample sizes and extended follow-up periods to demonstrate whether the intervention under investigation has an effect on long-term health outcomes. Such trials often have stringent inclusion and exclusion criteria and samples include typically lack of representation of true clinical populations with respect to underlying health status. They also include highly motivated trial participants who are likely more adherent than a real world population. Additional challenges to behavioral and social science efficacy research include the intervention's potential lack of relevance (either the intervention components and/or the delivery of the intervention) to real world practice settings.

T3: FROM GUIDELINES TO PRACTICE

T3 research is defined as research that adapts and implements evidence-based guidelines and best practices identified through T2 research. This phase aims to test interventions and/or procedures that have been previously found to be efficacious under ideal research conditions in real world settings.

Biomedical Sciences

Specific guidelines, practices, and procedures identified through rigorous efficacy studies in biomedical research must be tested in clinical or public health settings to determine the effect on the general public. Methodologies used for these types of T3 studies include randomized trials, but can also include quasi-experimental designs and comparative effectiveness research. Challenges at the T3 stage include complications of real world implementation such as local contextual factors related to multiple settings, populations, and pathways. Only those guidelines, practices, and procedures that show effectiveness in real world settings should be moved forward for full implementation to impact the public's health.

Behavioral and Social Sciences

The T3 stage for behavioral and social scientists who develop and evaluate these types of interventions focuses on whether efficacious interventions and findings can be generalized to multiple real world settings and populations. The translational goal for T3 research testing behavioral interventions is to identify those policies, programs, and packages of intervention that are ready for clinical and/or population implementation. In the behavioral and social sciences, this involves two types of research: effectiveness research and dissemination and implementation research.

Effectiveness research involves testing the impact of interventions that are implemented in heterogeneous settings and populations on health outcomes. Examples of questions asked in effectiveness research include: Does this efficacious intervention work when implemented in an entire health care system? Can an intervention developed with middle-class youth be adapted for urban minority youth in public schools? What is the cost-effectiveness of an intervention as it is being tested in a population-based setting?

Dissemination research refers to "the systematic study of processes and factors that lead to widespread use of an evidence-based intervention by the target population," whereas implementation research "seeks to understand the processes and factors that are associated with integration of evidence-based interventions within a particular setting" (Bowen et al., 2009; Colditz, 2012, pp. 3–22). The two are integrally linked in that they seek to understand methods by which to best implement evidence-based interventions and policies in real world settings. The type of question answered in this research includes, "What contextual processes and strategies are most likely to result in the adoption and use of efficacious innovations in specified contexts?"

Products from T3 behavioral and social sciences research include tools for clinical and community practitioners to incorporate into daily practice. Challenges in this type of research relate to the multiple and complex barriers that can occur when implementing a health behavior change intervention in real world settings. At this stage, methodological tradeoffs in study design, implementation, and evaluation are made to enhance the external validity, scalability, and reach of the intervention. For example, use of non-randomized study designs, such as quasi-experimental, observational, and cross-sectional studies may be more feasible and appropriate in diverse community settings, despite the potential for limiting internal validity. Intervention fidelity may be difficult to maximize and evaluate. Also, adoption of interventions after the research program has ended does not always happen, owing to multiple issues including staff turnover, institutional commitment, and lack of resources (Pagoto, 2011).

T4: FROM EFFECTIVENESS TO POPULATION OUTCOMES

The T4 phase is defined as the evaluation of practices, upon implementation and dissemination, on health outcomes at the community and population level.

Biomedical Sciences

In the biomedical sciences, T4 research could be called post-evaluation surveillance, as this phase often involves monitoring the general public for changes in outcomes as a result of full implementation of interventions. Both harms and benefits can be the focus of T4 research, as in other stages. Research methods used in this stage include regular and frequent surveillance of important health outcomes in the general public such as disease counts, symptoms and side effects, unintended harms, and quality of life. A primary challenge with conducting T4 research is accurate attribution of the outcome measured to the specific intervention that was implemented, due to the use of non-randomized designs. Other challenges include defining the population to be monitored and the specific outcomes that are hypothesized to change, and actually having population values for those outcomes at the time they are needed and in the desired region.

Behavioral and Social Sciences

T4 research in the behavioral and social sciences places emphasis on assessing the diffusion of behavioral and social interventions into the general public. The types of questions that a behavioral or social scientist might ask during the T4 stage are: To what extent is the behavior of interest reduced or enhanced within a given practice setting? How is the intervention diffusing through the public's understanding and use? What are the best, most powerful ways to communicate to all relevant levels of the general public about a new screening tool? What are the social forces that work against acceptance of a specific health promotion activity in a particular country?

T4 behavioral and social science research focuses on the widespread implementation of programs and policies and the evaluation of their impact on population health. The research methodologies used in this stage of behavioral and social science research include surveillance methods, observational and comparative data monitoring at the level of state, country, or region, and other forms of policy evaluation and observational research. The multiple challenges to this type of research are similar to those of other disciplines and include establishing causal inference between observed changes in the outcome(s) and the specific intervention(s) of focus, cost of implementing a new intervention in a population and savings that could occur, harms that might be due to the new intervention, and sustainability of new interventions over years or decades.

CASE STUDY: THE 5 As MODEL FOR TREATING TOBACCO USE AND DEPENDENCE

Treatment for tobacco use provides an important example to illustrate the role of social and behavioral sciences, specifically the use of health behavior change research methods, in the translational research continuum. In recent decades, there have been dramatic decreases in smoking rates across the U.S. adult population. This has been achieved through application of comprehensive tobacco treatment clinical services, community programs, and policies that included multi-pronged, multi-sectorial strategies targeting prevention and treatment. Behavioral and social-science-based clinical interventions, including the 5 As model for treating tobacco use and dependence (Fiore et al., 2000), have played a central role in this public health success (Fiore et al., 2008). The 5 As is an evidence-based, patient-centered counseling approach that includes sequential strategies for providers to use with their smoking patients: "Ask" all patients about their tobacco use; "Advise" all patients who identify as smokers to quit; "Assess" the patient's willingness to quit; "Assist" the patient to identify counseling or pharmacologic treatment options and make appropriate prescriptions and referrals for individuals ready to make a quit attempt; and "Arrange" follow-up contacts to support patients receiving evidence-based pharmacologic treatment or counseling. Since the model was originally introduced in 1989 (National Cancer Institute [NCI]) as the 4 As (Glynn & Manley, 1989), there has been a wealth of research conducted using it. The 4 As were changed to the 5 As, adding the "assess" step with the release of the first smoking cessation clinical practice guidelines (Agency for Healthcare Policy and Research, 1996). In the following paragraphs, we use the development, implementation, and dissemination of the 5 As model to illustrate our translational framework.

Beginning in the late 1970s and early 1980s, there was a growing recognition of the potential of health care providers as behavior change agents to achieve reduction in smoking rates. Several studies investigated the prevalence of physician advice and counseling for smoking cessation (Anda, Remington, Sienko, & Davis, 1987; CDC, 1993; Ockene, 1987; Orleans, George, Houpt, & Brodie, 1985), followed by a series of studies testing approaches to encourage providers to assist patients in their efforts to quit smoking (Russell, Wilson, Taylor, & Baker, 1979; Schauffler & Parkinson, 1993) (T2). In 1983, the National Cancer Institute funded five randomized controlled trials (Cohen, Stookey, Katz, Drook, & Smith, 1989; Cummings et al., 1989; Kottke, Brekke, Solberg, & Hughes, 1989; Ockene et al., 1991; Wilson et al., 1988) that tested the efficacy of physician-delivered tobacco treatment, together demonstrating that this approach is effective. The findings from the five studies were synthesized to develop the 4 As model and to begin to decipher the theoretical underpinnings of effective counseling approaches, the synthesis and theoretical work being an extension of the T1 phase. The role of health care providers was further explored in additional T2 studies as part of the multi-site NCI-funded Community Intervention Trial for Smoking Cessation (COMMIT) trial (COMMIT Research Group, 1991) that aimed to reduce smoking among adults through interventions delivered by health care providers, worksites and community organizations, cessation resources, and media and community events. In COMMIT, a review of available evidence and expert consensus culminated to support the "4 As" approach (Ask, Advise, Assist, Arrange), that was then incorporated into COMMIT comprehensive intervention activities (Ockene, Lindsay, Berger, & Hymowitz, 1990), which had a beneficial impact on smoking rates.

The nonlinearity of the research process utilized in the case study example described above is important to note. An inductive use of evidence supported the theoretical elements of effective provider tobacco treatment counseling (T1) and the efficacy of this type of approach (T2). The sum of this work established a proof of concept, that this counseling approach can result in increased smoking cessation when implemented under ideal circumstances (Cohen et al., 1989; Cummings et al., 1989; Kottke et al., 1989; Ockene et al., 1991; COMMIT Research Group, 1995; Wilson et al., 1988). An important culmination of this work includes evidence-based guidelines that recommend the 5 As in routine clinical practice from organizations such as the U.S. Preventive Services Task Force (2009), and the Public Health Service (Fiore et al., 2000).

T3 research of the 5 As research has focused on tools and delivery models to implement the intervention approach by physicians and other health care professionals. A 2010 systematic review by Papadakis and colleagues identified 37 trials conducted in 10 countries testing such smoking cessation tools and models in primary care settings (Papadakis et al., 2010). The outcomes of these studies focused on success in achieving smoking abstinence (i.e., effectiveness) and provider performance in delivery of each of the 5 As components (i.e., implementation). Tools and models tested were targeted at patients (e.g., tailored print materials), providers (e.g., performance feedback), practices (e.g., reminder systems and decision supports), and systems (e.g., provider incentives). This review concluded that multicomponent strategies targeting more than one level are most effective in achieving provider adherence to 5 As delivery and patient smoking cessation.

The role of T4 research is to determine the utilization and utility of the 5 As in actual practice. Several observational studies assessed the extent to which the 5 As and its components are delivered by a variety of health care providers in diverse practice settings and the impact of delivery on cessation rates (Chase, McMenamin, & Halpin, 2007; Geller et al., 2008, 2011; Halpin Schauffler, Mordavsky, & McMenamin, 2001; Lopez-Quintero, Crum, & Neumark, 2006; Manfredi & LeHew, 2008; Quinn et al., 2009). For example, Chase and colleagues conducted a study which involved a random sample telephone survey of 563 Medicaid enrollees identified as smokers or recent past smokers who self-reported receipt of each of the 5 As components by a health care provider in the past year. Results indicated high rates of being asked about smoking status (87%) and being advised to quit (65%), with reports of receipt of each subsequent step declining. Only 9% reported receipt of all 5 As components. This pattern is typically found in studies assessing receipt of the 5 As components in the real world. In addition, this body of research has identified disparities in receipt of smoking cessation counseling according to patient attributes such as socioeconomic characteristics, race, and ethnicity (Houston, Scarinci, Person, & Greene, 2005; Lopez-Quintero et al., 2006).

CONSIDERATIONS AND RECOMMENDATIONS FOR TRANSLATIONAL HEALTH BEHAVIOR CHANGE RESEARCH

Translational behavioral and social research is essential for improving health and quality of life; informing policy, payment systems, and health care reform; and improving cost-effectiveness. The framework presented for translational behavioral and social research in this chapter is adapted from current thinking in biomedical research that can be a general guide both for defining the types or "Ts" of translational research, and for understanding the process by which translational research evolves over time. To advance translational research, it is critical that the behavioral and social sciences achieve consensus on how to define the stages of translational research, and adopt common language and understanding with regard to health behavior research methodology. It is also imperative that the field continues to evolve. We offer the following considerations and recommendations for translational research.

Translational behavioral research is iterative, rather than linear. In the behavioral and social sciences, a nonlinear approach to the research process occurs across the phases of the research continuum. The 5 As model illustrates that the research process often is not a linear one, and in fact may be thought of as an inductive process, which is consistent with the biomedical sciences. For example, the development of the final 5 As model was influenced by observational studies and randomized trials that contributed to our understanding of the roles of providers and the theoretical underpinnings of the counseling approach. Findings from effectiveness, implementation, and diffusion studies can and should be used to inform the next generation of basic behavioral investigation and efficacy trials. The nature of behavioral and social research is such that we must continuously evolve and use new findings to inform basic questions needing further exploration, allowing a shift back and forth from big questions to small questions.

Renewed focus on basic research focusing on theoretical and conceptual frameworks is needed. In the biomedical realm, a substantial amount of research funding is dedicated to basic research. This is less so in the behavioral and social sciences (National Institutes of Health, 2009). Basic research is critical in informing the success of each of the subsequent translational research steps and the long-term success of behavioral and social products. Understanding the theoretical underpinnings of behavior change and the subsequent application of this theoretical base to intervention design and implementation allow for a corresponding structured evaluation that can demonstrate how and why interventions are effective (or not), highlight potential gaps or limitations of the application of existing behavior change theories, and provide insights on the development of new theories to predict and change health behaviors. Theoretical approaches are broad enough for application to a variety of populations, behaviors, and outcomes and allow for tailoring and modification specific to each research question, setting, and population of interest. As theories can be evaluated, evidence-based theories on health behavior are particularly valuable for translational research. In contrast, behavioral and social health interventions that lack a theoretical base are often developed without thoughtful consideration of how and why an intervention may work. For example, theory-based interventions carefully consider the relation between risk factors, mediators, and outcomes in the design of health behavior change interventions. Theory-based interventions provide a rationale structure for the proposed intervention as well as corresponding structured evaluation that allows for testing of the intervention and the theory. In atheoretical interventions, it is often unclear how and why such interventions worked, and how and why interventions did not work. As such, atheoretical interventions that demonstrate efficacy may be limited in their applicability to other populations and settings. In fact, evidence indicates that behavioral and social science interventions based on theory have stronger impact than those that lack a theoretical base (Glanz & Bishop, 2010). However, considerable gaps exist between theory, research, and practice (Glanz & Bishop, 2010). To illustrate, recent reviews and opinion pieces related to the dissemination and implementation of evidence-based programs (Flay et al., 2005; Glasgow & Emmons, 2007; Green, Ottoson, Garcia, & Hiatt, 2009; Rabin, Glasgow, Kerner, Klump, & Brownson, 2010) note the lack of theoretically driven research. Future behavioral and social research should utilize and explicitly describe the theoretical or conceptual framework guiding the research questions, study design, analysis, and conclusions.

Behavioral and social research should clearly distinguish between goals of efficacy and effectiveness research. Behavioral and social science research is most similar to biomedical research at the efficacy stage. However, the distinction between efficacy and effectiveness research is not always clear in the behavioral and social sciences. Behavioral intervention implementation often includes elements that utilize "ideal" (i.e., efficacy) and "real world" (i.e., effectiveness) components. For example, an intervention may be designed to occur within a "real world setting," such as a school or worksite, and include intervention components that fit within the existing infrastructure of the setting, yet elements of the intervention may be delivered by highly trained research staff. Without particular attention to the specific goals of a given research study (i.e., efficacy or effectiveness) and subsequently designing the study to achieve those goals, the interpretation of results is difficult and thus the real world impact of the study's findings will be difficult to understand.

Implementation science methodologies should be advanced. Effectiveness research has a long-standing tradition in the behavioral and social sciences. While elements of implementation research, such as inclusion of systematic process evaluation, have been historically conducted in behavioral and social studies, it is only recently that implementation science has emerged as a discipline in and of itself. There has been a push toward greater focus on implementation outcomes with promulgation of the RE-AIM framework (Glasgow, 2008; Glasgow, Vogt, & Boles, 1999) and for intervention evaluation and strategic training and research initiatives aiming to promote implementation research (Department of Health and Human Services, 2010; National Cancer Institute & Division of Cancer Control and Population Sciences, 2012; UNC Center for Health Promotion and Disease Prevention, 2012; U.S. Department of Health and Human Services, National Institutes of Health, & Office of Behavioral and Social Sciences Research, 2012; U.S.

Department of Health and Human Services & National Cancer Institute, 2006). Effectiveness research and implementation research aim to demonstrate different outcomes. In effectiveness research, the focus is on health improvements. In implementation research, the focus is on measures related to intervention implementation, including adoption, fidelity, and sustainability. However, these types of research are not mutually exclusive, and effectiveness and implementation outcome measures can be assessed within research studies that aim to establish best approaches for locally adapting efficacious interventions.

With the recent emphasis on implementation research and establishing best practices for adoption and sustainability of evidence-based behavioral interventions in diverse real world settings, there is also a need to better understanding characteristics of organizations and settings in which interventions are delivered and how they impact the success of dissemination and implementation. This necessarily includes identifying, measuring, and understanding factors that make an organization function well and characteristics of organizations that help or hinder full operations and achievement of its mission. Findings from a recent review indicated that measurement methodologies for these types of organizational characteristics are sadly lacking; without appropriate measurement tools, we cannot conduct the types of research that are needed in this field (Emmons, Weiner, Fernandez, & Tu, 2012).

Behavioral and social research and its products must be integrated into a larger biomedical context. Behavioral and social science interventions are not often intended to be delivered in isolation, but rather in connection with biomedical treatments and clinical (and non-clinical) settings. Separating behavioral from biomedical sciences is artificial, as many medical advances must be implemented using behavioral interventions. The 5 As model, for example, is effective in clinical environments that support and encourage its use through systems that routinely identify patient smoking status and prompt clinician delivery of brief interventions to prescribe or recommend pharmacologic treatment and resources for referral to more intensive treatment. The "Assist" component of the 5 As model is intended to link patients with effective cessation treatments and community-based resources, including pharmacologic treatment. A greater emphasis on T3 and T4 research that tests behavioral implementation and dissemination strategies for efficacious biomedical interventions is needed to maximize the impact of biomedical advances on human health.

CONCLUSIONS

Behavioral and social sciences play an important role in translational research across scientific disciplines. For example, implementation of many tests, drugs, and devices requires understanding of behavioral and social factors, such as individual cognitions, behaviors, and lifestyle influences, associated with individuals' ability to purchase and/or properly use such drugs and devices. Using theory-driven and methodologically sound research methods is critical to understanding, measuring, and intervening on behavioral and social factors to promote adherence to medical tests, drugs, and devices and other health-promoting behaviors that will ultimately contribute to improvement and promotion of health at the population level.

The framework presented here is not new; rather it is adapted from a broader historical context regarding translational research. The Five Phases of Research in cancer prevention and control were first articulated in the 1980s by Greenwald and Cullen at the National Cancer Institute (Greenwalk & Cullen, 1985). These original phases included hypothesis generation, methods development, controlled intervention trials, studies in defined populations, and demonstration projects. In this framework, the emphasis was placed on interventions and the transition from research to practice was viewed as an "orderly sequence." This linear approach was updated over time to better reflect the real world circumstances in which research progresses (Best et al., 2003; Hiatt & Rimer, 1999).

In order to maximize the potential of behavioral and social sciences in preventing and reducing the most significant health problems that affect our population, we must continue to improve the translation of our behavioral and social research from basic conception to population benefit. The proposed framework integrates common definitions and understanding of translational research in the behavioral and social sciences in a manner consistent with current approaches to defining translational research in the biomedical sciences and highlights the importance of all phases of translational research for improving population health.

REFERENCES

Agency for Healthcare Policy and Research. (1996). *Smoking cessation clinical practice guideline no. 18.* Washington, DC: Agency for Healthcare Policy and Research, U.S. Department of Health and Human Services.

Anda, R. F., Remington, P. L., Sienko, D. G., & Davis, R. M. (1987). Are physicians advising smokers to quit? The patient's perspective. *Journal of the American Medical Association, 257*(14), 1916–1919.

Best, A., Hiatt, R. A., Cameron, R., Rimer, B. K., & Abrams, D. B. (2003). The evolution of cancer control research: An international perspective from Canada and the United States. *Cancer Epidemiology, Biomarkers & Prevention, 12*(8), 705–712.

Bowen, D. J., Sorensen, G., Weiner, B. J., Campbell, M., Emmons, K., & Melvin, C. (2009). Dissemination research in cancer control: Where are we and where should we go? *Cancer Causes & Control, 20*(4), 473–485.

Centers for Disease Control and Prevention (CDC). (1993). Physician and other health care professional counseling of smokers to quit: United States, 1991. *Morbidity and Mortality Weekly Report, 42,* 854–857.

CDC. (2010). *Distinguishing public health research and public health nonresearch policy.* Retrieved from http://www.cdc.gov/od/science/integrity/docs/cdc-policy-distinguishing-public-health-research-nonresearch.pdf

Chase, E. C., McMenamin, S. B., & Halpin, H. A. (2007). Medicaid provider delivery of the 5A's for smoking cessation counseling. *Nicotine & Tobacco Research, 9*(11), 1095–1101.

Cohen, S., Stookey, G., Katz, B., Drook, C., & Smith, D. (1989). Encouraging primary care physicians to help smokers quit: A randomized, controlled trial. *Annals of Internal Medicine, 110*(8), 648–652.

Colditz, G. A. (2012). The promise and challenges of dissemination and implementation research. In R. C. Brownson, G. A. Colditz, & E. K. Proctor (Eds.), *Dissemination and implementation research in health: Translating science to practice* (pp. 3–22). New York, NY: Oxford University Press.

Collins, F. S. (2012). *Congressional justification of the NIH fiscal year (FY) 2013 budget request, annual performance report and plan.* Retrieved from http://officeofbudget.od.nih.gov/pdfs/FY13/FY2013_Overview.pdf

COMMIT Research Group. (1991). Community Intervention Trial for Smoking Cessation (COMMIT): Summary of design and intervention. *Journal of the National Cancer Institute, 83*(22), 1620–1628.

COMMIT Research Group. (1995). Community intervention trial for smoking cessation (COMMIT): II. Changes in adult cigarette smoking prevalence. *American Journal of Public Health, 85*(2), 193–200.

Contopoulos-Ioannidis, D. G., Alexiou, G. A., Gouvias, T. C., & Ioannidis, J. P. (2008). Medicine. Life cycle of translational research for medical interventions. *Science, 321*(5894), 1298–1299.

Creswell, J. W., Klassen, A. C., Plano Clark, V. L., & Smith, K. C., for the Office of Behavioral and Social Sciences Research. (2011). *Best practices for mixed methods research in the health sciences.* Retrieved from http://obssr.od.nih.gov/mixed_methods_research

Cummings, S. R., Richard, R. J., Duncan, C. L., Hansen, B., Vander Martin, R., Gerbert, B., & Coates, T. J. (1989). Training physicians about smoking cessation: A controlled trial in private practice. *Journal of General Internal Medicine, 4*(6), 482–489.

Department of Health and Human Services. (2010). *Dissemination and implementation research in health (R01): PAR-10-038 2010*. Retrieved from http://grants.nih.gov/grants/guide/pa-files /PAR-10-038.html

Emmons, K. M., Weiner, B., Fernandez, M. E., & Tu, S. P. (2012). Systems antecedents for dissemination and implementation: A review and analysis of measures. *Health Education & Behavior, 39*(1), 87–105.

Fiore, M. C., Bailey, W. C., Cohen, S. J., Dorfman, S. F., Goldstein, M. G., Gritz, E. R., ... Wewers, M. E. (2000). *Treating tobacco use and dependence. Clinical practice guideline*. Rockville, MD: U.S. Department of Health and Human Services, Public Health Services.

Fiore, M. C., Jaen, C. R., Baker, T. B., Bailey, W. C., Benowitz, N. L., Curry, S. J., ... Wewers, M. E. (2008). *Treating tobacco use and dependence: 2008 update. Clinical practice guideline*. Rockville, MD: U.S. Department of Health and Human Services.

Flay, B. R., Biglan, A., Boruch, R. F., Castro, F. G., Gottfredson, D., Kellam, S., ... Ji, P. (2005). Standards of evidence: Criteria for efficacy, effectiveness and dissemination. *Prevention Science, 6*(3), 151–175.

Geller, A. C., Brooks, D. R., Powers, C. A., Brooks, K. R., Rigotti, N. A., Bognar, B., ... Zapka, J. (2008). Tobacco cessation and prevention practices reported by second and fourth year students at US medical schools. *Journal of General Internal Medicine, 23*(7), 1071-1076.

Geller, A. C., Brooks, D. R., Woodring, B., Oppenheimer, S., McCabe, M., Rogers, J., ... Winickoff, J. P. (2011). Smoking cessation counseling for parents during child hospitalization: A national survey of pediatric nurses. *Public Health Nursing, 28*(6), 475–484.

Glanz, K., & Bishop, D. B. (2010). The role of behavioral science theory in development and implementation of public health interventions. *Annual Review of Public Health, 31*, 399–418.

Glasgow, R. E. (2008). What types of evidence are most needed to advance behavioral medicine? *Annals of Behavioral Medicine, 35*(1), 19–25.

Glasgow, R. E., & Emmons, K. M. (2007). How can we increase translation of research into practice? Types of evidence needed. *Annual Review of Public Health, 28*, 413–433.

Glasgow, R. E., Vogt, T. M., & Boles, S. M. (1999). Evaluating the public health impact of health promotion interventions: The RE-AIM framework. *American Journal of Public Health, 89*(9), 1322–1327.

Glynn, T. J., & Manley, M. W. (1989). *How to help our patients stop smoking. A National Cancer Institute manual for physicians* (No. NIH Publication 89-3062). Washington, DC: U.S. Department of Health and Human Services, Public Health Service, National Institutes of Health.

Green, L. W., Ottoson, J. M., Garcia, C., & Hiatt, R. A. (2009). Diffusion theory and knowledge dissemination, utilization, and integration in public health. *Annual Review of Public Health, 30*, 151–174.

Greenwalk, P., & Cullen, J. W. (1985). The new emphasis in cancer control. *Journal of the National Cancer Institute, 74*, 543-551.

Halpin Schauffler, H., Mordavsky, J. K., & McMenamin, S. (2001). Adoption of the AHCPR Clinical Practice Guideline for Smoking Cessation: A survey of California's HMOs. *American Journal of Preventive Medicine, 21*(3), 153–161.

Hiatt, R. A., & Rimer, B. K. (1999). A new strategy for cancer control research. *Cancer Epidemiology, Biomarkers & Prevention, 8*(11), 957–964.

Houston, T. K., Scarinci, I. C., Person, S. D., & Greene, P. G. (2005). Patient smoking cessation advice by health care providers: The role of ethnicity, socioeconomic status, and health. *American Journal of Public Health, 95*(6), 1056–1061.

Khoury, M. J., Gwinn, M., & Ioannidis, J. P. (2010). The emergence of translational epidemiology: From scientific discovery to population health impact. *American Journal of Epidemiology, 172*(5), 517–524.

Kottke, T., Brekke, M., Solberg, L., & Hughes, J. (1989). A randomized trial to increase smoking intervention by physicians. *Journal of the American Medical Association, 261*(14), 2101–2106.

Lopez-Quintero, C., Crum, R. M., & Neumark, Y. D. (2006). Racial/ethnic disparities in report of physician-provided smoking cessation advice: Analysis of the 2000 National Health Interview Survey. *American Journal of Public Health, 96*(12), 2235–2239.

Manfredi, C., & LeHew, C. W. (2008). Why implementation processes vary across the 5A's of the Smoking Cessation Guideline: Administrators' perspectives. *Nicotine Tobacco & Research, 10*(11), 1597–1607.

National Cancer Institute & Division of Cancer Control and Population Sciences. (2012). *Implementation science: Integrating science, practice and policy*. Retrieved from http://cancercontrol.cancer.gov/is/

National Institutes of Health. (2009). *NIH science of behavior change: Meeting summary*. Retrieved from https://commonfund.nih.gov/pdf/SOBC_Meeting_Summary_2009.pdf

National Institutes of Health, Office of Behavioral and Social Sciences Research. (2001). *Qualitative methods in health research*. NIH Publication No. 02-5046. Bethesda, MD: Office of Behavioral and Social Sciences Research, National Institutes of Health.

Ockene, J. (1987). Physician-delivered interventions for smoking cessation: Strategies for increasing effectiveness. *Preventive Medicine, 16*(5), 723–737.

Ockene, J. K., Kristeller, J., Goldberg, R., Amick, T. L., Pekow, P. S., Hosmer, D., … Kalan, K. (1991). Increasing the efficacy of physician-delivered smoking interventions: A randomized clinical trial. *Journal of General Internal Medicine, 6*(1), 1–8.

Ockene, J. K., Lindsay, E., Berger, L., & Hymowitz, N. (1990). Health care providers as key change agents in the community intervention trial for smoking cessation (COMMIT). *International Quarterly of Community Health Education, 11*(3), 223–237.

Office of Behavioral and Social Sciences Research & National Institutes of Health. (2013). *Behavioral and social sciences (BSSR) definition*. Retrieved from http://obssr.od.nih.gov/about_obssr?BSSR _CC/BSSR-definition/definition.aspx

Orleans, C. T., George, L. K., Houpt, J. L., & Brodie, K. H. (1985). Health promotion in primary care: A survey of U.S. family practitioners. *Preventive Medicine, 14*(5), 636–647.

Pagoto, S. L. (2011). The current state of lifestyle implementation research. Where do we go next? *Translational Behavioral Medicine, 3*(1), 401–405.

Papadakis, S., McDonald, P., Mullen, K. A., Reid, R., Skulsky, K., & Pipe, A. (2010). Strategies to increase the delivery of smoking cessation treatments in primary care settings: A systematic review and meta-analysis. *Preventive Medicine, 51*(3–4), 199–213.

Quinn, V. P., Hollis, J. F., Smith, K. S., Rigotti, N. A., Solberg, L. I., Hu, W., & Stevens, V. J. (2009). Effectiveness of the 5-As tobacco cessation treatments in nine HMOs. *Journal of General Internal Medicine, 24*(2), 149–154.

Rabin, B. A., Glasgow, R. E., Kerner, J. F., Klump, M. P., & Brownson, R. C. (2010). Dissemination and implementation research on community-based cancer prevention: A systematic review. *American Journal of Preventive Medicine, 38*(4), 443–456.

Russell, M. A., Wilson, C., Taylor, C., & Baker, C. D. (1979). Effect of general practitioners' advice against smoking. *British Medical Journal, 2*(6184), 231–235.

Schauffler, H., & Parkinson, M. (1993). Health insurance coverage for smoking cessation services. *Health Education Quarterly, 20*(2), 185–206.

Shadish, W. R., Cook, T. D., & Campbell, D. T. (2002). *Experimental and quasi-experimental designs for generalized causal inference*. Boston, MA: Houghton Mifflin.

Sung, N. S., Crowley, W. F., Jr., Genel, M., Salber, P., Sandy, L., Sherwood, L. M., … Rimoin, D. (2003). Central challenges facing the national clinical research enterprise. *Journal of the American Medical Association, 289*(10), 1278–1287.

UNC Center for Health Promotion and Disease Prevention. (2012). *Training institute for dissemination and implementation research in health*. Retrieved from http://conferences.thehillgroup.com/OBSS Rinstitutes/TIDIRH2011/index.html

U.S. Department of Health and Human Services, National Institutes of Health, & Office of Behavioral and Social Sciences Research. (2012). *5th Annual NIH conference on the science of dissemination and implementation: Research at the crossroads*. Retrieved from http://conferences.thehillgroup.com /obssr/di2012/index.html

U.S. Department of Health and Human Services & National Cancer Institute. (2006). *The NCI strategic plan for leading the nation: To eliminate the suffering and death due to cancer*. Bethesda, MD: U.S. Department of Health and Human Services, National Institutes of Health, National Cancer Institute.

U.S. Preventive Services Task Force. (2009). *Counseling and interventions to prevent tobacco use and tobacco-caused disease in adults and pregnant women: Reaffirmation recommendation statement*. AHRQ Publication No. 09-05131-EF-1. Retrieved from http://www.uspreventiveservicestaskforce .org/uspstf09/tobacco/tobaccors2.htm

U.S. Preventive Services Task Force. (2012). The guide to clinical prevention services 2012. Retrieved from http://www.ahrq.gov/clinic/pocketgd1011/pocketgd1011.pdf

Waldman, S. A., & Terzic, A. (2010). Clinical and translational science: From bench-bedside to global village. *Clinical and Translational Science, 3*(5), 254–257.

Weathington, B. L., Cunningham, C. J. L., & Pittenger, D. J. (2010). *Research methods for the behavioral and social sciences*. Hoboken, NJ: John Wiley & Sons.

Wilson, D. M., Taylor, D. W., Gilbert, J. R., Best, J. A., Lindsay, E. A., Willms, D. G., & Singer, J. (1988). A randomized trial of a family physician intervention for smoking cessation. *Journal of the American Medical Association, 260*(11), 1570–1574.

Woolf, S. H. (2008). The meaning of translational research and why it matters. *Journal of the American Medical Association, 299*(2), 211–213.

Zerhouni, E. (2003). Medicine. The NIH Roadmap. *Science, 302*(5642), 63–72.

Index